UROGYNECOLOGY FEMALE PELVIC RECONSTRUCTIVE SURGERY
Just the Facts

Sam Siddighi, MD

Fellow
Urogynecology, Female Pelvic Medicine and Reconstructive Surgery
Department of Obstetrics and Gynecology
Good Samaritan Hospital
Cincinnati, Ohio

Jeffrey S. Hardesty, MD

Assistant Professor and Chief of Benign Gynecology and Urogynecology
Loma Linda University School of Medicine
Loma Linda, California

McGraw-Hill
Medical Publishing Division

New York   Chicago   San Francisco   Lisbon   London   Madrid
Mexico City   Milan   New Delhi   San Juan   Seoul
Singapore   Sydney   Toronto

UROGYNECOLOGY AND FEMALE PELVIC RECONSTRUCTIVE SURGERY
Just the Facts

1 2 3 4 5 6 7 8 9 0   QPD/QPD   0 9 8 7 6

ISBN 0-07-144799-7

This book was set in Times New Roman by International Typesetting and Composition.
The editors were Anne M. Sydor, Christie Naglieri, and Mary E. Bele.
The production supervisor was Catherine H. Saggese.
Project management was provided by International Typesetting and Composition.
Quebecor Dubuque was printer and binder.

This book is printed on acid-free paper.

Library of Congress Cataloging-in-Publication Data

Siddighi, Sam.
    Urogynecology and female pelvic reconstructive surgery : just the facts / Sam Siddighi,
Jeffrey S. Hardesty.— 1st ed.
        p. ; cm.
    Includes bibliographical references and index.
    ISBN 0-07-144799-7
    1. Urogynecology. 2. Pelvis—Surgery. 3. Generative organs, Female—Surgery. I.
Hardesty, Jeffrey S. II. Title.
    [DNLM: 1. Pelvis—surgery. 2. Gynecologic Surgical Procedures. 3. Reconstructive
Surgical Procedures. 4. Urologic Surgical Procedures. WP 155 S568u 2006]
RG484.S53 2006
618.1'059—dc22

                                                                2005056236

This book is dedicated to my mom for being a survivor.
I also want to express my deepest gratitude to all my teachers and mentors,
without whom this book would not be possible.

Sam Siddighi, MD

CONTENTS

CONTRIBUTORS

Marianna Alperin, MD, Fellow, Department of Obstetrics and Gynecology, Division of Gynecologic Specialties, Section of Urogynecology, University of Pittsburgh, Clinical Fellow, Magee-Women's Hospital, Pittsburgh, Pennsylvania

Kevin C. Balli, MD, Assistant Professor, Department of Gynecology and Obstetrics, Loma Linda University Medical Center, Loma Linda, California

Barry S. Block, MD, Associate Professor, Department of Gynecology and Obstetrics, Loma Linda University Medical Center, Loma Linda, California

Sandra J. Bosman, MD, Resident Physician, Department of Gynecology and Obstetrics, Loma Linda University Medical Center, Loma Linda, California

Jessica Bracken, MD, Resident Physician, Bethesda North Hospital, Cincinnati, Ohio

Murray E. Brandstater, MBBS, PhD, Professor and Chairman, Department of Physical Medicine and Rehabilitation, Loma Linda University Medical Center, Loma Linda, California

Sandy Chuan, MD, Resident, Loma Linda University Medical Center, Loma Linda, California

Dean E. Dagermangy, MD, Resident Physician, Department of Gynecology and Obstetrics, Loma Linda University Medical Center, Loma Linda, California

Elizabeth Dameff, MD, MPH, Department of Family Medicine and Obstetrics and Gynecology, Kaiser Permanente, Fontana, California

J. Linn Daudel, MD, MBA, Resident Physician, Department of Gynecology and Obstetrics, Loma Linda University Medical Center, Loma Linda, California

Tricia L. Fynewever, MD, Resident Physician, Department of Gynecology and Obstetrics, Loma Linda University Medical Center, Loma Linda, California

Rajiv B. Gala, MD, Assistant Professor, Department of Obstetrics and Gynecology, University of Texas Southwestern, Dallas, Texas

Dobie Giles, MD, MS, Fellow, Female Pelvic Medicine and Reconstructive Surgery, Mayo Clinic Scottsdale, Scottsdale, Arizona

Yvonne G. Gollin, MD, Assistant Professor, Department of Obstetrics and Gynecology, Loma Linda University Medical Center, Loma Linda, California

Bogdan A. Grigorescu, MD, Fellow, Pelvic and Reconstructive Surgery, Department of Obstetrics and Gynecology, Albert Einstein College of Medicine, Bronx, New York

Jeffrey S. Hardesty, MD, Assistant Professor and Chief of Benign Gynecology and Urogynecology, Loma Linda University School of Medicine, Loma Linda, California

Elaine Hart, MD, Instructor, Loma Linda University Medical Center, Loma Linda, California

Lindsey Huber, Fourth Year Medical Student, Loma Linda University School of Medicine, Loma Linda, California

Tricia Lin Kam, MD, Department of Obstetrics and Gynecology, Loma Linda University Medical Center, Loma Linda, California

Henry Kim, MD, Resident Physician, Department of Physical Medicine and Rehabilitation, Loma Linda University Medical Center, Loma Linda, California

John J. Kim, MD, Assistant Professor, Department of Obstetrics and Gynecology, Loma Linda University Medical Center, Loma Linda, California

Steven D. Kleeman, MD, Assistant Professor, University of Cincinnati, Associate Director of Urogynecology and Pelvic Reconstruction, Good Samaritan Hospital, Cincinnati, Ohio

Justin Thien Lee, MD, Urogynecology and Pelvic Reconstructive Surgery Fellow, Department of Obstetrics and Gynecology, Albany Medical Center, Albany, New York, Urogynecology and Pelvic Reconstructive Surgery Fellow, Women's Continence Center of Greater Rochester, Rochester, New York

Fatta B. Nabah, MD, FAAN, Clinical Fellow, National Institutes of Health, Bethesda, Maryland

John Occhino, MD, Resident Physician, Good Samaritan Hospital, Cincinnati, Ohio

Mayank Pandya, MD, Department of Obstetrics and Gynecology, Geisinger Medical Center, Danville, Pennsylvania

Rachel N. Pauls, MD, Fellow, Division of Urogynecology and Reconstructive Pelvic Surgery, Good Samaritan Hospital, University of Cincinnati, Clinical Instructor, Good Samaritan Hospital, Cincinnati, Ohio

Christopher M. Rooney, MD, Fellow, Urogynecology and Pelvic Reconstruction, Good Samaritan Hospital, Cincinnati, Ohio

Sam Siddighi, MD, Fellow, Female Pelvic Medicine and Reconstructive Surgery, Department of Obstetrics and Gynecology, Good Samaritan Hospital, Cincinnati, Ohio

Stacey L. Snowden, MD, Resident Physician, Tacoma Family Medicine, Department of Family Medicine, University of Washington School of Medicine, Tacoma, Washington

Uchechi A. Wosu, MD, MSc, Department of Obstetrics and Gynecology, University of Massachusetts, Worcester, Massachusetts

Sujata Yavagal, MD, Assistant Professor, Albany Medical Center, Albany, New York

FOREWORD

I am honored to be asked to write the foreword for the book, *Urogynecology and Female Pelvic Reconstructive Surgery: Just the Facts*. I feel that this book not only will be useful to resident physicians and fellows, but also for physicians practicing in the area of obstetrics and gynecology, urology, family medicine, and potentially colorectal surgery. Over the last decade it has become quite apparent that the prevalence of female pelvic floor dysfunction is quite high. Conservative estimates indicate that approximately 40% of women will sometime in their lives suffer from pelvic floor dysfunction that significantly impacts their quality of life. For this reason, it has become an intricate part of the everyday practice of obstetricians/gynecologists as well as other practitioners.

This book is a thorough yet quick and easy to understand summary of this specialty. It addresses all aspects of urogynecology and female pelvic medicine. It begins with a section on pelvic anatomy and epidemiology. It is then followed by a detailed section on the evaluation of pelvic organ prolapse and incontinence with appropriate testing. Nonsurgical as well as surgical modalities are discussed in a succinct and easy to comprehend, step-by-step fashion. There are specific sections on colorectal disorders and pregnancy issues pertaining to urogynecology, medications utilized in the field, as well as sexuality and female sexual dysfunction. The book ends with a unique chapter containing a time line of the field of gynecologic urology and detailed discussion of the application process for fellowship in a subspecialty of obstetrics and gynecology. A table containing detailed information about programs in female pelvic medicine and reconstructive surgery (FPMRS) is included. Every chapter has board-type review questions, answers, and explanations. A USMLE-type final examination can also be found at the end of the book.

All sections of the book are intended to be short, concise, and to the point. Dr. Siddighi has accumulated a group of young authors, most of whom are still in residency or fellowship training. The experienced clinician, as well as the resident or fellow in training will find this book to be a quick reference for a variety of pelvic floor disorders. While this area of gynecology is constantly changing, Dr. Siddighi, Dr. Hardesty, and their contributors must again be credited for very up-to-date information.

Mickey M. Karram

The field of urogynecology or recently renamed, female pelvic medicine and reconstructive surgery (FPMRS), is an exciting and growing subspecialty of Obstetrics and Gynecology. Currently, the care of the pregnant female patient and her unborn fetus (maternal fetal medicine or MFM), the female patient with genital tract cancer (gynecologic oncology), and the female patient who is unable to achieve pregnancy (reproductive endocrinology and infertility or REI) is provided by subspecialists with advanced training in the aforementioned fields. Now for more than a decade, the obstetrician-gynecologist is able to seek advanced, specialized training in FPMRS to provide care for the female patient who is afflicted with conditions that occur mostly after pregnancy and which deteriorate with aging. FPMRS treat conditions such as urinary incontinence, fecal incontinence, pelvic organ prolapse, and other conditions of the female lower urinary tract and pelvic floor.

Currently, there is a lot of interest in the field of FPMRS because of the rising demand. This interest will continue to grow into the future. The "baby boomers" are aging. According to the National Center for Health Statistics and various other sources, the life expectancy for a woman was 79.8 years in 2001 and it is rising. Today 13% of people are over age 65 and that number will increase by 25% by the year 2030. It is estimated that 7 million new surgeries and 2 million repeat surgeries for pelvic dysfunction will be necessary every year by the year 2030. Fifty percent of women will have a bladder control problem during their lifetimes. Currently, one in every nine woman undergoes surgery for pelvic organ prolapse or urinary incontinence by age 80. Even nulliparous college women who are not usually thought of as having pelvic dysfunction or incontinence may experience these problems. Additionally, there is increased awareness among physicians of specialties other than obstetrics and gynecology about incontinence, pelvic organ prolapse, and pelvic dysfunction. Therefore, more referrals are being made to gynecologists, female urologists, and urogynecologists. More women are also coming forth with their symptoms, perhaps, because of greater awareness, less shame, and increased physician screening.

In the past, "turf" battles have existed between urologists and gynecologists because of confusion over which specialty should manage certain conditions of the lower urinary and genital tracts. The "turf" politics are not unique to our two specialties (e.g., ENT vs. facial plastic surgery, OMFS vs. facial plastic surgery, general surgery and colorectal surgery, and so forth). The "turf" politics have resulted in fragmentation of our and other specialties. They have also made it difficult to develop a board examination for the subspecialty of FPMRS. It makes no sense to have such resistance since effective management of these patients requires a multidisciplinary approach. Consider the following facts:

1. Historically, Gynecology and Urology were closely associated and one developed through the other (see historical time line in Chapter 51, Essential Information About Female Pelvic Medicine and Reconstructive Surgery and Application to OB/GYN Subspecialty Fellowships in the United States, section describing Marion Sims and Howard Kelly).
2. "Embryologically, anatomically, and functionally, the lower urinary tract and genital tract are intimately associated." (W. Glenn Hurt. In: The Master's Techniques in Gynecologic Surgery, *Urogynecologic Surgery*. 2nd ed. Philadelphia, PA: Lippincott William & Wilkins; 2000:6.)
3. Neither gynecologists nor urologists alone are fully trained in the field of FPMRS. To become a urologist for females, graduating urology seniors must strengthen their knowledge and experience of genital anatomy and receive training in pelvic prolapse surgery and management of certain vulvar and vaginal conditions. Similarly, graduating senior gynecologists must strengthen their knowledge of the management of urinary incontinence (also fecal incontinence), and receive additional training in the recognition, evaluation, and management of certain conditions of the bladder and ureter below the pelvic brim.
4. According to the statistics already mentioned, there is absolutely no need for turf battles since there is plenty of business for all those interested in managing problems of the lower urinary tract and pelvic floor. However, there is a shortage of well-trained physicians to take care of the countless numbers of patients with these disorders.

The good news is that things are beginning to change. There are 23 nationally accredited programs in FMPRS, which are certified by both the American College of Obstetrics and Gynecology and the American Board of Urology. Currently, the top centers in the country manage lower urinary tract and pelvic floor dysfunction via a multidisciplinary approach which involves FPMRS specialists, female urologists, colorectal surgeons, gastroenterologists, physical therapists, trained physicians assistants and nurse practitioners, and others related to and/or trained in the specialty.

With the statistics being as such, there is no wonder why industry has such an interest in FPMRS. New pharmaceutical drugs, surgical instruments, anatomical models, incontinence products, tissue augmenting materials, pelvic floor dysfunction evaluation devices, and centers for behavioral and physical rehabilitation of the pelvis are emerging. The National Institutes of Health have noticed this need and have provided significant funding for research in this area. The Urinary Incontinence Network (UITN), which consists of investigators from nine centers and the Pelvic Floor Disorders Network (PFDN), which consists of investigators from seven centers across the United States is currently ongoing. The results of these trials will provide valuable information. In the near future, the field of obstetrics and gynecology will require more practitioners who are well trained in FPMRS, and therefore job security and strong income potential for the fellowship trained urogynecologist.

This book is ideal for the senior resident in obstetrics and gynecology or urology and the community generalist in the above fields who has an interest in evaluating and managing these benign pelvic conditions. The book can also serve as a quick review for the fellow training in the FPMRS. The book is meant to be a thorough yet succinct review of the literature in FPMRS combined with the opinions of experts. It is hoped that it can serve as a study guide for future residents and fellows seeking specialization in this field of study.

Time and money was not spent to include photographs and figures to each of the chapters because many good photographs are already in existence in the literature. I would like to direct the readers of this book to some of the references in the literature cited in the bibliographies of each chapter and to atlases such as Michael Baggish and Mickey Karram's *Gynecology and Pelvic Surgery Atlas*, and surgical videos from the American Urogynecologic Society (AUGS) and Society of Gynecologic Surgeons (SGS). A series of excellent surgical videos are also available at website pelvicmed.com. The strengths of this book are the following:

1. Easy to read and understand
2. Thorough yet not too lengthy
3. Current and up to date
4. Provides interesting facts about topics in FPMRS
5. Has tables and summaries not found anywhere else in the literature
6. Contains detailed descriptions of surgical techniques with useful surgical pearls
7. Contains chapters on topics that are scattered and briefly mentioned in the literature (e.g., selective cesarean, female sexuality, female sexual dysfunction, essential information about female pelvic medicine and reconstructive surgery, and application to OB/GYN subspecialty fellowships in the United States, and so forth)
8. It is the *only book* that has United States Medical Licensing Examination (USMLE)-type board questions, answers, and detailed explanations about all of the essential topics in FPMRS
9. Contains USMLE-type questions at the end of each chapter as well as a comprehensive final examination at the end of the book
10. Provides an unbiased summary of several review sources and countless peer-review papers

We hope the reader of this book will find it a useful addition to his or her collection of medical books. Good luck and see you at AUGS or SGS.

Sam Siddighi, MD
Jeffrey S. Hardesty, MD

ABOUT THE AUTHORS

Sam Siddighi graduated from New York Medical College and completed his residency in the Department of Gynecology and Obstetrics at Loma Linda University Medical Center. Currently, he is a fellow at one of few ABOG and ABU accredited fellowships in Female Pelvic Medicine and Reconstructive Surgery, Good Samaritan Hospital. He has received invaluable training under the mentorship of world-renowned urogynecologist and fellowship director, Mickey Karram and chairman of the Department of Obstetrics and Gynecology, Michael Baggish. Dr. Siddighi also gained extensive experience writing USMLE and board-type questions, as a research associate for the national testing and review center, Kaplan, during the year 2001. Additionally, he developed skills necessary in writing and editing medical review books through his interactions with Professor Elmar Sakala (author of *Board Review Series [BRS] in Obstetrics and Gynecology, High-Yield in Obstetrics and Gynecology*). Dr. Siddighi also coauthored the National Medical Series (NMS) in *Obstetrics and Gynecology*, 5th ed. in 2005.

Jeffrey S. Hardesty graduated from Loma Linda University School of Medicine in 1980 and finished his OB/GYN residency training at that institution in 1985. He then served as a full-time missionary physician in Penang, Malaysia. During the 8 years he worked in Malaysia, he was able to perform nearly 5000 deliveries as well as perform 10+ gynecologic surgeries each week. This wealth of clinical experience has been an important asset since his return to the teaching staff of LLU OB/GYN department in 1993. During his first 2 years at LLU, he did an apprenticeship in urogynecology and pelvic reconstructive surgery under the tutelage of Dr. Kenneth McGill who pioneered this field at Loma Linda. He then did a preceptorship with Dr. Donald Ostergard in 1995. Dr. Hardesty enjoys teaching vaginal surgery, participating in family activities, and going on annual medical mission trips to such places as Mexico, Nepal, and New Guinea.

1 ANATOMY RELEVANT TO FEMALE RECONSTRUCTIVE PELVIC SURGERY: PART I

Sam Siddighi

INTRODUCTION

- The pelvic floor has three functional layers:
  - Fascia (e.g., endopelvic fascia)—attaches and surrounds all pelvic organs (bladder, uterus, rectum).
  - Muscle (aka levator ani + coccygeus or *pelvic diaphragm*)—slow-type muscles which are constantly contracted and may contract further during increased intra-abdominal pressure.
  - Perineal membrane (PM) (aka urogenital diaphragm, muscles that make up the perineal body [PB], and striated urethral sphincter). When the perineum is viewed from dorsal lithotomy position, the PM consists of all of the soft tissues between the two ischiopubic rami, ischial tuberosities, and tip of the coccyx.
- The levator ani muscles create a dome-shaped pelvic floor at rest and a flat pelvic floor during strain.
- *Active muscular hammock*—proper function of pelvic muscles and their nerves is important to maintain proper orientation and active support of the pelvic organs. In other words, the load bearing is provided by pelvic muscles.
- The connective tissue (e.g., fascia), on the other hand, serves to hold and stabilize the organs.
- If the muscles do not function properly, then the fascial attachments of the pelvic viscera stretch over time and may break.
- The parietal fascia, which attaches to the skeletal muscles of the pelvis, is made of dense, structured collagen bundles; has low vascularity and few active fibroblasts.
- The visceral fascia, which encapsulates the smooth muscle coat of the pelvic organs, is made up of loose collagen, elastin, smooth muscle, and adipose; it is rich in vascularity.
- The viscera are anchored to parietal fascia by their visceral fascia, which not only serves to encapsulate them but also to attach them to the pelvic sidewall via visceral endopelvic fascia (aka fascia endopelvina). *The visceral and parietal fascia are continuous.* Endopelvic fascia also serves as the pathway for visceral nerves, vessels, and lymph drainage from the pelvic organs.
- The viscera of interest in the pelvis are the uterus, cervix, vagina, rectum, and bladder along with the input and output channels of the bladder, the ureters, and the urethra, respectively. The vagina and its support system are key to understanding pelvic prolapse. When the vaginal support system is normal, the bladder, urethra, cervix, and rectum will be normally situated.
- The vagina can be conceptualized as a fibromuscular, flattened, cylindrical tube with three attachment systems (discussed in Chap. 2, Anatomy Relevant to Female Reconstructive Pelvic Surgery: Part II).
- Unlike some side-view anatomic depictions of the pelvis, the vagina is not oriented vertically with its apex pointing cephalad. Instead, it has almost a horizontal axis and points posteriorly. Therefore, an increase in abdominal pressure does not evert the vagina directly, but instead pins it against the pelvic floor.
- Because of its support system and anatomic orientation, the vagina can only prolapse apically, anteriorly, or posteriorly, never laterally.
- Contraction of the pelvic floor compresses the vagina toward the symphysis pubis.
- The layers of the vagina are in sequence: nonkeratinizing stratified squamous epithelium → loose connective tissue (lamina propria) → fibromuscular layer → adventitia. Note that the outer part of the histologic fibromuscular layer and adventitia are referred to during surgery as the *pubocervical septum.*; however, *this is not true fascia. Therefore pubocervical septum (PCS)* is a better name.

BONES AND LIGAMENTS OF THE PELVIS

- Bony pelvis = two hip bones + sacrum-coccyx. Hip bones (aka ossa coxae or innominate bone) have three parts which meet at the acetabulum: ilium (superior portion) + ischium (inferior and posterior portion) + pubis (inferior and anterior). Note that the two halves of the pubis are connected at the symphysis by four ligaments (anterior, posterior, superior, and inferior [aka arcuate ligament]). The arcuate ligament is the strongest and most important of these four and is important in prevention of diastasis (>10 mm separation) during pregnancy.
- Borders of the greater sciatic foramen = sacrotuberous ligament (inferior and posterior border) + sacrospinous ligament (inferior border) + ischium (anterior border) + sacroiliac ligament (superior border) + sacrum (posterior border). The *largest branch of the internal iliac*, posterior division (superior gluteal artery), exits through the greater sciatic foramen. The inferior gluteal (branch of internal iliac, anterior division) also exits through this foramen. The anterior border of the greater sciatic foramen is vertical in orientation and is parallel to the path of the internal iliac artery after bifurcation of the common iliac artery.
- Just below the sacrospinous ligament is the lesser sciatic foramen through which course tendons of the obturator internus muscles which attach to the femur. Directly on top of the sacrospinous ligament lies the coccygeus muscle, which runs from the lateral borders of the coccyx and sacrum to the ischial spines.
- Obturator foramen —oval window made of half ilium and half pubis. Boundaries are superior = superior pubic ramus + body of pubis, inferior = ischium, anterior = inferior pubic ramus + ischial ramus, posterior = ischium + pubis. It is sealed by a dense sheath, the obturator membrane except at its most lateral, posterior, and superior border where the obturator vessels and nerve exit. Originating from the obturator foramen edges and the obturator membrane lies the obturator internus muscle and obturator externus muscle inside and outside the pelvis, respectively. Both of these muscles attach to the femur.
- Cooper's ligament—running posterolaterally from the pubic tubercles is a ridge of pubic bone which is continuous with the arcuate line of the iliac bone all the way to the sacral promontory. This iliopectineal line (aka pectin pubis) marks the circumference of the pelvic inlet (below the level of this line lies the true pelvis). Cooper's ligament lies on the most anterior portion of this line, is lateral to the pubic tubercles, and lies inside the superior pubic ramus. It is the attachment site of sutures during a Burch retropubic urethropexy.

MUSCLES, FASCIA, AND IMPORTANT LANDMARKS OF THE PELVIS

- The pelvis is a basin with four walls and a floor:
  ○ Front wall—back of symphysis pubis
  ○ Back wall = sacrum (centrally) + piriformis × 2 (laterally)
  ○ Two sidewalls—obturator internus muscle
  ○ Floor is made of levator ani muscles (pubococcygeus and iliococcygeus) and the coccygeus muscle (which lies over the sacrospinous ligament).
- Sidewalls in more detail from inside toward outside = obturator internus muscle and fascia → obturator membrane → obturator externus muscle and fascia.
- Front wall in more detail: The bodies of the pubic bones are connected in the midline via the arcuate ligament. The adductor longus is attached here. The inferior pubic rami are continuous with the ischial rami. The adductor brevis and gracilis are attached to the superior portion of the inferior pubic ramus. The adductor magnus spans the inferior pubic ramus and the ischial ramus.
- *Arcus tendineus levator ani* (ATLA) (or tendinous arch of levator ani or levator arcus, or *muscle* white line). A thickening of obturator internus parietal fascia from pubic bone (posterior, lateral, and superior on the pubic bone) to ischial spine from which the levator ani originates. ATLA ≠ arcus tendineus fascia pelvis (ATFP). Do not forget that part of the obturator internus exists below the level of ATLA and forms the lateral border of the ischiorectal fossa (see further).
- *Arcus tendineus fascia pelvis* (or fascia arcus, *fascial* white line). The parietal fascia covering of the levator ani muscles is thickened into a strong band on the surface of muscle; it spans from the lower one-sixth of the pubic bone (i.e., 1 cm from inferior margin of bone) and about 1 cm from the midline at one end to the ischial spine at the other. The ATFP and ATLA are fused at the ischial spine. ATFP is the connection site of several important structures.
- Pubococcygeus has medial and lateral fibers which are continuous.
  ○ The medial fibers of pubococcygeus arise from the superior ramus of the pubic bone and meet medial fibers from the opposite side forming the *levator cruri*. The *puborectalis* is the most medial and inferior portion of the pubococcygeus. The pubococcygeus and its puborectalis form the levator hiatus. The levator hiatus (aka genital hiatus or urogenital hiatus) is the space between the levator cruri through which course the urethra, vagina, and rectum.
  ○ Contraction of the pubococcygeus creates the anorectal angle, which is believed to contribute to fecal continence. The medial fibers of the pubococcygeus

and puborectalis muscles have attachments to the rectum and vagina (the pubovisceral portion). This portion is damaged during traumatic vaginal birth.

○ The lateral fibers of the pubococcygeus arise from the anterior portion of the obturator internus muscle (anterior ATLA) and meet fibers from the opposite side in front of the anococcygeal raphe (aka median raphe) and form the *levator plate*. The levator plate ($\approx$3.5 cm in length) is horizontally oriented in a standing person.

• Iliococcygeus is a thin muscle that arises from the posterior portion of the obturator internus (posterior ATLA) and its most posterior fibers slope inferiorly to the coccyx. Its posterior fibers also meet sister fibers from the opposite side at the anococcygeal raphe. Some of these fibers also attach directly to the rectum.

• The anterior fibers of the iliococcygeus also blend with the longitudinal coat of the rectum, between the internal and external anal sphincter. The medial portion of the pubococcygeus surrounds the lower one-third of the vagina.

• Muscles of the levator ani are innervated on pelvic side by sacral efferents (S2, S3, S4) and on perineal side by branches of the pudendal nerve.

• The levator ani is always contracted (i.e., has baseline tone) because of Type I (slow-twitch fibers), but can also contract further voluntarily (Type II, fast-twitch fibers).

• Normally, constant contraction of the levator ani keeps the levator hiatus closed by compressing the urethra, vagina, and rectum against the pubic bone while pulling the pelvic floor and viscera upward (cephalic direction). When these muscles relax, during defecation and micturition, or are damaged, the levator hiatus opens leaving the vagina and viscera supported by their fascia only.

• If the levator ani are damaged and do not function for long periods of time then the fascia stretches and breaks leading to pelvic organ prolapse.

THE PERINEUM

• Just inferior to the levator ani muscles are the spaces and structures of the perineum.

• The perineum is a diamond-shaped area. The anterolateral borders are the (ischiopubic rami + ischial tuberosities) $\times$ 2 and the posterolateral borders are the two sacrotuberous ligaments. A line drawn between the ends of the ischial tuberosities bisects the diamond shape into two triangles. The anterior triangle is the urogenital triangle and the posterior is the anal triangle. Halfway down the bisecting line is a crucial structure called the perineal body (aka central tendon of the perineum).

• Ischiorectal fossa (aka ischioanal fossa). Boundaries are anteriorly and laterally = ischial tuberosity and inferior part of obturator internus muscle, medially = anal

canal and external anal sphincter, posteriorly = sacrotuberous ligament and underside of the gluteus maximi muscles. The floor of the fossa is made up of the perineal side of the levator ani muscles. The anterior horn of the ischiorectal fossa extends into the urogenital triangle deep into the PM. The ischiorectal fossa contains mostly fibrofatty tissue, internal pudendal vessels and nerves which lie along its lateral border, and cutaneous nerves (S2, S3, S4). The internal pudendal vessels and nerves give off the inferior rectal vessels and nerves (posteriorly) and the perineal and labial vessels and nerves (anteriorly, inside urogenital triangle).

• *Perineal body.* PB is a thick pyramidal-shaped area ($\approx$3.5 cm) with the base of the pyramid (superficial) and the apex deep at a level where the lower one-third of the vagina becomes the middle one-third. PB is responsible for closure of the vaginal introitus. The base of the pyramid is where the two superficial transverse perineal muscles, the two bulbocavernosus muscles, and the external anal sphincter meet. The apex is where internal structures such as the levator ani muscles and the rectovaginal septum attach to the PB.

• Note that the other muscles inside the urogenital triangle are the paired ischiocavernosus muscles which are parallel to the ischiopubic ramus and are attached at the ischial tuberosity (posteriorly) and the crus of the clitoris and pubic arch (anteriorly).

• Based on magnetic resonance imaging (MRI) studies, patients with stress urinary incontinence have a greater likelihood of having attachment defects of the levator ani to the PB. If the levator ani muscles do not function properly, normal anatomic relationships cannot be maintained.

• *Perineal membrane* (formerly called urogenital diaphragm). A triangular supporting fibromuscular membrane that spans between the two ischiopubic rami and lies at the level of the hymen. It is the connection site of many crucial structures. The vagina and urethra perforate the PM as well as attach to it. The PM is also connected to the PB around the vagina. Deep or cephalad to the PM (anteriorly) lies the urogenital-sphincter complex (see Chap. 2, Anatomy Relevant to Female Reconstructive Pelvic Surgery: Part II).

BIBLIOGRAPHY

DeLancey JOL. Anatomy of the female bladder and urethra. In: Bent AE, Ostergard DR, Cundiff GW, Swift SE, eds. *Ostergard's Urogynecology and Pelvic Floor Dysfunction.* 5th ed. Philadelphia, PA: Lippincott Williams & Wilkins; 2003:3–18.

Divekar P, Keith LG. Pubic symphysis diastasis during pregnancy. *The Female Patient.* Vol 29, No 9. Sept. 2004:24–34.

Hurt WG. Retropubic urethropexy or colposuspension. In: Hurt WG, ed. *The Master's Techniques in Gynecologic Surgery, Urogynecologic Surgery.* 2nd ed. Philadelphia, PA: Lippincott Williams & Wilkins; 2000:82.

Kilgore LC, Shingleton HM. Recognizing injuries to the urinary tract. In: Sanz LE, ed. *Gynecologic Surgery.* 2nd ed. Cambridge, MA: Blackwell Science; 1995:317–323.

Moore KL. The pelvis and perineum. In: Moore KL, ed. *Clinically Oriented Anatomy.* 3rd ed. Baltimore, MD: Lippincott Williams & Wilkins; 1992:243–322.

Netter FH. *The Atlas of Human Anatomy.* East Hanover, NJ: Novartis; 1989:334–394.

Richardson AC. Paravaginal repair. In: Hurt WG, ed. *Urogynecologic Surgery.* Gaithersburg, MD: Aspen Publishers; 1992:73–80.

Rogers RM Jr. Anatomy of pelvic support. In: Bent AE, Ostergard DR, Cundiff GW, Swift SE, eds. *Ostergard's Urogynecology and Pelvic Floor Dysfunction.* 5th ed. Philadelphia, PA: Lippincott Williams & Wilkins; 2003.

Shull BL, Benn SJ, Huehl TJ. Surgical management of prolapse of the anterior vaginal segment: an analysis of support defects, operative morbidity, and anatomic outcome. *Am J Obstet Gynecol.* 1994;171:1429–1439.

Thompson JD. Operative injuries to the ureter: prevention, recognition, and management. In: Rock JA, Thompson JD, eds. *Te Linde's Operative Gynecology.* 8th ed. Philadelphia, PA: Lippincott-Raven; 1997:1135–1173.

Walters MD, Weber AM. Anatomy of the lower urinary tract, rectum, and pelvic floor. In: Walters MD, Karram MM, eds. *Urogynecology and Reconstructive Pelvic Surgery.* 2nd ed. St Louis, MO: Mosby; 1999:3–13.

Wei JT, De Lancey JOL. Functional anatomy of the pelvic floor and lower urinary tract. In: Weber A, ed. *Incontinence 2004.* Philadelphia, PA: Lippincott Williams & Wilkins; 2004:3–17.

QUESTIONS

1. A 54-year-old gravida 5, para 5, comes to your office complaining of constant pressure and bulge inside her vagina for the past year. She has no significant past medical or surgical history. Her obstetrical history is remarkable for five vaginal deliveries of which one was a forceps-assisted delivery. The largest of the five babies she delivered weighed 4500 g and was via unassisted, spontaneous vaginal delivery. You perform a speculum examination and notice prolapse of the anterior vaginal wall 1 cm past the hymen and lack of the superolateral sulcus, bilaterally. The vaginal apex and the posterior wall appear well supported. The primary structure(s) responsible for prevention of this patient's prolapse is/are _____.
   (A) ATFP
   (B) Attachments to the ATFP
   (C) Pubocervical septum
   (D) Obturator internus muscles
   (E) Levator ani muscles

2. During defecation the _____.
   (A) Levator ani muscles relax and the levator hiatus opens.
   (B) Levator ani muscles contract and levator hiatus opens.
   (C) Type I fibers contract and the anorectal angle increases.
   (D) Type II fibers contract and the anorectal angle decreases.

3. A 42-year-old gravida 3, para 3, presents to your office because of a bulge inside her vagina and lower back pain, which has been bothersome for the past 2 years. She is in good health. She had a tubal ligation 10 years ago. The Gellhorn pessary has relieved her symptoms for the past few months; however, she is tired of the inconvenience of pessary use and wants definitive surgical repair. She denies urgency, frequency, nocturia, dysuria, and symptoms of stress incontinence. Upon careful speculum examination, her uterus is well supported and the posterior compartment and the perineum are unremarkable. The anterior vagina is pink, moist, and well ruggated. There is loss of the anterosuperior sulcus on the right side. Also, the prolapse bulges to the level of the hymen on Valsalva. On physical examination, her stress test is negative with a full bladder and Q-tip test does not demonstrate hypermobility. No incontinence is demonstrated even after reduction of the cystocele. You decide to perform laparoscopic paravaginal repair. You place sutures from the pubocervical septum to a _____.
   (A) Thickening of fascia overlying the obturator internus
   (B) Thickening of fascia overlying the levator ani muscles
   (C) Band-like structure 3.5 cm from midline on the pubic bone at one end to the ischial spine at the other end
   (D) Structure spanning the PB to the ischial spine
   (E) Ligament connecting the pubis to the ischium

4. During a posterior colpoperineorrhaphy, the rectovaginal septum (RVS) is sutured to the PB. This is a key step in reconstructive surgery of the posterior compartment because the PB _____.
   (A) Is the meeting point of five muscle groups that maintain the integrity of the perineum
   (B) Is a pyramid–shaped structure
   (C) Provides continuous support to the posterior wall of the vagina from the perineum to the sacrum

(D) Is attached to the PM at several locations

(E) Is made of dense fibromuscular tissue with little vascularity

ANSWERS

1. *(E)*. Proper function of pelvic muscles and their nerves is important to maintain proper orientation and active support of the pelvic organs. The connective tissue (e.g., fascia), on the other hand, serves to hold and stabilize the organs.

   If the muscles do not function properly either because of damage from childbirth or from denervation injury, then the fascial attachments of the pelvic viscera stretch over time and may break. The levator ani muscles are always tonically contracted to some degree by Type I (slow fibers), but can also contract further voluntarily (Type II, fast fibers). Normal constant contraction of the levator ani keeps the levator hiatus closed by compressing the urethra, vagina, and rectum against the pubic bone while simultaneously pulling the pelvic floor and viscera upward (cephalic direction). When these muscles relax, during defecation and micturition, or are damaged, the levator hiatus opens leaving the vagina and viscera supported by their fascial attachments. Therefore, initial management of pelvic organ prolapse and long-term success of surgical repairs requires strengthening of the levator ani muscles by Kegel exercises or electrostimulation.

2. *(A)*. Normally, constant contraction of the levator ani muscles keeps the levator hiatus closed by compressing the urethra, vagina, and rectum against the pubic bone while pulling the pelvic floor and viscera upward (cephalic direction). When these muscles relax, during defecation and micturition, or are damaged, the levator hiatus opens leaving the vagina and viscera supported by the fascia. (C) is incorrect because contraction of the Type I fibers of puborectalis contributes to the anorectal angle which is thought to contribute to fecal continence. Additionally, contraction of the Type II fibers increases the anorectal angle.

3. *(B)*. The ATFP (or fascia arcus or *fascial* white line) is the parietal fascial covering of the levator ani muscles, which is thickened into a strong band on the surface of muscle. It spans from the lower one-sixth of the pubic bone about 1 cm from the midline (not 3.5 cm) at one end to the ischial spine at the other. The structure which starts at the PB and joins the ATFP before reaching the ischial

spine is called the arcus tendineus rectovaginalis (ATFRV) (see Chap. 2). There is no *ligament* between the pubis and ischium.

4. *(C)*. As described in Chap. 2, Anatomy Relevant to Female Reconstructive Pelvic Surgery: Part II, the PB is continuous with the sacrum as follows: PB → Rectovaginal Septum (RVS) [anterior wall] and Pubocervical Septum (PCS) [posterior wall] → cardinal uterosacral ligament [apex of vagina] → sacrum. The PB is the meeting point of three muscle groups (the bulbocavernosus muscles, the superficial transverse perinea, and the external anal sphincter). The levator ani muscles are also connected to the apex of the PB. The fact that the PB is pyramid shaped does not explain why this structure is key in a posterior colporrhaphy. The PB has little vascularity and the fact that it is made up of fibromuscular tissue does not explain its importance in posterior repair. The PM is connected to the PB around the vagina; however, this fact does not explain why attachment of the RVS to the PB provides strong support.

2 ANATOMY RELEVANT TO FEMALE RECONSTRUCTIVE PELVIC SURGERY: PART II
Sam Siddighi

SUPPORT OF THE PELVIC VISCERA

LEVEL I SUPPORT

Level I support is also known as DeLancey I, upper vagina or proximal vagina.

- This support network, which is thickened visceral fascia, is made up of the uterosacral (aka sacrouterine ligament) and cardinal ligaments (aka transverse cervical ligament or Mackenrodt's ligament) and act like suspension cables to hold the lower uterus, cervix, and upper vagina over the levator plate. The uterine and cervical attachments are called parametria, while the upper vaginal attachment is referred to as paracolpium.
- "Flap-valve"—As intra-abdominal pressure increases, the levator cruri contract and the urogenital hiatus closes. This allows transmission of pressure perpendicularly to the vagina and rectum against a horizontal levator plate.
- At the pelvic wall, the paired *cardinal ligaments* fan out and attach to the parietal fascia of the obturator internus, the piriformis, the anterior border of the

greater sciatic foramen, and the ischial spines. The internal iliac vessels have a vertical axis in this area and give off the uterine vessels which course through the cardinal ligaments. Near the cervix, the cardinal ligaments concentrate, narrow, and attach to the capsule of the cervix forming the *pericervical ring*. The cervix is at the level of the ischial spines. The pubocervical septum and the rectovaginal septum (RVS) are also in continuity at the pericervical ring.

- Therefore, reconstruction of the pericervical ring structure is essential after a hysterectomy so as to provide support for the anterior and posterior vaginal walls and the vaginal apex.
- The paired *uterosacral ligaments* (also dense visceral fascia) are considered by some as the most posterior portion of the cardinal ligaments. The uterosacral ligaments arise from the pericervical ring and attach posteriorly to presacral fascia (at the level of S2, S3, S4).
- The paracolpium can be appreciated as the lateral fornices on speculum examination.
- In a normally supported patient, level I support does not determine the resting position of the cervix.
- Detachment of the cardinal-uterosacral complex from the pericervical ring can result in apical prolapse, posthysterectomy vaginal vault prolapse (aka posthysterectomy cuff prolapse), uterine descensus, or enterocele (is a true hernia containing small bowel).
- An enterocele or cul-de-sac hernia occurs when the pericervical ring is disrupted and the RVS and pubocervical septum are no longer in continuity at the apex.
- The term enterocele is not appropriate preoperatively because accurate diagnosis is made only during surgery or with the use of radiologic methods.

LEVEL II SUPPORT

Level II support is also known as DeLancey II, mid-vagina; horizontal orientation.

ANTERIOR WALL
- In the standing patient, the orientation of the upper two-thirds of the vagina, bladder, and rectum is horizontal because of two parallel, trapezoid-shaped fascial *platforms* that are surgically referred to as pubocervical septum (aka pubocervical septum) and RVS (aka rectovaginal (RV) septum or fascia of Denonvilliers) [most distal portion].
- The pubocervical septum is the visceral fascia of the anterior vaginal wall and is fused with the vaginal epithelium.
- Both of these septi attach laterally to the arcus tendineus fascia pelvis (ATFP). The visceral fascia connecting between pubocervical septum and ATFP is

called endopelvic fascia (aka fascia endopelvina, paravaginal fascia, or transverse visceral septum), and measures up to 2 cm at the most proximal location of level II. Within this paravaginal fascia exits the periurethral vascular plexus (PVP).

- Proximally, the pubocervical septum fuses with the pericervical ring.
- Distally, the pubocervical septum forms a fascial hammock underneath the bladder, urethrovesical junction, and proximal urethra and attaches to the most inferior portion of the pubic arch and the perineal membrane (PM) (see Urethral Support).
- On speculum examination, the anterolateral vaginal sulci represent attachment of the pubocervical septum to the ATFP.
- Detachment of endopelvic fascia from the ATFP (aka paravaginal support defect) is responsible for anterior wall prolapse (formerly called displacement cystocele). This is in contrast to *central cystocele* where there is failure of the pubocervical septum centrally in the vaginal wall resulting in anterior prolapse.
- Defects in level II can also result in urethral hypermobility (proximal urethral support defects) and posterior wall prolapse (formerly called rectocele). The former terms should not be used to describe these conditions because the most accurate diagnosis can only be made during surgery or by radiologic means.

POSTERIOR WALL
- Unlike the pubocervical septum, the RVS is an embryologically distinct layer formed from fusion of peritoneum of the cul-de-sac underneath the posterior vaginal wall fibromuscular layer. A layer of adventitia separates the muscular layer of the rectum from the RV septum except at the perineal body (PB). RVS provides a platform between the posterior vaginal wall and the rectum.
- Tears or breaks in the RVS result in rectoceles.
- The most distal end of the RVS attaches to the apex of the PB. Disruption of this connection results in hypermobility of the perineum.
- Distally and laterally, the RVS merges with the parietal fascia of the iliococcygeus, below the level of the ATFP. In other words, the distal half of the RVS inserts onto a second thickening of parietal fascia of the iliococcygeus called the *arcus tendineus fascia rectovaginalis (ATFRV)*. This structure is actually connected to the ATFP, but travels distal to the ATFP in an inferior-oblique direction to attach to the apex of the PB.
- On speculum examination, the ATFRV creates the posterolateral sulcus in the nulliparous vagina.
- The proximal end of the RVS attaches to the cul-de-sac peritoneum. This inner end also attaches to the

uterosacral ligament. It is believed that the proximal portion of the RVS is not fascia but just folds of peritoneum whereas the distal portion is fascia. Therefore, one can say that the PB is connected to the sacrum because a continuous line of attachment exists from the PB through the RVS to the sacrum (via the uterosacral ligament).
- Lateral attachments. At its proximal end, the RVS is attached to ATFP (which is thickened parietal fascia of the iliococcygeus) via the endopelvic fascia.

LEVEL III SUPPORT

Level III support is also known as DeLancey III, lower vagina or distal; vertical orientation.
- At this level the vagina is directly connected to the surrounding structures without any intervening endopelvic fascia. Therefore, there is *fusion of visceral fascia* of the vagina (fibers of Luschka) and rectum with the *parietal fascia* of the pubococcygeus and puborectalis muscles.
- Level III also consists of attachments of the pubocervical septum to the PM (anteriorly) and RV septum to apex of the PB (posteriorly). These attachments stabilize the lower third of the vagina, the urethra, and the rectum.
- At this level, the visceral structures (lower one-third vagina, urethra, and anal canal) travel 3–4 cm past the levator hiatus and are vertically oriented.
- The puborectalis causes the 90° anorectal junction angle.
- Damage to level III support contributes to anterior and posterior prolapse, gaping introitus, urethrocele, and a hypermobile perineum.

THE URETHRA

URETHRAL LAYERS

- The female urethra is ≈4 cm long and ≈0.6 cm in diameter.
- The proximal urethra rests on top of the pubocervical septum. As the urethra courses distally it becomes invested within the pubocervical septum.
- Intrinsic smooth muscle of the urethra (the circular layer only) is continuous with the bladder smooth muscle but is embryologically distinct.
- Layers of the urethra starting from the lumen are: epithelium → loose connective tissue (lamina propria) → submucosa → thick longitudinal muscle → thin circular muscle→sphincter urethrae (if proximal urethra) or compressor urethrae/urethrovaginal sphincter (if distal urethra).
- During micturition, the thick longitudinal muscle contracts, shortening the urethra.

- The distal end of the urethral epithelium is of squamous type while the proximal end is of transitional type. The location of the squamous-transitional junction depends on a person's age, hormonal status, and possibly sexual activity. In reproductive years the junction is closer to the bladder (and sometimes covering the trigone), while in menopause it is the opposite.
- The submucosal layer is highly vascular and maintains a tight urethral lumen seal when arterial blood is under sufficient pressure. The urethral artery, which runs within the trigonal plate, sends tiny branches into the submucosa. This layer is also rich in glands but primarily along the dorsal side (or vaginal side) of the urethra. The glands are possible sites of formation of suburethral diverticula.

URETHRAL SUPPORT

- Like the vagina, the proximal urethra also has its own fascial attachments to the ATFP and muscular attachments to the medial border of the levator ani (aka pubovaginalis portion of the pubococcygeus muscle). The muscular connection to the levator ani maintains a high position of the urethrovesical angle.
- Detachment of the paravaginal fascia from ATFP is associated with stress urinary incontinence (as well as anterior prolapse).
- The normal resting tone of the levator ani maintains the normal position of the urethrovesical junction and proximal urethra while the paravaginal fascia (aka endopelvic fascia) stabilizes it.
- During micturition, the levator ani relax, allowing the urethrovesical junction to move inferiorly and posteriorly to the limit of its paravaginal fascial attachments (i.e., decrease in the urethrovesical angle).
- Therefore, the urethrovesical junction and the proximal urethra are mobile structures (proven by fluoroscopic studies) and lie within the adventitia of anterior vagina. The pubourethral ligaments, which are just lateral to the most proximal end of the urethra span from pubocervical septum to the posterior, inferior pubic symphysis. These bilateral ligaments are thought to contribute to continence.
- Slightly more than the distal third of the urethra, however, is fixed because the urethra is attached to the pubic bones via the PM and the urogenital sphincter complex (see further).
- In a normal person, during increases in intra-abdominal pressure (e.g., valsalva), the urethrovesical junction and proximal urethra are compressed against the stable, firm platform of the pubocervical septum causing occlusion. If, however, the platform of pubocervical septum were unstable and overly elastic, then stress incontinence could result.

- Coughing causes contraction of the levator ani which elevates and moves the urethrovesical junction anteriorly, stabilizing the pubocervical platform. Coughing also causes contraction of the urogenital sphincter complex. The common former belief that increase in intra-abdominal pressure is transmitted to the *intra-abdominal portion of the urethra*, causing occlusion is unsupported by urethral pressure studies because:
    1. Urethral pressure during cough is greatest in distal rather than proximal urethra.
    2. Pressure in the distal urethra exceeds intra-abdominal pressure.
    3. Rise in urethral pressure occurs before rise in cough pressure, suggesting a reflex contraction in anticipation of maximal cough pressures.

UROGENITAL SPHINCTER COMPLEX

- The urogenital-sphincter complex is also known as striated urogenital sphincter muscle, striated circular muscle, striated sphincter, or rhabdosphincter. These are three striated muscles which are immediately adjacent to the urethra and function as a unit. These muscles lie behind (just deep to) the PM.
- For the purpose of description, the most proximal end of the urethra at the internal urethral meatus is defined as 0%, while the distal end of the urethra where urine emerges during micturition (external meatus) is defined as 100%. The portion of the urethra through the bladder base is referred to as 0–20%. Here, continence is maintained by the intrinsic urethral sphincter (trigonal ring + circular smooth muscle of urethra).
- *Sphincter urethrae* muscle almost completely surrounds the urethra from 20% to 60% along its length. The gap is bridged by the trigonal plate (see below). Contraction causes occlusion of the urethra from 20% to 60% along its length.
- From 60% to 80% along the length of the urethra lie two bandlike muscles. The band that surrounds and fuses with the vaginal wall is called the *urethrovaginal sphincter*. The other band which attaches the urethra to the ischiopubic ramus is called the *compressor urethrae*. These two muscles overlap on the ventral side of the urethra. Contraction of these two muscles causes compression of the distal urethra. Along the lateral vaginal wall and between the cruri of the urethrovaginal sphincter and compressor urethrae lie the transverse vaginal muscles. In the past, these groups of muscles were erroneously grouped into the *deep transverse perineal muscle*. Note: 80–100% along the urethra does not contribute to continence and its only function is to aim urine.
- The urogenital sphincter complex is usually tonically contracted but is able to contract more vigorously by reflex or at will. Normally, the urethral closure pressure is maximal near the mid-urethra.
- This group of muscles contributes to continence since their removal after a radical vulvectomy results in incontinence. In these patients, the urethral support and the internal urethral pressure are unchanged yet they have incontinence.

THE BLADDER AND THE RETROPUBIC SPACE

- The normal bladder is a hollow viscus that fills without increase in pressure during the filling phase; and contracts during emptying phase.
- Its embryologic origin is the urogenital sinus.
- Anterior to bladder is the *retropubic or space of Retzius* (cave of Retzius). The boundaries are: anterior = symphysis pubis, lateral = pubic bone and obturator internus muscle, superior = superior ramus of pubic bone, inferior = pubocervical septum, pubourethral ligaments, pubovesical ligaments, urethrovesical angle, proximal urethra, and the extraperitoneal part of the bladder. Note: pubovesical ligaments ≠ pubourethral ligament. Pubovesical ligaments are fibrous connective tissue + outer longitudinal muscle of the bladder which attach to the pubic symphysis and the ATFP. These may be involved in vesical neck opening.
- The space of Retzius also contains: (1) loose adipose tissue, (2) directly behind the pubic symphysis and in the midline are a symmetric network of vessels called the anterior vesical and retropubic vessels which are both branches of the internal pudendal artery, (3) veins of Santorini (rich venous plexus in the paravaginal fascia [endopelvic fascia] traveling parallel to each other and perpendicular to the ATFP; they arise from the vaginal and internal pudendal vessels), and (4) the obturator neurovascular bundle going into the obturator canal. An *anomalous (aka aberrant, accessory) obturator artery and vein* are usually also encountered leaving the obturator neurovascular bundle near the canal and traversing laterally and superiorly to connect with the inferior epigastric system near the top of the pubic bone. The inferior epigastric vessels connect to the external iliac vessels. The aberrant obturator vessels are within 4–5 cm of the pubic tubercle and cross over Cooper's ligament. Therefore they must be recognized before placing stitches during Burch retropubic urethropexy. Additionally, there is an *unnamed vein* at the lower edge of the bladder which runs parallel to it (this is a constant landmark).
- *Vesical neck:* region of the bladder base where the urethral lumen joins bladder wall.

- The urethra at the bladder neck is not only held in place, but also may be occluded there by the sphincteric action of two bands of opposing U-shaped muscle fibers. The thicker Heiss's loop (aka detrusor loop) goes around the anterior vesical neck urethra and opens posteriorly. The thinner loop, which is made of circular *sphincter urethrae* muscle, almost completely surrounds the urethra from 20% to 60% along its length. The gap is bridged by the trigonal plate intermediate fibers of the bladder wall, goes around the posterior vesical neck urethra and opens anteriorly. Together, these U-shaped muscle fibers make up the trigonal ring at level of the internal urethral meatus; the ring contributes to the intrinsic urethral sphincter. The trigonal plate is also a band of trigonal tissue that only lies at the posterior (dorsal) aspect of the urethra and goes below the level of the trigonal ring to a level 80% along the length of the urethra. Urethral artery courses within the dorsal aspect of the trigonal plate.
- Layers of bladder wall: transitional epithelium (urothelium) mucosa → loose CT submucosa (lamina propria) → detrusor muscle layers (3) → visceral peritoneum (superior and upper posterior surface only).
- The three ill-defined smooth muscle layers gain more definition as they travel from the dome toward the base of the bladder, especially at the bladder neck. The layers are: outermost = longitudinal, intermediate = oblique and circular, and innermost = large mesh-like pattern of fibers.
- The outer longitudinal muscle fibers attach the bladder to the pubic symphysis anteriorly. Contraction of these fibers may contribute to bladder neck opening.
- The inner longitudinal muscle fibers are continuous with inner longitudinal layer of the urethra.
- The intermediate layer does not continue into the urethra but fuses with the trigonal muscles.
- *Trigone:* embryologically distinct (is mesonephric in origin and not urogenital sinus), triangular area in bladder base whose corners consist of the entrance of the pair of distal ureters and the proximal urethra. The ureteral openings are 3 cm apart and are slitlike. The openings are usually separated by a ridge of raised tissue called the interureteric ridge.
- The trigone has two layers:
  1. The predominant *superficial layer* is continuous with longitudinal fibers of distal ureters, the trigonal ring, and the longitudinal smooth muscle layer of the urethra; the superficial layer contains mostly noradrenergic receptors (causing contraction simultaneous with intrinsic urethral sphincter).
  2. *Deep layer* fuses with detrusor muscle and attaches to intravesical portion of the ureter called Waldeyer's sheath; this layer has mostly cholinergic receptors (causing contraction simultaneous with bladder wall).

- During voluntary levator ani contractions, the bladder base moves upward and forward (i.e., anterior and superior). However, during straining, the bladder base moves downward and backward (posterior and inferior).

THE ANAL SPHINCTER COMPLEX

- As you move distally from the sigmoid colon along the rectum toward the anal sphincter, there is an increase in the *inner circular layer of smooth muscle* as well as the outer longitudinal layers.
- The outer layer becomes concentrated on the anterior wall of the rectum then attaches to the PB; similarly, it becomes concentrated on the posterior wall of the rectum and attaches to the coccyx.
- The distal end of inner circular layer forms the internal anal sphincter which is responsible for majority of resting anal tone. It is controlled by the autonomic nervous system.
- Just inferior and outside the internal anal sphincter lies the external anal sphincter which is attached to the PB (anteriorly) and to the coccyx (posteriorly).
- The striated external anal sphincter also has baseline tonic contraction but can also be voluntarily contracted just like the levator ani muscles.
- The anal sphincter is made up of (1) internal anal sphincter, (2) puborectalis (of levator ani), and (3) the external anal sphincter; (2) and (3) appear and contract as a unit.
- Fecal incontinence may result because of denervation of the levator ani and external anal sphincter as well as physical disruption of the external anal sphincter. Anorectal angle may also contribute to continence.

THE URETERS

- The ureters start from the renal pelvis and go down and insert into the bladder, spanning a distance of about 25–30 cm. The upper half lies directly on the psoas muscle and receives its blood supply from the aorta and the renal arteries. The lower half or pelvic ureter receives its blood supply from the aorta and common and internal iliac arteries.
- Pelvic ureter (the ureters narrow at the pelvic brim). Path: at or close to the bifurcation of the common iliac arteries, the ureter crosses over the artery and lies medial to branches of anterior division of the internal iliac arteries. At this level the ureter is also medial and parallel to the infundibulopelvic ligament then passes underneath the infundibulopelvic ligament. This is the second most common site of injury to ureters in gynecologic surgery.

- Further down, the ureter travels 1–1.5 cm lateral to the border of the uterosacral ligaments.
- Then enters the cardinal ligament, lying only 1.5 cm lateral to the cervix, and crosses underneath the uterine artery ("water under the bridge") and moves medially just over the lateral fornices of the vagina to enter the bladder trigone. The junction of the uterine artery and ureter is the first most common site of injury to ureters in gynecologic surgeries.
- The ureter has only one smooth muscle layer which has a helical pattern along the entire length but becomes longitudinal at its distal end so it can insert into the superficial layer of the trigone.
- The ureters narrow again as they enter the bladder. The intravesical portion of the ureter is 1.5 cm in length and consists of the intramural and submucosal segments.
- The most distal part of the ureter and the intramural segment of the ureter have an additional layer called Waldeyer's sheath. It fuses proximally with the helical smooth muscle layer of the ureter, while it fuses distally with the deep layer of the trigone.

ARTERIAL SUPPLY OF STRUCTURES RELEVANT TO FEMALE RECONSTRUCTIVE PELVIC SURGERY

- The somatic (e.g., levator ani) and visceral pelvic structures receive the majority of their blood from branches of the internal iliac artery.
- Sacrum: (1) lateral sacral artery: branch of internal iliac, *posterior division* (note: the other arteries of the posterior trunk are iliolumbar artery and superior gluteal artery) (2) middle sacral artery: direct branch from aorta.
- Ureters: (1) aorta (2) renal artery (3) small arteries of the posterior abdominal wall (4) gonadal artery (5) **common iliac artery** (6) **internal iliac artery** (7) **inferior vesical artery**. The bolded arteries are important for the blood supply of the ureters below the pelvic brim.
- Bladder: (1) superior vesical artery: branch of internal iliac, anterior division (usually a branch of umbilical artery) (2) inferior vesical artery: branch of the internal iliac, anterior division, which supplies the bladder neck, urethrovesical junction, and the inferiormost ureters.
- Urethra: internal pudendal artery → deep perineal artery → urethral artery.
- Uterus: (1) uterine artery: a branch of the internal iliac, anterior division, it crosses over the ureters in the cardinal ligament and ascends within the broad ligament to reach the uterus. Its tubal branches anastomose with branches of ovarian artery (2) branches of the ovarian artery, which directly arise from the aorta (3) Sampson's artery: branch of the external iliac artery which supplies the round ligament of the uterus.

- Cervix and upper vagina: (1) branches of the uterine artery, vaginal branches, supply the cervix and upper vagina (2) twigs from middle rectal artery (branch of internal iliac) (3) anastomoses with lower vaginal branches.
- Middle and lower vagina: (1) vaginal branches of the internal pudendal artery (2) twigs from the middle rectal artery (3) anastomoses with upper vaginal branches.
- Perineum: (1) superficial perineal artery → transverse perineal artery: branch of internal pudendal artery (this is a branch of the internal iliac which exits pelvis through lesser sciatic foramen to enter the ischiorectal fossa and courses in the internal pudendal canal [aka Alcock's canal]) (2) inferior rectal artery: branch of internal pudendal also.
- Vulva and labia: perineal artery and posterior labial artery (both are branches of superficial perineal [which is a branch of the internal pudendal artery]).
- Erectile tissue, Bartholin's gland, and clitoris: the deep perineal artery gives rise to artery of Bartholin's gland and dorsal artery of clitoris, and is a branch of internal pudendal artery.
- Rectum: (1) middle rectal artery (aka hemorrhoidal artery): branch of the internal iliac, anterior division. Anastomoses with superior rectal artery (2) superior rectal artery: branch of the inferior mesenteric artery (which arises from the aorta) (3) inferior rectal artery: branch of the internal pudendal artery.
- Veins in the pelvic cavity usually follow the arteries but there is great variation. Eventually, the veins drain into the internal iliac vein.
- The rectum has its surrounding venous plexus which drain into the rectal veins.
- The bladder has its surrounding veins of Santorini and also veins which receive blood from the clitoris. These drain into the vesical veins.

BIBLIOGRAPHY

Baggish MS, Karram MM. Atlas of Pelvic Anatomy and Gynecologic Surgery. Philadelphia, PA: W.B. Saunders; 2001: 177–184.

DeLancey JOL. Anatomy of the female bladder and urethra. In: Bent AE, Ostergard DR, Cundiff GW, Swift SE, eds. *Ostergard's Urogynecology and Pelvic Floor Dysfunction.* 5th ed. Philadelphia, PA: Lippincott Williams & Wilkins; 2003:3–18.

Hurt WG. Retropubic urethropexy or colposuspension. In: Hurt WG, ed. *The Master's Techniques in Gynecologic Surgery, Urogynecologic Surgery.* 2nd ed. Philadelphia, PA: Lippincott Williams & Wilkins; 2000:82.

Kilgore LC, Shingleton HM. Recognizing injuries to the urinary tract. In: Sanz LE, ed. *Gynecologic surgery.* 2nd ed. Cambridge, MA: Blackwell Science; 1995:317–323.

Moore KL. The pelvis and perineum. In: Moore KL, ed. *Clinically Oriented Anatomy*. 3rd ed. Baltimore, MD: William & Wilkins; 1992:243–322.

Netter FH. *The Atlas of Human Anatomy*. East Hanover, NJ: Novartis; 1989:334–394.

Richardson AC. Paravaginal repair. In: Hurt WG, ed. *Urogynecologic Surgery*. Gaithersburg, MD: Aspen Publishers; 1992:73–80.

Rogers Jr. RM. Anatomy of pelvic support. In: Bent AE, Ostergard DR, Cundiff GW, Swift SE, eds. *Ostergard's Urogynecology and Pelvic Floor Dysfunction*, 5th ed. Philadelphia, PA: Lippincott Williams & Wilkins; 2003.

Shull BL, Benn SJ, Huehl TJ. Surgical management of prolapse of the anterior vaginal segment: an analysis of support defects, operative morbidity, and anatomic outcome. *Am J Obstet Gynecol* 1994;171:1429–1439.

Walters MD, Weber AM. Anatomy of the lower urinary tract, rectum, and pelvic floor. In: Walters MD, Karram MM, eds. *Urogynecology and Reconstructive Pelvic Surgery*. 2nd ed. St Louis, MO: Mosby; 1999:3–13.

Wei JT, De Lancey JOL. Functional anatomy of the pelvic floor and lower urinary tract. In: Weber A, ed. *Incontinence 2004*. Philadelphia, PA: Lippincott Williams & Wilkins; 2004:3–17.

QUESTIONS

1. A 52-year-old gravida 5, para 4, sab 1, presents to you complaining of severe loss of urine with straining. She has not had much benefit from duloxetine. After evaluation you diagnose her with urodynamic stress urinary incontinence. She is now interested in minimally invasive surgery to correct her incontinence. Prior to explaining the risks of the vaginal approach, suburethral tension-free vaginal type sling procedure, you review, all of the layers that the trocar passes through before emerging at the stab sites in the suprapubic area. The _____ has the lowest risk of injury by the trocar during this procedure.
   (A) Veins of Santorini
   (B) Bladder
   (C) Pubocervical septum
   (D) Aberrant obturator vessels
   (E) Pubourethral ligament

2. If a histologic cross section were made through cadaveric urethra at 25% along the urethral length, on its lateral side, one would encounter ___ distinct layers of muscle.
   (A) 1
   (B) 2
   (C) 3
   (D) 4
   (E) 5

3. If a histologic section were made through a cadaveric urethra at 25% along the urethral length, on its dorsal side (i.e., vaginal side), the last layer of tissue one encounters is the _____.
   (A) Compressor urethrae
   (B) Sphincter urethrae
   (C) Circular muscle of urethra
   (D) Trigonal plate

4. The urethrovesical junction and the proximal urethra are mobile structures. From fluoroscopic studies we know that the bladder moves _____ and _____ during micturition.
   (A) Superiorly and posteriorly
   (B) Superiorly and anteriorly
   (C) Inferiorly and posteriorly
   (D) Inferiorly and anteriorly
   (E) Posteriorly and laterally

5. The pericervical ring is a crucial structure because it serves as the attachment point of several important support structures. Detachment of the pubocervical septum from this ring results in _____.
   (A) Uterine descensus
   (B) Anterior prolapse—lateral detachment
   (C) Anterior prolapse—central failure
   (D) Apical prolapse
   (E) Enterocele

QUESTIONS 6–10

Match the word or description below either with its synonym or the best word(s) to describe it.
   (A) Fascia endopelvina
   (B) Fascia of Denonvilliers
   (C) Interureteric ridge
   (D) Urogenital diaphragm
   (E) White line
   (F) ATLA
   (G) ATFRV
   (H) ATLP
   (I) Retzius
   (J) Heiss
   (K) Waldeyer
   (L) Arcuate
   (M) Mackenrodt
   (N) Level I
   (O) Anal triangle
   (P) Levator plate

6. Anatomic misnomer that refers to a muscle layer sandwiched between two layers of fascia
7. The cardinal ligament
8. Lies anterior-superior to the pubovesical ligament
9. Segment of tissue which reinforces ureteral attachment to the bladder
10. Distal portion of a trapezoid-shaped septum formed by fusion of cul-de-sac peritoneum

ANSWERS

1. *(D)*. Although the aberrant obturator vessels are located within the retropubic space, they are far lateral and superior to where the trocar emerges during the vaginal approach of the tension-free vaginal tape sling procedure. Bladder perforation is a known risk of this procedure and has incidence of 4–6% and can be recognized intraoperatively with cystoscopy. Perforation of the pubocervical septum is a requirement of this procedure. Similarly, due to its location, the pubourethral ligaments can be pierced by the trocar. Injury to the veins of Santorini during this procedure results in bleeding.

2. *(C)*. One encounters three muscle layers surrounding the urethra (on its lateral side), starting from the lumen toward the outside. The first layer is the thick longitudinal muscle followed by the thin circular muscle and finally the sphincter urethrae (which exists at 20—60% along the length of the urethra).

3. *(D)*. No muscle layers surround the urethra on its dorsal side. In fact, on its dorsal side, the layers of the urethra are: epithelium → loose CT (lamina propria) → submucosa → trigonal plate. The sphincter urethrae muscle almost completely surrounds the urethra except on its dorsal side where the gap is bridged by the trigonal plate. The compressor urethrae and urethrovaginal sphincter are only located on the ventral side of the urethra. The longitudinal and circular muscles of the urethra are bridged on the dorsal aspect of the urethra by the trigonal plate.

4. *(C)*. The normal resting tone of levator ani maintains the normal position of the urethrovesical junction and proximal urethra. During micturition, the levator ani relax allowing the urethrovesical junction to move inferiorly and posteriorly to the limit of its paravaginal fascial attachments. In other words, during voiding, the bladder moves downward and back.

5. *(D)*. This question is best answered by the process of elimination. The lower uterus is supported by the cardinal-uterosacral complex, which meet around the pericervical ring. Uterine prolapse is unlikely because there is no mention cardinal-uterosacral ligament detachment. Anterior prolapse—lateral refers to paravaginal detachment of the pubocervical septum from the ATFP (not the pericervical ring). Anterior prolapse—central refers to anterior vaginal wall bulging due to failure of the pubocervical septum itself rather than its detachment. Enterocele refers to apical prolapse which contains small bowel. There is no mention of this in the question.

ANSWERS 6–10

6. *(D)* 7. *(M)* 8. *(I)* 9. *(K)* 10. *(B)*. The urogenital diaphragm is an incorrect name because it implies that a layer of muscle (formerly known as the deep transverse perineal muscle and adjacent sphincter muscle of the urethra) is sandwiched between two layer of fascia (the superior and inferior fascia of the urogenital diaphragm). The urogenital diaphragm is now called the PM. The cardinal ligament, the transverse cervical ligament, and the ligament of Mackenrodt are all synonyms. The space of Retzius lies anterior to the bladder. Waldeyer's sheath is a layer of tissue that reinforces ureteral attachment to the bladder. It fuses proximally with the helical smooth muscle layer of the ureter, while distally it fuses with the deep layer of the trigone. The RV septum, also known as the RVS or fascia of Denonvilliers, is an embryologically distinct layer formed from fusion of peritoneum from the cul-de-sac underneath the posterior vaginal wall fibromuscular layer.

3 # FUNCTION AND PHYSIOLOGY OF THE LOWER URINARY TRACT AND PELVIC FLOOR IN WOMEN

Marianna Alperin and Sam Siddighi

INTRODUCTION

Lower urinary tract dysfunction can lead to a multitude of clinical presentations, depending on the cause. Often problems are multifactorial, involving the interplay between anatomic changes, pathology of the nervous system, age-related factors, and comorbid conditions. Urinary incontinence is the most common presentation encountered, with the prevalence that increases with age. (see Chap. 4).

Pelvic floor disorders cause such morbidities as pelvic organ prolapse (POP), urinary incontinence, fecal incontinence, and disorders of evacuation of urinary and gastrointestinal systems. Pelvic floor dysfunction is a major health issue with women having 11.1% risk of undergoing an operation for POP or urinary incontinence in their lifetime.

Increasing the understanding of the disorders of lower urinary tract and changes in the pelvic anatomy will allow for the better choice of surgical procedure and medical therapy.

BASIC ANATOMY OF LOWER URINARY TRACT AND PELVIC FLOOR

BLADDER

- It is a hollow, muscular organ which consists of the dome and the *trigone* (the base).
- Two ureteral orifices and the internal urethral orifice constitute the three corners of the trigone. Superficial muscle of the trigone is continuous with proximal urethra.
- The lining of the bladder consists of transitional epithelium (urothelium) and supportive connective tissue (lamina propria).
- The smooth muscle of the bladder wall is termed *detrusor.*
- See Chap. 2 for more details.

URETHRA

- The dimensions of the female urethra on average are 4 cm in length and 6 mm in diameter.
- The lining of the urethra consists of stratified squamous epithelium, except at the bladder neck where it becomes transitional. It is supported by the lamina propria as well.
- The smooth muscle of the urethra together with the detrusor muscle at the base of the bladder form *intrinsic urethral sphincter.*
- The striated muscle of the urethra and skeletal muscle of the pelvic diaphragm constitute *extrinsic urethral sphincter.*
- The principles underlying the function of a sphincter are watertight apposition of the urethral lumen, compression of the wall around the lumen, structural support to keep the proximal urethra from moving during increases in pressure, a means of compensating for

abdominal pressure changes (pressure transmission), and neural control. Thus, normal sphincteric function is the result of an integrated interaction among all these factors.

PELVIC FLOOR

- The uterosacral/cardinal ligament complex, the levator ani muscles, and the endopelvic fascia support the pelvic organs. These structures attach the pelvic organs to the bony pelvis and form a continuous and interdependent organ complex.
- The levator ani muscle complex forms a broad hammock upon which the pelvic viscera lie. It consists of four parts: puboperineus, pubococcygeus, puborectalis, and iliococcygeus muscles.
- The levator ani and coccygeus muscles that are attached to the inner surface of the minor pelvis form the muscular floor of the pelvis. With their corresponding muscles from the opposite side, they form the *pelvic diaphragm.*
- *Urogenital diaphragm* is a musculofascial structure present over the anterior pelvic outlet below the pelvic diaphragm.
- The *perineal body* (PB) is a pyramidal fibromuscular structure in the midline between the anus and the vagina.
- The *puboperineus* muscle arises from the pubic bone immediately lateral to the pubic symphysis and inserts into the PB in front of the rectum.
- The *pubococcygeus* and the *puborectalis* muscles form a U shape as they originate from the pubic bone on either side of the midline, insert into the anal sphincter complex, and pass behind the rectum to form a sling. The pubococcygeus muscle can be appreciated during physical examination of the pelvis as a bulky muscular ridge on both lateral sidewalls of the vagina, superior to the hymen.
- The *iliococcygeus* muscle arises laterally from the arcus tendineus levator ani (ATLA) and forms a horizontal sheet that spans the opening in the posterior region of the pelvis, on which the pelvic organs rest.
- The fascial components of the pelvic floor include parietal and visceral fascia. Parietal fascia covers the skeletal muscles of the pelvic floor and attaches them to the bony pelvis. Visceral fascia, termed *endopelvic fascia*, exists throughout the pelvis. Uterosacral and cardinal ligaments represent condensations of the endopelvic fascia.
- Urethral support is provided by a coordinated action of anterior vagina, fascia, and muscles. This musculofascial support provides a hammock upon which the urethra is compressed during increases in intra-abdominal pressure.

- The anterior vagina is supported by lateral fibrous connections to the levator ani muscles. These connections form the *arcus tendineus fasciae pelvis* (ATFP). ATFP originates at the pubic bone and insert into the ischial spine. These bilateral structures provide support needed to suspend the urethra on the anterior vaginal wall.

FUNCTION OF THE LOWER URINARY TRACT

- Two main functions of lower urinary tract are storage of urine and its expulsion—micturition. To accomplish these, lower urinary tract consists of the urinary bladder, which serves as reservoir and the bladder outlet and urethra, which function as a sphincter.
- During bladder filling, detrusor pressure remains nearly constant because of a special property of the bladder smooth muscle and connective tissue known as *accommodation*. When accommodation is impaired, low bladder *compliance* results.
- During micturition, the sphincter relaxes and the bladder contracts and empties. When the lower urinary tract fails to maintain its storage function, urinary incontinence ensues.

FUNCTION OF THE PELVIC FLOOR

- The main function of the pelvic floor is to provide continence and prevent POP.
- The normal levator ani maintains tone in the upright position to support the pelvic viscera. Voluntary squeezing of the muscles of the pelvic floor counteracts increases in the intra-abdominal pressure.
- The anterior vaginal wall supports the urethra by its lateral attachment to the levator ani muscles and to the endopelvic fascia.
- The normal tone and integrity of the levator muscles maintain the normal dimensions of the urogenital hiatus, which is measured from the external urethral meatus to the posterior hymen.

NEURAL CONTROL OF THE LOWER URINARY TRACT AND PELVIC FLOOR

It is impossible to understand the physiology of the lower urinary tract without learning about neural pathways that play an integral role in storage of urine as well as micturition.

SENSORY INNERVATION

- Afferent impulses of the bladder wall originate from mechanoreceptors that respond to stretch and free nerve endings in the bladder mucosa that respond to pain and temperature.
- The impulses travel in the pelvic nerves and relay on the interneurons in the posterior gray horn of the spinal cord from where the secondary neuron travels through the spinothalamic tract to the *pontine micturition center* (PMC).
- Afferent impulses originating at the trigone and urethra relay mostly to the cerebral cortex.

MOTOR INNERVATION

- Parasympathetic and sympathetic nervous systems (SNS) exert opposite effect on the bladder and the urethra.
- The preganglionic parasympathetic nerves from S2, 3, 4, travel in the pelvic nerve and synapse in the cholinergic ganglia in the pelvic plexus and the wall of the bladder. Parasympathetic nervous system (PNS), through its effect on the cholinergic receptors in the bladder and urethra, excite the detrusor and inhibit urethral smooth muscle. Parasympathetic nerves from S2, 3, 4 provide major motor innervation to the detrusor muscle.
- The preganglionic sympathetic nerves from T10 to L2 communicate with the corresponding chain ganglia after which postganglionic neurons travel in the hypogastric nerve and synapse in the adrenergic ganglia in the pelvic plexus. SNS via its effect on beta-adrenergic receptors inhibits detrusor and stimulates urethral smooth muscle via alpha-adrenergic receptors.
- Somatic motor innervation to the external urethral sphincter and pelvic floor muscles is provided by the Onuf's nucleus, which is located in the anterolateral horn of the sacral spinal cord (S2, S3, S4). The fibers travel through the pudendal nerve.

CENTRAL CONTROL

- *Suprapontine region.* The parietal lobes and thalamus receive and coordinate detrusor afferent stimuli, the frontal lobes and basal ganglia provide modulation with inhibitory signals, thus *providing tonic inhibitory systems in the brain that suppress parasympathetic excitatory outflow to the bladder*. Damage to central inhibitory pathways can unmask primitive voiding reflexes and trigger bladder overactivity.

- *Pontine micturition center (PMC).* It is located in the ventral periaqueductal gray area of the pons and is the area of integration and control of afferent and efferent impulses from the urinary bladder.
- *Pontine continence center (PCC).* It is located in the lateral region of the pons' reticular formation. Its impulses provide a tonic excitation to the motor neurons of Onuf's nucleus, thus pelvic floor muscles and striated urethral sphincter maintain a baseline tone.
- When PMC is stimulated it activates sacral inhibitory interneurons, which, in turn, inhibit motor neurons to the external urethral sphincter and pelvic floor muscles. Urethral pressure is thus decreased and pelvic floor muscles relaxed. By simultaneously stimulating parasympathetic innervation of the detrusor, PMC causes increase in bladder pressure. These events allow micturition to take place.

PHYSIOLOGY OF FILLING AND STORAGE

- Due to the unique properties of its smooth muscle and connective tissue, the bladder is an extremely compliant organ. Secondary to bladder compliance, the intravesicular pressure increases minimally during bladder filling.
- In response to afferent neurons excitation during advanced filling, SNS inhibits detrusor contractions by relaxing the smooth muscle through beta-adrenergic receptors. At the same time sympathetic inhibition of parasympathetic ganglionic transmission in the pelvic plexuses and activation of the urethral smooth muscle through alpha-adrenergic receptor takes place. These processes facilitate storage of urine.
- Bladder stretch receptors communicate with PCC, which also increases SNS efferent activity, as well as activates Onuf's nucleus motor neurons to amplify tone of the striated muscles in the urethra and pelvic floor.

PHYSIOLOGY OF MICTURITION

- Micturition is a complex series of finely tuned and integrated neuromuscular events that involve anatomic and neurologic mechanisms. Alterations in any of these components may result in dysfunctional voiding and/or urinary incontinence.
- Voiding is a voluntary act, control of which starts in the frontal lobe of cerebral cortex. The cerebral cortex stops its inhibitory influence on the PMC when micturition is appropriate.

- When bladder capacity is reached, the bladder afferent nerve signals activate PMC which, in turn, stimulates PNS efferents, thus activating detrusor muscle. PMC simultaneously inhibits SNS output to the urethral smooth muscle and efferent somatic output to the striated muscles.
- In order to achieve micturition, the above neurologic pathways cause relaxation of the external urethral sphincter and pelvic floor muscles decreasing urethral pressure and at the same time elicit detrusor contraction. Voluntary interruption of the stream is accomplished by a sudden contraction of the striated periurethral musculature, which, through a reflex mechanism, shuts off the detrusor contraction, aborting micturition.

CONTINENCE

- Urethral closure pressure must be greater than bladder pressure, both at rest and during increases in abdominal pressure, to retain urine in the bladder.
- The resting tone of the urethral muscles maintains a favorable pressure relative to the bladder pressure.
- During activities such as coughing, when bladder pressure increases several times higher than urethral pressure, a dynamic process increases urethral closure pressure to enhance urethral closure and maintain continence.
- The vesical neck and urethra must be compressed to a closed position when abdominal pressure exceeds urethral pressure. The stiffness of the supportive layer under the bladder neck provides a backstop against which abdominal pressure compresses the urethra.

PATHOPHYSIOLOGY OF URINARY INCONTINENCE

INCONTINENCE

When evaluating patients with incontinence, the first step is deciding if underlying etiology is genitourinary or not. Please see Chap. 6, Evaluation for Urinary Incontinence in the Office and Indications for Referral to a Specialist, for definitions and details.

Genitourinary causes of incontinence can be divided into several broad categories:
1. Disorders related to the filling and storage:
   - Urodynamic stress urinary incontinence (USUI)
   - Urge incontinence
     ◦ Nonneurogenic detrusor overactivity
     ◦ Neurogenic detrusor overactivity

- Mixed incontinence
- Overflow incontinence
2. Incontinence caused by fistula formation:
   - Vesical
   - Ureteral
   - Urethral
3. Congenital causes of incontinence:
   - Ectopic ureter
   - Bladder extrophy
   - Epispadias

Nongenitourinary causes of urinary incontinence include impairment of the functional status, neurologic disease, cognitive decline, environmental factors, medications, as well as metabolic disorders.

URODYNAMIC STRESS URINARY INCONTINENCE (USUI)

- USUI is the most common cause of urinary incontinence in younger women and is second only to urge incontinence in older women. SUI is suspected when patient complaints of involuntary leakage with exertion, sneezing, or coughing. The diagnosis of SUI is made when leakage is demonstrated during increases in intra-abdominal pressure.
- There are two main causes of stress incontinence: Impaired urethral support from the pelvic endofascia and muscles (hypermobile urethra type [HMU, HMI]) and poor function of the urethra itself (ISD)
- Normal function of the urethral support system requires the contraction of the levator ani muscle, which supports the urethra through the endopelvic fascia. During a cough, the levator ani muscle contracts simultaneously with the diaphragm and abdominal wall muscles to build abdominal pressure. This levator ani contraction helps to tense the suburethral fascial layer thereby enhancing urethral compression. Functionally, the levator ani muscle and the endopelvic fascia play an interactive role in maintaining continence and pelvic support. If levator ani muscle tone is lost or decreased, the support provided by the muscle to resist intra-abdominal pressures generated by standing or any other provocation is diminished. Resulting hypermobility of the vesicourethral segment alters pressure transmission to the urethra during increase in intra-abdominal pressure, impairs the efficiency of the sphincteric musculature, and debilitates compression by the suburethral layer. In HMU anatomy of the sphincter is normal, but it has lost some of its efficacy due to excessive mobility and loss of support.
- Successful surgeries that correct stress incontinence do so by reinforcing or repairing the connective tissue (via a support hammock underneath the urethra) or by improving urethral function so as to counteract intrinsic sphincteric deficiency. The urethra sits on top of and is invested by the fibromuscular layer of the anterior vaginal wall (known surgically as the pubocervical septum or endopelvic fascia). In essence, the endopelvic fascia forms a hammock underneath the urethra. Additionally, the urethra is supported at its midportion by the pubourethral ligament. Normally, the urethra is compressed against this backboard during stress (e.g., cough) and becomes occluded. If the hammock is deficient, the urethra is not compressed and urine leaks during stress. Additionally, if the hammock is intact but the urethral function is poor (i.e., intrinsic sphincter deficiency [ISD]), the urethra is unable to occlude completely (lack of coaptation) and thus leakage occurs.
- The hammock theory gives a better explanation of the continence mechanism than historical explanations. Urethral hypermobility is a sign that the hammock is deficient (either broken or stretched). The retropubic location of the urethra and the idea of *zone of intra-abdominal pressure* is no longer the explanation for the mechanism of SUI. Studies have reported that hypermobility of the urethra persists following successful mid-urethral sling procedures. Therefore, when the hammock is deficient (thus rendering the urethra hypermobile), stress allows displacement of the urethrovesical junction, pressure transmission to the bladder, but not equally to the urethra. Since the urethra cannot be compressed against a stable backboard, urine loss occurs.
- ISD is the inability of the urethra to occlude. It can result from trauma, neuromuscular changes due to age, and mucosal atrophy in postmenopausal women. Unlike the stress-maneuver-related leakage of USUI, ISD can cause incontinence even without an increase in intraabdominal pressure.

URINARY URGENCY INCONTINENCE (UUI)

- UUI is caused by involuntary contractions of the detrusor during filling phase. Several etiologies exist, including nonneurogenic (previously known as idiopathic) detrusor instability, detrusor instability secondary to disruptions of neural control mechanisms, and bladder outlet obstruction (BOO). Overactive bladder (OAB) is characterized by sensory urgency.
- Principal abnormality in the cases of nonneurogenic detrusor instability seems to lie in pathologically enhanced cell coupling, which could mediate the spontaneous tone and tetanic contractions.
- Neurologic diseases affecting cerebral cortex can cause urge incontinence by interfering with the normal inhibition of detrusor muscle by PNS. Damage to the cerebrum can hamper the balance between facilitatory mechanisms and tonic inhibitory influence of the PMC, causing upregulation of excitatory pathways,

which, in turn, will lead to detrusor overactivity and urge incontinence.
- Neurologic lesions affecting spinal cord above the sacral region result in sphincter activity that is not coordinated with the detrusor contractions leading to functional obstruction, which causes overstimulation of the bladder afferent neurons inducing detrusor overactivity and urge incontinence.
- BOO can lead to urge incontinence by causing increased tension at the bladder neck. A rise in pressure at the bladder neck causes an increase in muscular tension, which, in turn, leads to increased afferent signals from tension receptors. The positive feedback to the detrusor muscle from such signals can lead to increased neural stimulation, which is possibly responsible for the decrease in electrical resistance between detrusor smooth muscle cells, causing uninhibited contractions of this muscle and thus urge incontinence.
- In patients with OAB, UUI is caused by sensory urgency characterized by decreased bladder capacity without detrusor motor instability and without loss of compliance. OAB is a progressive disease and urgency and frequency can precede development of overt urge incontinence.

MIXED INCONTINENCE (MUI)
- Components of both stress urinary incontinence and urge incontinence are present simultaneously. MUI is usually more severe than either of the former.

OVERFLOW INCONTINENCE
- Loss of urine is due to either chronic urinary retention secondary to BOO, impaired contractility of the detrusor, or impairement in sensation.

PATHOPHYSIOLOGY OF PELVIC ORGAN PROLAPSE

- Summary of POP pathophysiology: damage to levator ani muscle and nerve → decreased muscle tone and strength (Type I, slow-twitch) → muscle disuse atrophy → muscle descent and widened levator hiatus → now intra-abdominal pressure is unopposed thus places added forces on tissue → connective tissue stretches and tears over time → POP results (anterior vs. posterior vs. apical prolapse results depending on where defects have resulted).
- POP is a complex disease process with multifactorial etiology. Risk factors for POP include pregnancy, vaginal childbirth, menopause, chronic increase in intra-abdominal pressure, and pelvic floor muscle weakness.

- Prolapse can involve the anterior vaginal wall (e.g., cystocele and/or urethrocele) due to midline or paravaginal defect, the apical vagina (uterine descensus or vaginal vault prolapse), the posterior vaginal wall (enterocele and/or rectocele), or a combination of these sites.
- The normal tone and integrity of the levator muscles maintain support of pelvic organs. Striated muscles are susceptible to injury when forcibly lengthened, which will lead to the weakening of the levator ani muscle and associated POP. Once muscles are weakened, support of the pelvic organs shifts to the connective tissues, thus increasing stress on the pelvic ligaments and fascial condensations, eventually leading to their detachment from the bony pelvis or the organs they support.
- Nerves that supply these muscles are not as forgiving as these muscles. They may be irreparably damaged. For example, child birth traumas causing neuropathies will lead to the denervation of the muscles of the pelvic floor, causing ineffective contractions and loss of basal tone. Since the weight-bearing of the pelvic organs is provided by the pelvic floor muscles, the support shifts again onto the connective tissues.

BIBLIOGRAPHY

Benson JT, Walters MD. Neurophysiology of the lower urinary tract. In: Walters MD, Karram MM, eds. *Urogynecology and Reconstructive Pelvic Surgery*. 2nd ed. St Louis, MO: Mosby; 1999.

Blaivas JG, Olsson CA. Stress incontinence: classification and surgical approach. *J Urol*. 1988;139:727–731.

Cucchi A. Sequential changes in voiding dynamics related to the development of detrusor instability in women with SUI. *Neurourol Urodyn*. 1999;18(2):73–80.

DeLancey JO. Structural support of the urethra as it relates to stress urinary incontinence: the hammock hypothesis. *Am J Obstet Gynecol*. 1994;170(6):1713–1720.

DeLancey JOL. Structural aspects of the extrinsic continence mechanism. *Obstet Gynecol*. 1988;72(3 Pt 1):296–301.

DeLancey JOL. Anatomy of the female bladder and urethra. In: Ostergard DR, Bent AE, eds. *Urogynecology and Urodynamics*. 3rd ed. Baltimore, MD: Williams & Wilkins; 1991.

DeLancey JOL. The anatomy of the pelvic floor. *Curr Opin Obstet Gynecol*. 1994;6(4):313–316.

Fitzgerald MP, Mueller E. Physiology of the lower urinary tract. *Clin Obstet Gynecol*. 2004;47:18–27.

Herzog AR, Fultz NH. Prevalence and incidence of urinary incontinence in community-dwelling populations. *J Am Geriatr Soc*. 1990;38(3):273–281.

McGuire EJ. The innervation and function of the lower urinary tract. *J Neurosurg*. 1986;65(3):278–285.

Olsen AL, Smith VJ, Bergstrom JO, et al. Epidemiology of surgically managed pelvic organ prolapse and urinary incontinence. *Obstet Gynecol.* 1997;89(4):501–506.

Sui GP, Coppen SR, Dupont E, et al. Impedance measurements and connexin expression in human detrusor muscle from stable and unstable bladders. *BJU Int.* 2003;92:297–305.

Walters MD, Weber AM. Anatomy of the lower urinary tract, rectum, and pelvic floor. In: Walters MD, Karram MM, eds. *Urogynecology and Reconstructive Pelvic Surgery.* 2nd ed. St Louis, MO: Mosby; 1999.

QUESTIONS

1. A 36-year-old para 0, healthy woman presents for her annual gynecologic examination. While performing a digital pelvic examination, an examiner notices a small bulge above the hymen and lateral to the vagina on the right, palpation of the other side reveals the same findings. The most likely structure palpated by the examiner is:
   (A) Puboperineus muscle
   (B) PB
   (C) Cardinal ligament
   (D) Pubococcygeus muscle
   (E) ATFP

2. A 44-year-old woman para 3, presents with complaints of leaking urine when she does her aerobics exercises. This is interfering with her daily life. On physical examination you notice a second degree cystocele and hypermobility of the urethra. Most likely etiology for her incontinence is:
   (A) Disruption of the urethral sphincter
   (B) Uninhibited contractions of detrusor muscle
   (C) Altered pressure transmission to the urethra
   (D) Loss of sensation of bladder fullness
   (E) Enhanced bladder sensation

3. A 57-year-old woman presents with complaints of urinary frequency, occasional urgency, and loss of urine with coughing and sneezing. Her symptoms have worsened in the last 6 months and incontinent episodes are interfering with her usual activities. You decide to start with cystometry assessment. You do not see an increase in intravesicular pressure despite filling the bladder with 300 cc of sterile H_2O. This observation is secondary to:
   (A) Bladder accommodation
   (B) Bladder perforation
   (C) Low bladder compliance
   (D) Pelvic floor laxity

4. A 68-year-old woman with long-standing hypertension is admitted to the neurology floor after suffering an extensive stroke involving areas of the brain superior to the pons. In regard to the function of the patient's lower urinary tract, you would expect her to suffer mostly from:
   (A) Urinary retention
   (B) Urge incontinence
   (C) GSI
   (D) Overflow incontinence

5. A 42-year-old para 3, presents complaining of difficulty voiding. Your assistant is setting the patient up for the evaluation of her voiding pattern. During the process of micturition the following has to occur to ensure proper voiding:
   (A) Inhibition of detrusor muscle and activation of urethral smooth muscle by PNS
   (B) Activation of detrusor muscle and inhibition of urethral smooth muscle by SNS
   (C) Inhibition of detrusor muscle and inhibition of urethral smooth muscle by PNS
   (D) Activation of detrusor muscle and inhibition of urethral smooth muscle by PNS
   (E) Inhibition of detrusor muscle and activation of urethral smooth muscle by SNS

ANSWERS

1. *(D).* The pubococcygeus muscles form a U shape as they originate from the pubic bone on either side of the midline, insert into the anal sphincter complex, and pass behind the rectum to form a sling. The pubococcygeus muscle can be appreciated during physical examination of the pelvis as a bulky muscular ridge on both lateral sidewalls of the vagina, superior to the hymen.

   The puboperineus muscle arises from the pubic bone immediately lateral to the pubic symphysis and inserts into the PB in front of the rectum.

   The PB is a pyramidal fibromuscular structure in the midline between the anus and the vagina.

   The cardinal ligaments attach cervix and parametria to the bony pelvis and form a continuous and interdependent organ complex with uterosacral ligaments and levator ani muscles.

   ATFPs originates at the pubic bone and insert into the ischial spine. These bilateral structures provide support needed to suspend the urethra on the anterior vaginal wall. They are not palpable on the digital pelvic examination.

2. *(C).* This presentation is a typical scenario for someone with GSI. Normal function of the urethral support

system assures continence especially when intra-abdominal pressure is increased, for example, during exercise, or when coughing, sneezing, or laughing. This levator ani contraction helps to tense the suburethral fascial layer, thereby enhancing urethral compression. If levator ani muscle tone is lost or decreased, the support provided by the muscle to resist intra-abdominal pressures generated by standing or any other provocation is diminished. Resulting hypermobility of the vesicourethral segment alters pressure transmission to the urethra during increase in intra-abdominal pressure resulting in incontinence. The fact that the patient has cystocele tells us about the laxity of her pelvic floor caused by the loss of normal support, which very commonly leads to the combination of POP and stress incontinence.

Disruption of the urethral sphincter, which can result from trauma, will lead to its deficiency. Unlike the stress-maneuver-related leakage of GSI, ISD can cause incontinence without an increase in intra-abdominal pressure. The patient did not complain of the loss of urine without provocation.

Uninhibited contractions of detrusor muscle result in urge sensation and UUI, which is defined as the unwanted urine leakage that happens shortly after the sudden, intense desire to urinate. UUI is often accompanied by increased urinary frequency and nocturia. OAB can be also secondary to sensory urgency that is also characterized by a strong urge to urinate and incontinence when unable to suppress this urge. In patients with OAB, urge incontinence is caused by sensory urgency characterized by decreased bladder capacity without detrusor motor instability and without loss of compliance.

Impairment of sensation of bladder fullness results in overflow incontinence, which tends to happen independently of activity level.

3. *(A).* Cystometry is a test of bladder function in which pressure and volume of fluid in the bladder is measured during filling, storage, and voiding. A cystometrogram is a plot of bladder pressure versus bladder volume.

During bladder filling, detrusor pressure remains nearly constant because of a special property of the bladder smooth muscle and connective tissue known as accommodation.

Bladder perforation, even though can theoretically take place, is not a known complication of cystometry.

When accommodation is impaired, low bladder compliance results and increase in detrusor pressure during filling cystometry can be observed.

Laxity of the pelvic floor occurs when the muscles and the fascia that provide support to pelvic organs are weakened. This will not affect detrusor pressure.

4. *(B).* Suprapontine region includes the parietal lobes, the thalamus, the frontal lobes, and basal ganglia. Parietal lobes and the thalamus receive and coordinate detrusor afferent stimuli, the frontal lobes and basal ganglia provide modulation with inhibitory signals, thus providing tonic inhibitory systems in the brain that suppress parasympathetic excitatory outflow to the bladder. Damage to the cerebrum can hamper the balance between facilitatory mechanisms and tonic inhibitory influence of the PMC, causing upregulation of excitatory pathways, which, in turn, will lead to detrusor overactivity and urge incontinence.

Urinary retention can be due to BOO. BOO can be secondary to extensive prolapse, can occur postoperatively or be due to bladder stone or tumor. Retention can also be secondary to diminished ability of detrusor to contract, which can be seen, for example, in cases of diabetic neuropathy.

GSI is the most common cause of urinary incontinence in younger women and is second only to urge incontinence in older women. GSI is suspected when patient complains of involuntary leakage with exertion, sneezing, or coughing. The diagnosis of GSI is made when leakage is demonstrated during increases in intra-abdominal pressure. Two main causes of stress incontinence include impaired urethral support from the pelvic endofascia and muscles and failure of urethral closure due to ISD, which can occur secondary to trauma, neuromuscular changes due to age, and mucosal atrophy.

Overflow incontinence is due to either chronic urinary retention secondary to BOO, impaired contractility of the detrusor, or impairment in sensation.

5. *(D).* PNS and SNS exert opposite effect on the bladder and the urethra.

SNS via its effect on beta-adrenergic receptors inhibits detrusor and stimulates urethral smooth muscle via alpha-adrenergic receptors. These occur during the storage phase of the lower urinary tract cycle.

PNS, through its effect on the cholinergic receptors in the bladder and urethra, excite the detrusor and inhibit urethral smooth muscle. Parasympathetic nerves from S2, 3, 4 provide major motor innervation to the detrusor muscle. When bladder capacity is reached, the bladder afferent nerve signals activate PMC that, in turn, stimulates PNS efferents, thus activating detrusor muscle. PMC simultaneously inhibits SNS output to the urethral smooth muscle and efferent somatic output to the striated muscles, which causes relaxation of the striated urethral muscle and pelvic floor.

4 EPIDEMIOLOGY: URINARY INCONTINENCE, FECAL INCONTINENCE, AND PELVIC ORGAN PROLAPSE (POP)

Stacey L. Snowden and Sam Siddighi

INTRODUCTION

- One of the greatest accomplishments gained in studying the epidemiology of disease is the increase in awareness of those who are affected.
- More and more studies are showing that problems with urinary incontinence, fecal incontinence, and pelvic organ prolapse (POP) are actually common ailments faced by women today.
- In 2001, the average life expectancy for women was 79.8 years. As the world's population continues to grow and mature, the prevalence of these complications is projected to increase as well.
- The following are some general statistics and risk factors commonly implicated in subsequent development of urinary incontinence, fecal incontinence, and POP. The reasons why there is often a wide range of incidence and prevalence quoted in the literature is because:
  - There are not many studies of high epidemiologic quality.
  - Existing studies differ in their study methods.
  - Existing studies differ by how they define incontinence and prolapse.
- Awareness of the contributing risk factors and populations at greater risk can help guide clinicians to detect and subsequently treat patients with these symptoms.
- The risk factors are arranged in a helpful mnemonic, SO MARC, to better remember contributing factors: smoking, obesity, menopause, age, race, and childbirth/congenital factors.

TOP 10 THINGS TO REMEMBER ABOUT THIS CHAPTER

1. As a chronic illness, POP, overactive bladder (OAB), and urinary incontinence affect more women than diabetes, heart disease, or arthritis. Additionally, more money is spent on incontinence than on essential hypertension or breast cancer.
2. The average life expectancy for women was 79.8 years in 2003.
3. Currently one out of eight people is over 65. By 2030, 25% of the population will be over 65 years.
4. Lifetime risk for undergoing surgery for POP = 11.1% (approximately one in nine women by age 80). This risk may be increased to 16% if patient has had a hysterectomy.
5. In 2000, it was estimated that $32 billion was spent on diagnosis, treatment, and care, for patients with urinary incontinence.
6. More than equal to 50% of money spent on urinary incontinence was for incontinence consequences rather than for diagnosis or treatment.
7. In one study, 54% of women with urinary incontinence symptoms also had bowel symptoms. Yet only 12.2% of these women mentioned fecal incontinence symptoms before being prompted by specific questioning.
8. The age distribution of *women seeking care* for pelvic floor disorders (PFD) is as follows: *60–69 >70–79 >50–59 >>40–49 >80–89 >30s*.
9. The age distribution of *consults done* for PFD are as follows: *70–79 >80–89 >60–69 >>50s >40s >30s*.
10. Stress incontinence is more prevalent among younger women (40s); mixed incontinence is more prevalent among older women (60s).

GENERAL EPIDEMIOLOGIC DEFINITIONS

- *Prevalence*—total number of cases of a disease at a specific time.
- *Incidence*—number of new cases of a disease in a specific amount of time usually designated as one year.
- *Odds ratio*—compares the incidence of disease in those persons with an existing risk factor with the incidence of people without the disease who did not have an existing risk factor present. An odds ratio of 1 indicates that there is no significant difference.

URINARY INCONTINENCE

- Prevalence of urinary incontinence:
  - Ambulatory women aged 15–64 years = 10–30%
  - Women >60 years of age and living in the community = 10–40%
  - Women living in nursing homes = >50% experience urinary incontinence
- Mobility was shown to be a greater predictor of maintaining continence.
- Incontinence is not just a disease affecting older individuals. One study found that 28% of nulliparous college athletes have loss of urine during athletic activity.
- Only one in four women will seek medical advice for incontinence. Why?

○ Many women believe that it is a normal conse-quence of aging.
○ Many self-treat with store-bought incontinence products.
○ Others are embarrassed to discuss their symptoms.
○ Some believe that it is not treatable.
○ Many fear surgery.
○ Some health care providers do not screen for it.

SMOKING

• Women who smoke are approximately two to three times more likely to have urinary incontinence. (Current smokers and former smokers)
• A smoking history is implicated in the development of all types of urinary incontinence.
• Women who smoke are susceptible to chronic obstructive pulmonary disease (COPD) and may gen-erate high bladder pressures as a result of coughing.

OBESITY

• Increases in body mass index (BMI) have shown an increase in symptoms of urinary incontinence, partic-ularly stress incontinence.
• One study showed a reduction of stress incontinence from 61% to 12% following bariatric surgery for weight reduction.

MENOPAUSE

• Studies have inconsistently demonstrated any increase in urinary dysfunction after undergoing menopause.
• Estrogen use is more common among women with incontinence than among continent women. (See Chap. 34).
• However, in women given estrogen replacement therapy, there was a subjective decrease in sensory symptoms of urinary incontinence. Estrogen may increase the sensory threshold of the bladder and increase its relaxation.
• Improvement in urinary symptoms is better with local estrogen (cream, suppository, tablet, ring) than with systemic estrogen.
○ High-affinity estrogen receptors have been found on tissues of the urinary tract including the urethra, blad-der trigone, and pubococcygeus muscle. Some argue that estrogen helps maintain vascularity of vaginal and urinary tissues. It also increases the response of the urethral alpha-adrenergic receptors.
○ The decreases in urethral vascularity and urethral length seen with estrogen deficiency may lead to decreases in resting urethral pressure. Estrogen thickens the urethral mucosa which helps in its occlusion (coaptation).

○ Urogenital atrophy increases the risk of infections of the urinary tract. Estrogen prevents atrophy and keeps the vaginal pH more acidic; this helps decrease prolif-eration of potentially pathologic bacteria.

PREGNANCY

• Patients may experience urinary incontinence during pregnancy, which resolves shortly after birth to sev-eral months postpartum. (See Chap. 29).

AGE

• The mean age at which the different forms of urinary dysfunction present are as follows:
○ Stress incontinence = 48 years
○ Mixed incontinence = 55 years
○ Urge incontinence = 61 years
• The *overall prevalence* of incontinence in U.S. women (39.6 million people) in 2001:
○ With the following distribution: stress>mixed>urge
• The overall patterns of incontinence also appear to change with *increasing age*:
○ Women under age 60: stress>mix>urge>other
○ Women over age 60: mix>urge>stress>other

RACE

• Urinary incontinence:
○ Stress: Caucasian women>African-American women and Caucasian women>Asian women
○ Urge: African-American women>Caucasian women
• Asian women appear to have a decreased prevalence of urinary incontinence, possibly because of the increased amount of collagen found in their pelvic fascial supports. This may also be due to differences in the manner of voiding (i.e., squatting in Asian countries vs. sitting in Western countries).

CHILDBIRTH

• Numerous studies suggest a higher prevalence of uri-nary dysfunction in parous women versus nulliparous women. This may be related to damage sustained to the muscles and nerves of the pelvic floor.
○ *Stress incontinence* shows the strongest association with increased parity and vaginal delivery.
○ *Urge incontinence* showed minimal to no associa-tion with increased parity. However, cesarean deliv-ery may increase slightly the chance for future urge incontinence.

HYSTERECTOMY

- Studies have inconsistently shown that having a hysterectomy is a risk factor for developing urinary incontinence.
- The route of simple hysterectomy (vaginal, abdominal, or laparoscopic) does not appear to influence subsequent development of urinary incontinence.
- When comparing total versus subtotal abdominal hysterectomies, there was no significant difference in subsequent development of urinary incontinence 1 year after surgery.

FECAL INCONTINENCE

- Prevalence of fecal incontinence varies significantly by description used to define a clinically significant unwanted loss of stool, or incontinent episode.
- Most common definition: episodes of unwanted fecal loss that occurs one or more times per week, or episodes that require sanitary napkin use.
- The prevalence of anal incontinence in women was found to be approximately 4.5%, including those who had unwanted loss of gas or stool greater than once a week.
- Elderly women in the community had an even higher prevalence of fecal incontinence, with 3.7–18.4% reporting fecal incontinence at that time.
- Women in nursing homes had the highest prevalence of fecal incontinence, *with a prevalence of* up to 50%.

GENDER

- Fecal incontinence affects women approximately 1.3 times more than men.
  - This may relate to the increased probability of structural damage resulting from childbirth.
  - Lower anal squeeze pressures, or the pressures surmounted under voluntary contraction, are seen in women with increasing age.

MENOPAUSE

- Neither estrogen deficiency nor hormone replacement therapy has been shown to influence development or prevention of fecal incontinence.
- Estrogen receptors have been found in the external anal sphincter.

AGE

- The prevalence of fecal incontinence in women increases with age.

CHILDBIRTH

- Pregnancy itself does not significantly play a role in the development of anal incontinence.
- Damage to pelvic structures during vagina delivery appears to contribute to development of flatal and fecal incontinence (see Chap. 30, "Selective" Cesarean Section for Prevention of Pelvic Floor Disorders, Pros and Cons).
  - Symptoms of fecal incontinence were seen in 5% of primiparas and 4% of multiparas after vaginal delivery but in none of the cesarean delivery patients.
  - In another study that followed 259 women delivered at one hospital, none of the 31 delivered by cesarean section reported fecal incontinence compared to 13% of primiparas who delivered vaginally.
  - In another study, 62% of those with sphincter tears complained of fecal incontinence 8 years after vaginal delivery versus only 25% who delivered vaginally but who did not have evidence of sphincter disruption.
  - Resting anal sphincter pressures decrease after vaginal delivery up to 6 months. Squeeze anal sphincter pressures also reduced but not as much as resting pressures.
  - After vaginal delivery about 6% develop new fecal incontinence but this rises to about 50% in vaginal deliveries complicated by anal sphincter rupture.
  - Vaginal deliveries subsequent to delivery with sphincter rupture and fecal incontinence results in recurrent fecal incontinence in 39% and permanent fecal incontinence in 4%.
  - Use of midline episiotomy increases the risk of anal sphincter damage during delivery.

DOUBLE INCONTINENCE: URINARY + FECAL INCONTINENCE

- It is extremely important to consider other comorbidities when evaluating women for urinary incontinence, specifically fecal incontinence.
  - 54% of women with urinary tract symptoms also had bowel symptoms.
  - Only 12.2% of these women mentioned fecal incontinence symptoms before being prompted by specific questioning.
  - Fecal impaction causes urinary incontinence.
  - More data are necessary.

PELVIC ORGAN PROLAPSE

- Affects approximately 10–30% of the adult female population.
- POP is the third most common reason cited for hysterectomy.
- For women >50 years of age, 2.7–3.3 surgeries per 1000 women will be performed for POP.
- Distribution of prolapse in women ages 18–86 years, based on POP quantification (POPQ) system:
  - Showed a bell shape curve of distribution:
    - Stage 2>stage 1>>>(stage 0, stage 3, stage 4)

MENOPAUSE

- Menopausal women have been shown to be at high risk for development of POP.
- It is unclear if it is the estrogen deficiency of menopause that contributes to POP, or if advancing age plays a greater role in etiology.

AGE

- Incidence of POP roughly doubles with each decade in women aged 20–59 years.
- The incidence of POP requiring surgery also demonstrated a dramatic increase with each successive decade.

RACE

- Risk of POP: African-American and Asian<Caucasian <Hispanic.
  - African-American women show the lowest risk for uterine prolapse.
  - Hispanic women appear to have the highest risk.
  - Studies have demonstrated differences in the collagen content between Asian women and Caucasian women.
  - African-Americans have narrow pubic arches (android or anthropoid type of pelvis) which is more protective against POP when compared to the gynecoid pelvis.
- Though differences in the degree of fascial support between races have been reported, the impact on development of POP is still under investigation.

CHILDBIRTH

- Vaginal delivery appears to contribute significantly to the development of POP.
- An almost 11-fold increased risk is seen in women with four or more vaginal deliveries when compared to nulliparous women.

- Weight of infant delivered vaginally also appears to contribute to POP:
  - For every 1 pound increase in the birth weight of a vaginally delivered infant, a 10% increase in development of POP was seen.

CONGENITAL FACTORS

- Women with prolapse tended to have:
  - An abundance of weaker type III collagen in their tissues
  - Higher degree of joint hypermobility
- Collagen vascular diseases have been implicated.
  - However, one study of women with Ehlers-Danlos syndrome showed no relationship between joint hypermobility and POP, indicating that joint hypermobility is not a predictor of severity of prolapse.
  - Marfan's is also associated with POP.
- A positive relationship between spina bifida and presence of POP has been identified. Though only a few case reports have described this association, it is an important consideration.
  - One study found a 28% incidence of spina bifida occulta in women with POP (as opposed to a 10% incidence of spina bifida occulta in control population of women without POP).
  - An evaluation for underlying spina bifida occulta may be warranted, especially in nulliparous women who have severe prolapse.

HYSTERECTOMY

- The lifetime risk of developing POP in a hysterectomized patient may be as high as 16%.
- The route of hysterectomy (laparoscopic, abdominal, or vaginal) does not appear to influence the risk of POP after surgery.
- When comparing total versus subtotal abdominal hysterectomies, there was no significant difference in subsequent development of POP 1 year after surgery.
- Initial indication for hysterectomy has been shown to influence outcome.
  - Women who underwent hysterectomy to treat uterine prolapse had higher rates of developing POP after surgery than women who received hysterectomies for other reasons.
- Incidence of women developing severe POP after hysterectomy is 2–3.6 per 1000 woman-years.
- Rates as high as 15 per 1000 woman-years were seen in women who received hysterectomies due to initial complaints of POP.

PELVIC ORGAN PROLAPSE + URINARY + FECAL INCONTINENCE

- 62% of women with POP also reported stress urinary incontinence (SUI).
- 63% women with stress incontinence also had POP.
- Physical examination should evaluate for both conditions if surgical intervention is considered, since 20% of women who have surgery for POP also have concomitant surgery to correct urinary incontinence.
- The lifetime risk (at age 80) of undergoing surgery for prolapse or genuine stress incontinence (GSI) is 11.1% (one out of every nine women).
  ○ Risk of surgery by age: 70–80 years = 11.1%, 60–69 = 7.5%, 50–59 = 4.7%.
  ○ Of these women ≈30% will have repeat surgery in their lifetime.
- The prevalence of fecal incontinence in women with POP was found to be ≈26%.
- The presence of rectal prolapse showed a significant association with the development of fecal incontinence.
- Fecal or flatal incontinence occurs in 20% of patients with urinary incontinence.

ECONOMIC IMPACT

- Studies are limited to the exact economic cost of urinary incontinence, fecal incontinence, and POP.
- Direct cost: the cost surmounted to actually diagnose, treat, rehabilitate, and care for patients with these symptoms.
- Indirect cost: costs that accumulate from loss of patient productivity, cost to family members/friends who help care for the patient, and other ailments that arise secondary to incontinence (pressure ulcers, and the like).
- The total economic cost of urinary incontinence:
  ○ In 1994, it was estimated to be $16.4 billion.
  ○ By the year 2000, the estimate nearly doubled to $32 billion.
- The majority of these costs do not come from money spent on diagnosis or treatment, but from the cost of providing laundry, pads, and absorbent products.

BIBLIOGRAPHY

Bai SW, Jeon MJ, Kim JY, et al. Relationship between stress urinary incontinence and pelvic organ prolapse. Int Urogynecol J Pelvic Floor Dysfunct. 2002;13(4):256–260.

Brubaker L. Epidemiology of pelvic floor disorders. In: Weber AM, Brubaker L, Schaffer J, et al., eds. *Office Urogynecol.* 2004;1–10.

Bump RC, Mattiasson A, BoK, et al. The standardization of terminology of female pelvic floor dysfunction. *Am J Obstet Gynecol.* 1996;175:10–17.

Dietz HP, Eldridge A, Grace M, et al. Pelvic organ descent in young nulligravid women. *Am J Obstet Gynecol.* 2004;191(1):95–99.

Diokno AC, Estanol MV, Mallett V. Epidemiology of lower urinary tract dysfunction. *Clin Obstet Gynecol.* 2004;47(1):36–43.

El-Toukhy TA, Hefni M, Davies A, et al. The effect of different types of hysterectomy on urinary and sexual functions: a prospective study. *J Obstet Gynecol.* 2004;24(4):420–425.

Gimbel H, Zobbe V, Andersen BM, et al. Total versus subtotal hysterectomy: an observational study with one-year follow-up. *Aust N Z J Obstet Gynecol.* 2005;45(1):64–67.

Graham CA, Mallet VT. Race as a predictor of urinary incontinence and pelvic organ prolapse. *Am J Obstet Gynecol.* 2001;185(1):116–120.

Graves EJ, Kozak LJ. Detailed diagnoses and procedures. National Hospital Discharge Survey, 1996. *Vital Health Stat.* 1998;13:1.

Hagstad A, Janson PO, Lindstedt G. Gynaecological history, complaints, and examinations in a middle-aged population. Maturitas. 1985;7(2):115.

Hannestad YS, Rortveit G, Sandvik H, et al. A community-based epidemiological survey of female urinary incontinence: the Norwegian EPINCONT study. Epidemiology of Incontinence in the County of Nord-Trondelag. *J Clin Epidemiol.* 2000;53(11):1150–1157.

Hendrix SL, Clark A, Nygaard I, et al. Pelvic organ prolapse in the Women's Health Initiative: gravity and gravidity. *Am J Obstet Gynecol.* 2002;186(6):1160–1166.

Hu TW, Wagner TH, Bentkover JD, et al. Costs of urinary incontinence and overactive bladder in the United States: a comparative study. *Urology.* 2004;63(3):461–465.

Khan IJ. Urinary Incontinence: behavioral modification therapy in older adult. Clin Geriatr Med. 2004;20(3):499–509.

Luber KM. "Office Evaluation and Urodynamic Testing." *ACOG District IX Annual Meeting,* October 12, 2003, Santa Rosa, CA.

Milsom I, Stewart W, Thuroff J. The prevalence of overactive bladder. *Am J Manag Care.* 2000;6(11):S565–S573.

Ng SC, Chen YC, Lin LY, et al. Anorectal dysfunction in women with urinary incontinence or lower urinary tract symptoms. *Int J Gynecol Obstet.* 2002;77(2):139–145.

Olsen AE, Smith VJ, Bergstrom JO, et al. Epidemiology of surgically managed pelvic organ prolapse and urinary incontinence. *Obstet Gynecol.* 1997;89(4):501–506.

Parmentier H, Damon H, Henry L, et al. Frequency of anal incontinence and results of pelvic viscerography in 291 women with pelvic organ prolapse. *Gastroenterol Clin Biol.* 2004;28(3):226–230.

Samuelsson EC, Victor FT, Svardsudd KF. Five-year incidence and remission rates of female urinary incontinence in a Swedish population less than 65 years old. *Am J Obstet Gynecol.* 2000;183(3):568–574.

Swift, SE. Epidemiology of pelvic organ prolapse. In: Bent AE, Ostergard DR, Cundiff GW, et al., eds. *Ostergard's Urogynecology and Pelvic Floor Dysfunction.* 5th ed. Philadelphia, PA, Lippincott Williams & Wilkins; 2003;35–42.

Weber AM, Walters MD. Epidemiology and social impact of urinary and fecal incontinence. In: Karram MM, Walters MD, eds. *Urogynecology, Reconstructive Pelvic Surgery.* 2nd ed. Philadelphia, PA: Lippincott Williams & Wilkins; 1999;25–33.

Wilson L, Brown JS, Shin BP, et al. Annual direct cost of urinary incontinence. *Obstet Gynecol.* 2001;98(3):398–406.

Wagner TH, Hu TW. Economic costs of urinary incontinence. *Urology.* 1998;51:355–361.
National Center for Health Statistics (www.cdc.gov/nchs)

QUESTIONS

1. A 45-year-old woman presents to your office stating she has noticed intermittent unwanted loss of urine over the past few months. Considering only her age, what additional findings would she most likely describe in her history?
    (A) "I suddenly feel the urge to urinate, but I cannot make it to the bathroom in time."
    (B) "Sometimes I lose small amounts of urine when I sneeze, but I also notice large amounts of urine loss at times when I am just resting."
    (C) "Every time I cough, I find I lose a little bit of urine."
    (D) "I feel like I lose a little bit of urine all the time, nothing really makes it better or worse."

2. A 53-year-old gravid 3, para 2, abortus1, female presents to your office with symptoms of unwanted loss of urine over the past few months. She is significantly overweight with a BMI of 31, and has recently begun walking four times a week. She has a 30-pack-year history of smoking, but quit 10 years ago after recommendations from primary physician. Her only medications include estrogen replacement therapy, which she began 6 months ago for hot flashes, and a medication to control her cholesterol. What type(s) of incontinence is she most likely experiencing?
    (A) Urge incontinence
    (B) Overflow incontinence
    (C) Stress incontinence
    (D) Mixed incontinence

3. A 64-year-old gravid 5, para 3, abortus 2, female presents to your office with increased "heaviness" in vaginal area with activity. She states it has been increasingly painful to walk short distances, especially after strenuous bowel movements. On examination you find that her cervix extends to 0.75 cm beyond the hymenal plane with Valsalva. Approximately what percentage of women with similar symptoms as described above, also experience urinary incontinence and fecal incontinence, respectively?
    (A) 30% and 40%
    (B) 60% and 25%
    (C) 25% and 40%
    (D) 60% and 45%

4. Of the following simple hysterectomies, which route offers the least risk of development of urinary incontinence?
    (A) Total abdominal hysterectomy
    (B) Vaginal hysterectomy
    (C) Laparoscopic hysterectomy
    (D) Route of hysterectomy inconsequential.

ANSWERS

1. *(C)*. The previous descriptions are classic for the different types of urinary incontinence: urge, mixed, stress, and overflow, respectively. This question emphasizes the importance that symptoms of stress incontinence appear at a younger age than mixed or urge incontinence. Women with stress, mixed, and urge incontinence had mean ages of onset at age 48, 55, and 61, respectively. Had the question addressed women aged 55–60, further descriptions of a sudden urge to void, or loss of full amount of bladder contents would have been more likely.

    A woman's age at the onset of symptoms may then be an important consideration clinically, as it appears that younger women suffer from stress incontinence more commonly, which can be initially treated with exercise and minimally invasive techniques.

2. *(C)*. Stress incontinence. This patient's history of smoking and increased BMI is important to note as they both increase risk of developing urinary incontinence, specifically stress incontinence.

    Cigarette smokers were two to three times more likely to develop all forms of urinary incontinence than nonsmokers, including prior smokers. It has been noted that higher bladder pressures are generated with coughing in women who smoke, suggesting that symptoms of incontinence may be related to bladder pressures overcoming the pressures maintained by the urethral sphincter.

    An increased BMI was found to positively correlate with urinary incontinence, stress incontinence in particular. Encouraging patients to lose weight appears to be of considerable benefit, as weight loss alone may induce resolution of incontinence without any other intervention. One study looking at women with surgically induced weight loss showed that 75% had resolution of urinary incontinence at 1 year. Upon urodynamic testing, decreases in bladder pressures and pressures transmitted to urethra with coughing were seen, as well as decreases in urethral mobility.

Neither the estrogen deficiency of menopause nor the use of hormone replacement therapy has been shown to significantly contribute to the development of urinary incontinence.

3. *(B)*. Studies have demonstrated that up to 62% of women with POP had confounding SUI.

The prevalence of anal incontinence in women with POP was found to be 26%. Approximately one out of every four women with prolapse also experience symptoms of fecal incontinence.

These statistics further emphasize the necessity to address other possible comorbidities such as urinary and fecal incontinence, when a person presents with significant POP.

4. *(D)*. A recent article showed that the specific route by which simple hysterectomies are performed did not influence development of urinary incontinence at 6 months after surgery.

Some studies actually show that hysterectomies may actually decrease symptoms of urinary incontinence; however, these results have not consistently been demonstrated.

Additionally, the specific route of by which simple hysterectomies are performed does not appear to influence development of POP either. However, a greater rate of POP was seen in women who received hysterectomy for an initial complaint of uterine prolapse. In women who received hysterectomies due to initial complaints of POP, rates as high as 15 per 1000 woman-years were seen.

5 EVALUATION OF PELVIC ORGAN PROLAPSE (POP)

Sam Siddighi

COMMONLY USED TERMS AND NEW DEFINITIONS

- *Cystocele*—protrusion of anterior vaginal wall. It implies that there is a dysfunction with the bladder or that bladder base is on the other side of the prolapse. The term *anterior vaginal wall prolapse* is preferred unless ancillary tests (e.g., colporectocystourethrography [CRCU], magnetic resonance imaging [MRI], voiding cystourethrogram [VCUG]) have been performed for some other reason or it is diagnosed at surgery. Anterior vaginal wall prolapse may be used for cystoceles, urethroceles, and anterior enteroceles. The term *cysto- urethrocele* means anterior vagina wall prolapse + urethral hypermobility. For differentiation between paravaginal, central, transverse, and distal cystoceles, see Chap. 16.
- *Rectocele*—protrusion of the posterior vaginal wall. It implies that the rectum (i.e., fibromuscular layer) is in direct apposition to the vaginal epithelium. The term *posterior vaginal wall prolapse* is now preferred unless imaging confirms the above. Often it can be difficult to distinguish a high rectocele from a posterior enterocele during physical examination. These can be distinguished by CRCU, MRI, or during surgical repair.
- *Enterocele*—prolapse in the apex of vagina containing peritoneum ± bowel (thus a true hernia). It is more likely to occur in a hysterectomized patient. The term *enterocele* implies certainty of the aforementioned contents on the other side of the prolapse. The term *apical prolapse* is preferred unless ancillary testing is done to confirm the above. Apical prolapse can be used to describe an apical defect or posterior enterocele.
  - Traction—most common type; enterocele resulting from posterior cul-de-sac being pulled down vagina by prolapsing uterus or vaginal vault.
  - Iatrogenic or acquired—5–25% of cases; surgeries for incontinence or prolapse resulting in deviation of the normally horizontal axis of the upper vagina. For example, this is the reason a Burch urethropexy should be accompanied with a procedure that addresses the vaginal apex (e.g., uterosacral ligament plication).
  - Pulsion—enterocele resulting from repetitive, chronic increases in the intra-abdominal pressure which herniates cul-de-sac peritoneum (and possibly bowel) through the rectovaginal septum (RVS) in direct juxtaposition to vaginal epithelium.
  - Congenital—is rare and due to congenitally deep pouch of Douglas which can result when the anterior and posterior peritoneums of the cul-de-sac fail to fuse. This can result in an enterocele posterior to the vault of the vagina. May result because of inherited weakness in connective tissue or neurologic condition at birth (spina bifida).
  - *Anterior enterocele* versus *transverse cystocele*—both result from a transverse defect in the pubocervical septum. In other words, separation of the pubocervical septum from the cervix and the broad ligament. In anterior enterocele, hernia sac or small bowel protrudes through this separation while in transverse cystocele, the bladder protrudes through this separation. Transverse cystoceles usually result after previous surgery for vaginal apex (e.g., sacrocolpopexy).
  - *Simple enterocele* versus *complex enterocele*—*simple* denotes an enterocele that exists with the cuff of vagina well-supported; *complex* denotes an enterocele which is associated with vaginal vault prolapse. Can be differentiated on MRI.
- *Uterine prolapse (aka uterine descensus)*—the cervix and uterus descend down the vagina.

- *Vault prolapse (aka posthysterectomy vault prolapse)*—prolapse of vaginal cuff in a hysterectomized patient. The apical or most proximal vagina protrudes down the vagina.
- *Vaginal vault prolapse versus enterocele*—it is possible to have a well-supported vagina apex in the presence of posterior enterocele. These two are often difficult to differentiate by physical examination alone but shortening of the posterior vaginal wall is more consistent with vault prolapse. An imaging study is necessary if a definite diagnosis is required prior to surgery.
- *Complete procidentia*—prolapse of the cervix and uterus well beyond the introitus. Pelvic organ prolapse quantification (POP-Q) or Baden-Walker quantification of the severity of POP is preferred.

RISK FACTORS

(See Chap. 4, Epidemiology: Urinary Incontinence, Fecal incontinence, and Pelvic Organ Prolapse.)
- Vaginal parity (damage to pelvic floor muscle and nerve)
- Neuropathy (spina bifida, spinal cord accident)
- Excessive, chronic valsalva or coughing (e.g., chronic constipation, chronic obstructive pulmonary disease [COPD])
- Lifestyle (occupation or recreational activity with repetitive straining)
- Obesity
- Ascites
- Smoking
- Prior surgery
- Estrogen status
- Advancing age
- Inherited connective tissue disorders (Ehlers-Danlos, Marfan's)
- Genetics (differences between races, different pelvis types)

PROPOSED MECHANISM FOR THE DEVELOPMENT OF POP

(See Chap. 3, Function and Physiology of the Lower Urinary Tract and Pelvic Floor in Women.)
- Damage to levator ani muscles and nerves → decrease muscle tone and strength (Type I, slow-twitch) → muscle disuse atrophy → muscle descent and widened levator hiatus → now intra-abdominal pressure is unopposed thus places added forces on tissue → connective tissue stretches and tears over time → POP results (anterior vs. posterior vs. apical prolapse results depending on where defects have resulted).

EVALUATION OF POP

HISTORY

- As with any medical problem, evaluation of POP should begin with a thorough history followed by a directed physical examination.
- It is important to note any previous evaluation and/or treatment.
- In patients with symptoms of POP, the following information must be obtained:
  ○ There is a wide range of symptoms associated with POP.
    - Feeling that everything is falling out
    - Feeling of protrusion, bulge, or mass in vagina, especially with valsalva (esp. if more severe POP)
    - Feeling that she is bearing down or has pelvic pressure (esp. if less severe POP)
    - Feeling of low back pain (ironically, more often in mild POP), chronic pelvic pain, bilateral groin pain
    - Difficulty with sex, dyspareunia, or partner complaining of inability to fully penetrate
    - Rectal tenesmus, splinting to defecate (classic rectocele symptom), inability to evacuate rectum
      • Constipation by itself is not a symptom of rectocele but is associated with it.
    - Voiding dysfunction, splinting to urinate, unusual positions to void (leaning, bending), lying down for a bit to reduce prolapse before attempting to void, or incontinence
    - Vaginal bleeding or discharge due to vaginal erosions or ulcerations due to friction in severe POP (such ulcers are common on posterior vagina and posterior fourchette)
  ○ What is the duration of the symptoms?
  ○ If not mentioned already, does she have any associated urinary and fecal symptoms. The following are examples:
    - Stress urinary incontinence (SUI) may accompany anterior prolapse (which may resolve as prolapse worsens).
    - Voiding dysfunction and urinary retention may accompany advanced POP.
    - Difficulty with evacuation or fecal incontinence may accompany posterior prolapse.
  ○ What is its effect on the patient's quality of life (QoL)?
    - Tools such as the incontinence impact questionnaire (IIQ) and pelvic floor impact questionnaire (PFIQ) are useful in assessing the impact of these conditions on the patient's life.
    - *Which symptom is the most bothersome*?
    - Does the patient desire treatment for the condition? If yes, does she have a strong preference for conservative management or surgery?

- Patient characteristics that favor surgery over conservative management are severe prolapse, young age, and previous pelvic surgery.
  - The physician's biases and preferences also play a role in the type of management chosen.
- *Medical history*: diabetes mellitus, chronic cough (COPD), asthma, chronic constipation, restricted mobility (e.g., severe arthritis, quadriplegic), and urinary tract infections (UTIs).
- *Neurologic history*: multiple sclerosis (e.g., may cause urinary retention and overflow incontinence), history of cerebrovascular accident (CVA), tumor, dementia, Parkinson's, lumbar disc disease, and neuropathy.
- *Obstetric history*: gravidity and parity number and type of deliveries (cesarean, spontaneous vaginal, forceps), lacerations (third or fourth degree), episiotomies, and desire or lack of desire for future childbearing is important as many experts perform surgery only on those who have completed childbearing.
- *Gynecologic history*: menopause/hormone therapy, contraceptive method, pain, neoplasm.
  - In premenopausal women symptoms may get worse during menses.
- *Surgical history*: especially gynecologic (hysterectomy or previous prolapse surgery), previous anti-incontinence surgeries, or radical surgery.
  - *Important to obtain records and operative reports if available*
  - Prior surgeries may have resulted in trauma to the genitourinary (GU) and gastrointestinal (GI) tract
  - Notice surgical scars and document.
- Medications may have urinary side effects or that cause constipation.

PHYSICAL EXAMINATION

OBSERVATION
- Simple observation can give the clinician information on the patient's general health, mobility, gait, and cognitive limitations.
- If possible, observe the patient ambulate.
- Abnormalities may suggest underlying neurologic or spinal injury.
- Obese patients may have a harder time with some management options.
- Look for scars and correlate them to the surgical history, inquire about any not mentioned in the patient's history.

NEUROLOGIC EXAMINATION

- *Mental status, gait, and coordination* should be evaluated (rule out dementia, delirium, normal pressure Hydrocephalus [NPH], brain tumor).

- Pelvic neurologic examination should be done early in examination so the patient is still alert to the sensation of touch.
- Motor function of lower extremities: flex/extend hips, knees, ankle, feet (inversion/eversion) against resistance.
- All reflexes should be checked bilaterally: patellar, ankle, plantar, and...
  - Bulbocavernosus reflex—tapping of clitoris or stroking the labium majus, causes contraction of bulbocavernosus and ischiocavernosus. If reflex is not seen visually, it may be felt by placing finger just inside the hymenal ring. This test is not used often because it is not present in 20% of normal women and is occasionally difficult to assess.
  - Anal reflexes (aka "anal wink")—stroking skin next to anus causes contraction of external anal sphincter. Rarely used because of the above reasons.
  - Warning the patient before eliciting these reflexes may result in conscious inhibition.
  - If these reflexes are intact, then both sensory and motor reflex arcs of S_2-S_3 is intact.
- Sensory (S_2-S_4) of lower extremities: symmetry, light touch and pinprick sensation on perineum and sacral dermatomes, pain.

GYNECOLOGIC EXAMINATION

- It is important to document vulvar, vaginal, urethral, and other pelvic changes as well (e.g., posterior vaginal ulcers from friction).
- A *diaper rash* may indicate chronic urine contact with perineal and vulvar skin.
- Atrophy of vaginal tissues suggests atrophy of the urethral as well as periurethral tissue since they all share common embryologic structure (urogenital sinus). Signs of atrophy include thin pale skin, agglutinated labia, and sparse pubic hair.
- Vaginal discharge or vaginitis may mimic urinary incontinence.
- Look for perineal scars from previous episiotomy or laceration repairs.

ASSESSMENT OF POP

- POP assessment is best accomplished on a conscious patient. We do not have data on how general anesthesia affects quantification of POP.
- Assessment of symptomatic POP *with or without urinary symptoms* may proceed in the following manner:
  1. Patient arrives at clinic with full bladder and voiding diary. Take history and perform stress test.

2. She empties bladder in private (texas hat or ± uroflowmetry device).

3. $U_{dipstick}$, urinalysis (UA), urine culture and sensitivity ± (UC&S), postvoid residuals (PVR) (this is a convenient time to perform catheterized PVR and to use this urine sample for testing).

4. Neuro examination, POP-Q (on empty bladder), Q-tip test, pelvic muscle strength, bimanual, rectovaginal examination performed.

5. Simple cystometry (eye ball bladder filling is recommended by many experts).

6. Stress test with POP *not reduced* →→if negative→→ stress test with POP reduced → if negative → stress test in standing and POP reduced.

7. Patient voids (± uroflow or pressure-flow studies):
   - Complex cystometry, uroflowmetry, pressure-flow studies, and radiologic imaging (kidney-ureter-bladder x-ray [KUB], cystogram, MRI, and the like) are usually not necessary for evaluation of POP but many academic centers will perform some of the above prior to surgery.

- Examination may be started in lithotomy position but if the prolapse is less than the maximum the patient has experienced or less than her symptoms would suggest, the examination should be repeated in erect or standing position.
- In premenopausal women, the examination may be deferred to just before or during menses when symptoms can be worse.
- The examination should be performed at rest and then with strain. Intensity and type of straining (Valsalva vs. cough) should be documented.
- Points gh and pb of the POP-Q are evaluated first while examining the external genitalia.
- Type of vaginal speculum (e.g., graves bottom blade) or retractor (e.g., Sims) should be documented.
- Retract posterior vaginal wall to visualize the anterior vaginal wall and vice versa.
- The apex may be visualized and evaluated with the intact speculum.
- Fullness of the bladder should be noted.
- Measuring device (for POP-Q) should be documented (proctoscopy swab stick with markings at every centimeter, ring forceps with centimeter etched in, clear plastic rulers, and so forth).
- Although not routinely done, ancillary testing to characterize the contents of the prolapse (or to establish what is on the other side of the prolapse) may be accomplished with one of the following:
  - Digital, rectovaginal examination
  - CRCU, MRI, CT (computerized tomography), or ultrasound
  - Cystoscopy, proctoscopy

QUANTIFICATION OF POP

- A comparison of POP-Q and Baden-Walker (aka halfway scoring system) (see Table 5-1).
- Both of these systems need to be understood as the Baden-Walker will not be completely abandoned and the POP-Q will not be utilized by all.
- Baden-Walker or halfway scoring system:
  - Indicates which type(s) of prolapse (cystocele, rectocele, uterine, vault, or enterocele) and its/their extent of protrusion
  - Grade 0—no prolapse
  - First degree/grade 1—leading edge of prolapsed structure(s) descends halfway to the introitus
  - Second degree/grade 2—leading edge prolapsed structure(s) descends to the introitus
  - Third degree/grade 3—leading edge of prolapsed structure(s) are up to halfway outside the vagina
  - Fourth degree/grade 4—leading edge of prolapse structure(s) protrudes more than halfway outside the vagina
  - Each defect is given its own prolapse grade (e.g., "the patient has a grade 2 cystocele, a grade 1 uterine prolapse, and grade 2 rectocele")
- POP-Q (adopted by ICS, AUGS, SGS in 1996).
- Tic-tac-toe or 3×3 grid notation: upper row consists of Aa, Ba, and C; lower row consists of Ap, Bp, and D; and middle row consists of gh, pb, and tv (see Fig. 5-1).
- Upper rows focus on anterior vaginal wall; lower rows focus on posterior vaginal wall.
- Middle row is obtained *during rest* (without strain).

TABLE 5-1 Methods of Describing Pelvic Organ Prolapse

PELVIC ORGAN PROLAPSE-QUANTIFICATION (AKA POP-Q)	BADEN-WALKER (AKA HALFWAY SYSTEM)
Exact value for severity of POP (cm/staging)	Approximation of severity of POP (grade/degree)
Standardization useful for research purposes and for accurate written and verbal communication between physicians	Still used for verbal communication between physicians. Some experts believe level of detail is sufficient for clinical care.
Eliminates ambiguity by using hymen instead of vaginal *introitus* and other ambiguous terms	Easier to learn/teach and less time consuming
Used at many academic centers	Still used by many authorities

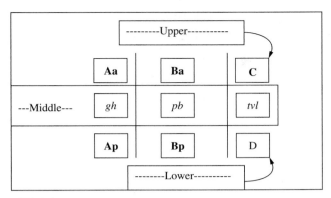

FIG. 5-1

- ○ *gh*—genital hiatus is the distance from urethral meatus to hymen (posterior, midline); gh and pb are the first measurements of POP-Q.
- ○ *Pb*—perineal body (PB) is the distance from hymen (posterior, midline) to anus (opening); gh and pb are the first measurements of POP-Q.
- ○ *Tvl*—greatest length of vagina when prolapse is reduced completely.
- Upper and lower rows are obtained during maximum straining.
  - ○ *Aa*—imaginary point on anterior vaginal wall, in the midline, which is 3 cm proximal to hymen. Values can be −3 to +3 cm relative to the hymen. Example, in a patient without prolapse, Aa = −3 cm, whereas in a patient with complete procidentia, Aa = +3 cm.
  - ○ *Ba*—distance from hymen to the most distal or dependent edge of the anterior vaginal wall. Values can be −3 cm up to a value ≤+C.
  - ○ *C*—distance from hymen to most distal edge of cervix or leading edge of vaginal apex (in hysterectomized).
  - ○ *Ap*—imaginary point on posterior vaginal wall, in the midline, which is 3 cm proximal to posterior hymen. Values are −3 to +3 cm; analogous to Aa but is on posterior vaginal wall.
  - ○ *Bp*—distance from hymen to the most distal or dependent edge of the posterior vaginal wall. Values can be −3 cm up to a value ≤+C; analogous to Ba but is on posterior vaginal wall.
  - ○ *D*—is omitted in hysterectomized patients. Symbolizes the distance from hymen to the posterior fornix. This point is only included to differentiate uterine prolapse (due to anatomical defects) from a well-supported uterus with a long cervix.
- *Bp (pulsion)*: If you're able to differentiate between an enterocele and a rectocele on physical examination then use *pulsion*. Sometimes an enterocele may be

encountered in posterior vaginal wall and/or small bowel may be appreciated within the rectovaginal space. If after rectovaginal examination, one can digitally palpate loops of bowel or visualize peristaltic activity then *pulsion* may be added in front of the value of Bp.
- Based on the POP-Q, a stage can be assigned to the prolapse as follows (Note *B* means either Ba or Bp):
  - ○ Stage 0 —no prolapse
  - ○ Stage 1—most distal edge of prolapse, B or C <−1 cm
  - ○ Stage 2—most distal edge of prolapse, B or C between −1 and +1
  - ○ Stage 3—most distal edge of prolapse, B or C between +1 and tvl −2
  - ○ Stage 4—most distal edge of prolapse, B or C between tvl −2 and tvl
- Why was the "−3" used as the reference point in the POP-Q? On the average, it is the location of the urethrovesical junction.
- What does *point D* represent? Attachment level of the uterosacral and cardinal ligaments.
- The following is not quantified by POP-Q: width or transverse dimension of prolapse or genital hiatus, volume of prolapse, characterization of defects leading to prolapse (see Table 5-1), and assessment of rectal prolapse.

CORRELATING POP WITH ANATOMIC DEFECTS

(See Chap. 16, Urethral Augmentation for Correction of Stress Urinary Incontinence: Bulking Procedures and Artificial Urinary Sphincter.)
- Defects in the support system (usually ≥ 2 defects) occur at multiple sites.
- Preoperative assessment of pelvic support defects is not without error. Many times, support defects are discovered during surgery and thus need to be addressed.
- Incomplete correction of weakened or defective regions during POP surgery may lead to recurrence of POP.
- Apical, anterior, and posterior prolapses are associated with each other. 67% of patients with any prolapse have prolapse of other areas as well: concomitant anterior prolapse (7%), posterior prolapse (30%), or multiple compartment prolapse (30%).

BIMANUAL EXAMINATION

- Do not forget to assess uterine size and contour (if not hysterectomized), pelvic masses, and tenderness.
- Examine the patient after the bladder is emptied as this allows better evaluation of the uterus and adnexae.

ANORECTAL EXAMINATION ·

- "Dovetail sign" suggests anterior separation of the external anal sphincter.
- Digitally evaluate the tone and integrity of the external anal sphincter and the rectovaginal septum.
- Flatal or fecal incontinence occurs in 20% of patients with urinary incontinence.
- Fecal impaction may be encountered.
- Good time to perform a fecal occult blood test and discuss compliance with colorectal cancer screening.

PELVIC MUSCLE STRENGTH

- Digitally evaluate the contractility of the pelvic muscles.
  - Insert index and middle fingers few centimeters inside the hymen, just adjacent to sidewalls and ask the patient to squeeze (1 s and 3 s squeezes).
  - Assess strength, duration, and symmetry.
- Often patients mistakenly perform valsalva, using abdominal and gluteal muscles instead of the pubococcygeus muscles.
  - Strong muscles: A patient with very strong contraction of these muscles will not benefit from physical therapy but may benefit from strengthening exercises.
  - Weak muscles: Referral to a physical therapist should be made if pelvic floor muscles are weak.
  - No strength: This suggests severe atrophy of the pelvic floor muscles and/or neuropathy. This patient may benefit from biofeedback or electrical stimulation.

EVALUATION OF ASYMPTOMATIC OR MINIMALLY SYMPTOMATIC POP

- Evaluate as described earlier in this chapter, but there is no need for treatment. Observation is sufficient.
- There is no evidence that pelvic floor exercises can prevent or slow the progression of POP.
- Nevertheless, patients may benefit from the following suggestions:
  - Adequate fluid intake
  - Increase fiber in diet
  - Avoid constipating foods and medications
  - Avoid excessive lifting (if lifting, use proper body posture)
  - Lose weight if obese
  - Stop smoking
  - Treat coexistent medical conditions (esp. COPD, asthma)
  - Kegels if pelvic muscles are weak

EVALUATION OF POP WITH URINARY AND/OR GASTROINTESTINAL SYMPTOMS

- The Big 3: Patients with POP may have coexistent dysfunction of the pelvic organs (bladder, bowel) and sexual dysfunction (discussed in Chap. 49).
- Up to 60–75% of women with advanced POP have incontinence.
- POP + urinary symptoms.
  - POP + overactive bladder (OAB) or urge incontinence symptoms
    - During sexual intercourse, orgasm may cause detrusor contractions and incontinence.
    - Try pessary, local estrogen, manage fluids, change diet (avoid caffeine, alcohol, acidic foods), bladder retraining, pelvic muscle exercise, bedside commode, anticholinergic medication.
    - Be careful when treating with anticholinergic medications because constipation will lead to excessive straining at defecation which can worsen prolapse and/or dislodge pessary.
    - Increased fiber, avoidance of iron, stool softeners, laxatives may be necessary to alleviate constipation.
  - POP + SUI symptoms
    - Usually, small amount of urine is lost immediately after strain.
    - Larger amounts of incontinence may suggest ISD (or if large amounts are lost few seconds after strain, this suggests urge incontinence).
    - SUI with POP usually occurs when prolapse is mild to moderate because severe prolapse may occlude urethra.
    - During sexual intercourse, vaginal penetration may cause incontinence.
    - Manage conservatively first: (1) local estrogen and choose appropriate pessary (e.g., ring with incontinence knob), Kegels, fluid management, scheduled voiding or (2) pessary + periurethral bulking + above suggestions.
    - Surgery if conservative management fails or if patient desires it.
  - POP + voiding dysfunction
    - One-third of women with POP have obstructive voiding, especially as prolapse becomes advanced.
    - Straining to void may exacerbate prolapse thus making urethral occlusion worse.
    - Patient who initially had SUI symptoms may believe she is cured of it, as prolapse advances and causes distortion, compression, or kinking of the urethra (thus occluding it).
    - In some patients when the prolapse is reduced during POP evaluation, SUI is revealed. This is

referred to as *occult incontinence* (aka potential, latent, or masked incontinence).

- Similarly, if a patient with POP develops SUI after prolapse surgery, this is referred to as *de novo SUI*.
- Therefore, those with advanced prolapse (i.e., grade 3 or 4) should have it reduced via pessary, Sims speculum, ring forceps, vaginal packing, or large swabs with care not to occlude the urethra. Prolapse reduction may serve in counseling patients and for performing prophylactic surgery.
- Management of occult incontinence is controversial. Currently, we cannot scientifically predict which patients will have de novo SUI after prolapse surgery. Therefore, some experts perform a prophylactic anti-incontinence procedure along with surgery for prolapse.
- However, data for this is lacking. The National Institutes for Health (NIH)-funded, pelvic floor disorders network (PFDN) will be revealing.
- Advanced prolapse may also cause some degree of detrusor muscle dysfunction (in addition to urethral occlusion mentioned before).
- Evaluate patient with POP + voiding dysfunction as described earlier in this chapter.
- Positive stress test at low bladder volumes suggests more severe incontinence.
- *Patients with elevated PVR even after reduction of prolapse are at risk for voiding dysfunction* if an anti-incontinence operation such as sling is performed during prolapse surgery. Some experts would perform complex cystometry ± pressure-flow study to determine if the detrusor muscle is dysfunctional, if urethral obstruction is present, and to elucidate voiding mechanism utilized.
- Manage conservatively first: local estrogen and pessary (usually reduces PVR to normal, especially in patients with advanced POP [>90%]); if PVR remains elevated then intermittent self-catheterization is necessary.
- If patient wants surgery despite high PVRs after pessary reduction then she must be counseled about the possibility of long-term intermittent self-catheterization 2–3 times per day.
  - Recurrent UTIs (see Chap. 25, Lower Urinary Tract Infections and Asymptomatic Bacteriuria).
    - Treat with antibiotics for at least 7 days.
    - Repeat cultures in 2–3 weeks after treatment.
    - Local estrogen and pessary may resolve recurrent UTIs.
    - Prophylactic antibiotics may be necessary.
- POP + GI symptoms
  - GI symptoms have more stigma and embarrassment than urinary symptoms.

- Evaluate POP as described earlier in this chapter, paying close attention to the following on rectovaginal examination and neurologic examination:
  - Tissue irritation from chronic contact with stool or foul-smell
  - Perineal descent and PB integrity
  - "Dovetail" sign; most obstetrical anal sphincter disruptions occur at 12 o'clock position
  - Tone of anal sphincter: resting (tonic internal anal sphincter contraction) versus voluntary contraction (external anal sphincter muscle contraction for ≥10 s)
  - Fecal occult blood testing
  - Rectal prolapse—patients cannot differentiate between this and POP
  - Sensation (dull, sharp), reflexes (bulbocavernosus, anal wink)
- POP + constipation (major feature)
  - Must explain to patient because she may have a different definition of constipation. Ask about frequency of bowel movements, consistency of stool, and need to strain.
  - Treat constipation:
    - Change diet (increase fluids, increase dietary fiber)
    - Fiber supplements
    - Stool softeners
    - Laxatives (osmotics may be used regularly but irritant and cathartic should be used prn only)
    - Exercise
    - Avoid constipating agents (iron, calcium, nonsteroid anti-inflammatory drugs [NSAIDs])
    - If using anticholinergic medications change to long-acting or sustained release or discontinue if possible
  - Refer to GI:
    - Colon transit time study (prolonged?)
    - Defecation proctography or anal manometry (*puborectal muscle contraction instead of normal relaxation during defecation is treated by pelvic muscle retraining*)
- POP + fecal urgency symptoms
  - Urge to defecate is very strong and patient may not be able to make it to the bathroom on time; this may occur often; once it starts, patient may/may not be able to stop it; stress or hurry may provoke it.
  - Refer to GI:
    - Must rule out Crohn's disease or ulcerative colitis (e.g., fistulas in the perineum or vagina from Crohn's should not be treated surgically)
    - Colonoscopy with biopsy
    - If all objective tests are normal diagnosis may be irritable bowel syndrome (IBS)

○ POP + fecal incontinence symptoms
  ▪ Up to 26% of patients with POP may have fecal incontinence.
  ▪ Symptoms and signs: leaking of gas, liquid, or solid spontaneously or with activity (including sex); staining of stool on underclothes; need to wear a pad.
  ▪ Intrinsic bowel disease must be ruled out and/or treated.
  ▪ Perform pelvic muscle exercises.
  ▪ Evaluate with endoanal ultrasound if surgery is planned.
    • Overlapping sphincteroplasty may be performed with POP surgery without increase in morbidity.
    • However, long-term outcome for surgical cure of fecal incontinence is poor.
○ Rectal prolapse (see Chap. 22, Rectal Prolapse and Hemorrhoids).
  ▪ Treat constipation as described earlier.
  ▪ Refer to colorectal surgery or general surgery for rectopexy.

INDICATIONS FOR REFERRAL TO A SPECIALIST

• All physicians should screen patients for incontinence and PFDs because majority (>60%) of patients do not address these issues with their doctors or delay seeking treatment for an average of 5 years. Why?
  ○ Embarrassment
  ○ Discomfort
  ○ Feeling of isolation
  ○ False belief that symptoms are part of the normal aging process
• Usually, the patient with incontinence or POP first sees a gynecologist, family practitioner, internist, or urologist.
• The majority of referrals come from primary care physicians, internists, and family practitioners.
• The gynecologist is in an excellent position to workup and manage patients with PFD and incontinence since many women see their gynecologist for primary care as well as gynecologic care.
• Additionally, since operations for POP are frequently done in conjunction with other gynecologic procedures, having one doctor and one anesthetic trial may lead to better patient care.
• Barriers to gynecologist doing evaluation for incontinence include:
  ○ Discomfort with subject material
  ○ Lack of training in Female Pelvic Medicine and Reconstructive Surgery (FPMRS) during residency
  ○ Time constraints (evaluation may take extra 20–30 min of office time)

• If a gynecologist is interested in managing POP patients, he or she may ask the patient to complete a questionnaire (urogenital distress inventory [UDI], IIQ, pelvic floor distress inventory (PFDI), pelvic floor impact questionnaire (PFIQ), pelvic organ prolapse incontinence sexual questionnaire (PISQ), keep a voiding diary, and schedule her for a return visit to address this issue.
• If a gynecologist does not want to manage PFD or if cases are complicated, he/she should make a referral to a specialist.
• A specialist is a gynecologist or urologist who is adequately trained or experienced in the field of female pelvic medicine and reconstructive surgery (usually a urogynecologist, female pelvic medicine and reconstructive surgeon (FPMRS) or female urologist). Indications for referral to a specialist are as follows:
  ○ Failed conservative or medical therapy
  ○ Patient unsatisfied with current therapy and desires further evaluation
  ○ When considering surgical treatment (esp. if previous surgery failed)
  ○ Previous failed anti-incontinence surgery
  ○ Recurrent or refractory UTIs
  ○ Urinary retention or abnormal postvoid residual volume
  ○ Previous radical pelvic surgery or pelvic radiation therapy
  ○ Legal purposes (to document nerve damage after surgery or work-related injuries)
  ○ Symptomatic POP beyond the hymen
  ○ Neurologic disease such as multiple sclerosis or stroke concurrent
  ○ Hematuria without the presence of infection
  ○ Presence of a fistula or urethral diverticulum
  ○ Complex cases or uncertain diagnosis

BIBLIOGRAPHY

Abrams P, Cardozo L, Fall M, et al. The standardization of terminology of lower urinary tract function: report from the standardization sub-committee of the International Continence Society. *Neurourol Urodyn.* 2002;21:167–178.

Baden WF, Walker T, Lindsey JH. The vaginal profile. *Tex Med.* 1968;64:56.

Barber MD, Visco AG, Wyman JF, et al.; Continence Program for Women Research Group. Sexual function in women with urinary incontinence and pelvic organ prolapse. *Obstet Gynecol.* 2002;99:281–289.

Brinks CA, Well TJ, Smapselle CM, et al. A digital test for pelvic muscle strength in women with urinary incontinence. *Nurs Res.* 1994;43:352–356.

Bump RC, Mattiasson A, Bo K, et al. The standardization of terminology of female pelvic organ prolapse and pelvic floor dysfunction. *Am J Obstet Gynecol.* 1996;175:10.

Ellerkmann RM, Cundiff GW, Melick CF, et al. Correlation of symptoms with location and severity of pelvic organ prolapse. *Am J Obstet Gynecol.* 2001;185:1332–1338.

FitzGeral MP, Brubaker L. Variability of 24 hours voiding diary variables among asymptomatic women. *J Urol.* 2003;169:207–209.

FitzGerald MP, Kulkarni N, Fenner D. Postoperative resolution of urinary retention in patients with advanced pelvic organ prolapse. *Am J Obstet Gynecol.* 2000;183:1361–1364.

Gallentine ML, Cespedes RD. Occult stress urinary incontinence and the effect of vaginal vault prolapse on abdominal leak point pressures. *Urology.* 2001;57:40–44.

Halverson Al, Hull TL, Paraiso MF, et al. Outcome of sphincteroplasty combined with surgery for urinary incontinence and pelvic organ prolapse. *Dis Colon Rectum.* 2001;44:1421–1426.

Heit M, Culligan P, Rosenquist C, et al. Is pelvic organ prolapse a cause of pelvic or low back pain? *Obstet Gynecol.* 2002;99:23–28.

Heit M, Rosenquist C, Culligan P, et al. Predicting treatment choice for patients with pelvic organ prolapse. *Obstet Gynecol.* 2003;101:1279–1284.

Herzog AR, Diokno AC, Brown MB, et al. Two-year incidence, remission, and change patterns of urinary incontinence in non-institutionalized adults. *J Geront Med Sci.* 1990;45:M67-M74

Jackson SL, Weber AM, Hull TL, et al. Fecal incontinence in women with urinary incontinence and pelvic organ prolapse. *Obstet Gynecol.* 1997;89:423–427.

Moehrer B, Hextal A, Jackson S. Oestrogens for urinary incontinence in women. *Cochrane Database Syst Rev.* 2003;(2):CD001405.

Raz R, Stamm WE. A controlled trial of intravaginal estriol in postmenopausal women with recurrent urinary tract infections. *N Engl J Med.* 1993;329:753–756.

Rogers RM, Richardson CA. Clinical evaluation of pelvic support defects with anatomic correlations. In: Bent AE, Ostergard DR, Cundiff GW, et al., eds. *Ostergard's Urogynecology and Pelvic Floor Dysfunction.* 5th ed. Philadelphia, PA: Lippincott Williams & Wilkins; 2003:77–93.

Romanzi LJ, Chaikin DC, Blaivas JG. The effect of genital prolapse on voiding. *J Urol.* 1999;161:581–586.

Shull BL, Baden WF. Paravaginal defect repair for urinary incontinence: a six year experience. *Am J Obstet Gynecol.* 1989;160:1432–1440.

Shull BL, Benn SJ, Kuehl TJ. Surgical management of prolapse of the anterior vaginal wall segment: an analysis of support defects, operative morbidity, and anatomic outcome. *Am J Obstet Gynecol.* 1994;171:1429–1439.

Shull BL, Capen CV, Riggs M, et al. Bilateral attachment of the vaginal cuff to iliococcygeus fascia: an effective method of cuff suspension. *Am J Obstet Gynecol.* 1993;168:1669–1677.

Singh K, Reid WN, Berger LA. Assessment and grading of pelvic organ prolapse by use of dynamic magnetic resonance imaging. *Am J Obstet Gynecol.* 2001;185:71–77.

Spence-Jones C, Kamm MA, Henry M, et al. Bowel dysfunction: a pathogenic factor in uterovaginal prolapse and urinary stress incontinence. *Br J Obstet Gynaecol.* 1994;101:147–152.

Swift SE, Herring M. Comparison of pelvic organ prolapse in the dorsal lithotomy compared with the standing position. *Obstet Gynecol.* 1998;91:961–964.

Walters MD. Description and classification of lower urinary tract dysfunction and pelvic organ prolapse. In: *Urogynecology, Reconstructive Pelvic Surgery.* 2nd ed. St. Louis, MO: Mosby; 1999:35–44.

Weber AM. Symptomatic prolapse. In: Weber AM, Brubaker L, Schaffer J, et al., eds. *Office Urogynecology.* New York: McGraw-Hill; 2004:201–234.

Weber AM, Walters MD, Ballard LA, et al. Posterior vaginal prolapse and bowel function. *Am J Obstet Gynecol.* 1998; 179:1446–1450.

QUESTIONS

QUESTIONS 1–3

Match the statement below with the word that best describes it above. Each answer may be used once, more than once, or not at all.

(A) Transverse cystocele

(B) Anterior enterocele

(C) Complex enterocele

(D) Simple enterocele

(E) Complete procidentia

(F) Pulsion enterocele

(G) Traction enterocele

(H) Vaginal vault prolapse

(I) Apical POP

(J) Anterior POP

(K) Posterior POP

1. Separation of the fibromuscular layer of the anterior vagina from the pericervical ring leading to protrusion of bowel into the anterior vaginal wall

2. A hernia in the apex of the vagina resulting from chronic coughing

3. During physical examination, it may be difficult to know if a bulge in the posterior vaginal wall is a result of protruding rectum versus bowel

4. A 60-year-old gravida 4, para 4, presents to you because of pelvic pressure and low back pain which has been getting worse over the last year. She says she feels a protrusion from her vagina. Her past medical history is remarkable for diabetes mellitus, hypertension, and arthritis. Her surgical history is remarkable for trans vaginal hysterectomy-bilateral salpingo oophorectomy (TVH-BSO), anterior and posterior colporrhaphy 6 years ago. She has also had an appendectomy 20 years ago. She admits to smoking one pack per week and two glasses of wine with dinner each night. During examination, stroking of the skin of the labium majus does not produce reflex contraction of the bulbocavernosus muscle. Pelvic examination reveals an atrophic vagina with the following POP-Q: Aa = +3 cm, Ba = +6 cm; Ap and Bp = −2; C = 0 cm. On a subjectively full

bladder, the patient has a negative stress test with and without reduction in the standing position. The factor in the history and physical examination that is most important to your surgical management of POP is _____
(A) Lack of sacral reflex
(B) Vaginal atrophy
(C) Diabetes mellitus
(D) Previous surgical history
(E) Smoking

5. A 50-year-old gravida 3, para 3, presented to you a year ago with grade 2 anterior prolapse. She was managed conservatively with local estrogen cream and ring pessary. She now returns to you because she is tired of the pessary and wants definitive surgical correction. On pelvic examination, she has a grade 3 anterior prolapse and a grade 1 posterior and apical prolapse. On cystometric filling, she does not have stress incontinence in the supine position with valsalva at 150 mL. However, her stress test is positive at 150 mL, in sitting position, with prolapse reduced. Her maximum cystometric capacity is 550 mL. She voids 550 mL with PVR of 40 mL. The term that best describes this scenario is _____.
(A) Urodynamic stress incontinence
(B) Potential stress incontinence
(C) Urinary retention
(D) Low leak point pressure
(E) Stage I POP

ANSWERS

ANSWERS 1–3

1. *(B)*, 2. *(F)*, 3. *(K)*. Separation of the pubocervical fascia from the cervix and the broad ligament can result in a hernia. In an anterior enterocele, hernia sac or small bowel protrudes through this separation while in transverse cystocele, the bladder protrudes through this separation. Pulsion enteroceles result from repetitive, chronic increases in the intra-abdominal pressure which herniate cul-de-sac peritoneum (and possibly bowel) through the RVF in direct juxtaposition to vaginal epithelium. The term posterior vaginal wall prolapse is now preferred unless ancillary testing or imaging confirms which organ is in direct apposition to vaginal epithelium. Often it can be difficult to distinguish a high rectocele from a posterior enterocele during physical examination. These can be distinguished by CRCU or MRI.

4. *(D)*. Women who have failed previous surgery for prolapse have recurrent POP. According to some experts, this group of patients may be candidates for augmentation (e.g., graft). Approximately 20% of patients normally lack the bulbocavernosus reflex. Vaginal atrophy may be treated prior to surgery. Diabetes mellitus does not dictate surgical management, but it is associated with increased wound infection thus sugars should be controlled (<200). Smoking may interfere with wound healing but it does not change one's surgical management.

5. *(B)*. The above patient leaks urine in sitting position only when her prolapse is reduced. Thus she has potential or occult stress incontinence. There is not enough information in the clinical scenario to make the conclusion that she has urodynamic stress incontinence (i.e., she has to have stress test positive and lack of detrusor contraction on cystometry [CMG]). She does not have urinary retention since her PVR is low. Valsalva leak point pressures (VLPP) were not mentioned in the clinical scenario. The largest prolapsing compartment is anterior. Baden-Walker grade 3 (halfway outside vagina) does not correspond to POP-Q stage I prolapse (inside vagina).

6 EVALUATION OF URINARY INCONTINENCE IN THE OFFICE AND INDICATIONS FOR REFERRAL TO A SPECIALIST

John Occhino and Sam Siddighi

COMMON WORDS ENCOUNTERED IN THE LITERATURE OF URINARY INCONTINENCE

- *Urinary incontinence (UI)*—the complaint of any involuntary leakage of urine *severe enough to constitute a social or hygienic problem.* UI is a symptom, a sign, and a diagnosis.
  - *Stress urinary incontinence (SUI)*—the complaint of *immediate, small-in-amount, self-limited, involuntary* leakage of urine on effort (lifting, jumping, running, sneezing, laughing, or coughing). However, urine loss with events that increased intra-abdominal

pressure is not always SUI (see later in this section). SUI patients have normal bladder capacities and normal postvoid residuals (PVR).

- Hypermobile urethra incontinence (aka HUI, HMI, HMU): The urethra sits on top of and is invested within the fibromuscular layer of the anterior vaginal wall (aka pubocervical fascia or endopelvic fascia), which also forms a hammock underneath the urethra. Additionally, the urethra is supported at its mid portion by the pubourethral ligament. Normally, the urethra is compressed against this backboard during stress (e.g., cough) and becomes occluded. If the hammock is deficient, the urethra becomes hypermobile and is not compressed. This results in urine leakage during stress. HUI is demonstrated by the Q-tip test (hypermobility), perineal ultrasonography or fluoroscopy (closed urethrovesical junction (UVJ) at rest).

- Intrinsic sphincteric deficiency (aka ISD, type III urethra, low-pressure urethra, "lead-pipe" urethra): Although the urethral support hammock is intact (i.e., no urethral hypermobility), the urethra itself fails to function as a competent sphincter (i.e., open at rest) because of lack of one or more of the following essential urethral components: smooth muscle (tonic contraction at rest), striated muscle (voluntary contraction), autonomic and somatic innervation, connective tissue elasticity, mucosal coaptation, and submucosal venous plexus. ISD is suggested by leakage in the supine position and a positive empty bladder stress test (EBST+). It is best demonstrated by valsalva leak point pressure (VLPP <60 cm H_2O) and maximum urethral closure pressure (MUCP <20 cm H_2O) testing (i.e., complex cystometry with urethral pressure profile). ISD may result from congenital weakness as a consequence of defects in muscle, tissue structure, or innervation (e.g., smooth or striated muscle disorder, epispadias or myelomeningocele) or can result from any of the following:
  - Previous anti-incontinence surgery
  - Radical pelvic surgery
  - Trauma
  - Radiation (pelvic x-ray, x-ray therapy [XRT], and the like)
  - Spinal cord lesion (sacral spinal cord [sc])
  - Childbirth
  - Chronic catheter drainage
  - Aging
  - Hypoestrogenism
- *Urinary urgency incontinence (UUI) or OAB-wet*—the complaint of involuntary leakage accompanied by or immediately preceded by urgency. These patients typically have large volume leaks with complete bladder emptying that is difficult to stop or occasionally have frequent small losses between voids. Occasionally, increases in intra-abdominal pressure may provoke detrusor contraction(s) which may cause incontinence. Therefore rises in the intra-abdominal pressure cause a *delayed* (5–10 s rather than immediately after cough) continuous leakage of urine. These patients have small bladder capacities but normal PVR.

- *Overactive bladder-dry (OAB-dry)*—urgency + frequency without incontinence.
- *Mixed urinary incontinence (MUI)*—the complaint of involuntary leakage associated with urgency and also with exertion, effort, sneezing, or coughing. Although both stress and urge incontinence exist, one factor often predominates. The severity of incontinence is also greater in these patients (i.e., episodes and volumes). PVR is normal.
- *Continuous urinary incontinence*—the complaint of continuous leakage.
- *Bypass urinary incontinence*—uncommon cause of incontinence; continuous urine loss due to an anatomic problem which disrupts the integrity of the urinary tract. Examples include *fistulas* (vesicovaginal, vesicouterine, urethrovaginal, ureterovaginal), *urethral diverticula* (postvoid dribbling symptoms), *ectopic ureter* (which empties distal to internal urethral sphincter mechanism), and *epispadias* (an opening by the separation of the labia minora and a fissure of the clitoris).
- *Functional urinary incontinence*—urine loss due to inability to reach the bathroom in time, inability to remove clothing (either because many layers or lack of manual dexterity), mentally recognize the need to go to the bathroom, or inability to access bathroom.
- *Transient incontinence*—when UI is a presenting symptom of another medical condition (e.g., diabetes mellitus [DM], congestive heart failure [CHF], Interstitial Cystitis (IC) and may remit when the medical condition is treated. Other conditions, most of which are reversible, are summarized by the acronym DIAPPERS. The following can make the elderly susceptible to UI:
  - *Delirium*—differentiate from dementia
  - *Infection*—elderly may be asymptomatic; bacterial endotoxins inhibit alpha-adrenergic receptors
  - *Atrophy*—effect of estrogen on incontinence is unclear
  - *Pharmaceutical*—do not forget over the counter medications in addition to prescription medications
  - *Psychiatric*—factitious disorder, hypochondria, to gain attention
  - *Excess urine output and endocrine*—e.g., CHF/edema and DM or hypercalcemia, respectively
  - *Restricted mobility*—arthritis, gait difficulty
  - *Stool impaction*—fecal impaction cause UI

○ *Overflow urinary incontinence*—urine loss due to bladder hyposensation or loss of detrusor contraction which results in overdistension of the bladder, urinary retention, incontinence, and other urinary symptoms (dribbling, SUI and, constant wetness). These patients have high bladder capacity, high PVR, and are prone to recurrent urinary tract infections (UTIs). They may be treated by clean, intermittent self-catheterization, alpha-adrenergic blockers, bethanechol, or even surgical therapy. There are numerous causes of overflow incontinence:

- Medications (anticholinergic, calcium channel blocker, alpha-adrenergic agonists, beta-adrenergic agonists)
- Neuropathy (vitamin B_{12} deficiency, tabes dorsalis, herniated disk, peripheral neuropathy)
- Endocrine (hypothyroid, DM)
- Decreased compliance states (radiation, interstitial cystitis, recurrent UTIs)
- Outflow obstruction (pelvic organ prolapse [POP], pelvic neoplasm [large fibroid, large adnexal mass], previous incontinence surgery, involuntary contraction of pelvic floor muscle [from pain, infection, and the like.])

• *Supine incontinence*—leakage of urine while lying on the back.

• *Supine empty bladder stress test (EBST +)*—observation of urine leakage from the urethra during positional changes or spontaneous increases in intraabdominal pressure during pelvic examination in lithotomy position. This suggests ISD.

• *Nocturia*—the complaint that the individual has to wake at night ≥2 time(s) to void. Besides OAB, nocturia may be due to shifting of interstitial fluids, diuretic or other medication taken before bedtime, large fluid intake before bedtime, and reduction of antidiuretic hormone (ADH).

• *Nocturnal enuresis*—bed-wetting or complaint of loss of urine occurring during sleep. This must be differentiated from SUI caused by coughing or turning in bed while asleep.

• *Polyuria*—urine output ≥2800 mL in a day for adults.

• *Urgency*—the complaint of a sudden compelling desire to pass urine, which is difficult to defer. Two good examples: (1) strong urge or need to void but may not reach the bathroom on time, (2) strong need to void when nervous, in hurry, or under stress.

• *Frequency*—voiding more than 7–8 times per day or voiding more often than every 2 hours.

• *Hesitancy*—when an individual describes difficulty in initiating micturition resulting in a delay in the onset of voiding after the individual is ready to pass urine. This may occur with urethral obstruction from advanced POP.

• *Dysuria*—the feeling of pain or discomfort when passing urine. Besides UTI, suprapubic pain and chronic pelvic pain with urgency may be due to interstitial cystitis.

• *Urodynamic stress incontinence (USUI)*—involuntary leakage, observed during bladder filling cystometry and occurring with increased intra-abdominal pressure in absence of detrusor contraction. The term "genuine" stress incontinence or GSUI is no longer used.

• *Urodynamic detrusor overactivity incontinence (UDOI)*—a urodynamic observation characterized by incontinence due to involuntary detrusor contractions during the filling phase which may be spontaneous or provoked. The following terms are no longer used: uninhibited bladder, motor urge incontinence, reflex incontinence, detrusor instability, and detrusor hyperreflexia.

○ *Nonneurogenic detrusor overactivity*—formerly detrusor instability

○ *Neurogenic detrusor overactivity*—formerly detrusor hyperreflexia

• *Overactive bladder (OAB)*—term coined by industry for purpose of coding and medication prescription; it includes any or all of the following: urgency, frequency, nocturia, and urge incontinence. The more types of OAB symptoms a patient has, the greater the chance that she has detrusor overactivity on complex cystometry.

HISTORY TAKING

• As with any medical problem, evaluation of UI should begin with a thorough history followed by a directed physical examination.

• History for evaluation of incontinence serves three main purposes: (1) to find and treat reversible causes of incontinence, (2) to determine its effect on quality of life, (3) to determine its severity (i.e., conservative management is chosen for mild symptoms while surgical options may be explored for severe symptoms).

• Any previous evaluation and/or treatment is important.

• Patient history alone is only 50–70% specific and sensitive in the diagnosis of UI and is poor at differentiating one type of incontinence from another.

• All patients should be screened for PFD, including UI, especially in the postpartum period.

○ It is very important to use language the patient will understand.

○ For example, some patients may confuse stress incontinence with emotional stress leading to incontinence rather than increased intra-abdominal pressure as its cause.

• A large number of women will develop new onset UI, therefore, is important to rescreen all returning patients.

○ Screening questionnaires, like the pelvic floor distress inventory (PFDI), urogenital distress inventory (UDI), incontinence impact questionnaire (IIQ), pelvic floor impact questionnaire (PFIQ), or pelvic organ prolapse/urinary incontinence sexual function questionnaire (PIS-Q), medical, epidemological, and social aspects of aging questionnaire (MESA) questionnaire may be used to help screen patients for pelvic floor dysfunction and incontinence.

- In patients with symptoms of UI, the following information must be obtained:
  - What is the patient's main complaint?
  - What is the duration of the symptoms?
    - Abrupt onset → e.g., allergic or infectious
    - Gradual onset → e.g., if after oophorectomy may be related to estrogen deficiency
  - When and how often does it occur?
  - Does she wear a pad?
  - Does she leak during sexual intercourse?
  - What is its effect on the patient's quality of life (QoL)?
    - For example, a patient may leak urine only once a week during exercise and yet be willing to do almost anything to get this resolved as it has a great impact on her QoL (i.e., decrease in physical and social functioning, vitality, and an increase in psychological consequences).
    - On the other hand, a woman may soak eight pads per day but is not bothered by it.
    - The goal of the IIQ and PFIQ is assessment of life impact of UI and POP.
  - Does the patient desire treatment for the condition? If so, does she have a strong preference for one management over another (conservative vs. surgical)
- Focus on any condition that may be contributing to and/or causing the patient's UI (e.g., constipation).
- *Social history*: smoking (associated with both stress and urge incontinence), occupational stress (heavy lifting), recreational or athletic stress (chronic, repetitive straining).
- *Family history*: prevalence of UI is higher in family members of incontinent women.
- *Medical history*: DM (e.g., poorly controlled causes polyuria and nocturia), diabetes insipidus, thyroid disease, *lung diseases* (chronic cough, chronic obstructive pulmonary disease [COPD], asthma), chronic constipation, restricted mobility (e.g., severe arthritis, quadriplegia), CHF (edema, mobilization of third-space fluid at night), UTI, radiation (which may have rendered urethra rigid and fibrotic).
- *Neurologic history*: Does she have a history of any of the following? Multiple sclerosis (e.g., may cause urinary retention and overflow incontinence), history of cerebrovascular accident (CVA), tumor, dementia, Parkinson's, lumbar disc disease, neuropathy, upper motor neuron lesion.
- *Urologic history*: urgency, frequency, dysuria, UTI, hematuria, voiding dysfunction (i.e., urinary retention, hesitancy, slow urinary stream, straining to void, interrupted urinary stream, feeling of bladder still being full).

- *Urinary diary (aka urolog, 24 hours, 3 days, or 7 days)* is an inexpensive and helpful adjunct because histories may be unreliable or misleading.
  - Information such as fluid intake (type, amount, and time; e.g., weight reduction programs require large fluid intake; also belief that drinking water to "flush the system"), voids day versus night, leakage and associated or precipitating factors, sense of urgency, maximum voided amount, and pad usage. Texas hat may be placed in commode to help with urine measurement.
  - 24-hour diary is good for evaluation of frequency and nocturia.
  - 3-day diaries are most commonly used and have a high degree of correlation to a 7-day diary.
  - Diaries require tremendous patient motivation.
  - Patients with detrusor overactivity incontinence may have more difficulty keeping track of voids and leakage episodes.
  - Urinary diaries have an observed therapeutic effect that is greater than placebo during pharmaceutical drug trials. The act of keeping track of the above may have behavioral modification benefits.
  - A few examples are as follows:
    - 75–150 mL (small) frequent voids with urge sensation → rule out OAB
    - 350–550 mL (large) infrequent voids and stress symptoms → rule out SUI
    - Patient takes >4 L of fluid per day → rule out diabetes insipidus
    - Voiding small volumes almost every hour during day only → rule out psychologic condition
- *Obstetric history*: gravida and para, number and type of deliveries (cesarean, spontaneous vaginal, forceps), lacerations (third or fourth degree), episiotomies, and desire or lack of desire for future childbearing is important, as many experts will not perform surgery on those who have not completed childbearing.
- *Gynecologic history*: prolapse, menopause/hormone therapy, pain, neoplasm (fibroids or large ovarian masses may push on the bladder, reduce bladder capacity, and may cause urgency and frequency symptoms).
- *Surgical history*: especially gynecologic (hysterectomy or prolapse surgery), previous anti-incontinence surgeries, or radical surgery.
  - *Important to obtain records and operative reports if available.*
  - Prior surgeries may have resulted in trauma to the lower urinary tract which may have caused uninhibited urethral relaxation.
  - Notice surgical scars.

- *Sexual history*: is she sexually active? satisfaction, incontinence during intercourse, dyspareunia.
- *Colorectal history*: bowel function, fecal or flatal incontinence.
- Medications may have urinary side effects. Elderly Americans are taking an average of four drugs daily.
  - Frequency, polyuria, urgency: diuretics, caffeine, alcohol, cholinergic agonists (e.g., bethanechol, cisapride)
  - Retention and overflow incontinence: anticholinergics, alpha-adrenergic agonists, anti-Parkinson agents, narcotics, calcium channel blockers, beta-blockers, antipsychotics
  - SUI: alpha-adrenergic blockers (e.g., prazosin, doxazosin), antihypertensives, neuroleptics, phenothiazines, benzodiazepines (e.g., diazepam)
  - Indirect effects (i.e., can worsen severity of incontinence): angiotensin converting enzyme (ACE) inhibitors (cough), iron and narcotics (constipation), anxiolytics (sedation and sphincter relaxation), nonsteroid anti-inflammatory drugs (NSAIDs), (constipation)

PHYSICAL EXAMINATION

OBSERVATION

- Simple observation can give the clinician information on the patient's general health, mobility, gait, and cognitive limitations.
- If possible, observe the patient ambulate.
- Abnormalities may suggest underlying neurologic or spinal injury.
- Obese patients have greater magnitude of stress on their bladder and may have a harder time with some management options; both SUI and OAB are more prevalent in obese women.
- Peripheral edema and nocturia may be due to mobilization of third-space fluids at night.
- Look for scars and correlate them to the surgical history, inquire about any not mentioned in the patient's history.
- Look for urine loss at all times during the physical examination.

NEUROLOGIC EXAMINATION

- *Mental status, gait, and coordination* should be evaluated (rule out [r/o] dementia, delirium, Normal Pressure Hydrocephalus [NPH], brain tumor).
- Pelvic neurologic examination should be done early in examination so the patient is still alert to the sensation of touch.

- *Motor* function of lower extremities: flex/extend hips, knees, ankle, feet (inversion/eversion) against resistance.
- All *reflexes* should be checked bilaterally:
  - Watch for hyperreflexia in patellar reflex—indicates upper motor neuron lesion (e.g., stroke, multiple sclerosis [MS]).
  - Positive plantar reflex (Babinski) means upper motor neuron lesion—stroking of reflex hammer across foot causes fanning of toes and dorsiflexion of big toe instead of normal response of flexion of all toes.
  - Bulbocavernosus reflex (aka *clitoral-anal*—S2-S3)—tapping of clitoris or stroking the labium majus causes contraction of bulbocavernosus and ischiocavernosus. If reflex is not seen visually, it may be felt by placing finger just inside the hymenal ring. This test is not used often because it is not present in 20% of normal women and is occasionally difficult to assess.
  - Anal reflexes (aka *anal wink*—S2-S5) stroking skin next to anus causes contraction of external anal sphincter. Rarely used because of the earlier mentioned reasons.
  - If these reflexes are intact, then both sensory and motor reflex arc of S_2-S_3 is intact.
- *Sensation* (S_2-S_4) of lower extremities: symmetry, light touch, and pinprick sensation on perineum and sacral dermatomes, pain.
- Normal perineal nerve function is important because abnormalities lead to higher failure rates after surgery. Electromyograph (EMG) may be helpful for this purpose.

GYNECOLOGIC EXAMINATION

- Though you may primarily be screening for incontinence, it is important to look for vulvar, vaginal, urethral, and other pelvic changes.
- A *diaper rash* may indicate chronic urine contact with perineal and vulvar skin.
- Atrophy of vaginal tissues suggests atrophy of the urethral as well as periurethral tissue since they all share common embryologic structure, urogenital sinus. Local estrogen therapy is not a direct treatment for stress incontinence, but it does help improve irritative symptoms, promotes stronger, thicker vaginal and urethral tissues, and potentiates alpha-adrenergic response when combined with an agonist.
- Vaginal discharge or vaginitis may mimic UI.
- Suburethral mass, tenderness, or extrusion of discharge may suggest presence of urethral diverticulum.
- Suprapubic tenderness or costovertebral angle tenderness suggest infection or stone.

- Presence of urine in vagina may hint at some type of a genitourinary (GU) fistula.
- Initial examination may be done with the patient in the stirrups (rather than supine) to assess for prolapse and leakage, especially with valsalva.
- If patient does not leak have patient stand or squat, then repeat stress test.
- Shield yourself to prevent soiling with urine during involuntary leakage with valsalva.
- Look for perineal scars from previous episiotomy or laceration repairs.
- Speculum examination should be performed in the usual fashion and you may want to do a pap smear if she is not a referred patient.
- Bimanual examination should assess uterine size (if present), pelvic masses, and subjectively assess vaginal length, especially in patients with previous surgery.
- Vaginal support should be evaluated for the presence of anterior prolapse (cystocele), posterior prolapse (rectocele), or apical prolapse (enterocele, uterine or vault prolapse). Note that it may be difficult to differentiate between cystocele and urethrocele because they usually coexist. Use POP-Q (standard) or Baden-Walker classification to assess degree of prolapse (see Chap. 5, Evaluation of Pelvic Organ Prolapse [POP]).
- Patients with POP may have distortion, compression, or kinking of urethra which occludes it and may mask UI. This is referred to as *occult incontinence* (aka potential, latent, or masked incontinence). Therefore, those with advanced prolapse (i.e., grade 3 or 4) should have it reduced (via pessary, Sims speculum, ring forceps, or large swabs with care not to occlude the urethra so as to simulate the effect of surgery) and then asked to cough or valsalva with the bladder full to see if SUI is now present.
- Remember two things about occult incontinence testing: (1) do not occlude the urethra as this will create false negative results, and (2) be careful not to push down on the levator ani as this will paralyze the levator muscles, lead to relaxation of the bladder outlet, and therefore false-positive occult incontinence.
- Currently, some experts perform a prophylactic sling along with surgery for prolapse to avoid de novo SUI in a patient who has occult incontinence. However, the data for this are lacking. The pelvic floor disorders network (PFDN) and other studies will shed light on this matter.
- Anorectal examination
  - Digitally evaluate the tone and integrity of the external anal sphincter. Flatal or fecal incontinence occurs in 20% of patients with UI.
  - Fecal impaction—UI improves after resolution of fecal impaction in elderly institutionalized patients.
  - Good time to perform a fecal occult blood test and discuss compliance with colon cancer screening.

- Pelvic muscle strength
  - Digitally evaluate the contractility of the pelvic muscles.
    - Insert index and middle fingers inside vagina and ask the patient to squeeze or do a Kegel squeeze (both 1s and 3 s squeezes).
    - Often patients mistakenly perform valsalva, use abdominal and gluteal muscles instead of the pubococcygeus muscles.
  - Strong muscles: A patient with very strong contraction of these muscles will not benefit from physical therapy but may benefit from strengthening exercises.
  - Weak muscles: Referral to a physical therapist should be made if pelvic floor muscles are weak.
  - No strength: This suggests severe atrophy of the pelvic floor muscles and/or neuropathy. This patient may benefit from biofeedback or electrical stimulation.
- Many clinicians evaluate urethral hypermobility in patients with symptoms of stress incontinence via the *Q-tip test.*
  - Initially introduced by Crystle.
  - By standard, >30 degrees movement of the Q-tip is considered hypermobile urethra (HMU), but there is no clear cutoff between normal and abnormal as there is overlap between asymptomatic, parous women and women with SUI.
  - Procedure: (1) cleanse with antibacterial solution or iodine, (2) place 2% lidocaine gel-impregnated cotton swab in bladder. Decrease in resistance means you are past bladder neck. Location of Q-tip is very important as bladder placement or midurethral placement changes values, therefore, (3) after insertion into the bladder, Q-tip should be withdrawn slowly until resistance is felt. This is the bladder neck or UVJ! The Q-tip portion should be just beyond the UVJ.
  - Disadvantage is that (1) it can be uncomfortable for patients, (2) it is misunderstood: urethral hypermobility does not automatically mean SUI.
  - The degree of movement of the swab, from the horizon, between rest and valsalva are measured using protractor or orthopedic goniometer.
  - There is nothing magical about the number "30." By changing the criteria to >40 degrees, one reduces the false-positive rate while only slightly reducing the true-positive rate. By increasing the criteria angle to 80 degrees, one reduces false-positive to zero but sacrifices true-positive rate (20%).
  - This test is positive in women with advanced POP (stage 3 or 4) and usually positive in stage 2.
  - However, this test is not significantly affected by bladder volume.
  - There is good intraobserver (≈85%) and interobserver correlation (≈90%) for this test.

○ Correlates well with bladder neck movement measured by perineal ultrasound.

○ This test is unnecessary if surgery is not going to be performed.

○ The Q-tip test does not predict surgical outcome.

○ *A patient with symptoms of SUI and a negative Q-tip test has a 50% higher failure rate for Burch urethropexy.*

• Q-tip testing for documentation of urethral hypermobility replaced beaded chain urethrocystoscopy as it is less expensive and does not involve exposure to radiation.

• *Stress test* (CST = cough stress test, VST = valsalva stress test): This test objectively demonstrates SUI.

○ This test is best done after simple cystometry because: (1) exact bladder volume is known and (2) if uninhibited detrusor contractions were found, then positive stress test is not as reliable (since coughing may provoke detrusor contractions leading to delayed loss of urine after cough).

○ The patient is asked to strain and hold, then cough vigorously in lithotomy or erect position (preferred) while the bladder is subjectively full (>250 mL otherwise test is unreliable; stress test is more convenient at maximum bladder capacity).

○ This test is improved if the patient lacks urgency and if intravesical pressure is measured during stress test to rule out delayed, provoked bladder contractions as cause of leakage.

○ Immediate (or simultaneous with cough or valsalva) loss of urine indicates a positive stress test.

○ This test cannot be considered negative unless performed in erect (or standing position), POP reduced, cough, and with a full bladder. A negative test objectively rules out stress incontinence.

○ For convenience, some practitioners will do stress test in the following sequence until urine leakage is observed: dorsal lithotomy + valsalva →→ if negative →→ dorsal lithotomy + cough →→ if negative→→ standing + valsalva →→ if negative →→ standing + cough.

• Bonney test (aka Marshall test; Read test, and Marchetti test are similar): either examiner's fingers or instrument placed on either side of the urethra (stay away from medial to prevent occlusion of urethra!) and bladder neck is elevated to a retropubic position. Then, while patient is standing or erect, she is asked to strain then cough. If this test eliminates SUI, it is considered positive. This test has high false-positive rate (no urine left in the bladder or urethra accidentally occluded).

• Radiologic assessment (ultrasound either vaginal, or perineal, or cystourethrograph) may also be utilized to accurately demonstrate urethral mobility, bladder neck descent, funneling, and pathology (e.g., urethral diverticulum, obstruction, fistula, reflux) (see Chap. 12, Radiologic Imaging of Pelvic Floor and Lower Urinary Tract).

• Videocystourethrography allows assessment of anatomy, as described earlier, plus functional changes simultaneously (see Chap. 12, Radiologic Imaging of Pelvic Floor and Lower Urinary Tract).

• Urethrocystoscopy allows direct visualization of the UVJ and lack of coaptation as the cystoscope is withdrawn may be appreciated (see Chap. 11, Urethrocystoscopy).

BASIC OFFICE TESTING

• Clean catch, midstream urine or catheterized urine specimen for urinalysis (UA), culture, and sensitivity.

• Some practitioners will first perform an office dipstick urinalysis. If it is indicative of UTI or hematuria then a UA and culture and sensitivity (UC&S) are sent. The dipstick has extremely high specificity (97%) and negative predictive values (99%).

○ UTI screening is important because many elderly patients may be bacteriuric and not have any symptoms.

○ Additionally, symptoms of UTI (especially if recent in onset) can masquerade or mimic OAB symptoms or (UUI). *Escherichia coli* and other gram negative bladder pathogens secrete toxins that cause transient detrusor overactivity. If patient has UTI, it must be treated and patient re-evaluated in several weeks.

○ Hematuria in the absence of infection warrants cytology and cystoscopy for evaluation of bladder carcinoma. Further workup with ultrasound and intravenous pyelogram (IVP) may also be necessary (see Chap. 12, Radiologic Imaging of Pelvic Floor and Lower Urinary Tract).

○ Recurrent UTIs may need evaluation with cystoscopy, renal ultrasound, or IVP (rule out stone, cancer, congenital anomaly, and the like).

• Renal function.

○ Blood urea nitrogen (BUN), creatinine, glucose, calcium may be ordered if suspect chronic obstructive uropathy or polyuria in absence of medication-related causes.

• Measure postvoid residual (PVR) urine volume by ultrasound or catheterization (see Chap. 8, Urodynamics II: Tests that Evaluate Bladder Emptying).

PERINEAL PAD TESTING

• One hour International Continence Society (ICS) protocol: an absorbent, preweighed pad is worn by

patient for a 1-h period (also 24 h test is possible), patient drinks 500 mL of fluid over 15 min, and engages in the following for 30 min: walking, climbing stairs, sitting, then standing 10 times, coughing 10 times, running in place for 1 min, bending 5 times, hand-washing for 1 min. After the test, the pad may be sealed in plastic bag and sent to be weighed once more.
- Test result may be overestimated because of miscalculation, sweat, and vaginal discharge.
- Test-retest reliability is okay.
- But sensitivity is poor between pad weight gain and incontinence severity.
- It does not identify cause of incontinence (urge vs. stress; urethral vs. other).
- Oral phenazopyridine (Pyridium) may help, as it turns urine red-orange. However, it may turn other body fluids into this color and has high false-positive rate. Healthy continent women may test positive 50% of time.
- Pad test is a research tool.

SIMPLE CYSTOMETRY

(See Chap. 7)
- Authorities in the field believe that simple filling cystometry or "eye-ball" urodynamics should be performed during basic evaluation of incontinence.
- Typical order of events is as follows: (1) patient comes in with full bladder, (2) stress test is performed (3) voids into texas hat in private, (4) PVR is obtained by catheterization and urine tested, (5) *simple cystometry* is performed.
- Some physicians may not perform simple cystometry if they plan on managing incontinence medically or by behavioral modification.
- Certain physicians may not perform complex urodynamics on uncomplicated patients even if they plan to perform surgery. Why? (1) Urodynamic testing may not be cost-effective if the probability of SUI is high (>80%). (2) Even complex urodynamic testing may detect only 60% of uninhibited detrusor contractions.
  - Example: the patient voids only six times per day, lacks symptoms of OAB, has mild asymptomatic pelvic prolapse, has normal PVR, and a positive stress test. In this case simple cystometry may not be done by certain practitioners.
- However, many experts at academic centers will perform complex urodynamics on patients whom they plan to take to the operating room.
- The indications for complex urodynamic testing (electronic) are the following:

- Mixed incontinence symptoms
- History of urge incontinence but normal simple cystometry
- Urge incontinence refractory to therapy
- Failed previous surgery for incontinence (i.e., recurrent incontinence)
- History of pelvic radiation
- History of radical pelvic surgery
- Neurologic disorders
- Frequency, urgency, and pain syndromes refractory to therapy
- Nocturnal enuresis refractory to therapy
- Continuous incontinence (rule out fistula)
- Severe incontinence
- Voiding dysfunction
- Elevated PVR
- Decreased bladder capacity
- POP beyond hymen
- Positive EBST (EBST+ is suggestive of intrinsic sphincter deficiency [ISD])
- Fixed urethra (not hypermobile)

DIAGNOSIS

- After completion of the evaluation, a presumptive diagnosis should be made.
- As stated earlier, it is important to understand the patient's desire for treatment and present her with the available treatment options.
- Approximately 60% of patients with mild to moderate SUI will respond to conservative therapy, therefore this should be tried first (see Chap. 13, Conservative Management of Incontinence and Pelvic Organ Prolapse).
  - Behavior modification (drinking and diet modification, bladder retraining drills, change exercise routines)
  - Biofeedback assisted therapy (sensors or probes send information regarding pubococcygeus muscle activity and relay this to patient in the form of audio or video)
  - Occlusive/mechanical devices (trial of pessary [Cook continence ring, incontinence ring, Introl], urethral plug for 1–2 weeks)
  - Medications (advise that different drug types and doses are available and that it may take 4-6 weeks to see results)
  - Pelvic floor muscle exercising (Kegel alone, vaginal cones, perineometer) ± physical therapist
  - Neuromodulation (e.g., electrical stimulation with vaginal/rectal probes)
  - Treatment of reversible causes: (UTI→ antibiotics (abx); atrophy→ local estrogen every other night for

2–3 weeks, then 1–2 times per week; stool impaction→ deimpact, enemas; medication side-effects→ discontinue, reduce dose, or switch and watch for drug interactions; hypercalcemia→ determine cause and treat with diuretics or bisphosphonates; hyperglycemia→ determine cause, oral hypoglycemic agent, insulin; excess fluid intake→ modify intake, decrease caffeine and acidic food intake, delirium→ determine cause and treat; injury→ treat injury; immobility→ modify living environment, commode, catheterize)
- Complex urodynamic evaluation may be necessary as mentioned previously.

INDICATIONS FOR REFERRAL TO A SPECIALIST

- All physicians should screen patients for incontinence and PFD because majority (>60%) of patients do not address these issues with their doctors or delay seeking treatment for an average of 5 years. Why?
  ◦ Embarrassment
  ◦ Discomfort
  ◦ Feeling of isolation
  ◦ False belief that symptoms are part of the normal aging process
- Usually, the patient with incontinence first sees a gynecologist, family practitioner, internist, or urologist.
- The majority of the referrals come from primary care physicians, internists, and family practice physicians.
- The gynecologist is in an excellent position to workup and manage patients with PFD and incontinence since many women see their gynecologist for primary care as well as gynecologic care.
- Additionally, since anti-incontinence operations are frequently done in conjunction with other gynecologic procedures, having one doctor and one anesthetic trial may lead to better patient care.
- Barriers to gynecologist doing evaluation for incontinence include
  ◦ Discomfort with subject material
  ◦ Lack of training in female pelvic medicine and reconstructive surgery (FPMRS) during residency
  ◦ Time constraints (evaluation may take extra 20–30 min of office time)
- If a gynecologist is interested in managing incontinence patients, he/she may ask the patient to complete a questionnaire (UDI, IIQ, PFDI, PFIQ, PISQ), keep a voiding diary, and schedule her for a return visit to address this issue.
- If a gynecologist does not want to manage PFD or if cases are complicated, he/she should make a referral to a specialist.

- A specialist is a gynecologist or urologist who is adequately trained or experienced in the field of FPMRS (usually a urogynecologist, female pelvic medicine and reconstructive surgeon (FPMRS) or female urologist). Indications for referral to a specialist are as follows:
  ◦ Failed conservative or medical therapy
  ◦ Patient unsatisfied with current therapy and desires further evaluation
  ◦ When considering surgical treatment (esp. if previous surgery failed)
  ◦ Previous failed anti-incontinence surgery
  ◦ Recurrent or refractory UTI
  ◦ Urinary retention or abnormal PVR
  ◦ Previous radical pelvic surgery or pelvic radiation therapy
  ◦ Legal purposes (to document nerve damage after surgery or work-related injuries)
  ◦ Symptomatic POP beyond the hymen
  ◦ Neurologic disease such as MS or stroke concurrent
  ◦ Hematuria without the presence of infection
  ◦ Presence of a fistula or urethral diverticulum
  ◦ Complex cases or uncertain diagnosis

BIBLIOGRAPHY

Abrams P, Blaivas JG, Stanton SL, et al. The standardization of terminology of lower urinary tract function. *Scand J Urol Nephrol.* 1988;114(Suppl): 5–19.

Abrams P, Cardozo L, Fall M, et al. The standardization of terminology of lower urinary tract function: Report from the Standardization Sub-committee of the International Continence Society. *Neurourol Urodyn.* 2002;21:167–168.

Bent AE, Richardson DA, Ostergard DR. Diagnosis of lower urinary tract disorders in postmenopausal patients. *Am J Obstet Gynecol.* 1983;145:218–222.

Bergman A, Bhatia NN. Urodynamics: effect of urinary tract infection on urethral and bladder function. *Obstet Gynecol.* 1985;66:366–371.

Bergman A, Koonings PP, Ballard CA. Negative Q-tip test as a risk factor for failed anti-incontinence surgery. *J Reprod Med.* 1989;34(3):156–160.

Crystle CD, Charme LS, Copelane WE. Q-tip test in stress urinary incontinence. *Obstet Gynecol.* 1971;38:313–315.

DeLancey JOL. Structural support of the urethra as it relates to urinary incontinence: the hammock hypothesis. *Am J Obstet Gynecol.* 1994;170:1713–1723.

Fantl JA, Bump RC, McClish DK. Mixed urinary incontinence. *Urology.* 1990;38:273–281.

Fantl JA, Wyman JF, McClish DK, et al. Efficacy of bladder training in older women with urinary incontinence. *JAMA.* 1991;265(S):609–613.

Fantl JA, Hurt WG, Bump RC. Urethral axis and sphincteric function. *Am J Obstet Gynecol.* 1986;155:554–558.

Fine PM, Antonini TG, Appell RA. Clinical evaluation of women with lower urinary tract dysfunction. In: Weber A, ed. *Clinical Obstetrics and Gynecology, Incontinence.* Philadelphia, PA: Lippincott Williams & Wilkins; 2004:44–52.

Handa VL, Jensen JK, Ostergard DR. Federal guidelines for the management of urinary incontinence in the United States: which patients should undergo urodynamic testing. *Int Urogynecol J Pelvic Floor Dysfunct.* 1995;6:198–203.

Harvey MA, Versi E. Predictive value of clinical evaluation of stress urinary incontinence: a summary of the published literature. *Int Urogynecol J Pelvic Floor Dysfunct.* 2001;12:31–37.

Jensen JK, Nielsen FR, Ostergard DR. The role of patient history in the diagnosis of urinary incontinence. *Obstet Gynecol.* 1994;38:904–910.

Karram MM, Bhatia NN. The Q-tip test: standardization of the technique and its interpretation in women with urinary incontinence. *Obstet Gynecol.* 1988;71:807–811.

Karram MM, Culligan P, Fleischman SJ. The role of the Ob/Gyn in evaluating and managing urinary incontinence. *OBG Management.* April 2002;(Suppl):1–11.

McClennan MT, Bent AE. Supine empty stress test as a predictor of low Valsalva leak point pressure. *Neurourol Urodyn.* 1998;17:121–127.

Mcguire EJ, Fitszpatrick CC, Wan J, et al. Clinical assessment of urethral sphincter function. *J Urol.* 1993;150:1452–1454.

Nager CW, Albo ME. Testing in women with lower urinary tract dysfunction. In: Weber A, ed. *Clinical Obstetrics and Gynecology, Incontinence.* Philadelphia, PA: Lippincott Williams & Wilkins; 2004;53–55.

Nergardh A, Boreus LO, Holme T. The inhibitory effect of coli-endotoxin on alpha-adrenergic receptors functions in the lower urinary tract: an in vitro study in cats. *Scand J Urol Nephrol.* 1977;11:219–224.

Ouslander J, Leach G, Abelson S, et al. Simple versus multichannel cystometry in the evaluation of bladder function in an incontinence geriatric population. *J Urol.* 1988;140:1482–1486.

Resnick NM, Yalla SV, Laurino E. The pathophysiology of urinary incontinence among institutionalized elderly persons. *N Engl J Med.* 1989;320:1–7.

Resnick NM. Geriatric incontinence. *Urol Clin North Am.* 1996;23:55–74.

Sand PK, Brubaker LT, Novak T. Simple standing incremental cystometry as a screening method for detrusor instability. *Obstet Gynecol.* 1991;77:453–457.

Sand PK, Ostergard DR. *Urodynamics and the Evaluation of Female Incontinence, a Practical guide.* London: Springer; 1995.

Swift SE, Yoon EA. The test retest reliability of the cough stress test in women with urinary incontinence. *Obstet Gynecol.* 1999;94:99–102.

Weinberger MW. Differential diagnosis of urinary incontinence. In: Bent AE, Ostergard DR, Cundiff GW, et al., eds. *Ostergard's Urogynecology and Pelvic Floor Dysfunction*, 5th ed. Lippincott Williams & Wilkins; 2003:61–68.

Wyman JK, Elswick RK, Wilson MS, et al. Relationship of fluid intake to voluntary micturitions and urinary incontinence in women. *Neurourol Urodyn.* 1991;10: 463–473.

Yarnell JWG, Voyl GJ, Richards CJ, et al. The prevalence and severity of urinary incontinence in women. *J Epidemiol Community Health.* 1981;35:71–74.

QUESTIONS

1. Match the following terms with their correct definitions:
   - SUI ___
   - UUI ___
   - Bypass UI ___
   - Functional UI ___
   (A) Involuntary leakage of urine accompanied by or immediately preceded by a strong urge to void
   (B) Continuous leakage of urine due to an abnormality which disrupts the integrity of the urinary tract
   (C) Urine loss due to the inability to reach the bathroom in time, the inability to remove clothing, or the inability to access a bathroom
   (D) Immediate, small-in amount, self-limited, involuntary leakage of urine with effort

2. A 38-year-old female, gravida 3, para 2, presents to your office with complaints of leaking urine after a motor vehicle accident in which she sustained neurologic damage. On physical examination, she has lost sensation to the posterior, medial aspect of her legs and her perineum, however retains sensation to the anus. Damage to which of the following nerves is likely the cause of her loss of sensation?
   (A) L4-S1
   (B) S1-S3
   (C) S2-S4
   (D) S3-S4

3. A 28-year-old female is referred to your office by her primary gynecologist for complaints of postvoid dribbling. On further questioning, she states it has gotten worse over the past 6 months and she also has dyspareunia and dysuria. On review of her records, you notice that she has been treated for UTI five times in the past year. On physical examination, you notice a palpable anterior vaginal wall mass and expression of purulent material from the urethra upon palpation of the mass. The most likely diagnosis is:
   (A) Vesicovaginal fistula
   (B) Urethral diverticulum
   (C) Foreign body
   (D) Infectious urethritis

4. A 63-year-old woman, gravida 4, para 4, presents with complaints of leakage or urine when she coughs and sneezes as well as multiple episodes of nocturnal enuresis. On physical examination she has a small cystocele and vaginal epithelium is within normal limits for her age. Her neurologic examination is within normal limits. Her urine dipstick is normal. She has a small amount of loss of

urine when coughing with a full bladder in the supine position and her Q-tip test straining angle is 40 degrees. Her PVR volume is 20 mL. Thus far, her diagnosis is most consistent with:

(A) Overflow incontinence

(B) Mixed incontinence

(C) Genuine stress urinary incontinence (GSI)

(D) Detrusor instability

(E) Bypass UI

5. A 58-year-old female complains of continuous leakage of urine. She has a medical history significant for breast cancer status post mastectomy and local radiation. She had a vaginal hysterectomy at age 49. Physical examination reveals atrophic vaginal epithelium and a grade 2 cystocele and rectocele. She has been treated for three UTIs in the past 2 years. Her PVR volume is 15 mL. Which of the following in her history and physical examination is an indication for complex urodynamic testing?

(A) Continuous leakage of urine

(B) History of radiation therapy

(C) History of vaginal hysterectomy

(D) Presence of cystocele and rectocele

(E) History of UTI

(F) Her PVR urine volume

6. The single *most* important evaluation for the diagnosis of SUI is ___.

(A) Q-tip test

(B) Stress test

(C) Bonney test

(D) Cystoscopy

(F) Cystometry

ANSWERS

1. Definitions
   - SUI → D
   - UUI → A
   - Bypass UI → B
   - Functional UI → C

2. *(C)*. As seen in the dermatome map (Fig. 6-1) in the following section, dermatomes S2-S4 cover the posterior, medial aspects of the lower limbs as well as the perineum, the area noted in this patient.

   L4-S1 (A) would contain the posterior and lateral aspects of the lower limbs and would not cover the perineum. S1-S3 (B) is very close to our patient's affected area; however, the S1 dermatome covers the posterior begins to cover the lateral aspect of the legs.

S3-S4 (D) would cover the perineum; however, would not include this patient's loss of sensation on her legs.

A focused neurologic examination should be done on all patients evaluated for incontinence; however, a more broad examination may be indicated in those women with known neurologic injuries. Sensation to touch may be tested using a Q-tip. The bulbocavernosus reflex tests S2-S3 nerve roots. This is done by tapping the clitoris or stroking the labia majus which causes contraction of the bulbocavernosus and ischiocavernosus muscles. The anal reflex (anal wink) test S2-S5 nerve roots, and is elicited by stroking the skin next to the anus which causes contraction of the external anal sphincter. It is of note that these reflexes are rarely tested in clinical practice, though, if they are both intact, it indicates that both sensory and motor reflex arcs of S2-S3 is intact.

3. *(B)*. All of this patient's findings point to the presence of a urethral diverticulum.

   The origin of acquired urethral diverticula has been attributed to obstruction and subsequent rupture of the periurethral glands into the urethral lumen with epithelialization over the opening resulting in a diverticulum. Infection and recurrent obstruction of the neck of the bladder cavity causes various symptoms as well as enlargement of the diverticulum. The periurethral glands exist over the entire length of the urethra, Skene's glands are the largest, and most distal of these glands. Urethral diverticula occur mostly in the area of these glands, thus are found most commonly in the distal end of the urethra.

   Patients may complain of the following symptoms: recurrent UTI, pelvic pain, incontinence, postvoid dribbling, dyspareunia, dysuria, urinary frequency and urgency, nocturia, a feeling of incomplete bladder emptying or a multitude of other nonspecific lower urinary tract symptoms. An anterior vaginal wall mass may be noted on physical examination, which, upon palpation, may be quite tender and express purulent discharge through the urethra. Adjunctive radiographic studies such as voiding cystourethrography, ultrasound, and MRI may be used to confirm the diagnosis and evaluate the size of the diverticulum in relation to the urethral lumen.

   A vesicovaginal fistula (A) is a subtype of female urogenital fistula. It is an abnormal fistulous tract (connection) extending between the bladder and the vagina that allows the continuous involuntary discharge of urine into the vaginal vault.

   Vesicovaginal fistulas (VVF) in developing countries, are due to prolonged obstructed labor. In the U.S. the majority of VVF develop after inadvertent injury after surgery. The uncontrolled leakage of urine into the

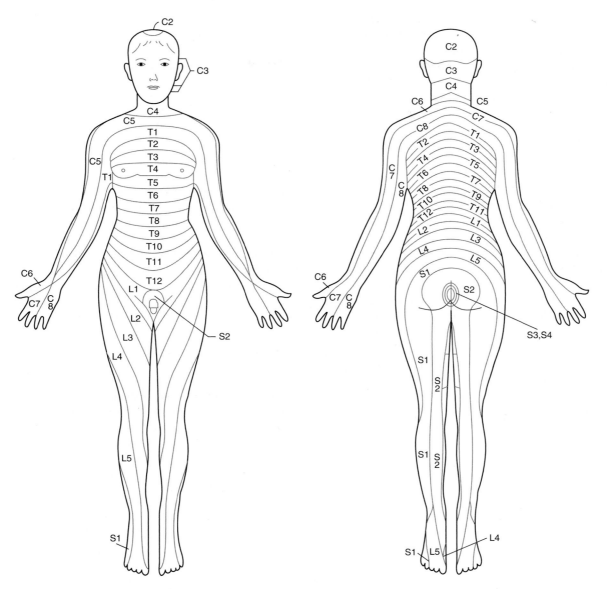

FIG. 6.1 Dermatome Map of Human Body

vagina is the hallmark symptom of patients with this disorder.

Patients may complain of UI or an increase in vaginal discharge following pelvic surgery or pelvic radiotherapy with or without antecedent surgery. The drainage may be continuous; however, in the presence of a very small fistula, it may be intermittent. Increased postoperative abdominal, pelvic, or flank pain; prolonged ileus, and fever should alert the physician to possible urinoma or urine ascites and mandates evaluation. Recurrent cystitis or pyelonephritis, abnormal urinary stream, and hematuria should also initiate a workup.

A vesicovaginal fistula can be diagnosed by injecting sterile milk or methylene blue dye through a catheter into the bladder and observe whether the dye progresses through the bladder and into the vagina. Radiologic studies including intravenous urogram as well as cystoscopy can be quite helpful in the evaluation, diagnosis, and location of the fistula.

A urethral foreign body (C) is very rare, and would typically cause more obstructive symptoms in this patient if it were present. Vaginal foreign bodies are more common but would cause vaginal discharge and rarely have associated urinary symptoms.

Infectious urethritis (D) is divided into two classifications: gonococcal and nongonococcal. Patients classically complain of dysuria and may have concurrent vaginal discharge, though up to 60% cases may be asymptomatic. Sample of the discharge should be taken for evaluation of gonococcus and appropriate treatment can be administered upon diagnosis.

4. *(B)*. The clinical picture in this patient is most consistent with mixed incontinence. The patient has leaking with coughing and sneezing which are classic symptoms of GSI. Nocturnal enuresis (and nocturia, not mentioned in this patient's history) is usually associated with detrusor overactivity/instability. On examination, this patient has no neurologic abnormalities noted. Leakage of urine with cough in the supine position was demonstrated on examination and again is consistent with GSI. The patient also has HMU because her Q-tip test straining angle was 40 degrees, and normal is less than 30 degrees. Her PVR volume is within normal limits. No single type incontinence could be responsible for all of her symptoms and thus she is correctly diagnosed with mixed incontinence.

5. The indication for urodynamic testing are as follows:
   - Mixed incontinence
   - History of urge incontinence but normal simple cystometry
   - Urge incontinence refractory to therapy
   - Failed previous surgery for incontinence (i.e., recurrent incontinence)
   - History of pelvic radiation
   - History of radical pelvic surgery
   - Neurologic disorders
   - Frequency, urgency, and pain syndromes refractory to therapy
   - Nocturnal enuresis refractory to therapy
   - Continuous incontinence (rule out fistula)

- Severe incontinence
- Voiding dysfunction
- Elevated PVR
- Decreased bladder capacity
- POP beyond hymen
- Positive EBST (EBST+ is suggestive of ISD)
- Fixed urethra (not hypermobile)

(A) Radiation therapy to the pelvis is an indication; however, our patient only had local radiation to the breast for her breast cancer. Her history of vaginal hysterectomy is not an indication for testing, only radial pelvic surgery necessitates urodynamic testing. Her cystocele and rectocele are minor and their presence is not an indication for testing. Recurrent UTIs are an indication, but three UTIs in 2 years would not be considered recurrent. Lastly, she has a normal PVR volume.

6. *(B)*. The Q-tip test can be positive (>30 degree deflection from horizontal) in patients with and without stress incontinence. It does not have adequate sensitivity or specificity and is no longer recommended as part of the basic evaluation. Similarly, the Bonney test is no longer utilized because of the high false-positive rate. In academic centers, cystoscopy is done only after diagnosis of incontinence is made and surgery is planned or if there is an indication for it (see Chap. 11, Urethrocystoscopy). Cystometry is essential to the diagnosis of SUI. Two pieces of information are valuable once a patient is suspected of having stress incontinence: (1) confirmation that detrusor contractions are not responsible for the incontinence (i.e., mixed or urge) and (2) to know at what bladder volume (minimum = 150 mL and maximum = maximum cystometric capacity) the patient demonstrates stress incontinence. A patient who demonstrates a positive stress test in supine position and on a nearly empty bladder has severe SUI (i.e., positive EBST).

7   URODYNAMICS PART I: EVALUATION OF BLADDER FILLING AND STORAGE

Sam Siddighi

- *Urodynamics* studies that quantify bladder and urethral function over time while *reproducing the patient's symptoms*. They may consist of any or all of the following: cystometry, uroflowmetry, pressure-flow studies, urethral pressure profilometry, videourodynamics, ambulatory urodynamics, and electromyography.
- The following two facts are very important because urodynamics is not an exact science:
  - Patient has symptoms but urodynamics are normal → does not mean she does not have pathology.
  - Urodynamics are abnormal but patient has no symptoms → does not mean she has pathology.

CYSTOMETRY

Cystometry is also known as urethrocystometry, cystometrogram, CMG.
- A urodynamic test that measures pressure-volume relationships of the bladder, assesses bladder activity, evaluates bladder sensation, capacity, detrusor contraction and stability, and derives bladder compliance.
- *Simple (single-channel) cystometry* (aka "eye ball" urodynamics, simple office bladder filling) 60–84% sensitivity. The positive predective value (PPV) for urodynamic stress urinary incontinence (USUI) on complex cystometry is 82%. It is an inexpensive, simple office bladder filling using a small catheter with an empty 60 cc syringe filled with water elevated 15 cm above the level of the pubic symphysis. It is better if the patient is standing. As the bladder is filled in a retrograde fashion, barring valsalva or cough, rises in the meniscus signify detrusor contractions. You may also use a 3-way Foley catheter and CVP manometer to perform simple cystometry. The disadvantages of simple cystometry are twofold: (1) the intra-abdominal pressure cannot be measured and (2) any bladder contractions that increase pressure less than 15 cm H_2O cannot be detected. Occasionally these small bladder contractions may cause symptoms of overactive bladder (OAB).
- Symptoms of stress incontinence predominate + simple cystometry + cough stress test + normal postvoid residuals (PVR) = 88–97% sensitive for detection of urodynamic stress incontinence (i.e., diagnosed by complex cystometry).
- However, symptoms of stress incontinence *alone* are not reliable, because (1) two-thirds of people with OAB complain of symptoms of stress incontinence, (2) ≈20% of those with urodynamic stress incontinence have symptoms of urge incontinence, and (3) out of 100 women with symptoms of stress incontinence, only 65 had urodynamic confirmation of SUI.
- Nevertheless, simple cystometry may be as good as complex cystometry in a population with a high prevalence of detrusor abnormalities (e.g., elderly).
- *Complex cystometry* (aka multichannel, subtracted, or electronic cystometry) is the gold standard for diagnosing detrusor overactivity, urinary urgency incontinence (UUI), mixed urinary incontinence, and urodynamic stress incontinence. It utilizes a combination of several electronic pressure catheters (abdominal, bladder, urethral) with/without flow studies, fluoroscopy, and electromyography to evaluate lower urinary tract function.
  - Urodynamic stress incontinence—any leakage during provocative maneuvers in the absence of bladder contractions or true bladder pressure rises
  - Detrusor overactivity—involuntary urinary leakage associated with a strong urge to urinate and cystometry demonstrates a rise in true detrusor pressure, spontaneously, or with provocation
- Patients with three or more symptoms of bladder overactivity (see Chap. 6, Evaluation of Urinary Incontinence in the Office and Indications for Referral to a Specialist) have >80% chance of having detrusor overactivity by urodynamic testing.

TABLE 7-1 Pros and Cons of Urodynamic Testing

ARGUMENTS FOR URODYNAMIC TESTING	ARGUMENTS AGAINST URODYNAMIC TESTING
Accurate diagnosis is important for preoperative counseling, quoting percent failure and setting realistic expectations	Does not correlate with outcomes after surgery, therefore one cannot rely on any values
May help in selecting type of surgery	Unlikely to change surgeon's management plan
Reimbursement rates have risen for testing	If done routinely, may not be cost-effective
Urodynamic machines can be affordable ($8000–$100,000) and testing takes only 30 min to perform	Requires training and time to utilize and interpret
May enhance patient satisfaction	Puts patients in uncomfortable, unnatural environment which may not represent her daily life
Most specialists and experts will test prior to surgery	Young, healthy, multiparous with hypermobile urethra type of SUI do not need testing

- Accurate diagnosis is important not only to take appropriate management steps, but also to set realistic expectations for the patient. Someone with *mixed incontinence or detrusor overactivity has a ≥30% higher failure rate after continence surgery.*
- The disadvantages of complex cystometry are threefold: (1) there is no standardization of cystometric methodology and instrumentation from medical center to medical center, (2) it only measures bladder activity during a short period of time and under artificial conditions, (3) complex cystometry does not correlate with outcomes after incontinence surgery, therefore it may not be clinically significant. Doing complex cystometry on every patient prior to surgery does not improve outcome and therefore may not be cost-effective. (Table 7-1)

CYSTOMETRIC PARAMETERS

BLADDER FILLING

- In a normal bladder, there is hardly any rise in bladder pressure throughout most of the filling cycle. A steady rise in pressure indicates low bladder compliance (e.g., interstitial cystitis).
- Normal resting bladder pressure is 8–12 cm H_2O in supine position (standing position = *add* 5–10 cm H_2O).
- During phase I of bladder filling, there is only a small rise (2–8 cm H_2O, average rise = 6 cm H_2O). Phase II is marked by almost no rise in pressure during further bladder filling, because of the bladder's intrinsic elastic properties or compliance. During phase III, there is a rapid rise in pressure due to the limits of bladder capacity.
- Any significant rise in pressure from baseline to capacity, usually ≥5 cm H_2O but surely a rise >15 cm H_2O signifies poor bladder compliance (see later in this section).
- According to the new International Continence Society (ICS) guidelines, pressure increases in the bladder do not have to exceed 15 cm H_2O to be considered an involuntary detrusor contraction. Pressure rise of <15 cm H_2O which reproduces the patient's symptoms are pertinent because 10% are associated with UUI and 85% are associated with urgency.
- Patients with *OAB* will have detrusor contractions during normal filling volumes with or without leakage. The term *detrusor hyperreflexia* refers to detrusor overactivity due to a neurologic condition, whereas *detrusor instability* refers to an idiopathic cause of bladder overactivity. These terms are no longer used.
- In a normal, healthy woman, voiding should be under voluntary control even in phase III. Normal women are aware of the urge to void before a bladder contraction occurs and are able to suppress detrusor contractions.
- In a patient with severe neurological disorder, chronic uninhibited detrusor contractions >40 cm H_2O place the patient at risk for vesicoureteral reflux and possible renal damage in the long run.

BLADDER AND ABDOMINAL PRESSURES

- Since both intra-abdominal and/or bladder contractions can increase the pressure inside the bladder, we need to calculate the true bladder pressure or *detrusor pressure or P_{det}* = Intravesical pressure or P_{ves} (pressure inside the bladder whether created by bladder wall or extrinsic pressures) minus intra-abdominal pressure or P_{abd} (estimated from vaginal, rectal, or rarely extraperitoneal pressure recording). Formula: $P_{det} = P_{ves} - P_{abd}$.
- P_{det} at rest is 0 cm H_2O in both supine and standing positions.
- Increases in intra-abdominal pressure are seen as positive deflections in the P_{abd} (vaginal or rectal pressure transducer), P_{ves} (bladder pressure transducer), and P_{ure} (urethral pressure transducer), but not in P_{det}.
- Vaginal catheters ($P_{vag} = P_{abd}$) are preferred for measurement of intra-abdominal pressure because they are

more comfortable, easier to maintain, cleaner, and usually lack artifacts caused by rectal peristalsis and insertion of pressure catheter into stool. However, vaginal peristaltic activity can also be a source of confusion and should be distinguished from valsalva activity. During vaginal peristalsis, one does not see pressure changes in P_{ves} and simultaneous mirror image dips in P_{det} will occur.

- Rectal catheters ($P_{rect} = P_{abd}$) may be more accurate in a patient with severe pelvic relaxation.
- Artifacts:
  ○ Movement of intra-abdominal catheter.
  ○ The intra-abdominal pressure may decrease gradually throughout cystometry as the patient becomes less anxious. This may cause an artifactal increase in detrusor pressure over time.
  ○ Intra-abdominal pressure will also decrease with inspiration.
  ○ Contractions of the rectum or vagina.
- In conclusion, one must be careful when evaluating a rise in P_{det} because the increase in pressure may not be a reflection of detrusor pressure but rather a drop in intra-abdominal pressure.

BLADDER VOLUMES AND SENSATION

- *Bladder sensation* is a subjective measurement and is obtained by noting the *volume* inside the bladder during filling, when the patient is asked:
  1. *First sensation* (usually 0–100 mL)
  2. Normal desire to void (usually 200–400 mL)
  3. Strong desire to void or *fullness*
  4. Maximum cystometric capacity (400–600 mL)
  5. Urgency (bladder volume that evokes fear of leakage and/or pain). Pain during bladder filling or voiding is never normal. On the other hand, absence of filling sensation is also abnormal.
- Hypersensation or low compliance bladder—the bladder sensation volumes, capacity, and compliance are all decreased in conditions which result in fibrosis and decreased bladder elasticity: interstitial cystitis, post-radiation cystitis, tumor, cystitis, and neurogenic conditions.
- OAB and emotion-provoking situations can also result in a low compliance bladder. OAB will be discussed in detail in another chapter.
- Hyposensation, detrusor areflexia, and acontractile bladder—acontractile bladder should be distinguished from detrusor areflexia. The latter term is reserved for cases due to a neurologic condition. Bladder sensation volumes, capacity, and compliance are all increased in acontractile bladder. The detrusor muscle may fail to contract when these patients want to void. Therefore, they are at risk for recurrent cystitis.

- Hyposensation is not always pathologic and is sometimes taught or learned (avoiding urination in "unclean" places, busy professionals lacking time at work to void regularly) or it may be due to replacement of bladder smooth muscle by collagen because of aging. In one study, one-third of women with bladder capacities >800 mL by bladder diaries were urodynamically normal.
- Acontractile bladder and overflow incontinence can be associated with certain conditions such as causes of bladder outlet or urethral obstruction, immediate postpartum and postoperative states, neuropathies (e.g., diabetes mellitus [DM], hypothyroid), neurologic conditions (e.g., multiple sclerosis [MS], pernicious anemia, tabes dorsalis, herpes genitalis), and radical pelvic surgery.
- To determine whether the cause of hyposensation is due to neurologic injury, one can employ the bethanechol supersensitivity test. A denervated bladder will have an exaggerated response to 2.5–5.0 mg of subcutaneous bethanechol and should respond in ≈15 minutes by increasing P_{det} by >15 cm H_2O. Note: bethanechol is contraindicated in asthma, peptic ulcer, gastrointestinal (GI) obstruction, bradycardia, hypotension, and Parkinson's. Atropine is the antidote for bethanechol toxicity.
- Additionally, in patients with spinal cord injuries, instillation of 50–100 mL of ice water can cause bladder contractions mediated through the sacral reflex arc.

BLADDER CAPACITY

- There are three types of *bladder capacity*:
  ○ *Functional bladder capacity* is the physiologic capacity obtained from voiding diary or by asking patient to drink large amount of fluid and hold it until she feels the most sensation to void. Then, it is obtained by addition: amount voided + PVR.
  ○ *Maximum cystometric capacity* is the greatest volume obtained during cystometry. It is the volume voided when the patient has a *strong urge to void*, in other words, when the patient can no longer delay voiding, yet there is no pain. This volume is usually between 400–550 mL.
  ○ *Anesthetic bladder capacity* is the greatest volume obtained from bladder during general or regional anesthesia.

COMPLIANCE

- Compliance is a gradual increase in bladder pressure without subsequent decrease (as in a bladder contraction). It is a measure of the instrinsic elastic properties and may be modified by any bladder condition (e.g., interstitial cystitis decreases bladder compliance). It can be derived from the formula, Δ volume/Δ true bladder pressure = $\Delta V/\Delta P_{det.}$ Most neurologically intact women have compliance $\geq$130 mL/cm H_2O.

- A compliance of <20 mL/cm H_2O is abnormal!

METHODS OF CYSTOMETRY

- During cystometry, the patient must be unsedated, off medications, unanesthetized, and completely aware of her surroundings.
- In the descriptions that ensue, the **words given in bold** describe methods used commonly in urogynecologic practices today.
- Filling media: **sterile water, saline, radiographic contrast**, carbon dioxide, and air. CO_2 is not used frequently because: (1) certain voiding test and measurements are unable to be performed since CO_2 is a compressible gas (e.g., stress test, bladder volume), (2) it dissolves in urine forming carbonic acid (causes detrusor overactivity), and (3) it is not physiologic. CO_2 however, has the advantage being clean, easy, and quick to perform. Air is not used because of the possibility of air embolism.
- Media temperature: **body temperature.** *Room temperature* is adequate. Cold media induces more detrusor contractions and may be perceived as first sensation of coolness rather than first sensation of pressure. Warm (38°C), cold, or icy fluid may also be used.
- Patient position: **Sitting in inclined chair or semierect** (urodynamic chair) is usually preferred. Standing is the best position and should be used if patient's symptoms are not reproduced during cystometry in semierect position. Supine position may need to be used in those who cannot tolerate other positions (e.g., elderly, neurologic disorders). Lithotomy position is uncomfortable and may create anxiety during this lengthy examination.
- Bladder filling technique: **Retrograde filling** using **transurethral catheter** by gravity or a pump to instill fluid. Orthograde filling (i.e., water load + diuretics) is more physiologic but takes more time to perform.
- Bladder filling rate: (1) slow = 10 mL/min (used in neurologic disorders), (2) **medium** = 10–100 mL/min, (3) **fast** = >100 mL/min (is the most effective in provoking bladder contractions).
- Catheters used: In simple cystometry, use three-way Foley catheter. In complex cystometry, can use (1) fluid-filled balloon catheters (cheap, easy, and disposable) or (2) **microtransducer catheters** with two channels (advantage: small [3–12 Fr], flexible,

sensitive; disadvantage: expensive and may produce artifacts).

- Zeroing: All channels are set at zero after catheter tip is placed in water and is flushed to remove air bubbles. Therefore, the bladder catheter is **zeroed to atmospheric pressure** before it is inserted. Then it is tested with a cough.
- Provocative maneuvers: walking, heel bouncing, hand washing, **straining**, **coughing**, walking in place, and listening to running water.
- Transducer placement and calibration: Orientation of the microtransducer catheter can alter pressure readings. Therefore, consistent, lateral orientation of urethral microtransducer should be used. Transducer contact with the bladder wall (esp. empty bladder) will cause a false elevation of pressure recording in P_{ves} and P_{det}, but not in P_{ure}. One must also be sure that intra-abdominal pressure is picked up well in the vaginal or rectal pressure transducer; and be aware that pressure transmission between organs can be equal one minute and unequal the next. When unequal pressure transmission is suspected, perform valsalva-inspiration-Valsalva maneuver or a series of coughs and observe simultaneous slow changes or tiny pressure spikes, respectively, in P_{det}.
- **Summary of actual procedure**: full bladder $\rightarrow$ void $\rightarrow$ measure **PVR** $\rightarrow$ pelvic support examination $\rightarrow$ fill bladder with only 150 mL fluid $\rightarrow$ connect, calibrate, and flush catheter $\rightarrow$ abdominal pressure transducer into vagina (supine position) $\rightarrow$ dual microtransducer catheter into bladder then sitting position $\rightarrow$ cough test should show deflection in vesical, abdominal, and urethral pressure graphs, but not in the true bladder (P_{det}) graph $\rightarrow$ as you fill the bladder, ask bladder sensation, perform provocative maneuvers (at 250 mL or maximum cystometric capacity obtain VLPP), observe urethra for urine loss throughout entire procedure $\rightarrow$ may perform voiding studies (including uroflowmetry and pressure-flow studies).

VIDEO AND AMBULATORY CYSTOMETRY

Video and ambulatory cystometry is also known as continuous urodynamic monitoring.

- Video cystometry—using a radio-opaque filling medium to fill the bladder while performing complex cystometry and observing bladder function on a screen. Allows visualization of the movements and funneling of the bladder neck, retrograde movement of urine from urethra into the bladder, and detection of bladder or urethral diverticula. Its disadvantages are cost, radiation use, training, and personnel required to operate the equipment.

- Ambulatory cystometry—small complex cystometric system (with small catheters, 3 Fr) connected to a portable computer that is worn over the patient's shoulder for several hours. The patient can go home with it. This technology may also use a specialized pad with electronic urine-loss detection system. These technologies allow the patient to perform ordinary activities and may reflect the physiologic functioning of the bladder. However, ambulatory cystometry is expensive, time consuming, requires expertise, and is difficult to interpret; it also has questionable validity.
- Ambulatory cystometry has demonstrated the following about the bladder:
  1. Voiding pressures measured during ambulatory cystometry are higher than pressures measured in complex cystometry.
  2. 30% of people who have *normal* bladder cystometry experience detrusor contractions with ambulatory monitoring. Therefore, some degree of bladder contractions is present and may be normal.
  3. Discomfort, conscious and unconscious inhibition of detrusor contractions play a role during office cystometry.
- Ambulatory cystometry may be utilized for a patient with history that is highly suggestive of detrusor overactivity but uninhibited contractions have not been documented on complex cystometry.
- Currently, none of the two aforementioned techniques have absolute indications. They can be performed on patients with complicated neurologic conditions or when conventional methods have not provided adequate information.

The indications for complex urodynamic testing (electronic) are the following:
- Symptoms and physical examination do not correspond (e.g., complaint of urine leakage on minimal exertion but stress test is negative on full bladder)
- Positive empty-bladder supine test (EBST+ is suggestive of intrinsic sphincteric deficiency [ISD])
- Fixed urethra (not hypermobile)
- Continuous or severe incontinence
- Mixed incontinence symptoms
- History of urge incontinence but normal simple cystometry
- Urge incontinence refractory to therapy (although cystoscopy is more important)
- Frequency, urgency, and pain syndromes refractory to therapy
- Nocturnal enuresis refractory to therapy
- History of pelvic radiation
- Failed previous surgery for incontinence (i.e., recurrent incontinence)
- History of radical pelvic surgery
- Neurologic disorders

- Voiding dysfunction
- Elevated PVR
- Decreased bladder capacity
- POP beyond hymen

BIBLIOGRAPHY

Abrams P, Cardozo L, Fall M, et al. The standardization of terminology of lower urinary tract function: report from the Standardization Subcommittee of the International Continence Society. *Neurourol Urodyn.* 2002;21(2):167–178.

Glazener CM, Lapitan MC. Urodynamic investigations for management of urinary incontinence in adults. *Cochrane Database Syst Rev.* 3:CD003195,2002.

Handa VL, Jensen JK, Ostergard DR. Federal guidelines for the management of urinary incontinence in the United States: which patients should undergo urodynamic testing. *Int Urogynecol J Pelvic Floor Dysfunct.* 1995;6:198–203.

Kadar N. The value of bladder filling in the clinical detection of urine loss and selection of patients for urodynamic testing. *Br J Obstet Gynaecol.* 1988;95:698–704.

Karram MM. Urodynamics: cystometry. In: Walters MD, Karram MM, eds. *Urogynecology and Reconstructive Pelvic Surgery.* 2nd ed. St Louis, MO: Mosby; 1999:55–67.

Kim YH, Kattan MW, Boone TB. Correlation of urodynamic results and urethral coaptation with success after transurethral collagen injection. *Urology.* 1997;50:941–948.

Nager CW, Albo ME. Testing in women with lower urinary tract dysfunction. In: Weber A, ed. *Incontinence 2004.* Philadelphia, PA: Lippincott Williams & Wilkins; 2004:55–57.

Ouslander J, Leach G, Abelson S, et al. Simple versus multichannel cystometry in the evaluation of bladder function in an incontinent geriatric population. *J Urol.* 1988;140:1482–1486.

Sand PK, Ostergard DR. *Urodynamics and the evaluation of female incontinence.* London: Springer-Verlag; 1995.

Slack M, Culligan P, et al. Relationship of urethral retro-resistance pressure to urodynamic measurements and incontinence severity. *Neurourol Urodyn.* 2004;23(2):109–114.

Summitt RL, Stovall TG, Bent AE, et al. Urinary incontinence: correlation of history and brief office evaluation with multichannel urodynamic evaluation in genuine stress incontinence. *Obstet Gynecol.* 1993;81:430–433.

Swift SE, Ostergard DR. Evaluation of current urodynamic testing methods in the diagnosis of genuine stress incontinence. *Obstet Gynecol.* 1995;86:85–91.

Theofrastous JP, Swift SE. Urodynamic testing. In: Bent AE, Ostergard DR, Cundiff GW, Sweift SE. *Ostergard's Urogynecology and Pelvic Floor Dysfunction.* 5th ed. Philadelphia, PA: Lippincott Williams & Wilkins; 2003:115–124.

Wall LL, Wiskind AK, Taylor PA. Simple bladder filling with cough stress test compared with subtracted cystometry for the diagnosis of urinary incontinence. *Am J Obstet Gynecol.* 1994;171(6):1472–1479.

Weber AM, Walters MD. Cost-effectiveness of urodynamic testing before surgery for women with pelvic organ prolapse and stress urinary incontinence. *Am J ObstetGynecol.* 2000;183(6):1338–1347.

QUESTIONS

1. The statement which best describes a person at her maximum bladder capacity __.
   - (A) While having a conversation with her friend, Sally suddenly ran off and returned a few minutes later explaining that she had to go to the bathroom because she was afraid she was about to wet her pants.
   - (B) If you were watching your favorite television show, you would wait until the next commercial break to go to the bathroom.
   - (C) A patient is having conversation with you as you fill her bladder in a retrograde fashion. She tells you that the current bladder volume is hurting her.
   - (D) While returning from a long road trip and only miles from home, Jane pulls over at the side of the road to void.

2. You are analyzing result of multichannel cystometry from one of your patients. You notice that as bladder volume increased from 200 to 300 mL, P_{det} increases by 25 mm H_2O. The condition which is most representative of this patient's bladder compliance is ____.
   - (A) Spinal cord injury
   - (B) Long-standing diabetes mellitus
   - (C) Acute cystitis
   - (D) Interstitial cystitis
   - (E) Bladder augmentation

3. In an otherwise healthy patient without any past surgical history and straightforward SUI, you decide to perform surgery without doing urodynamic testing. The argument which would best support your decision is that complex cystometry _____.
   - (A) Has low sensitivity for detection of SUI
   - (B) Has low specificity for detection of SUI
   - (C) Is expensive and inconvenient
   - (D) Has no improved outcome after incontinence surgery in uncomplicated patients
   - (E) Is performed in an artificial setting and therefore is not representative of the patient's natural setting

4. During cystometry in which carbon dioxide gas is used as the filling medium, many detrusor contractions are observed in a woman who has not had any symptoms of bladder overactivity. The best explanation for this is _____.
   - (A) Carbon dioxide gas is compressible and more readily allows observation of normally occurring bladder contractions
   - (B) Carbon dioxide gas forms carbonic acid which irritates the detrusor
   - (C) Carbon dioxide gas forms oxygen radicals which injure the detrusor
   - (D) Carbon dioxide gas can permeate bladder vessels and create decreased compliance
   - (E) Carbon dioxide gas cools as it expands and low temperatures can provoke bladder contraction

5. A 62-year-old gravida 5, para 5, presents to your office complaining of leakage of urine when she coughs, laughs, sneezes, or gets up from a chair. This has been happening for many years and she is embarrassed to tell you that she has to wear adult diapers at all times. She also tells you that occasionally, she has an urge to void when she hears the sound of water emerging from a faucet and goes to the bathroom three to four times every night. Her past medical history is remarkable for long-standing diabetes mellitus for which she takes two different tablets everyday. Her past surgical history is remarkable for a Kelly plication in Mexico 10 years ago. Her pelvic examination is unremarkable other than a low resistance urethra to Q-tip, positive Q-tip angle test, and positive stress test. The next best step in the management of this patient is _____.
   - (A) Simple cystometry
   - (B) Multichannel cystometry
   - (C) Periurethral bulking agent injection
   - (D) Burch retropubic urethropexy
   - (E) Tension free vaginal tape sling

6. Select the word that best fits the following analogy: ECG: 24-hour Holter monitor → complex cystometry: _____
   - (A) Simple cystometry
   - (B) Videocystometry
   - (C) Ambulatory cystometry
   - (D) Detrusor contraction
   - (E) Compliance

ANSWERS

1. *(D)*. A maximum bladder capacity is demonstrated by statement (D) because Jane has to void and cannot delay it until the next convenient time (which would be when she arrived at home). Another example of maximum bladder capacity is demonstrated by a person who is watching her favorite TV show, interrupts her program to void. A normal desire to

void is best demonstrated by statement (B) because the person is able to delay voiding until a more convenient time. Statement (A) describes *urgency*, since Sally ran off because of fear of leakage. Statement (C) also describes *urgency*, because the bladder volume has produced pain.

2. *(D)*. By calculating compliance (change in bladder volume divided by change in bladder pressure), you get 4 mL/cm H_2O. You know from this chapter that most neurologically intact women have a bladder compliance >130 mL/cm H_2O and that <20 cm H_2O is considered abnormal. Therefore, this patient has an extremely noncompliant bladder. Conditions such as postradiation cystitis, interstitial cystitis, and bladder carcinoma may create such low compliance. Acute cystitis can lower compliance but only transiently and not to the extent of the conditions described earlier. The other answer choices are examples of conditions which may increase bladder compliance.

3. *(D)*. Complex cystometry has not improved outcomes after incontinence surgery for patients with uncomplicated SUI.

    (A) and (B) are incorrect because multichannel cystometry along with symptoms has both high sensitivity and specificity and is the gold standard for diagnosing *urodynamic stress incontinence*. Although complex cystometry does add some cost, it is not extreme nor is it inconvenient. One of the criticisms of urodynamic testing is that it is less representative of the patient's natural situation since results are obtained in an unnatural setting (voiding on command, instrumentation, knowledge of being observed, and so forth). This is not, however, the best reason to abstain from performing cystometry prior to surgery.

4. *(B)*. The best explanation for this phenomenon is that CO_2 gas combines with H_2O to form H_2CO_3 and this dissociates into H^+ ions (acids) which are irritating to the bladder. Statement (C) is incorrect. Oxygen radicals are formed from peroxide (H_2O_2) not carbon dioxide. The fact that carbon dioxide is compressible does not explain why there are more contractions observed in this patient. Ice cool filling media can provoke bladder contractions, and this may contribute to some extent. However, answer (B) is the best answer.

5. *(B)*. A patient who has a complicated history (symptoms of OAB in addition to stress symptoms), history of prior continence surgery (Kelly plication), and possible neurologic influence on bladder function (long-standing diabetes mellitus) should undergo multichannel cystometry. Simple cystometry is not enough. This patient has indications for complex cystometry. Procedures such as injecting the urethra or surgeries may be premature at this point.

6. *(C)*. A Holter monitor is a form of an ECG that is worn by the patient and taken home. Similarly, the ambulatory cystometry is a form of complex or electronic cystometry that the patient can wear and take home so that her voiding function is continuously monitored.

8 URODYNAMICS II: TESTS THAT EVALUATE BLADDER EMPTYING

Sam Siddighi

POSTVOID RESIDUAL

- Postvoid residual (PVR) is the volume of urine remaining in the bladder immediately after spontaneous completion of micturition. It may be misrepresentative of true bladder function if it is done in unfamiliar surroundings and under command.
- PVR is also inaccurate in the setting of vesicoureteral reflux (VUR) or bladder diverticula since some of the urine in the bladder came from outside the bladder and therefore does not really represent bladder function.
- PVR can be measured by a transurethral catheter or approximated by ultrasound (PVR = 0.52 × [anteroposterior dimension (cm) + transverse dimension (cm) + mid-sagittal dimension (cm)]). Ultrasound is 96% specific in detecting bladder volumes >100 mL.
- PVR can also be estimated by cystoscopy, radiography, or radioisotopes.
- High PVR is a result of increased bladder outlet resistance, decreased bladder contractility, or both.
- PVR increase with age, pelvic prolapse, and immediately after surgery.
- PVR must be performed before any incontinence surgery and is the first step in the suggested protocol for performing complex urodynamics.
- There is no universally accepted abnormal PVR lower limit.
- PVR is usually <60 mL (50–100 mL may be normal; >200 mL is abnormal). Nevertheless, it is more useful to indicate PVR as a percentage of total volume voided (i.e., *PVR/total voided volume*). A value of <20% is normal.
- If PVR is between 60 and 200, then it should be repeated (often several times) and correlated to the patient's clinical condition.

UROFLOWMETRY

MEASUREMENT OF URINARY FLOW (UROFLOWMETRY OR NONINVASIVE UROFLOWMETRY)

- Noninvasive test that measures urine volume over measured time in a relaxed patient voiding into a special commode. It is essential to create a private, tension-free setting and to ask the patient how representative the experience was in comparison to usual voiding. Noninvasive uroflowmetry (NIF) produces a graph of flow rate versus time. NIF can also be obtained simply via a stopwatch and a basin.
- Instrumentation (catheter will reduce peak flow rates), voiding on command (>25% of patients cannot), the knowledge of being observed, fast rates of bladder filling, and overfilling can significantly affect results obtained from NIF and pressure-flow studies (see Pressure-flow Studies). For example, voiding pressures are higher with physiologic bladder filling versus retrograde filling via a catheter.
- Ideally, uroflowmetry measures the relationship between detrusor contraction ($\uparrow$) and urethral resistance ($\downarrow$) during voiding. Detrusor contraction is altered by medications (e.g., bethanechol), neurologic conditions, conscious inhibition, and intrinsic detrusor muscle dysfunction (acontractile bladder). Similarly, urethral resistance is changed by medications (e.g., alpha-adrenergic agonists), atrophy (e.g., menopause), fibrosis (e.g., radiation), stroke (detrusor-sphincter dyssynergia), neuropathies (e.g., multiple sclerosis [MS] or spinal cord lesion), intrinsic obstruction (urethral strictures or tumor), and extrinsic urethral lesions (e.g., vaginal masses or pelvic prolapse).
- When performing uroflowmetry, one must specify patient environment, position (sitting, standing, supine), type of fluid voided (natural vs. saline), and diuresis (natural vs. stimulated with diuretics and water load).
- NIF is volume-dependent. Peak flow rates increase as initial bladder volumes or volume voided increase. NIF studies should be performed with at least 150 mL in the bladder.

UROFLOW PARAMETERS

- Voiding time = total duration of micturition (including interruptions). If there are no interruptions, then voiding time = flow time.
- Voided volume = area under the flow rate versus flow time curve. This can be directly measured from the total amount of urine voided into specialized container.

- Flow rate (Q) = volume of urine voided divided by time (mL/s) (usually 26 ± 14 mL/s).
- Maximum flow rate (Q_{max}) = maximum flow rate derived from the highest point on the flow rate (mL/s) versus time (s) graph. ($Q_{max} <15$ mL/s is *abnormal*.) This is the most important NIF parameter.
- Average flow rate (Q_{avg}) = total volume voided over total flow time (Q_{time}). Q_{avg} is only useful if flow is continuous and without terminal dribbling.
- All Q measurements are higher in women than men because of lower urethral resistance. Women have a shorter urethra and lack of prostate. The short urethra also allows P_{abd}, i.e., valsalva, to easily influence voiding parameters.
- On the other hand, patients with pelvic prolapse or some patients after stress incontinence surgery may have an obstructive pattern on NIF.
- NIF may be completely normal in stress incontinence and overactive bladder (OAB).
- There is a paucity of data regarding female uroflow parameters (e.g., Liverpool monograms), because most of the work has been done on men with outlet obstruction from benign prostatic hyperplasia (BPH).
- Rule of thumb: Normal female should void 200 mL over 15–20 s; it should depict a single, continuous, smooth bell-curve (with left skew, i.e., only one-third of total voiding time spent reaching Q_{max}); and Q_{max} should be >20 mL/s. Patients with $Q_{max} <15$ mL/s or $Q_{avg} <10$ mL/s may require further urodynamic testing.
- Normal voiding is initiated by voluntary, sustained detrusor contraction which can be suppressed. Additionally, during normal voiding, the urethra is relaxed from beginning to end of voiding.

UROFLOW PATTERNS (ON FLOW RATE VS. TIME GRAPH)

- Intermittent, multiple-peak pattern (roller-coaster)— voiding with multiple sharp decreases and increases of flow rate, but not down to 0. This type of pattern occurs with valsalva voiding and is associated with elevated PVR. The decreases in flow rate are caused by reflex contractions of the levator ani and the striated urogenital-sphincter muscle complex which occurs during valsalva. In this graph, Q_{max} is determined by choosing the highest peak which lasts for ≥ 1 s. Then, a uroflow graph in the shape of a triangle is made by drawing a continuous line from t = 0, q = 0 to Q_{max}, and a line from Q_{max} to location on the graph where voiding is finished.
- Intermittent, interrupted pattern—voiding with several instances of no flow (Q = 0) followed by some flow. Patients with detrusor-sphincter dyssynergia

(e.g., MS) have prolonged flow times, low peak flow rates, and high PVR.

- Hi-flow pattern—short voiding duration with high Q_{max} (e.g., instrinsic sphincteric deficiency [ISD]).
- Outlet obstruction pattern—long voiding duration with low Q_{max} (e.g., men with BPH or women with advanced POP).

PRESSURE-FLOW STUDIES

INTRODUCTION

- A study where uroflowmetry (i.e., flow rate vs. time graph) is conducted at the same time that complex cystometry is performed, and the graphs are correlated. Hence, the objective is to obtain the P_{det} graph and overlap it with the uroflow graph.
- This study is useful because voiding is not only a function of bladder contraction and urethral relaxation, but also is influenced by abdominal straining (P_{abd}) and urethral resistance. For example, an obstructed patient may have a normal voiding flow rate (on uroflow graph) because she makes up for it by increasing intravesical pressure via valsalva. On the other hand, a patient whose bladder is acontractile may have normal flow rates because of simultaneous sphincteric relaxation and valsalva.
- Parameters measured are defined by the International Continence Society:
  1. Premicturition pressure = baseline P_{det} prior to start of voiding
  2. Opening pressure = P_{det} at onset of urine flow
  3. Opening time = time from initial rise in P_{det} to onset of urine flow
  4. Maximum voiding pressure = Max P_{det} while patient is voiding
  5. Pressure at maximum flow rate = P_{det} at Q_{max}
  6. Contraction pressure = pressure at Q_{max} minus premicturition pressure
  7. After contraction = after the flow of urine ceases, there is a pressure increase
- Physics resistance formula, P/Q_{max}, should not be used to measure urethral resistance because the urethra is not a rigid, straight pipe with laminar flow.

METHODOLOGY

- Pressure-flow studies are usually performed after cystometry so that the P_{abd} catheter (intravaginal or intrarectal) can be utilized.
- Voided volume/time, patient environment, patient position (sitting, supine, or standing), filling (diuresis

or catheter), type of fluid, and the type of equipment used should be recorded. A two- or three-lumen, 4–7 Fr catheter maybe used (lumen 1 = filling, lumen 2 = P_{ves}, lumen 3 = P_u).
- Patient is asked to void to completion (into a specialized container and in private) and P_{abd}, P_{ves}, and P_{det} are measured (see Chap. 7, Urodynamics Part I: Evaluation of Bladder Filling and Storage). This way the examiner can assess whether P_{abd} (valsalva) is used in order to facilitate voiding.
- Some centers add electromyograph (EMG) electrodes during pressure-flow studies.
- During voiding, a reliable measure of detrusor contractions, the *isometric detrusor pressure* can be obtained by performing the stop test.
  Stop test: Sometimes pressure created by detrusor contraction is difficult to measure and is not seen on P_{det} (e.g., someone with zero urethral resistance). Therefore, during voiding effort either the patient is asked to stop her urinary stream (levator ani contraction) or her urethra is mechanically compressed with a finger. These maneuvers increases the patient's urethral closure pressure. Now the detrusor is contracting against a closed urethra and a pressure rise can be recorded. High values indicate good detrusor contraction, but low values are not helpful because detrusor contraction can be reflexively inhibited.

PRESSURE-FLOW PATTERNS

- Urethral overactivity pattern: urethra contracting or failing to relax during voiding. (1) Detrusor-sphincter dyssynergia: striated urogenital muscle complex contractions happen in phase with detrusor contractions and therefore you record very high voiding pressures (P_{det}) and intermittent interrupted flow pattern. (2) Subset of children with incontinence: child is neurologically intact, but flow of urine during voiding is interrupted by contraction of the levator ani.
- *Normal values:* Q_{max} >20 mL/s and P_{det} <20 cm H_2O.
- Outlet obstruction pattern: low flow rates and high detrusor pressures (P_{det}). Q_{max}<12 mL/s + P_{det} >20 cm H_2O at Q_{max}. Patients with obstructive voiding are at risk for ureteral and renal damage and may benefit from a renal ultrasound.
- Acontractile detrusor pattern or poor detrusor function: low flow rates and low P_{det}. These patients have to strain (increase P_{abd}) in order to void. This may be better appreciated by performing the stop test. (Note: normal detrusor contractions are more effective in producing voiding than increases in intra-abdominal pressure created by straining.)

USES OF UROFLOWMETRY AND PRESSURE-FLOW STUDIES

- Statistically, these tests are not as useful in women as in men because only 4% of lower urinary tract dysfunction in women is related to voiding dysfunction.
- The limitations of these studies are numerous: (1) there is no clear cut off between normal and abnormal values (lack of data in women), (2) lack of standardization (e.g., catheter size 6 Fr vs. 7 Fr vs. others) (3) expertise required for operation and interpretation, (4) nonphysiologic, stress-provoking, and uncomfortable testing environment, and (5) artifacts.
- Uroflowmetry is best used as a screening test in women with voiding dysfunction and may identify patients who may need more complex urodynamic testing; it can also measure disease progression and treatment in those patients.
- NIF and pressure-flow studies may by utilized in the following situations:
  1. *After* pelvic *surgery*, e.g., after a Burch urethropexy or suburethral sling, for patient who develops postoperative urinary retention with consistently elevated PVR (either caused by denervation injury from pelvic surgery or increased urethral resistance from suture or sling after stress incontinence surgery). The outlet obstruction pattern may indicate need to take down repair (urethrolysis).
  2. Pressure-flow studies may be done *before surgical correction* for stress incontinence to predict which patients are at risk for prolonged bladder catheterization (i.e., >7 days). Q_{max} <20 mL/s and those patients using valsalva during voiding are at risk for prolonged return to voiding.
  3. *Frequency/ urgency syndrome*, e.g., may be used to assess response before and after urethral dilation in patients with urethral syndrome.
  4. *Neurologic patients*: to establish baseline and measure improvement in voiding with therapy.

BIBLIOGRAPHY

Bhatia NN, Bergman A, Karram MM. Changes in urethral resistance following incontinence surgery. *Urology.* 1989;34:200.

Bhatia NN, Bergman A. Urodynamic predictability of voiding following incontinence surgery. *Obstet Gynecol.* 1984;63:85.

Bhatia NN, Bergman. Use of preoperative uroflowmetry and simultaneous urethrocystometry for predicting risk of prolonged postoperative bladder drainage. *Urology.* 1986;28: 440.

Chassagne S, Bernier PA, Haab F, et al. Proposed cutoff values to define bladder outlet obstruction in women. *Urology.* 1998;51:408–411.

Drach GW, Ignatoff J, Layton T. Peak urinary flow rate: observations in female subjects and comparison to male subjects. *J Urol.* 1979;122:215.

Karram MM. Urodynamics: voiding studies. In: Walters MD, Karram MM, eds. *Urogynecology and Reconstructive Pelvic Surgery.* 2nd ed. St. Louis: Mosby; 1999:69–79.

Lemack GE, Zimmern PE. Pressure flow analysis may aid in identifying women with outflow obstruction. *J Urol.* 2000;163:1823–1828.

Massey JA, Abrams PH. Obstructed voiding in the female. *Br J Urol.* 1988;61:36–39.

Nager CW, Albo ME. Testing in women with lower urinary tract dysfunction. In: Weber A, ed. *Incontinence 2004.* Philadelphia, PA: Lippincott Williams & Wilkins; 2004:57–60.

Sand PK, Ostergard DR. *Urodynamics and the Evaluation of Female Incontinence, a Practical Guide*: Springer-Verlag; 1995.

QUESTIONS

1. Uroflow and pressure-flow studies are not as useful as cystometry in evaluation of a female patient. Which of the following arguments support the use of these tests in women?
   - (A) There is no cutoff between normal and abnormal values in women.
   - (B) There is lack of standardization of both procedures in women.
   - (C) Lower urinary tract dysfunction as cause of voiding dysfunction is uncommon in women.
   - (D) After continence surgery in women, these tests may help to elucidate the reason for postoperative urinary retention.
   - (E) Prior to continence surgery in women, these tests can reliably predict who will require prolonged bladder catheterization.

2. A 48-year-old gravida 3, para 3, underwent anterior repair, uterosacral ligament colposuspension, and suburethral sling (TVT) yesterday. Prior to discharge from the hospital, *of the following listed options*, the best way to write a voiding trial order is by writing, "after second voiding attempt, _____."
   - (A) Discontinue indwelling catheter and discharge home if PVR <60 mL
   - (B) Discontinue indwelling catheter and discharge home if PVR <220 mL
   - (C) Discontinue indwelling catheter and discharge home if PVR/total voided volume × 100% is less than 20%
   - (D) Discharge home with indwelling catheter if PVR >80 mL
   - (E) Discharge home with indwelling catheter if PVR >60 mL and return to office in 2 days for voiding trial

QUESTIONS 3–5

Match the following uroflow parameters with the condition or situation which they would be associated. The answers may be used once, more than once, or not at all.

(A) Hypoparathyroid

(B) MS

(C) Third degree pelvic organ prolapse (POP)

(D) Valsalva

(E) ISD

3. Voided 200 mL in 7 s; Q_{max} = 75 mL/s
4. Voided 200 mL in 35 s with two episodes of no flow (Q = 0); Q_{max} = 18 mL/s
5. Uroflow pattern with multiple peaks, but flow never stops (Q ≠ 0); Q_{max} = 18 mL/s
6. The fact that _____ is a reason why urine flow rates during micturition are higher in women as compared to men.

(A) Women have wider urethras

(B) Women lack intrinsic internal obstruction

(C) Resistance = pressure/flow; women have higher voiding pressures

(D) In women, the urethra is a straight rigid pipe

(E) In women, urinary flow is turbulent rather than laminar

ANSWERS

1. *(D)*. Statements (A), (B), and (C) are reasons why uroflow and pressure-flow studies are not useful in women. Statement (E) is incorrect because pressure-flow studies before surgical correction of stress incontinence may help to predict which patients are at risk for catheterization past 7 days, but it is not reliable and consistent. Additionally, uroflow may be completely normal in patients with OAB or stress incontinence (the two conditions dealt with in urogynecology).

2. *(C)*. Although PVR is usually <60 mL and normally between 50 and 100 mL, there is no magic threshold. It is more useful to indicate PVR as a percentage of the total volume voided. Option (A) would miss many patients who would be at risk for urinary retention and may need to continue indwelling catheterization. Option (B) would prematurely discontinue indwelling catheters in patients who would be at risk for urinary retention. Option (D) and (E) would be placing indwelling catheters in more patients than may be necessary.

ANSWERS 3–5

3. *(E)*, 4. *(B)*, 5. *(D)*. Remember the rule of thumb: a normal female should void 200 mL in about 15–20 s and Q_{max} >20 mL/s. In question 3, the patient has voided 200 mL in very little time with a high flow rate (i.e., hi-flow pattern). In question 4, the patient has taken more time than normal to void and has had two episodes of zero flow. This intermittent, interrupted pattern is consistent with detrusor-sphincter dyssynergia (in MS, cerebrovascular accident [CVA], upper tract diseases, and the like). In question 5, a roller-coaster pattern and lower Q_{max} is consistent with someone who uses valsalva to void. Answer (A) is a distractor. Hypothyroidism (not hypoparathyroidism) and diabetes mellitus are conditions which are associated with acontractile bladders. As such, voiding duration would be expected to be longer and Q_{max} lower than normal. Third degree POP may cause kinking of the urethra which would cause obstruction. This would be appreciated best by a pressure-flow study which would show decreased Q_{max} (<15 mL/s) and increased P_{det} (>20 cm H_2O).

6. *(B)*. Urinary flow rates are higher in women because there is less total resistance since the urethra is shorter and there is lack of an internal structure (the prostate) to cause obstruction. Women do not have wider urethras or higher voiding pressures. The formula R = P/F is used in physics to describe laminar flow through a straight, rigid pipe. This is not true in humans. The urethra is distensible, slightly curved, and has turbulent flow. Furthermore, the fact that flow is turbulent does not explain why women have higher urine flow rates than men.

9 URODYNAMICS PART III: EVALUATION OF URETHRAL FUNCTION

Sam Siddighi

BACKGROUND

- In a person who is continent, pressure inside the urethra exceeds the pressure in the bladder except during micturition.
- The high-pressure state inside the urethra is a result of several factors: (1) the pelvic floor muscles (tonic

contraction at rest and reflexive contraction with increases in intra-abdominal pressure), (2) endopelvic fascial hammock (see later in this section), (3) the urethral muscles (smooth muscle [circular and longitudinal] and striated muscle complex [sphincter urethrae, compressor urethrae, and urethrovaginal sphincter]), (4) corresponding innervation, (5) vascular seal provided by the submucosal venous plexus, and (6) mucosal coaptation.

- The highest pressure in the urethra occurs at mid-urethra. Perhaps, this is true not only because of the aforementioned facts, but also because the urethra is supported at its mid-portion by the pubourethral ligament.
- The endopelvic fascial hammock (i.e., pubocervical septal support underneath the proximal urethra [DeLancey level II]) and the distal urethral attachment to the perineal membrane (DeLancey level III) contribute to continence and maintenance of urethral pressure.
- Urethral function can be assessed objectively via maximum urethral closure pressure (MUCP), leak point pressure (LPP), fluoroscopic visualization of the urethrovesical junction, and electromyograph (EMG). LPP and MUCP will be discussed in this chapter. EMG will be discussed in Chap. 10, Electrophysiologic Testing. Fluoroscopy will be discussed in Chap. 12, Radiologic Imaging of Pelvic Floor and Lower Urinary Tract.

URETHRAL PRESSURE PROFILE (UPP)

DEFINITION AND INTRODUCTION

- Upper urethral closure pressure profiles are graphic representation of the pressure within the urethra along its entire length. Normally it is a symmetric, bell-shaped curve. From this, it can be deduced that the highest pressure in the urethra occurs in the mid-urethra.
- There are few distinctions: storage phase UPP is the pressure within the urethra at rest, while voiding UPP measures the pressure within the urethra while voiding (may be used to determine pressure and site of urethral obstructions).
- Also static (at rest), dynamic (during cough, valsalva) or augmenting (while squeezing the levator ani and periurethral muscles to stop passage of flatus or urine). Augmenting increase MUCP and functional urethral length (FUL).
- Maximum urethral closure pressure (MUCP) = maximum urethral pressure (MUP) minus intravesical

pressure (P_{ves}). Of all the measurements obtained from UPP, MUCP is more useful. Formula: $MUCP = P_u$ (at max) $- P_{ves}$.
- The point of MUCP occurs at the mid-urethra.
- Both MUP and MUCP decrease with age. One study noted average MUP of 90 cm H_2O in *normal healthy* people in their mid 20s and 65 cm H_2O in those in their mid 60s.
- Functional urethral length (FUL) is the length of urethra along which the urethral pressure exceeds the intravesical pressure (this length is always smaller than the anatomic, total urethral length which is between 3 and 5 cm). This length can also be measured during stress.
- Pressure transmission ratio (PTR) = during stress (i.e., cough, valsalva), the increase in urethral pressure (P_u) divided by the increase in intravesical pressure (P_{ves}) and multiplied by 100%. This ratio ($\Delta P_u/\Delta P_{ves} \times 100\%$) can be calculated for any point along the FUL. Interestingly, PTR decrease as the strength of cough increases. The word *transmission* in PTR may be inaccurate because increase in urethral pressure during stress is due to muscle contraction which is an active process. During stress, the pressure increase in urethra occurs before increase in pressure in the bladder.
- Patients with stress incontinence have lower PTR (negative PTR), but there is no cutoff value to help distinguish continence from incontinence.
- UPP is done during cystometry. Usually six simultaneous, overlapping graphs are produced (6 lines of data) for example, line 1 = EMG, line 2 = P_{abd}, line 3 = P_{ves}, line 4 = P_u (aka intraurethral pressure), line 5 = P_{det} ($P_{ves} - P_{abd}$), and line 6 = P_{ucp} ($P_u - P_{ves}$). Lines 5 and 6 are calculated.

TECHNIQUES

- Urethral pressures can be measured using balloon catheters: (1) shows integrated, average pressures rather than point pressures, (2) does not give instant pressure rises during cough, and (3) deformation of balloon may cause artifacts.
- UPP can be obtained by perfusion techniques: (1) one- or two-channel catheters with side holes, (2) fluid or gas can be infused into side holes to prevent blockage, (3) sudden rises in urethral pressure can block side holes as urethral tissue collapses, thus resulting in artificially elevated pressures.
- Many centers obtain UPP via a *dual microtransducer system*. The distal catheter with its mounted transducer is placed inside the bladder while the more

proximal is withdrawn manually or mechanically through the urethra as the UPP is graphed.

STANDARDIZATION

To try to standardize UPP measurements, experts have advocated using the dual-sensor microtip transducer system and the following:

- Sitting position (supine, or standing). Note: there is an increase in MUCP as patient position is made more upright.
- Liquid infusion medium (or gas).
- A standard bladder volume (UPP increase with increasing bladder volumes).
- Zero catheter system to atmospheric pressure.
- Same catheter size (8–12 Fr), rigidity, type, and orientation (directed laterally, 3 and 9 o'clock position rather than vertically at 6 or 12 o'clock position, which artificially decreases or increases the UPP, respectively). Remember, we are not actually measuring pressure with this catheter but instead are measuring force. There is greater anterior/posterior force when the urethra undergoes coaptation.
- Same transducer position and distances along catheter.
- Rate of movement of the recording paper (e.g., 1 mm/s during static and cough and 5 mm/s during valsalva).
- Resting UPP: proximal transducer pulled out of bladder by a mechanical puller at a constant rate (1–40 cm/min) and the UPP graphed.
- Proximal transducer replaced into bladder and step 4 repeated, then UPP from the two trials averaged.
- Stress UPP: during stress (e.g., cough): steps 4 and 5 repeated with the patient coughing every 2 seconds with a consistent cough intensity.

SOME HELPFUL THINGS TO KEEP IN MIND DURING URODYNAMIC TESTING

- Realize that catheters reduce peak flow rates because of obstruction.
- Realize that certain things *lower LPP values*: small caliber catheter, larger bladder volumes, more upright position, spontaneous bladder contractions, decreased bladder compliance states.
- Realize that certain things *increase LPP values*: advanced prolapse, recordings from cough-induced LPP (vs. valsalva induced).
- Realize that urine leakage observation by naked eye maybe more sensitive than leakage observed on fluoroscopy.
- Minimize catheter movements as they cause artifacts and unexpected pressure readings.

- Realize that artifacts may be caused by vaginal/rectal peristalsis, breathing, and patient movements.
- Minimize catheter, wires, equipment, and observers so that the patient can be in a less artificial environment.
- Try to minimize observers during urodynamic studies.

EXAMPLES OF MULTICHANNEL CYSTOMETRY WITH UPP

EMG + *activity in EMG electrode*
P_{abd}, P_{ves}, P_u, P_{det}, *or* P_{ucp}
0 *no change in pressure or activity*
$\uparrow$ *increase in pressure or activity*
$\downarrow$ *decrease in pressure or activity*

- "Normal" person + valsalva or cough = EMG +, P_{abd} $\uparrow$, P_{ves} $\uparrow$, P_u $\uparrow$, P_{det} 0, P_{ucp} $\uparrow$ (increased curve shape in valsalva vs. spikes on top of curve in cough. Note you will see negative spikes in P_{ucp} in distal urethra. This is normal since this part of the urethra is below the level of pelvic diaphragm) $\uparrow$.
- "Normal" person + maneuver to stop passage of flatus = EMG +, P_{abd} 0, P_{ves} 0, P_u, P_{det} 0, P_{ucp} $\uparrow$.
- *Person with urethral diverticula or fistula* = EMG 0, P_{abd} 0, P_{ves} 0, P_u $\uparrow \downarrow \uparrow$, P_{det} 0, P_{ucp} $\uparrow \downarrow \uparrow$ (i.e., segment just before the fistula has increased pressure then a decrease in pressure over the defect, and finally an increase in pressure past the defect; also the overall P_{ucp} baseline is lower before than after repair of the defect). In planning surgery, if UPP indicates the diverticula are distal to area of MUCP, then marsupialization procedure is preferred and if the diverticula are proximal to area of MUCP, then removal of diverticula and closure may be a better procedure).
- *Uninhibited urethral relaxation* = EMG 0/+, P_{abd} 0, P_{ves} 0, P_u $\downarrow$ 0 $\downarrow\downarrow\downarrow$, P_{det} 0, P_{ucp} $\downarrow$ 0 $\downarrow\downarrow\downarrow$ (i.e., isolated episode of instability (– 0) followed by complete urethral relaxation (—); in this rare condition, the urethra relaxes in the absence of bladder contraction and results in urine loss).
- *Stress urinary incontinence* (SUI) (sitting patient at maximum cystometric capacity asked to cough then valsalva) = EMG +, P_{abd} $\uparrow$, P_{ves} $\uparrow$, P_u $\uparrow\downarrow$, P_{det} **0**, P_{ucp} $\downarrow$ (along entire urethra, there are negative pressure spikes on P_{ucp} during cough; during valsalva effort there is negative continuous P_{ucp}. *Note that there is activity in EMG because coughing causes reflex contraction of pelvic floor muscle*s).
- *Detrusor overactivity without incontinence* (patient is asked to cough, or other provocative maneuver, but no urine leak is observed) = EMG $\uparrow$, P_{abd} $\uparrow$, P_{ves} $\uparrow\uparrow$, P_u $\uparrow$, P_{det} $\uparrow$, P_{ucp} $\uparrow$ (there is a delay between cough (P_{abd}) and increase in P_{det}. There is no such delay in urodynamic stress incontinence)

- *Detrusor sphincter dyssynergia* (stroke patient is asked to void) = EMG 0 + 0 +, P_{abd} 0 0 0 0, P_{ves} ↑↑↑ 0, P_u 0 ↑ 0 ↑, P_{det} ↑↑↑ 0, P_{ucp} ↓↑↓↑ (other long-term findings in these patients are habitual contraction of striated urogenital muscle complex during voiding, increases in PVR, and bladder trabeculations observed on cystoscopy).

LIMITATIONS

- Does not always produce consistent and reproducible values even when only one method of measurement is utilized.
- The information gained from UPP during storage phase (no voiding) has limited value.
- There is marked overlap in values between healthy and dysfunctional states.
- Standardization and outcome studies using LPP are lacking.

POSSIBLE USES OF UPP

- May be useful in differentiating between intrinsic sphincteric deficiency (ISD) and urethral hypermobility types of stress incontinence. Most studies use MUCP >20 cm H_2O to exclude ISD. Also see LPP in the following section.
- This is controversial. But MUCP may help predict surgical success of different procedures; however, there is conflicting evidence. Surgeries that focus on correction of hypermobility (e.g., Burch retropubic urethropexy) may have higher success rate in patients with MUCP >20 cm H_2O. Procedures that occlude the urethra (sling, bulking agents, or artificial sphincters) may be better suited for patients with MUCP <20 cm H_2O.

LEAK POINT PRESSURE (LPP)

DEFINITION AND INTRODUCTION

- The lowest pressure in cm H_2O (either absolute or change in pressure from baseline) produced by straining (either valsalva [VLPP] or cough [CLPP]) that overcomes urethral resistance and produces urine leakage (either gross leakage or fluoroscopic evidence of leakage). The abdominal LPP is a simple, objective study that reveals the severity of stress incontinence. Usually, more severe incontinence tends to have lower LPP.
- Detrusor versus abdominal LPP: Detrusor LPP is measured by slowly filling the bladder until it is full and watching for leakage. The total pressure (P_{ves} + P_{abd}) when leakage occurs is known as the bladder LPP. During this study, P_{ves} should be kept <40 cm H_2O to prevent bladder injury. Measurement of abdominal LPP requires a catheter in the bladder. The technique is described in the following section.

- Valsalva versus cough LPP: As a provocative maneuver, valsalva is preferred because it can be gradually increased, and the lowest pressure value that results in leakage can be obtained. If leakage does not occur with valsalva then cough maneuver can be utilized to produce leakage. Though more intense pressures can be generated with coughing, it is more difficult to obtain the lowest pressure that results in leakage since coughing creates sudden uncontrolled pressure spikes.
- Abdominal LPP measurements can also be obtained without a catheter inside the bladder if the patient does not leak with valsalva or cough. With this method, the bladder is filled to maximum cystometric capacity (instead of 150–200 mL) and the abdominal pressure is measured via intravaginal or intrarectal pressure catheter. The LPP values are lower with this technique.
- Inconsistent or weak correlation exists between MUCP and LPP. We have found LPP more useful for predicting the severity of incontinence.

TECHNIQUES

- The dual-sensor microtip transducer system can be used.
- 6-Fr catheter placed inside bladder.
- Bladder filled to volume of 150–200 mL.
- Sitting position.
- Patient performs gradually more vigorous valsalva.
- Lowest pressure at which leakage occurs is noted and the change in pressure from baseline is called the abdominal LPP or ΔLPP.

POSSIBLE USES OF LPP

- LPP <60 cm H_2O is consistent with ISD or type III SUI (<60 cm H_2O has 90% sensitivity but 64% specificity for diagnosing low pressure urethra; lower LPP cutoffs decrease sensitivity but increase specificity). Procedures that partially obstruct the urethra (i.e., proximal urethral sling, urethral bulking injections, or artificial sphincter) are more likely to benefit patients with low LPP.
- LPP >100 cm H_2O + SUI is consistent with urethral hypermobility as cause of SUI. Patients with high LPP may benefit from suspension procedures (e.g., Burch retropubic urethropexy).
- LPP 60–100 cm H_2O are patients with features of both ISD and hypermobility. These patients may benefit from sling procedures and possibly suspension procedures.
- Mideurethral slings may be effective for both low and high LPPs.

LIMITATIONS

- Although the values (e.g., <60 cm H_2O) have been used to guide choice of procedure by some, there are insufficient data to make such recommendations.

- There is lack of standardization in terms of how to perform the LPP measurements. Many factors (see earlier section) can affect LPP values.
- Because of lack of standardization and limited prognostic information, LPP is not required as a routine test in patients with stress incontinence. The Urinary Incontinence Treatment Network Trial results will provide more answers in the near future.

URETHRAL RETRO-RESISTANCE PRESSURE (URP)

- URP—a simple and reproducible test for stress incontinence which measures the pressure required to open a closed urethra (i.e., *the pressure required to achieve and maintain an open sphincter*).
- Retrograde filling of bladder with saline is performed while a urethral plug maintains a seal in the distal urethra. Pressure is slowly increased until the internal urethral meatus opens and remains open.
- URP shows a consistent relationship with the severity of incontinence (i.e., URP values are lower with more severe incontinence).
- More research is needed on this subject.

BIBLIOGRAPHY

Karram MM, Miklos JR. Urodynamics: urethral pressure profilometry and leak point pressures. In: Walters MD, Karram MM, eds. *Urogynecology and Reconstructive Pelvic Surgery.* 2nd ed. St. Louis, MO: Mosby; 1999:81–94.

Kim YH, Kattan MW, Boone TB. Correlation of urodynamic results and urethral coaptation with success after transurethral collagen injection. *Urology.* 1997;50:941–948.

Nager CW, Albo ME. Testing in Women with lower urinary tract dysfunction. In: Weber A, ed. *Incontinence 2004.* Philadelphia, PA: Lippincott Williams & Wilkins; 2004:53–69.

Sand PK, Ostergard DR. *Urodynamis and the Evaluation of Female Incontinence.* London:Springer-Verlag; 1995.

Slack M, Culligan P, Tracey M, et al. Relationship of urethral retro-resistance pressure to urodynamic measurements and incontinence severity. *Neurourol Urodyn.* 2004;23(2):109–114.

Theofrastous JP, Swift SE. Urodynamic testing. In: Bent AE, Ostergard DR, Cundiff GW, Sweift SE, eds. *Ostergard's Urogynecology and Pelvic Floor Dysfunction.* 5th ed. Philadelphia, PA: Lippincott Williams & Wilkins; 2003: 115–140.

QUESTIONS

1. The combination of resting FUL, MUCP, respectively, most representative of patients with severe ISD is ____; ____.

   (A) 4 cm; 40 cm H_2O
   (B) 5 cm; 4 cm H_2O
   (C) 1 cm; 4 cm H_2O
   (D) 1 cm; 40 cm H_2O
   (E) 7 cm; 15 cm H_2O

2. A 46-year-old gravida 5, para 4, sab 1, has symptoms of stress incontinence. During cystometry, $P_u = 55$ cm H_2O and $P_{ves} = 50$. She undergoes suburethral sling procedure and is reevaluated 6 months postoperatively. Now $P_u = 40$ and $P_{ves} = 30$. The best explanation for this phenomenon is that there has been a(n) _____ after the surgical procedure.

   (A) Increase in the pressure transmission ratio (PTR)
   (B) Decrease in urethral closure pressure (P_{ucp})
   (C) Decrease in vesical pressure (P_{ves})
   (D) Decrease in detrusor pressure (P_{det})
   (E) Increased ratio of P_{ves} to P_u (P_{ves}/P_u)

3. You have performed multichannel cystometry on a patient whom you believe has an exaggerated guarding reflex because her MUCP is high (140 cm H_2O). To isolate the contribution of the striated urogenital-sphincter complex to the urethral closure pressure, you can _____.

   (A) Ask the patient to take a deep breath
   (B) Ask the patient to cough
   (C) Ask the patient to pretend to stop the flow of urine during micturition
   (D) Perform bilateral pudendal nerve block with local anesthetic
   (E) Give patient an alpha agonist

4. A 56-year-old gravida 3, para 3, presents to your office because of incontinence and pressure inside her vagina. After evaluation, you diagnose grade 3 anterior prolapse and stress incontinence. Prior to reduction of the prolapse, you obtain the following results during valsalva: $P_{abd} = 60$ cm H_2O, $P_{ves} = 65$ cm H_2O, $P_u = 200$ cm H_2O, calculated $P_{ucp} = 135$ cm H_2O, and there is no urine leakage. After reduction of the prolapse with a pessary and repeating what was done earlier, you may find _____ if she is at risk for de novo stress incontinence after surgical repair (all values are measured in cm H_2O).

   (A) $P_{ves} = 60$, $P_{abd} = 55$, $P_u = 0$
   (B) $P_{abd} = 55$, $P_{ves} = 60$, $P_u = 60$
   (C) $P_{ves} = 0$, $P_{abd} = 0$, $P_u = -60$
   (D) $P_{det} = 60$
   (E) $P_{ucp} = 60$

5. A 77-year-old gravida 2, para 1, therapeutic abortion (tab) 1, has a 10-year history of worsening stress incontinence. She has a history of neuropathy related to diabetes mellitus and has also had nocturia. She has not had any operations in the past. She has no POP.

The Q_{tip} angle is + 15 degrees, cystometry is negative for detrusor contractions, and the stress test is immediately positive (and simultaneous detrusor contractions are absent). LPP = 15 cm H_2O and MUCP = 5 cm H_2O. The best incontinence procedure for this patient is _____.

(A) Kelly plication
(B) Burch retropubic urethropexy
(C) Marshall-Marchetti-Krantz procedure (MMK)
(D) Needle suspension procedure
(E) Tension free vaginal tape sling

ANSWERS

1. *(C)*. A person with ISD had very low MUCP (<20 cm H_2O). This eliminates answers (A) and (D). Answer (E) is incorrect because the female urethra is anatomically only 3–5 cm (not 7 cm). Therefore, FUL is always less than the length of the anatomic urethra. Answer (B) is not possible because if there is ISD then the FUL must be much less than the highest value of anatomic urethra.

2. *(A)*. Prior to surgery, the patient's calculated P_{ucp} was 5 cm H_2O ($P_u – P_{ves} = 55 – 50$) and PTR was 1.1 ($P_u/P_{ves} = 55/50$). After surgery, the calculated P_{ucp} became 10 cm H_2O (40 – 30) and PTR became 1.33... (P_u/P_{ves}). Therefore, both P_{ucp} and PTR increased after surgery. Answer (D) is incorrect because this question has nothing to do with P_{det}. Answer (E) is incorrect because PTR is calculated P_u/P_{ves} and not its reciprocal value.

3. *(D)*. By performing bilateral pudendal nerve block, you eliminate the contribution of the striated urethral sphincter to the urethral pressure. Intra-abdominal pressure will decrease with inspiration. This has no effect on the urethral sphincter. Coughing will cause a reflexive increase in urethral pressure. Answer (C) is incorrect because that maneuver makes the patient squeeze the urethra which would increase the closure pressure. An alpha blocker (not agonist), baclofen, diazepam, and other muscle relaxants and anxiolytics would reduce the striated muscle component of urethral pressure.

4. *(A)*. Patients with POP may have kinking of the urethra which acts to obstruct it. These patients may develop de novo stress incontinence after repair of the POP as the urethra is no longer kinked and obstructed. After reduction of the prolapse with a pessary, you would encounter leakage of urine during valsalva. This means that the P_{ucp} would have to be a negative number. Answer (A) is the only answer in which P_{ucp} is negative (= $P_u – P_{ves} = 0 – 60 = –60$). (B) is incorrect because the calculated P_{ucp} would be 0. Answer (C) is incorrect because P_{abd} and P_{ves} are not 0 during valsalva. Answer (D) is incorrect because a patient with pure stress incontinence should have a large detrusor contraction. Answer (E) is incorrect because the value is positive. Additionally, note that in answer (A), P_{abd} is slightly lower than P_{ves} even though there is no detrusor contraction. This artifact is a result of unequal pressure transmission between the intra-abdominal pressure catheter and the intrabladder pressure catheter.

5. *(E)*. This patient has urodynamic stress incontinence due to ISD (LPP <60, MUCP <20, Q-tip negative). She would not benefit from procedures that decrease urethral hypermobility such as Burch and MMK are retropubic colposuspension procedure. Burch, MMK, Kelly, and suspension procedures are inappropriate for a patient with pure ISD. She would do better with a procedure that obstructs the urethra (i.e., bulking agent injection, sling, or artificial sphincter).

10 ELECTROPHYSIOLOGIC TESTING

Henry Kim and Murray E. Brandstater

INTRODUCTION

- Electrophysiologic studies play an essential role in the evaluation of patients with neuromuscular disorders.
- Pelvic floor dysfunction is often closely associated with neuropathic processes.
- Electrophysiologic tests can aid in the localization of the lesion as well as determining the age, severity, and prognosis of the lesion.

OVERVIEW OF ELECTROPHYSIOLOGIC STUDIES

- The most commonly performed electrophysiologic studies are nerve conduction study (NCS) and electromyography (EMG).
- It is important to note that the NCS and EMG are only able to detect lower motor neuron lesions in the peripheral nervous system (anterior horn cells in the spinal cord, roots, plexus, peripheral nerves, and neuromuscular junction).

• Evoked potential is less frequently employed. It is performed by stimulating a peripheral nerve and recording the response from central nervous tissues such as spinal cord and cortex. It may be abnormal in both upper and lower motor neuron lesions but its clinical use is limited because of difficulty in obtaining consistent responses.

NERVE CONDUCTION STUDY

• Applying external electric shock to a peripheral nerve generates the propagation of action potential. In the motor NCS, the action potential is recorded over the muscle innervated by the stimulated nerve. The potential recorded over the muscle is called compound muscle action potential (CMAP) and is also referred to as M-wave.
  ○ Two electrodes are used for stimulation, a cathode and an anode. Two paired electrodes, G1 (active) and G2 (reference), are attached on the skin over the muscle innervated by the stimulated nerve. G1 is usually placed over the center of the muscle belly (closest to the motor end-plate). A ground electrode is placed between the stimulating and recording electrodes in order to minimize artifact. When performing stimulation, cathode must be pointed to the active electrode (G1). The stimulating current is gradually increased to the point that the CMAP no longer increases in size (supramaximal stimulation).
• The main parameters of a CMAP that are analyzed in pelvic floor electrophysiologic test such as pudendal motor NCS are amplitude and latency.
  ○ Amplitude (mV): It reflects the number of muscle fibers that fire. Low amplitude is caused by either axon loss or conduction block. If axon is damaged, fewer numbers of muscle fibers are in contact with their nerve supply and fewer will fire resulting in low amplitude. Conduction block occurs when the axon is intact but *severe* demyelination blocks traveling impulse.
  ○ Latency (ms): It is the time required for the stimulus to initiate a CMAP. Demyelination slows propagation of impulse and results in prolonged latency.
  ○ Conduction velocity can be calculated in the motor NCS if the nerve is stimulated at two different points and the length of the nerve between the stimulations can be estimated. However, two point stimulations or estimating the length of the nerve is difficult in pelvic floor electrophysiologic test such as in pudendal motor NCS and conduction velocity is not routinely used in clinical practice.
  ○ In general, axon loss and conduction block cause low amplitude and demyelination results in prolonged latency.

• Axon loss generally carries a worse prognosis than demyelination in peripheral nerve injury. Severe demyelination may cause conduction block where the traveling action potential is blocked. However, conduction block is reversible and prognosis for recovery is good. Recovery from axon loss is also feasible depending on the severity of the injury but is generally less complete and more protracted.

ELECTROMYOGRAPHY

• EMG is performed by inserting a needle electrode directly into the muscle of interest. The electrical activities detected by the needle electrode are amplified, filtered to reduce electrical noise, and displayed on a computer screen. The electrical activities can also be heard through audio amplification.
• Three types of needle electrodes are currently available—monopolar, concentric, and single fiber. These are not used commonly in urogynecology.
  ○ Concentric needles are most frequently used today.
  ○ Monopolar needles tend to be less painful due to the Teflon coat but they are generally less favored because of the increased display of recording artifact.
  ○ Single-fiber EMG needles are specialized concentric needles designed to record potentials from single individual muscle fiber. These can be inserted into the anal sphincter or the urethral muscles. Single-fiber concentric needles are preferable to surface electrodes but are uncomfortable.
• Practically speaking, only striated muscles can be studied. Smooth muscle cannot be analyzed with the conventional electrophysiologic devices because of low current generation.
• Typical urodynamic studies involve crude measurements of muscle activity rather than localization of specific muscles.
• Needle EMG is more specific but more uncomfortable for the patient. For example, a 30-mm needle electrode can be inserted into or next to the striated urogenital muscle complex of the urethra in patients suspected of having detrusor-sphincter dyssynergia such as multiple sclerosis, stroke, and spinal cord injury.
• EMG is largely divided into the analysis of the spontaneous activity in relaxed muscle and the analysis of the motor unit action potential (MUAP) in voluntarily contracting muscle.
  1. Analysis of spontaneous discharges
     ○ Spontaneous discharges are best detected when the muscle is relaxed. Some spontaneous activities are normal. However, there are abnormal spontaneous activities such as fibrillation potentials and positive sharp waves.

○ Fibrillation potentials and positive sharp waves are spontaneous depolarization of a single muscle fiber that has lost its nerve supply. They are small potentials that usually fire in slow regular rate.

○ The presence of fibrillation potentials in the muscle indicates that the axon loss has occurred and the muscle fibers have lost the nerve supply (denervation). It also suggests that the lesion causing the axon loss is acute and ongoing. Fibrillation potentials disappear when the axons have recovered from the injury.

2. Analysis of MUAP:
   ○ MUAP morphology (amplitude, duration, and phase) and recruitment of motor unit pattern are analyzed.
   ○ Amplitude, duration, and phase
     ▪ The skeletal muscles are innervated by the axons originating from the anterior horn cells in the spinal cord. The motor unit is defined as one anterior horn cell, its axon, all of its neuromuscular junctions and the connected muscle fibers. When an action potential is created, all the muscle fibers in the motor unit are subsequently activated generating an MUAP.
     ▪ Three main parameters of MUAP are analyzed in needle EMG—amplitude, duration, and phase.
       • The amplitude and duration of MUAP represent the number of muscle fibers that fire in the motor unit.
       • Phases of the MUAP show the extent to which the muscle fibers in single motor unit fire at the same time—synchrony.
     ▪ When axon is lost or damaged, recovery from the injury occurs by the regrowth of the injured axon or collateral sprouting from the adjacent surviving axon. This process of reinnervation increases the number of muscle fibers that a given axon innervates. When there are a large number of muscle fibers that fire in a motor unit, the amplitude and the duration of the MUAP will increase. Since the large number of the muscle fibers may not fire at the same time, the phase of the MUAP will also increase.
     ▪ Detection of the abnormal MUAPs with large amplitudes, duration, and polyphasia signifies that the process of reinnervation has occurred. This process of reinnervation may take months to years to complete and its presence helps determine the age of the lesion. MUAPs with large amplitudes, long duration, and polyphasia suggest that the lesion is not acute and that it has been present for several months to years.
   ○ Recruitment of motor units:
     ▪ There are only two ways a muscle can increase its force of contraction—increasing the firing rate of the motor unit and bringing in additional motor units to fire (recruitment).
     ▪ As the force of contraction increases, firing rate of the motor units is increased and additional motor units are gradually activated.
     ▪ Recruitment refers to the successive activation of additional motor units to increase the force of muscle contraction.
     ▪ In conditions where axons are destroyed and the ability to recruit additional motor units is reduced, the muscle can only increase the firing rate of the motor units. In this situation, the recruitment pattern is reported to be reduced.
   ○ EMG is able to localize the lesions in the peripheral nervous system by detecting the muscles that have been denervated. It is also able to suggest the age of the lesion. Fibrillation potential indicates acute and ongoing lesion whereas MUAPs showing large amplitude, polyphasic, and long duration suggest old lesion.
   ○ EMG can also detect the direct muscle fiber damage that occurs in myopathy.
   ○ Instead of needle electrodes, surface electrodes can be used to record MUAPs. Surface electrodes are often used to monitor perineal muscle activity during urodynamic studies. The electrodes are placed on either side of anal orifice. Two electrodes are placed: the active (G1) is placed over the muscle under study and a reference (G2) placed at a slightly distant site. Surface electrodes are more convenient to use and cause less discomfort for the patients than needle electrodes. However, major limitations are that only the net electrical activity can be recorded and the individual MUAP cannot be analyzed. It is not possible to distinguish normal individual MUAPs from abnormal ones with surface electrode techniques.

PELVIC FLOOR ELECTROPHYSIOLOGY

The main electrophysiologic studies available for the study of female pelvic floor neurophysiology are sacral reflexes, pudendal NCS, sphincter needle EMG, and pudendal somatosensory evoked potentials.

SACRAL REFLEXES

• Reflex contraction of external anal muscle can be elicited by stimulation of urethra, bladder wall, or clitoris (urethral anal reflex, the bladder anal reflex, and the clitoral anal reflex). These reflexes can be analyzed electrophysiologically for abnormal or absent response. They are true reflexes with sensory afferent limb, intervening synapse, and motor efferent limb. Lesions anywhere along the reflex arc can result in abnormal response.
  ○ Urethral anal and bladder anal reflex

- The afferent pathways are hypogastric nerve to thoracolumbar cord for urethral anal reflex, and autonomic nerve to sacral cord for bladder anal reflex. The efferent limb is pudendal motor nerve for both.
- The test is performed using the Foley catheter ring electrode (two platinum wire rings placed 1 cm distal to the Foley balloon). The Foley catheter is used to carry and place the stimulating electrodes. It can be inserted to stimulate urethra or moved deeper into the bladder to stimulate the bladder. Surface electrodes placed near the anal mucocutaneous junction (external anal sphincter) on both sides are used to record the response.

○ Clitoral anal reflex
- The reflex arc involves somatic pathways with pudendal nerve participating as both afferent sensory and efferent motor limbs. The synapses are in the sacral cord.
- Prong electrodes are used to stimulate the clitoris. The responses are picked up at the external sphincter just as in the urethral anal and bladder anal reflexes.

○ Clinical application of sacral reflexes
- Sacral reflexes are normally suppressed during voiding. Inability to suppress the reflexes during voiding suggests upper motor neuron lesion in the suprasacral spinal cord.
- All the sacral reflexes are expected to be abnormal in cauda equina or conus medullaris lesions.
- Pelvic plexus lesions are usually seen after radical pelvic surgery or radiation therapy. The afferent and efferent pathways of the pudendal nerve in the clitoral anal reflex study are usually spared in these pelvic plexus injuries. The typical findings in the pelvic plexus lesions are abnormal urethra-anal and bladder-anal reflexes with preserved clitoral anal reflex.
- Pudendal nerve neuropathy is frequently seen with significant pelvic floor prolapse. Clitoral anal reflex is most profoundly affected because both afferent and efferent pathways are supplied by the pudendal nerve.

PUDENDAL NERVE MOTOR CONDUCTION STUDY

- The pudendal nerve originates from the lower division of lumbosacral plexus (anterior rami of S3 and S4). It exits the pelvis through the greater sciatic foramen and passes through Alcock's canal by the ischial spine.
- The pudendal nerve can be stimulated either transrectally (near Alcock's canal by ischial spine) or transvaginally. Transvaginal stimulation is generally more comfortable for patients.
- It is performed with St. Mark's pudendal electrode which is cleverly designed to allow mounting of electrodes

(both stimulating and recording) on the index finger of the disposable glove with adhesive sheet. It was originally developed for transrectal stimulation. The stimulating electrodes are attached at the tip of the finger permitting easy fingertip stimulation of the nerve while the recording electrodes are at the base of the finger in touch with external sphincter.
- The responses can also be recorded with separate surface electrodes placed on para-anal skin. Standard positioning of the recording electrodes on the para-anal skin (3–9 o'clock position for active and 6 o'clock position for reference in lithotomy position) allows more consistent and reproducible measurement of amplitudes.
- The pudendal nerve terminal motor latency (PNTML) has been found to be prolonged in fecal and urinary incontinence. Increases in pudendal distal motor latency has been found to occur in the first few days following vaginal delivery and normalizing within 2 months in two-thirds of women.
- The amplitude which reflects the total axon content and the actual strength of muscle contraction is also a valuable clinical parameter.

SPHINCTER NEEDLE ELECTROMYOGRAPHY

- The needle EMG of the external anal sphincter muscles is performed with the patient in the lithotomy position. Anesthetic cream is applied prior to the needle insertion. The ground plate is placed over bone such as iliac crest to reduce artifacts. The needle is inserted at the 3 and 9 o'clock position. At each insertion site, the needle is partially withdrawn and redirected superiorly, laterally, and inferiorly to sample different motor units.
- The urethral sphincter muscles can also be studied with needle EMG. The urethral sphincter may be approached either transvaginally or transperineally. The transvaginal route is less painful as the vaginal mucosa is less sensitive to needle insertion.
- Unlike the typical skeletal muscle, the skeletal muscle in the sphincter demonstrates continuous tonic activity, resting only at the onset of micturition or defecation. The fibrillation potentials which signify denervation of the muscle is best seen when the muscle is relaxed. Therefore, the identification of fibrillation potentials in the sphincter muscles can be challenging. Relaxing the muscles by having the patient attempting to void (with Foley catheter) can aid in recognizing fibrillation potentials.
- In the past, sphincter needle EMG was used to assist surgeons in locating damaged skeletal muscle of the external anal sphincter to aid in its repair. However, the endoanal ultrasound has largely replaced needle EMG in mapping external sphincter defect. Currently,

the main role of sphincter EMG is preoperative identification of irreparable sphincter neuropathy.

EVOKED POTENTIALS

- Following electrical stimulation of peripheral nerve, potentials are generated along the somatosensory pathways from the peripheral nerve to the cortex. The potentials recorded from central nervous tissue (spinal cord and cortex) are referred to as evoked potentials.
- The evoked potentials have small amplitudes and can only be identified against the background noise by computer averaging.

PUDENDAL NERVE SOMATOSENSORY EVOKED POTENTIAL

- Pudendal somatosensory evoked potential is obtained by applying stimulus adjacent to the clitoris.
- For the cortical recording, the active electrode is placed in the midline, 2 cm posterior to the halfway between the inion and the nasion (Cz1). The reference electrode is positioned in the upper mid-forehead (Fp). The electrodes are placed in the midline because the stimulation of the pudendal nerve activates the medial region of the contralateral cortex.
- The recording electrodes can also be placed over the spine for spinal cord response. However, the spinal responses are technically difficult to obtain in women.

- Pudendal somatosensory evoked potentials are primarily used to investigate suspected spinal cord pathology causing pelvic floor dysfunction such as in multiple sclerosis.

NEUROPHYSIOLOGY OF URINARY FUNCTION

- Frontal lobe is the site of conscious control of urinary voiding. It inhibits bladder contraction and voiding when socially undesirable. Infants have no control and reflexively urinate whenever bladder fills to a critical volume. Children are toilet trained at around age 2. They usually learn to walk and talk before being toilet trained suggesting that bladder control is a complex task.
- Pontine micturition center coordinates bladder contraction and sphincter relaxation. Normal micturition takes place when simultaneous bladder contraction and bladder outlet relaxation occur. This coordination requires intact connection between the pons and the sacral anterior horn cells (Onuf's nucleus) supplying the pelvic floor muscles via pudendal nerve (S2-S4). Voluntary interruption of the urination occurs with the contraction of the external sphincter muscles innervated by the pudendal nerve. The frontal lobe controls the timing of voiding by its influence on the micturition center. It is important to remind that the ability to inhibit bladder contractions is a cerebral event.
- The location of the neurological lesion would determine the type of bladder dysfunction (Table 10-1).

TABLE 10-1   Characterization of Voiding Problem by Location of Anatomic Lesion

LESION LOCATION	CLINICAL FEATURES	<>ELECTROPHYSIOLOGIC TESTS
Lesions above pontine micturition center (i.e., stroke, head trauma, Parkinson's disease, and brain tumor)	Loss of voluntary and involuntary inhibition of bladder contraction resulting in overactive bladder (detrusor hyperreflexia.) Coordinated bladder and sphincter activities are not affected.	Abnormal pudendal cortical evoked potentials Normal sacral reflexes with loss of suppression during voiding
Spinal cord lesions below the midbrain and above sacral cord	Detrusor hyperreflexia In some patients, coordinated bladder and sphincter activities are lost which can lead to bladder contraction against closed bladder outlet—detrusor sphincter dyssynergia. The high voiding pressure resulting from the dyssynergia may lead to hydronephrosis and chronic renal failure.	Normal sacral reflexes with loss of suppression during voiding
Sacral cord (conus medullaris)	Detrusor areflexia— acontractile bladder to high pressure poorly compliant bladder leading to overflow incontinence	Loss of sacral reflexes, abnormal pudendal conduction study and sphincter needle EMG
Cauda equina	Same as above	Abnormal sacral reflexes, pudendal NCS, and sphincter needle EMG
Pelvic plexus	Same as above	Abnormal urethral-anal and bladder- anal reflex with normal clitoral anal reflex
Pudendal nerve	Sensory loss in pudendal distribution Stress urinary incontinence and fecal incontinence	Abnormal clitoral anal reflex, pudendal NCS, and sphincter needle EMG

BIBLIOGRAPHY

Benson JT. *An AAEM Workshop: Pelvic Floor Neurophysiology.* Rochester, MN: American Association of Electrodiagnostic Medicine, Lippincott William and Wilkins October 1998.

Benson JT. Clinical neurophysiologic techniques in urinary and fecal incontinence. *Ostergard's Urogynecology and Pelvic Floor Dysfunction.* Philadelphia, PA: Lippincott Williams & Wilkins; 2003.

Benson JT. Electrophysiologic testing. In: Karram M.M., Walters M., eds. *Practical Urogynecology.* St. Louis, MO: Mosby; 1993.

Dumitru D. *Electrodiagnostic Medicine.* 2nd ed. Philadelphia, PA: Hanley & Belfus; 2002.

Fitzpatrick M, O'Herlihy C. The effects of labour and delivery on the pelvic floor. *Best Pract Res Clin Obstet Gynaecol.* 2001;15(1):63–79.

Hadley G. Pathophysiology of female voiding dysfunction. 4th Annual Seminar in Urology, Mammoth Lakes; 1994 Feb.

Preston D, Shapiro B. Electromyography and neuromuscular disorders, clinical-electrophysiologic correlations. Boston, MA: Butterworth-Heinemann; 1998.

QUESTIONS

1. The *most* common type of electrode used for EMG during multichannel cystometry is _____.
   - (A) Monopolar
   - (B) Concentric
   - (C) Surface
   - (D) Single fiber
2. A *true* statement about NCS is _____.
   - (A) It is particularly useful for evaluating upper motor neuron disorders.
   - (B) Axon loss results in smaller amplitude.
   - (C) Conduction block carries a poor prognosis as it is not reversible.
   - (D) Conduction block typically occurs when there is extensive axon loss.
3. A gravida 2, para 2, just delivered a baby weighing 4000 g by spontaneous vaginal delivery. When her pudendal nerve was stimulated with an electrical shock, the time to attain the MUAP was a few milliseconds longer than when the same test was performed before delivery. The best explanation is _____.
   - (A) Effect of progesterone withdrawal
   - (B) Decreased amplitude
   - (C) Increased latency
   - (D) Decreased propagation velocity
   - (E) Changed phase

4. A 63-year-old woman had a cerebrovascular accident 7 months ago. Now, voiding has become incomplete and ineffectual because of involuntary striated urethral sphincter activity. On further testing, she has elevated postvoid residuals and strong detrusor contractions when she attempts to void. The best test to diagnose this condition is _____.
   - (A) Pudendal somatosensory evoked potential
   - (B) EMG
   - (C) Sacral reflexes
   - (D) NCS
   - (E) Fibrillation potentials
5. During single-fiber concentric needle EMG of the striated urethral sphincter, increased activity can be seen during _____.
   - (A) Micturition
   - (B) Defecation
   - (C) Bladder filling
   - (D) Incontinence

ANSWERS

1. *(C).* Monopolar, concentric, and single fiber are all needle electrodes. These are not used often in the field of female pelvic medicine and reconstructive surgery (FPMRS). During complex cystometry, surface electrodes are placed near the external anal sphincter muscles. Surface electrodes may be helpful in measuring gross motor function to assess muscle groups which are active during micturition or bladder filling. These electrodes do not function if they become wet (during involuntary urine leakage).

2. *(B).* It is important to note that the NCS and EMG are only able to detect lower motor neuron lesions in the peripheral nervous system. Amplitude (mV) reflects the number of muscle fibers that fire. Low amplitude is caused by either axon loss or conduction block. If axon is damaged, fewer numbers of muscle fibers are in contact with their nerve supply and fewer will fire resulting in low amplitude. Conduction block occurs when the axon is intact but severe demyelination blocks traveling impulse.

3. *(C).* Studies have shown that there is an increase in PNTML after spontaneous vaginal delivery (60% of which recovered by 2 months; however, a third of those returning for follow-up *5 years after delivery* still may have evidence of nerve damage). Pregnancy itself caused no changes in PNTML.

Latencies were worse for forceps delivery, higher parity, and patients with longer second stage of labor. PNTML also correlate with increasing parity. Progesterone withdrawal does not change how fast the action potential is propagated. Amplitude (mV) reflects the number of muscle fibers that fire. Low amplitude is caused by either axon loss or conduction block. Conduction velocity can be calculated in the motor nerve conduction study if the nerve is stimulated at two different points and the length of the nerve between the stimulations can be estimated.

4. *(B)*. Detrusor sphincter dyssynergia (DSD) is a condition where there is a paradoxical contraction of the striated urethral sphincter muscles during voiding attempts. In a neurologically intact individual, the external sphincter relaxes when the detrusor contracts. DSD occurs in patients with neurological disorders such as multiple sclerosis and stroke. These patients have elevated residual urine volumes and trabeculations in the bladder on cystoscopy. EMG is the best way to diagnose this. Increased EMG activity (or persistence of EMG activity) is recorded during detrusor contractions (during voiding attempt), with intermittent urethral relaxation. The treatment is intermittent self-catheterization in addition to pharmacologic management (alpha blockers, baclofen, diazepam, and so forth).

5. *(C)*. During bladder filling and coughing, the striated urethral sphincter contracts as the patient attempts to hold fluid and inhibit voiding. On the other hand, during micturition or incontinence, the urethra is relaxed and thus urine is able to escape. During defecation, single-fiber EMG of the external anal sphincter (not the striated urethral sphincter) would show decreased activity.

11 URETHROCYSTOSCOPY

Uchechi Amy Wosu

Real-time evaluation of the urethra, bladder, and ureteral functioning has played an important role in obstetrics and gynecology. It is helpful in the investigation of chronic pelvic pain and incontinence revealing conditions such as interstitial cystitis, and urethral diverticula. Increasingly, this modality is becoming mainstream in the early detection of lower urinary tract injuries during gynecologic surgeries, especially pelvic reconstructive surgery.

In this chapter, the instrumentation, and components of a standard cystoscopic evaluation will be reviewed. The role of cystoscopy to evaluate urinary tract injury during gynecologic surgery, as well as pathologic findings seen on cystoscopy will also be discussed. Treatments using this technique and complications secondary to it are addressed.

INSTRUMENTATION

RIGID CYSTOSCOPY

The standard cystoscope is composed of three components: the telescope, the sheath, and the bridge.

THE TELESCOPE
- Required to transmit light to the bladder cavity as well as to provide an image for the examiner.
- The 30 degree lens provides the best view of the bladder base and the posterior wall. This lens is often used for diagnostic purposes and after operative procedures.
- The 70 degree lens is excellent for visualizing the anterior and lateral walls, and may be required in the presence of elevation of the urethrovesical junction.
- The 0 degree lens provides a straight ahead view, essentially for inspection of the urethra during urethroscopy.
- The 120 degree lens is not routinely used for female cystoscopy, but allows one to view the urethral opening into the bladder.

THE SHEATH
- The means by which the telescope and the distending media are introduced into the bladder.
- Various calibers are available, measured in the unit of French (Fr). They usually range from 17 to 28 Fr in adults. The smallest sheath is most easily tolerated for diagnostic purposes. Larger calibers are needed when performing operative cystoscopy and the placement of instruments via the sheath are required.
- The proximal end of the sheath has ports for the introduction and removal of the distending media.
- The distal end allows for the introduction of instruments for operative cystoscopy.

THE BRIDGE
- *The bridge* is the connector between the telescope and the sheath forming a watertight seal.

DISTENTION MEDIA
- *Distention media* comes in three types: nonconductive fluid, conductive fluid, and gas.

- Liquid media affords the advantage of washing away blood and debris that would otherwise limit visualization.
- Liquid media also allows the achievement of more physiologic bladder volumes.
- To achieve adequate flow of distending media, the height of the bag of media to be infused should be 80–100 cm above the patient's pubic bone.
- If absorption of a large amount of fluid into the vascular space is anticipated then an osmotic solution such as normal saline should be used. Systemic absorption of hypotonic solutions would lead to electrolyte imbalance.
- When electrocautery is needed, electrocautery may be used, a nonconducting fluid such as glycine or water is best.
- Carbon dioxide gas can be used which may be advantageous when bleeding is present. In such a case, blood would run down the walls rather than being dispersed in the media, obscuring the visual field. There are issues, however, with bubbling of the carbon dioxide gas, as well as bladder irritation from the formation of carbonic acid.

LIGHT SOURCES
- Provide adequate illumination via a fiberoptic or fluid-filled cable.
- A high-intensity light source such as xenon is appropriate for video monitoring.
- Fluid-filled cables tend to be more durable. Fiberoptic cables are flexible but more prone to damage.

FLEXIBLE CYSTOSCOPY

- Combines the optical systems and the irrigation-working channel in a single unit.
- The optical system is composed of one image-bearing fiberoptic bundle and two light-bearing bundles. These bundles are able to transmit light even when bent.
- Due to the flexibility of the fiberoptic bundles, a distal tip deflecting mechanism can deflect the tip as much as 290 degrees in a single plane.
- The image is not as clear as that obtained with the rigid cystoscope.
- Flexible cystoscopy can be more comfortable for the patient than rigid cystoscopy.

STANDARD CYSTOSCOPIC EVALUATION

Cystoscopy can be easily performed in the outpatient setting, namely, the office or an ambulatory clinic. The patient is placed in the lithotomy position. Usually, only topical anesthesia on the cystoscopic sheath is required at most to allow introduction of the cystoscope through the urethra into the bladder.

THE URETHRAL MUCOSA

- Visualized as the cystoscope passes through the urethra toward the bladder neck.
- Voiding causes the urethra to open widely.
- The urethrovesical junction normally closes with increases in abdominal pressure such as with coughing, or valsalva.

BLADDER MUCOSA

- The walls of the bladder are examined at each hour of an imaginary clock.
- Normal bladder mucosa on cystoscopy is pink and smooth, often with a glistening white hue.
- It is typical to see branched submucosal vasculature.

THE TRIGONE

- Shaped as an inverted triangle with the urethrovesical junction at the inferior apex, and the superior apices formed by the ureteral orifices.
- Reddened granular appearance, different from the bladder mucosa. On closer inspection, it is covered with a thickened white membrane, with a villous contour. This difference is accounted for, by different embryologic origins (mesonephric).
- The interureteric ridge is an elevation forming the superior boundary of the trigone.
- The ureteral orifices appear as slitlike openings on either side of the interureteric ridge. These slits open with the efflux of urine, signifying the patency of the ureters.

EVALUATION OF URINARY TRACT INJURY DURING PELVIC SURGERY

The urinary tract is in danger of injury during gynecologic surgery given its close proximity to pelvic organs. Early recognition can prevent major morbidity including renal damage and urogenital fistula formation. Cystoscopy is an excellent adjunct to gynecologic surgery to identify lower urinary tract injuries even before leaving the operating room.

It is fairly well established that cystoscopy should be used with complex reconstructive surgery of the pelvic floor (e.g., uterosacral ligament vault suspension), particularly those involving procedures for urinary incontinence (e.g., TVT or Burch). Many practitioners also use cystoscopy in the operating room with other gynecologic procedures when dissection in the area of the lower urinary tract is difficult, as would occur in the case of extensive pelvic adhesions. Performing cystoscopy during what is considered to be routine gynecologic surgery is still a matter of debate. Some clinicians advocate its use during all gynecologic surgeries, while others reserve it for particularly difficult cases in which they are concerned about lower urinary tract injury.

TYPES OF INJURY

THE BLADDER
- Can be injured as a result of perforation from sharp dissection, cautery, or inappropriate suture placement.

THE URETER
- The close proximity of the ureter to the ovarian and uterine vasculature makes ureteral injury such a concern. The ureter courses over the bifurcation of the iliac vessels at the pelvic brim. It also travels in the cardinal ligament passing beneath the uterine artery 1.5 cm lateral to the cervix at the level of the internal os? The ureter also passes medially over the anterolateral vaginal fornix before entering the bladder at the trigone.
- The ureter can be ligated, kinked, transected, burned, crushed, and devascularized from extensive dissection.
- A difficult surgery due to factors such as extensive pelvic adhesions from endometriosis, or distorted anatomic relationships from a large fibroid uterus increases the chance of ureteral injury.
- Ureter can be kinked after a uterosacral ligament vault suspension stitch that is placed too laterally.

IDENTIFICATION OF URINARY TRACT INJURY DURING PELVIC SURGERY

VAGINAL SURGERY
- The patient is in an ideal position for standard transurethral cystoscopy.

- One ampule (5 mL) of indigo carmine is given intravenously. This will stain the urine blue. A 30 or 70 degree endoscope is introduced transurethrally.
- The bladder mucosa is inspected in a systematic clockwise fashion, looking for any evidence of operative trauma such as intraluminal sutures or perforation. The ureteral orifices are then visualized.
- Without ureteral injury, a definite blue effluent would be seen emanating from the orifices approximately 5–10 minutes after the administration of indigo carmine. Sometimes some lasix may be needed to concentrate this.
- Delayed or absent efflux of urine from either ureter suggests injury.

ABDOMINAL PROCEDURE
- If an abdominal procedure is being performed, the patient can be repositioned in the dorsal lithotomy position which can be cumbersome and time consuming.
- *Suprapubic telescopy* can be performed, in which the telescope is introduced through a purposeful cystotomy.
  - The extraperitoneal dome of the bladder is entered.
  - A purse-string suture (chromic or delayed absorbable) is placed, and the purposeful cystotomy is made within it.
  - A 0 or 30 degree telescope is placed within the bladder through the cystotomy.
  - The purse-string suture is then cinched tightly. Inspection of the bladder mucosa and ureteral orifices is performed as mentioned in the earlier section.
  - After the telescope is removed, a Foley catheter can be introduced into the purposeful cystotomy through a separate skin stab wound for suprapubic drainage.
  - Alternatively, the purse-string suture is tied and imbricated, and a transurethral Foley catheter is placed.
  - See Chap. 33 for intraoperative repair of urinary tract injury.

DIAGNOSIS OF PATHOLOGY BY CYSTOSCOPY

Cystoscopy is helpful in the workup of a variety of issues often seen in gynecology, such as incontinence, recurrent urinary tract infections, or persistent symptoms of intractable dysuria. Urinary stones, urethral diverticula, fistulous tracts, cancer, and findings suggestive of interstitial cystitis can be diagnosed with office cystoscopy.

URETHRAL FINDINGS

- *Chronic urethritis*—associated with erythematous mucosa, possibly with exudates. Fronds or polyps may also been seen.
- *Urethral diverticula*—ostium along the lateral or posterior surface of the urethra. Exudate may be expressed from the ostium on palpation.
- *Urethral stricture*—this is seen as a narrowing of the urethra typically at the meatus.
- *Hypoestrogenism*—appears as pale epithelium.

CYSTOSCOPIC FINDINGS

- *Bacterial cystitis:* This would appear as normal urothelium to pink or peach-colored macules or papules. Edema and hypervascularity may also be present. As would be expected, symptoms include pain and burning with urination, urgency, and frequency.
- *Hemorrhagic cystitis:* On cystoscopy, this may appear as individual or confluent mucosal hemorrhages. A patient may present with hematuria and irritative voiding symptoms.
- *Radiation cystitis:* These are areas of hemorrhage surrounded by pale mucosa, fibrotic and hypovascular.
- *Interstitial cystitis:*
  - Interstitial cystitis is an inflammatory bladder condition of unknown etiology and is a diagnosis of exclusion, characterized by urinary frequency, nocturia, urgency, suprapubic pressure, and bladder pain.
  - This condition commonly affects women between the ages of 40 and 60 years.
  - To diagnose the condition, patients undergo *fill-refill* cystoscopy. The bladder is initially distended with 80–100 cm of water pressure for 1–2 minutes. To achieve adequate flow of distending media, the height of the bag of media to be infused should be 100 cm above the patient's pubic bone. The bladder is emptied, and then redistended to look for mucosal lesions.
  - The typical pathognomonic lesion is that of diffuse petechial hemorrhages, coalescing to form larger hemorrhagic areas. Lesions in severe forms of interstitial cystitis are velvety red patches or linear cracks seen with a granulating base, and surrounding vascular congestion.

- *Chronic inflammation:*
  - There is a pattern of appearance referred to as cystitis cystica. This appears as clear mucosal cysts found in multiple areas over the base of the bladder. These cysts are formed by subepithelial transitional cells which degenerate.
  - Another pattern seen on cystoscopy for chronic inflammation is referred to as cystitis glandularis. As discussed earlier, cysts are apparent at the bladder base, but are not clear and have a less uniform contour. There is an association between cystitis glandularis and adenocarcinoma.
- *Genitourinary neoplasms:* Histologic types range from transitional cell carcinoma, adenocarcinoma, and even squamous cell carcinoma which occurs more in association with a chronic indwelling catheter. Depending on the type and grade, neoplasms may appear as raised lesions with a feathery or papillary texture.
- *Auxiliary ureteral orifices:* The ectopic ureter enters the bladder slightly superior to the trigone near the other ureteral orifice.
- *Ureteroceles:* These present as herniation into the vesical cavity during efflux of urine.
- *Trabeculations:* With distention, smooth muscle ridges become prominent. They appear as interlaced cords, with intervening sacculations. This represents hypertrophied detrusor musculature seen with detrusor overactivity or bladder outlet obstruction.
- *Bladder diverticulum:* With high intravesical pressure, there is enlargement in the intervening sacculations seen with trabeculations. Neoplasms have been reported in the interior of these diverticula in 7% of cases.
- *Vesicovaginal fistulas:*
  - If there is a high index of suspicion that a vesicovaginal fistula has developed, cystoscopy is helpful in the diagnostic process.
  - Upon inspection, the edges of the fistulous tract appear edematous and hyperemic. The most common location of posthysterectomy fistulas is at the bladder base, superior to the interureteric ridge, corresponding to the level of the vaginal cuff.
  - 75% of vesicovaginal fistulas result from abdominal hysterectomies. Other etiologies include vaginal hysterectomy, urologic procedures, radiation, foreign bodies, cancer, and obstetric trauma.
  - Fistulous tracts can be small, or several centimeters in diameter. Patients may present with continuous watery vaginal discharge.
  - Up to 25% of vesicovaginal fistulas have concomitant ureterovaginal fistulas, which should be evaluated with retrograde ureteropyelography.

- *Vesicoenteric fistula:*
  - Fistula may have surrounding inflammation, and bulbous edema.
  - Fistulous tract is indiscernible in 60% of cases.
  - Etiologies are similar to those of vesicovaginal fistulas. In addition, severe inflammatory bowel disease (i.e., Crohon's) may result in a fistulous tract.
- *Bladder calculi:* Stones appear in a variety degrees of shapes, sizes, and colors accompanied by varying of mucosal inflammation.

TREATMENTS

- Cystoscopy is also used for treatment purposes. Bulking agents injected into the urethra are being used in an effort to address urinary incontinence. The material, often collagen, is injected at 3 and 9 o'clock position, distal to urethrovesical junction providing coaptation. This is an excellent way to address incontinence for the appropriately selected patient in the office setting.
- Injection of botulinum toxin into the posterior bladder wall for patients with persistent overactive bladder is also done cystosioptically; usually multiple injections are required per session.

COMPLICATIONS

- Minimal complications associated with cystoscopy.
- The most common complication postoperatively is urinary tract infection with an incidence of <4%. Prophylactic antibiotics may minimize this infection risk.
- After cystoscopy, pyridium may help reduce bladder irritation.
- The incidence of bacteriuria after outpatient cystoscopy is 2–7%. Most patients have no or very few symptoms, and it often resolves spontaneously. Neither meticulous aseptic technique, nor antibiotics reduces the incidence of infection. Nonetheless, many clinicians do prescribe a short course of antibiotics after the procedure. Appropriate prophylactic antibiotics should be given to patients at risk for subacute endocarditis.
- Bladder perforation can occur when the endoscope is not inserted under direct visualization, which occurs infrequently.
- Difficulty passing the endoscope through the urethra can cause trauma or a false passage.

SUMMARY

Cystoscopy is a fairly safe and easy procedure that is being used increasingly in obstetrics and gynecology.

It can provide early identification of lower urinary tract injuries in the operating room, thereby limiting postoperative morbidity. This procedure is also helpful in the office setting for the workup of issues such as incontinence, recurrent urinary tract infections and symptoms of persistent dysuria. Cystoscopy also lends itself to outpatient management of conditions such as urinary incontinence with the help of bulking agents. This versatile and safe procedure will most likely become more mainstream in the practice of obstetrics and gynecology.

BIBLIOGRAPHY

Aronson MP, Bose TM. Urinary tract injury in pelvic surgery. *Clin Obstet Gynecol.* 2002;45(2):428–438.

Bent A, Cundiff G. Cystourethroscopy. In: Baggish M, Karram M, eds. *Atlas of Pelvic Anatomy and Gynecologic surgery.* Saunders; 2001.

Cundiff GW, Bent AE. Endoscopic evaluation of the lower urinary tract. In: Walters MD, Karram MM, eds. *Urogynecology and reconstructive pelvic surgery.* 2nd ed. St. Louis: Mosby; 1999.

Ferro A, Byck D, Gallup D. Intraoperative and postoperative morbidity associated with cystoscopy performed in patients undergoing gynecologic surgery. *Am J Obstet Gynecol.* 2003;189(2):354–57.

Gilmour DT, Dwyer PL, Carey MP. Lower urinary tract injury during gynecologic surgery and its detection by intraoperative cystoscopy. *Obstet Gynecol.* 1999;94(5 Pt 2):883–89.

Kwon CH, Godberg RP, Koduri S, et al. The use of intraoperative cystoscopy in major vaginal and urogynecologic surgeries. *Am J Obstet Gynecol.* 2002;187(6):1466–1472.

Reuter MA, Reuter HJ. The development of the cystoscope. *J Urol.* 1998;159(3):638–640.

Weinberger MW. Cystourethroscopy for the practicing gynecologist. *Clin Obstet Gynecol.* 1998;41(3):764–776.

Yossepowitch O, Baniel J, Livine P. Urological injuries during cesarean section: intraoperative diagnosis and management. *J Urol.* 2004;172(1):196–99.

QUESTIONS

1. A 63-year-old para 3 has just undergone placement of one trocar arm during the tension-free vaginal tape procedure from the vaginal incision, through the retropubic space, and exiting the abdominal incision above the right pubic tubercle. During cystoscopy, to assure appropriate placement, the trocar

was noted to enter the bladder from the lateral wall at 8 o'clock and exit the bladder at 11 o'clock position. Which lens would afford the best view of this injury?

(A) 0 degree lens

(B) 70 degree lens

(C) 30 degree lens

(D) 120 degree lens

(E) None of the above

2. During diagnostic cystoscopy of a normal bladder, you would expect to see the following except:

(A) Smooth bladder mucosal surface with a glistening white hue.

(B) The trigone covered with a thickened white membrane, with a villous contour.

(C) Slitlike openings found on either side of the interureteric ridge.

(D) Numerous diffuse petechial hemorrhages that may coalesce to form larger hemorrhagic areas.

(E) None of the above.

3. Delayed or absent efflux of urine from the ureters on cystoscopy after a difficult hysterectomy can be seen with which of the following ureteral injuries?

(A) Burn injury due to electrocautery

(B) Extensive retroperitoneal dissection of the ureter

(C) Crush injury of a segment of ureter

(D) Transection of the ureter

(E) All of the above

4. A 44-year-old female has persistent complaints of urinary frequency, nocturia, urgency, suprapubic pressure, and bladder pain despite repeatedly normal urine cultures to evaluate her symptoms. You suspect interstitial cystitis and attempt to perform cystoscopy in the operating room to evaluate her bladder mucosa after bladder distention. As you attempt to fill her bladder, you notice that there is minimal flow of the distending media. You look at the height of the distending media fluid on the IV pole and note that it is at 30 cm above the patient. What is the appropriate height of the distending media to provide adequate flow?

(A) 20 cm above symphysis pubis

(B) 50 cm above symphysis pubis

(C) 100 cm above symphysis pubis

(D) 130 cm above symphysis pubis

(E) None of the above

5. You wish to take your 57-year-old patient with genuine stress incontinence, and grade 2 cystocele to the operating room to perform an anterior vaginal

wall repair, and tension-free vaginal tape procedure with cystoscopy. As you review the risks of the procedure, what would you describe as the most common complication attributable to cystoscopy alone?

(A) Bladder perforation

(B) Urinary tract infection

(C) Urethral disruption

(D) None of the above

Answers

1. *(B)*. 70 degree lens. The tension-free vaginal tape procedure is a minimally invasive mid-urethral sling procedure that has significantly emerged in the treatment of urinary stress incontinence. It affords the convenience of time, as it should only take approximately 15–20 minutes to perform barring any unforeseen difficulties. As such it is easily coupled with other pelvic floor procedures that a person may need without significantly adding to operating room time. If it is the only procedure needed, the patient can go home the same day and expect a short recuperation time. Complications include cystotomy, retropubic hematoma, and urinary retention. The procedure involves placing a prolene mesh beneath the mid-urethra. This is accomplished with the help of steel, curved trocars attached to each end of the mesh that guides the ends of the mesh from an anterior vaginal incision made beneath the mid-urethra, to abdominal incision sites above the pubic tubercles. While care is taken to keep the bladder out of the way of the course of steel trocars, cystotomy is a common complication. The location of bladder injury is usually the lateral walls of the bladder. There are often entry and exit holes corresponding to the course of the trocar. Due to this common complication, cystoscopy is performed after each trocar has been guided to the abdominal incision. The 70 degree lens affords the best view of the anterior and lateral walls of the bladder, making it an excellent choice to inspect for this sort of bladder injury. The 30 degree lens is good for the inspection of the bladder base and the posterior wall. The 120 degree lens is not routinely used for female cystoscopy, but allows one to view the urethral opening into the bladder. The 0 degree lens allows one to look straight ahead and is essential for urethroscopy, but not ideal for cystoscopy.

2. *(D)*. Normal bladder mucosa on cystoscopy is pink and smooth, often with a glistening white hue. It is also typical to see branched submucosal vasculature. The trigone is shaped as an inverted triangle with the urethrovesical junction at the inferior apex, and the superior apices formed by the ureteral orifices. Trigone itself has a reddened granular appearance, different from the bladder mucosa. On closer inspection, it is covered with a thickened white membrane, with a villous contour. This difference is accounted for by different embryologic origins. The interureteric ridge is an elevation forming the superior boundary of the trigone. The ureteral orifices appear as slitlike openings on either side of the interureteric ridge. These slits open with the efflux of urine. Diffuse petechial hemorrhages, coalescing to form larger hemorrhagic areas are one of the pathognomonic lesions seen in interstitial cystitis. Rare petechiae may be seen in normal patients usually caused by trauma from the cystoscope. Interstitial cystitis is an inflammatory bladder condition of unknown etiology, characterized by urinary frequency, nocturia, urgency, suprapubic pressure, and bladder pain. To diagnose the condition, general anesthesia is required to fill the bladder to its maximum capacity. In more severe forms of interstitial cystitis, velvety red patches or linear cracks are seen with a granulating base, and surrounding vascular congestion.

3. *(E)*. Approximately 82% of all urinary tract injuries are caused by operations in the pelvis. 75% of ureteral injuries occur during gynecologic surgery, and 75% of those are during abdominal procedures. The close proximity of the ureter to the ovarian and uterine vasculature makes ureteral injury such a concern in these procedures. The ureter courses over the bifurcation of the iliac vessels at the pelvic brim. It also travels in the cardinal ligament passing beneath the uterine artery 1.5 cm lateral to the cervix at the level of the internal os. The ureter also passes medially over the anterolateral vaginal fornix before entering the bladder at the trigone. Given these anatomic relationships, one must always be mindful during a hysterectomy, and other pelvic procedures about the location of the ureter to prevent injury. The ureter can be ligated, kinked, transected, burned, crushed, and devascularized from extensive dissection. A difficult surgery due to factors such as extensive pelvic adhesions from endometriosis, or distorted anatomic relationships from a large fibroid uterus, increases the chance of ureteral injury. To diagnose ureteral injury intraoperatively using cystoscopy, one ampule (5 mL) of indigo carmine is given intravenously. This will stain the urine blue. A 30 or 70 degree endoscope is introduced transurethrally. The ureteral orifices are then visualized. Without ureteral injury, a definite blue effluent would be seen emanating from the orifices approximately 5 minutes after the administration of indigo carmine. Delayed or absent efflux of urine from either ureter is cause for concern that an injury might have taken place. During abdominal procedures where the patient is not in the lithotomy position, suprapubic telescopy with visualization of the ureters to look for the efflux of urine is also valid. In this case, the endoscope is introduced into a purposeful, extraperitoneal cystotomy.

4. *(C)*. Interstitial cystitis is an inflammatory bladder condition of unknown etiology, characterized by urinary frequency, nocturia, urgency, suprapubic pressure, and bladder pain. This condition commonly affects women between the ages of 40 and 60 years. To diagnose the condition, patients undergo *fill-refill* cystoscopy. The bladder is initially distended with 80–100 cm of water pressure for 1–2 minutes. To achieve adequate flow of distending media, the height of the bag of media to be infused should be 100 cm above the patient's pubic bone. The bladder is emptied, and then redistended to look for mucosal lesions. The typical pathognomonic lesion is that of diffuse petechial hemorrhages, coalescing to form larger hemorrhagic areas. Lesions in severe forms of interstitial cystitis are velvety red patches or linear cracks seen with a granulating base and surrounding vascular congestion.

5. *(B)*. Cystoscopy is a quick benign procedure with minimal complications. The most common complication postoperatively is urinary tract infection with an incidence of <4%. Prophylactic antibiotics may minimize this infection risk.

The incidence of bacteriuria after outpatient cystoscopy is 2–7%. Most patients have no or very few symptoms, and it often resolves spontaneously. Neither meticulous aseptic technique nor antibiotics reduces the incidence of infection. Nonetheless, many clinicians do prescribe a short course of antibiotics after the procedure. Appropriate prophylactic antibiotics should be given to patients at risk for subacute endocarditis.

Bladder perforation can occur when the endoscope is not inserted under direct visualization, which occurs infrequently. Difficulty passing the endoscope through the urethra can cause trauma or a false passage.

12 RADIOLOGIC IMAGING OF PELVIC FLOOR AND LOWER URINARY TRACT

Lindsey Huber and Sam Siddighi

INTRODUCTION

- Radiologic studies remain one of the key components in the evaluation of the lower urinary tract. These studies help to detect abnormalities and dysfunctions.
- Traditionally, the plain film and intravenous pyelogram (IVP) have been the cornerstone radiographic tests that were conducted to diagnose problems of the lower urinary tract.
- Since the development of newer technologies, namely, computed tomography (CT) and magnetic resonance imaging (MRI), the clinician is now able to diagnose a broader variety of urologic and urogynecologic abnormalities.
- This chapter will briefly summarize the radiologic tests available to the clinician and how each should be utilized in the clinical setting in order to accurately diagnose a disease with minimal risk to the patient and at a minimal cost.
- Two useful radiologic studies for the evaluation of pelvic floor dysfunction and the lower genitourinary (GU) tract are MRI and CRCU (aka *colporectocystourethrography*). These are described in more detail at the end of this chapter.

THE PLAIN FILM

- The main purpose of the plain film of the abdomen is to screen for urinary calculi.
- This test could also unveil abnormal gas patterns in the gastrointestinal tract, masses, bony lesions, and calculi in suburethral diverticula.
- Advantages: (1) readily available and (2) inexpensive.
- Disadvantage: it exposes the patient to ionizing radiation.

SIMPLE CYSTOGRAPHY

- Cystography is the modality that is used most commonly to detect injury to the bladder from trauma or surgical procedure.

- It is also used to detect bladder diverticula or possible fistulas between the bladder and adjacent organs (e.g., vesicovaginal fistulas).
- Procedure
  - Obtain a postvoid residual (PVR) on a patient and then take a plain film.
  - Next, the bladder is filled under low pressure to capacity with a contrast medium either through the urethra or a suprapubic catheter and then another plain film is shot.
  - After the bladder is drained, another film is obtained in order to evaluate for extravasation of contrast medium.
  - Extravasation from an extraperitoneal leak will appear as an irregular mass around the site of injury and will remain there for a long period of time.
  - Leakage from intraperitoneal injury will appear in the entire abdominal cavity and will be absorbed quickly.
- Contraindication: acute urinary tract infection.
- Complication: (1) urinary tract infection, so prophylactic antibiotics are recommended, (2) contrast medium may cause detrusor overactivity, urethral spasm, mucosal irritation, vesicoureteral reflux or uncontrollable urine loss.

INTRAVENOUS PYELOGRAM

- The IVP continues to be the modality of choice to visualize the urinary tract.
- IVP is performed by injecting the patient with a contrast medium and then allowing it to travel through the patient's blood stream until it reaches the urinary system where several radiologic images are then taken in succession.
- The IVP provides detailed anatomic and functional information about the urinary tract.
  - Evaluation of ureteral obstruction
  - Urolithiasis
  - Fistula
  - Congenital anomalies
  - Detailing the course of the pelvic ureters when evaluating pelvic masses
  - Preexisting abnormalities (i.e., a nonfunctioning kidney or hydronephrosis)
  - Incidental abnormalities
    - Bladder and suburetheral diverticula
    - Residual urine
- Advantages: (1) relatively safe, (2) inexpensive, and (3) usually readily available to the clinician.
- Disadvantages:

○ In a situation of acute ureteral obstruction the opacification of the urinary tract is generally delayed for several hours or more because of the decrease in glomerular filtration and the increased water and sodium reabsorption in the proximal convoluted tubule.

○ A clinician may not be able to see calyceal dilation for anywhere from 24 to 48 hours after the onset of patient symptoms.

○ Some abnormalities appear as nonspecific (such as radiolucent filling defects). When this situation occurs, it becomes necessary to utilize other diagnostic imaging modalities to diagnose the patient's condition.

• Contraindications:
  ○ History of a severe reaction to contrast medium
  ○ Moderate to severe renal failure
  ○ Renal insufficiency: Patients with renal insufficiency may not be able to either excrete an adequate amount of contrast medium to opacify the urinary tract or the contrast medium itself has the potential to worsen the renal insufficiency. Therefore check BUN/creatinine prior to precedure.
  ○ Relative contraindications: mild renal insufficiency and congestive heart failure

• Alternatives to IVP are retrograde or anterograde pyelogram
  ○ Retrograde pyelogram:
    ▪ Performed by inserting a cone-tipped catheter into the ureteral orifice under fluoroscopic guidance and injecting contrast medium.
    ▪ This procedure can be valuable when there is a coexisting reason for cystoscopy.
    ▪ Disadvantages: (1) increased rate of infection, (2) systemic absorption if a large enough amount of contrast medium is injected under pressure.
    ▪ Contraindications: (1) known allergy to contrast medium, (2) recent lower urinary tract trauma, (3) recent surgery.
  ○ Anterograde pyelogram:
    ▪ Consists of placing the patient in a prone position and then inserting a 22- or 25-gauge needle into the collecting system under ultrasound or fluoroscopic guidance after intravenous (IV) contrast has been administered.
    ▪ This procedure is performed rarely for diagnostic purposes alone.
    ▪ Is usually performed when there is a coexisting indication for percutaneous puncture. It provides the clinician with an exceptional view of the renal collecting system.
    ▪ In the case of a suspected obstruction, the patient needs to undergo decompression before injection of the contrast medium in order to avoid overdistention or urosepsis.
    ▪ Disadvantage: increase in the rate of infection.

VOIDING CYSTOURETHROGRAPHY

• This is a dynamic procedure that enables a physician to evaluate the anatomy of the bladder and urethra.
• To extract the most information from this modality, it should be used in conjunction with an assessment of bladder function and capacity.
• It is used to detect possible suburethral diverticula, increased bladder volume, vesicoureteral reflux, and congenital abnormalities.
• This procedure is performed by filling the bladder with contrast medium through a catheter and then removing the catheter and obtaining a radiograph while the patient is actively voiding.
• Disadvantage: some patients may not be able to void in the laboratory setting.

POSITIVE-PRESSURE URETHROGRAPHY

• The positive-pressure urethrography is utilized as a diagnostic test to evaluate the urethra and search for possible suburethral diverticula that were not discovered by a voiding cystourethrography (VCUG).
• The procedure consists of using a Trattner catheter (which has two balloons with an opening in the lumen of the catheter between the balloons that the contrast medium can pass through).
• The proximal balloon is inserted into the bladder and the distal or sliding balloon is placed just outside of the external urethra meatus.
• This creates a temporary closed system that enables the contrast to fill the urethra and opacify the diverticulum.
• This is now mainly of historical importance because it is technically difficult to perform and is usually painful for the patient unless general anesthesia is used.

ULTRASOUND

• Ultrasound has become an increasingly important diagnostic tool of urinary tract diseases due to major technological advances.
• Advantages: (1) noninvasive, (2) relatively inexpensive, (3) does not require contrast medium, and (4) does not expose the patient to ionizing radiation.
• Disadvantages: (1) quality of the study varies greatly, (2) is operator dependent, and (3) does not provide any physiologic information.

- Ultrasound can be performed by various routes: transabdominal, transvaginal, transperineal, and transrectal.
  - The transabdominal ultrasound evaluates adynamic changes.
  - This is used to assess hydronephrosis, the renal parenchyma, renal calculi, measure PVR volumes, bladder tumors, suburethral diverticula, and anatomic defects associated with urge and stress incontinence.
  - This modality is very sensitive for detecting pelvicaliceal dilation; however, it cannot determine the degree of the obstruction or differentiate whether the hydronephrosis is due to an obstructive or nonobstructive process.
  - Disadvantage: it cannot delineate the course of the ureters as they travel retroperitoneally causing difficulties with visualization and localization of an obstruction below the ureteropelvic junction.
- The transvaginal ultrasound is best for visualizing structures of the lower urinary tract, diagnose suburethral diverticula, and measure bladder volume.
- The transperineal ultrasound can also be used to detect suburethral diverticula and to locate any calculi that are in the diverticula.
- Transanal ultrasound is useful for detecting defects in the internal and external anal sphincters which can lead to fecal incontinence.

ENDOLUMINAL SONOGRAPHY

- This modality provides the physician with a three-dimensional image that is useful for evaluating strictures, masses, stones, and normal anatomic variants of the upper urinary tract.
- This technique uses an ultrasound transducer placed in a small diameter catheter in order to assess the lumen of the urethra, ureter, and renal pelvis.
- The catheter can be positioned in the upper urinary tract by retrograde or anterograde route.

DOPPLER SONOGRAPHY

- A Doppler supplies the clinician with physiologic information about the urinary tract.
- This modality is utilized to diagnose ureteral obstruction and detect channels between the urethra and the diverticula.
- Advantage: it allows detection of acute ureteral obstruction before the onset of pelvicaliceal dilation. The Doppler detects ureteral obstruction by utilization of the transvaginal color transducer to relay information about the presence or absence of urine entering the bladder (ureteric jet phenomenon).

- Disadvantages: (1) geometric fluctuations in the jet frequency may result in prolonged or false positive studies, (2) technical problems, and (3) the requirement of greater operator experience.

VIDEOCYSTOURETHROGRAPHY

- Videocystourethrography is unique because the physician visualizes the urethral sphincter and bladder while recording urodynamic data.
- This modality combines the fluoroscopic VCUG with recordings of urine flow rate, vesicular, intraurethral, and intra-abdominal pressures.
- This is utilized to diagnose urethral diverticula and vesicoureteral reflux.
- Videocystourethrography is useful for the following: (1) failed incontinence surgery, (2) urologic disease, (3) voiding disorders, and (4) complex data with ambiguous results.
- This imaging technique is considered the gold standard in urodynamic examination.
- Disadvantages: (1) some women cannot void while standing, (2) the exposure to radiation, (3) high cost.
- A newer technique that may replace videocystourethrography in the future utilizes perineal ultrasound while recording urodynamic data. The major advantages of this modality are twofold: (1) the patient is sitting (allows evaluation of the lower urinary tract in its physiologic position) and (2) there is no exposure to radiation.

COMPUTED TOMOGRAPHY

- The helical CT is a relatively new tool for physicians and provides superb anatomic detail of not only the upper and lower urinary tract, but also structures that are adjacent to or far from the ureter.
  - CT is the study of choice for evaluation of the upper tract.
  - Images seen allow both direct cross-sectional views of the entire urinary tract, images in several different planes and the computer generates a three-dimensional picture.
  - CT obtains images quickly.
- Disadvantages: (1) cost, (2) exposure to radiation, (3) soft tissue not seen with as much detail as provided by MRI.
- During the evaluation of a patient, if IVP, sonogram, or retro- or anterograde pyelography fail to show the presence or cause of ureteral obstruction the next step in management is CT. Many clinicians would order a CT scan from the outset.
- One study using noncontrast-enhanced helical CT to investigate acute flank pain due to an unknown cause

found that in approximately 5 minutes, CT scan accurately determines the cause of ureteral obstruction or whether that cause relates to the urethra or is nonrenal.

- Helical CT is also useful for detecting stones.
  - Stones are one of the most common causes of acute flank pain and ureteral obstruction.
  - Stones are mostly composed of calcium and are radiopaque on plain film.
  - However, a small percentage of stones are composed of xanthine or uric acid and are radiolucent on plain film.
  - A helical CT can determine the exact location and size of a stone regardless of its composition.

COLORECTOCYSTOURETHROGRAPHY (CRCU)

- A radiologic technique introduced in France in 1965
- It is a type of fluoroscopic study in which images are obtained in the lateral projection under rest, strain, and contracted states
- Technique
  - Patient drinks two cups of barium fluid 1–2 hours before procedure.
  - Patient lies in supine position on a mobile x-ray table.
  - Bladder is catheterized and 50 cc of contrast is instilled.
  - Urethra is filled with 3 cc of barium sulfate cream.
  - Vagina is painted with thick barium paste (powder + water).
  - Rectum is filled with 50 cc of barium paste.
  - Radiopaque marker is placed on perineal body.
  - Static pictures: patient is in upright, sitting position on commode and x-ray pictures (lateral view) are taken with pelvic floor muscles at rest, contracted, and during strain.
  - Dynamic pictures: patient sits on commode, and x-ray video is taken during defecation and micturition.

- For evaluation of pelvic floor defects, standing position is better.

Normal pelvic floor

- Allows indirect visualization of pelvic floor muscles
- Allows visualization of anterior, apical, posterior pelvic organ prolapse (POP) and urethral mobility
  - *Urethral hypermobility* can be demonstrated by superimposing the rest and strain films of the urethrovesical junction. Patients with SUI have anterior and inferior movement of urethrovesical junction.
  - *Intrinsic sphincteric deficiency (ISD)* can be demonstrated when the urethrovesical junction is funnel-shaped at rest.
  - *Kinking* of the urethra with advanced anterior POP can be seen on CRCU.
  - *Anterior POP* can be seen directly on CRCU and may be underestimated on static pictures in comparison to dynamic pictures.
  - *Posterior POP* can also be seen directly on CRCU.
  - *Uterine prolapse, vaginal wall prolapse, and enterocele* can be seen on CRCU when there is widening of the vaginal line between the bladder and rectal echolucencies.
- Allows visualization of puborectalis muscle dysfunction
  - Normally, with relaxation of the puborectalis, the anorectal angle becomes obtuse (see Table 12-1).
  - In puborectalis muscle dysfunction, with relaxation of puborectalis, the anorectal angle remains acute.
- Allows visualization of improper sling position, suburethral diverticula, vesicovaginal fistula, and postsurgical stenosis of urethra
- Patients who successfully completed pelvic floor rehabilitation programs have greater
  - ↓ in anorectal angle (i.e., more acute angle)
  - ↓ in urethrovesical inclination
  - ability to lift bladder base and posterior rectal wall
- May be indicated for the following patients:
  - Failed previous UI or POP surgery
  - Postsurgical UI
  - Women whose physical examination is inadequate (e.g., elderly)

TABLE 12-1 Shape of Pelvic Floor and Related Structures at Various States of Contraction

	AT REST	CONTRACTION	STRAINING
Levator hiatus	Narrow	More narrowing	Open
Pelvic floor shape	Basin	Flat (moves up)	Rounded (moves down)
Bladder base	Above inferior portion of pubic symphysis	↑ and anterior rotation (i.e., up + forward)	↓ and posterior rotation (i.e., down + backward)
Puborectalis	Contracted	Contracted more	Relaxed
Anorectal angle	Acute angle (<90°)	More acute angle (<<90°)	Becomes obtuse (≥90°)

○ To gauge effectiveness of pelvic floor rehabilitation programs

MAGNETIC RESONANCE IMAGING

- The MRI has become another very important diagnostic tool for physicians. It
  ○ offers superior soft tissue contrast
  ○ has a high sensitivity for fluid detection
  ○ may be used when other modalities have not been able to delineate the problem
  ○ has an ability to visualize dynamic movements of the pelvic floor
  ○ provides direct, multi-planar images
  ○ is noninvasive
  ○ does not expose the patient to ionizing radiation
  ○ can provide detailed views at rest and strain (for UI and POP evaluation)
- Entire procedure requires 10–15 minutes in the MRI room.
- Images are obtained in supine position, with 3 seconds of suspended respiration for each image, and various degrees of strain for pelvic floor evaluation.
- Endovaginal or endorectal MRI with a vaginal/rectal coil provides excellent images of the urethra and pelvic floor.
- Disadvantages: (1) high cost (comparable to fluoroscopy); (2) inability to determine the cause of an obstruction (especially when due to small ureteral calculi); (3) upright position MRI is not widely available, (POP is worse when standing); (4) UI is a dynamic process, MRI cannot capture moving images; (5) ureter and renal pelvis can only be evaluated when urinary tract is filled with fluid (gadolinium is often necessary for better evaluation of the collecting system); (6) cannot evaluate renal or ureteral stones.
- An MRI provides accurate images of ureteral dilation, hydronephrosis, moderate to large size stones, blood clots, pelvic masses, acute hemorrhage, POP, pelvic floor musculature, urethral hypermobility, suburethral diverticula, preoperative evaluation of the bladder neck and urethra.
  ○ MRI can detect pelvic masses (carcinoma, ovarian cysts, ovarian solid tumors, hydrosalpinges, nabothian cysts, and fibroids).
  ○ MRI (especially with endovaginal coil) is superior to double balloon catheter positive pressure urethrography and VCUG for the diagnosis of suburethral diverticula because it is less invasive and give precise information about the location, size, number, and structure of diverticula.
  ○ MRI can be used to grade POP (0–4) based on three anatomic landmarks:
    - Pubococcygeal line (PCL) → distance from pubic bone to coccyx
    - H-line → width of levator hiatus (normal <6 cm)
    - M-line → amount of descent of the pelvic floor (descent of H-line) below PCL during straining (normal <2 cm)
  ○ MRI is highly sensitive for different types of POP.
    - MRI is highly sensitive (87%) for enteroceles (can differentiate simple vs. complex enteroceles and high rectocele vs. posterior enterocele).
    - MRI is extremely sensitive for cystoceles (100%).
    - MRI without opacification may miss 24% of rectoceles (however, by placing transmission gel or gadolinium into the rectum, sensitivity approaches 100%).
    - MRI is highly sensitive for uterine prolapse (87%) and is helpful because it gives three additional, important pieces of information: (1) How big is uterus? → vaginal versus abdominal approach. (2) Is there concomitant cancer? (3) Is there any concomitant upper tract dilation or ureteral kinking which may accompany high grade POP?
  ○ One study showed that 45% of patients with SUI have degeneration of levator ani muscles on MRI.
  ○ MRI is ideal for investigating the presence, location, and complications of suburethral diverticula because it clearly shows the course of urethra and periurethral anatomy.

CONCLUSION

- This chapter has briefly presented a summary of the variety of radiographic modalities that are currently available to physicians.
- An understanding of the appropriate studies is necessary in order to quickly and accurately diagnose urologic and urogynecologic disorders with the maximum benefit to the patient.
- The indications, limitations, sensitivity, specificity, and cost of each procedure need to be carefully considered by the physician before a plan of action is instituted.

BIBLIOGRAPHY

Benson JT, Kelvin FM. Dynamic cystoproctology. In: Blaivas J, ed. *Atlas of Urodyamics*. Baltimore, MD: Williams & Wilkins; 126.

Brubaker L, Heit MH. Radiology of the pelvic floor. *Clin Obstet Gynecol*. 1993;36:1.

Juras JC, Bourcier AP, Villet RM. Colporectocystourethrography: the dynamic investigation. In: Bourceir AP, et al., eds. *Pelvic Floor Disorders*. Philadelphia, PA: Elsevier Saunders; 2004: 164–175.

Kelvin FM, Maglinte D, Hornback, et al. Pelvic prolapse: assessment with evacuation proctography (defecography). *Radiology*. 1992;184:547.

Kelvin FM, Maglinte DDT, Benson JT. Dynamic cystoprocto-graphy: a technique for assessing disorders of the pelvic floor in women. *AJR Am J Roentgenol.* 1993;163:368.

Klarskov P, Jepsen PV, Dorhp S. Reliability of voiding colpo-cysto urethrography in female urinary incontinence before and after treatment. *Act Radiol.* 1988;26:685.

Rodriguez LV, Raz S. Dynamic magnetic resonance imaging in the evaluation of pelvic pathology. In: Bourceir AP, et al., eds. *Pelvic Floor Disorders.* Philadelphia, PA: Elsevier Saunders; 2004:83–190.

Vanbeckevoort D, Vn Hoe L, Oyen R. Pelvic floor descent in females: comparitive study of colpocystodefecography and dynamic MR imaging. *J Magn Reson Imaging.* 1999;9:373.

QUESTIONS

1. In a healthy, nulligravid woman the puborectalis and the bladder base during defecation are best described as _____ and _____, respectively.
   (A) Contracted and superior
   (B) Contracted and posterior
   (C) Relaxed and superior
   (D) Relaxed and inferior
   (E) Contracted and oblique

2. Based on MRI studies, the width of the levator hiatus in an individual *without* POP is ____.
   (A) 0.5 cm
   (B) 2 in.
   (C) 7 cm
   (D) 6 in.
   (E) 10 cm

3. Puborectalis muscle dysfunction can best be diagnosed by _____.
   (A) CRCU
   (B) MRI
   (C) IVP
   (D) Ultrasound
   (E) Plain x-ray

4. One of the main disadvantages of MRI in the field of female pelvic medicine and reconstructive surgery (FPMRS) is ____.
   (A) Low soft tissue contrast
   (B) High cost
   (C) Inability to obtain upright images
   (D) Inability to obtain dynamic images
   (E) Inability to obtain images of upper urinary tract

5. The study of choice if one was interested in evaluating POP by radiographic means would be _____.
   (A) Ultrasound
   (B) IVP
   (C) CT
   (D) Videocystourethrography
   (E) MRI

6. A 37-year-old woman is seen in the emergency department for severe flank pain that began 6 hours ago. She is afebrile and has no Costovertebral angle (CVA) tenderness. The patient has a history of urinary calculi. The initial best step in diagnosing this patient's condition is:
   (A) IVP
   (B) MRI
   (C) VCUG
   (D) Plain x-ray
   (E) CT

7. A 19-year-old woman is being seen for persistent dribbling of urine. She states that this has always been a problem but recently it has gotten worse and requires her to wear large pads that she has to change about four times a day. The dribbling occurs all of the time. The patient has tried various voiding schedules, but still experiences the same problem. The patient states that you are the first physician that she has seen for this problem. The best imaging modality to use at this time is:
   (A) Positive-pressure urethrography
   (B) Ultrasound
   (C) VCUG
   (D) IVP

ANSWERS

1. *(D).* During straining efforts or defecation, the puborectalis muscle relaxes, the levator hiatus opens, and the bladder moves inferiorly and posteriorly.

2. *(B).* The levator hiatus or the H-line is <6 cm in a *normal* female patient. Answers (C), (D), and (E) are larger than 6 cm. Answer (A) is too small of a measurement for the levator hiatus. Therefore, the answer is (B). Two inches is about 4.5 cm.

3. *(A).* CRCU allows visualization of puborectalis muscle dysfunction. Normally, with relaxation of the puborectalis, the anorectal angle becomes obtuse (see Table 12-1). In puborectalis muscle dysfunction, with relaxation of puborectalis, the anorectal angle remains acute.

4. *(D).* MRI has very high soft tissue contrast. Although it can be expensive, this is not a disadvantage specific for the field of FPMRS. Some centers have

upright MRI potential, although this techno-logy is not widely available. The upper tract can be visualized well as long as gadolinium is utilized. The main disadvantage of MRI is that currently it cannot obtain dynamic images, for example, video images of a patient while she is voiding.

5. *(E)*. MRI has very high sensitivity for the detection of anterior, posterior, and apical prolapses because of its high resolution for soft tissues. Videocystourethrography can be helpful during the evaluation of incontinence. CT is not as good as MRI for POP. Ultrasound and IVP are not good imaging modalities for POP.

6. *(D)*. The plain film of the abdomen is the initial screening tool for the evaluation of urinary calculi. The IVP can also be used to visualize urinary calculi, but it is not the initial choice. MRI would not be the modality of choice because of its inability to determine the cause of the obstruction and its high cost. VCUG is commonly used to investigate suburethral diverticula, vesicoureteral reflux, increased bladder volume, ureterocele, and primary megaureter. CT is an excellent tool for the evaluation of urinary calculi but is only used after plain film, IVP, ultrasound, retro- and anterograde pyelography have not unmasked the obstruction.

7. *(E)*. Of the listed options, IVP is the best. IVP remains the modality of choice for visualizing the urinary tract because it is safe, readily available, and inexpensive. IVP can easily diagnose a fistula, which is what this patient is describing. Ultrasound is mainly used to diagnose hydronephrosis, urinary calculi, renal parenchymal abnormalities, PVR volume, suburethral diverticula, and bladder tumors. MRI is used if IVP and other modalities have not been able to reveal the location of the fistula. VCUG is used to evaluate suburethral diverticula, vesicoureteral reflux, increased bladder volume, ureterocele, and primary megaureter. Positive-pressure urethrography is mainly used to investigate possible suburethral diverticula that are not visualized on VCUG.

13 CONSERVATIVE MANAGEMENT OF INCONTINENCE AND PELVIC ORGAN PROLAPSE

Sam Siddighi

INTRODUCTION

- Conservative or nonsurgical management is recommended by the Agency for Health Care Policy and Research, and should be attempted before surgery is contemplated because:
  - It is safer—nonsurgical management options do not have associated mortality but surgery does
  - Minimally invasive
  - Simple
  - It does not preclude surgery at a later time
  - Recurrences occur after surgery and repeat surgeries have higher morbidity and failure rate
  - Inexpensive
  - Although cure rate is not as high as for surgical therapies, patient satisfaction can be quite high
- Indications for nonsurgical therapy
  - Treatment of pelvic organ prolapse (POP), stress urinary incontinence (SUI), overactive bladder (OAB), urge incontinence, mixed incontinence, and fecal incontinence
  - Anyone with mild to moderate symptoms
  - Patient awaiting surgery for SUI
  - Patient not interested in surgical treatment of SUI or POP
  - Patient who has not completed childbearing
  - Patient who is not an ideal surgical candidate (elderly + multiple medical conditions)
- Motivation of the patient is crucial to the success of nonsurgical therapies.
- Many nonsurgical management protocols are based on expert opinion and accepted wisdom rather than on

prospective controlled trials. Therefore, more studies are necessary to guide our practice.
- Pharmacologic management of OAB, urinary urgency incontinence (UUI), mixed incontinence, and SUI will be discussed in Chap. 37, Medicines Used in Urogynecology.

LIFESTYLE MODIFICATION

- Weight reduction
  - Obesity is an independent risk factor for urinary incontinence—in one study, the prevalence of weekly SUI increased by 10% for every five units of BMI.
  - Both SUI and UUI are more prevalent in obese women.
  - Significant weight loss in morbidly obese results in decrease in SUI.
  - Weight reduction in overweight or obese patients may also help.
- Management of fluid intake
  - There is a positive relationship between fluid intake and severity of incontinence in women aged ≥55 with SUI.
  - Keeping a voiding diary helps manage fluid intake.
  - Recommended daily intake is six to eight glasses per day.
  - Do not take too much: some women believe excessive liquid intake (>3 L/day) is beneficial (e.g., exercise regimens and special diets).
  - Do not take too little: some women limit fluid intake to reduce incontinence, but this may produce concentrated urine, which can irritate the bladder.
  - Severe thirst and polydipsia may be from a metabolic disorder (hypercalcemia, diabetes mellitus [DM], and so forth).
  - Restrict fluids after 6 p.m. to reduce nocturia.
- Smoking cessation may help
  - Smoking is not confirmed as a risk factor for incontinence; however, nicotine is irritating to the detrusor muscle.
  - Smoking can aggravate chronic pulmonary disorders (e.g., COPD, asthma) which are risk factors.
  - Heavy smokers also have worse tissue regeneration and healing.

- Regular voiding pattern
  - Busy professionals should find time to empty their bladders regularly.
  - Avoid rushing to the toilet on a full bladder, this will cause accidents. It is better to go to the bathroom in a calm, controlled fashion.
- Reduce coffee, tea, chocolate, alcohol, carbonated beverages, artificial sweeteners (aspartame), and other foods with high acidity rating or caffeine (see Chap. 24, Management of Detrusor Overactivity)
  - Reduce caffeine gradually over several weeks to avoid withdrawal symptoms.
  - Acidity of these products may irritate the bladder.
- Reduce occupational or recreational activities that require repetitive, chronic straining, if possible
  - Job involves lifting heavy boxes or furniture all day.
  - Your favorite activity is shot-putting or weight lifting.
- Proper bowel care is important
  - There is a positive relationship between SUI and straining at stool and between SUI and constipation.
  - Take appropriate amounts of fluid and fiber in the diet (foods such as wheat bran, apple sauce, and prune juice).
  - Use laxatives and fiber supplements, if necessary to avoid constipation and fecal impaction.
  - Fecal impaction is associated with urinary incontinence and its management improves incontinence.

TREATMENT OF REVERSIBLE CAUSES

- Treat conditions of the lung (asthma, COPD) or conditions that provoke coughing (allergy, sinusitis) as they create episodes of repetitive increase in intra-abdominal pressure.
- Treat endocrine and metabolic disorders (DM, hypercalcemia).
- Treat underlying cause of delirium.
- If a patient is immobile, modify her environment (provide bedside commode) or make it easier for her to get to the toilet.
- Treat urinary tract infections (UTIs) as they mimic incontinence and OAB.
- Watch out for side effects of medications that the patient may be taking (e.g., prazosin prescribed for blood pressure can cause SUI). You may reduce dose or switch to a different medication.
- Treat atrophic vaginitis with local estrogen (cream, tablet, ring).

BLADDER RETRAINING

- Is effective for OAB, urge incontinence, mixed incontinence (also used for SUI).

- Goal is to re-establish cortical inhibition of the bladder emptying reflex.
- A behavior modification technique where a voiding schedule is implemented and intervals between urination are increased gradually.
  - Initially 1-hour interval between voiding attempts (or choose an interval more often than incontinence episodes)
  - Must void on schedule regardless of lack of urge to void
  - Increase voiding interval by 15–30 minutes about every week, if patient is ready
  - Goal to reach 2–4 hours between voiding attempts
- Urgency control strategies (relaxation and distraction techniques) and a defensive posture (quick pelvic muscle contractions) are learned.
- Desensitization techniques can also be practiced for those who have specific events (e.g., urge with sound of running water) that trigger incontinence.
- Bladder training is continued for 6 weeks, then patient can void on a more comfortable voiding schedule.
- May reduce incontinence episodes by 60%.
- Success is dependent on both patient and physician motivation.
- One prospective randomized study showed 80% reduction in urge incontinence episodes in the behavior modification group versus pharmacologic therapy group or placebo, after only four sessions of biofeedback-assisted behavior modification.
- Bladder retraining is different from timed voiding or prompted voiding.
  - Timed voiding: voiding schedule is preset and the difference is (1) no attempt is made to delay or suppress urge to void, and (2) voiding schedule is not progressively lengthened.
  - Prompted voiding: usually initiated in nursing home patients; patient is checked frequently by caregivers and is asked to use the toilet. She is praised for maintaining continence (dry underpants) and making attempts to void.
- As a rule of thumb, pharmacologic treatments combined with behavioral treatments are better than either one by itself.
  - Oxybutynin versus oxybutynin + bladder retraining → combination is more effective

PELVIC FLOOR MUSCLE EXERCISES

Pelvic floor muscle (PFM) exercises are also known as PFME or Kegel exercises.
- Introduced by Arnold Kegel in 1948.
- Effective for not only SUI but also for OAB, urge incontinence, mixed incontinence, fecal incontinence

- Goal: rehabilitation and strengthening of the muscles and nerves of the pelvic floor—the levator ani (especially the pubococcygeus muscle [PCM]) and the striated urethral sphincter.
- The PCM consist of 70% slow-twitch (Type I) which uses aerobic oxidative metabolism and 30% fast-twitch (Type II) which uses anaerobic glycolysis. On the other hand, the striated urethral sphincter is predominantly slow-twitch. These muscles can be hypertrophied by PFME.
- Some women may have tried *Kegels* and believe they do not work for them. To avoid resistance to these exercises, call them PFME instead of Kegels. It is likely that the Kegels did not work for them because they performed them incorrectly.
- Women will perform PFME incorrectly given simple, brief verbal instructions.
  - The instruction "squeeze as if you are trying to stop the flow of urine" is not sufficient.
  - Many women will utilize the wrong muscles (e.g., abdominal, gluteal, abductors).
  - Many women will valsalva.
- During pelvic examination, the patient can be taught to contract the correct muscles by palpating them and asking the patient to contract her vaginal muscles.
- Assess PFM before initiating PFME to establish a baseline.
  - Symmetry at rest and with contraction: parous women with SUI cannot hold muscle contraction as long as nulliparous, continent women can and often contract asymmetrically.
  - Areas of muscle defect or atrophy.
  - Can contraction elevate the bladder neck?
  - Normally, contraction should cause descent of the clitoris and retraction of vaginal introitus, perineal body, and anal sphincter; conversely, coughing should not produce perineal descent.
  - Assess tone of muscle (how much resistance is provided against two fingers placed in the vagina to the level of the first knuckles.
  - Rate PFM strength from 0 to 5 (0 = no contraction; 1 = flicker; 2 = a weak 2 second squeeze; 3 = fair squeeze with lift; 4 = a good squeeze, hold, and lift; 5 = strong squeeze, hold, lift, and repeatable).
    - 0–1 → will benefit from electrical stimulation (may benefit: PFME ± biofeedback assistance)
    - 2–3 → definite benefit from intensive PFME
    - 4–5 → possible benefit from PFME, biofeedback, electrical stimulation
- Adequate teaching, encouraging, and follow-up is necessary to perform PFME correctly and to achieve high success rates.
  - Study comparing rigorous or intensive exercise group (i.e., instruction on anatomy and physiology, digital and perineometric measures of muscle contraction, proper isolation of PFM, weekly 45 minute group exercise sessions) versus normal PFME group showed significantly better symptomatic improvement in the intensive group.
  - More frequent follow-up leads to higher success rate.
  - Consult a physical therapist as this can increase success rate.
  - More number of repetitions does not necessarily lead to improved results. Technique, adequacy, and perseverance are very important.
  - Elderly may need longer training interval.
- PFME regimens vary widely
  - 6 weeks to 6 months duration, 3 times a day for an hour each time, 35–300 repetitions a day (Kegel recommended 100–300 repetitions/day), 3–40 seconds squeeze hold
  - Recommended by the International Consultation on Incontinence: 3–4 times/week, 8–12 slow strong squeeze (hold 6–8 seconds) × 3 sets for 4–5 months
  - Must relax completely between contractions
  - Some may interpose 3–4 fast contractions ("quick flicks") between the slow squeezes
  - Patients should be encouraged to incorporate PFME into daily activities (driving, brushing teeth, and so forth)
  - Results may be seen in 2–3 months
- Too much PFME is not good → may lead to pelvic muscle spasm (coccygodynia—see Chap. 47, Dyspareunia and Chronic Pelvic Pain of Urinary Tract Origin), and urinary and defecatory dysfunction.
- PFME has been shown to reduce incontinence episodes by 65–90%.
  - PFME helps the patient develop the ability to produce a strong, timely closing force on the urethra (by pressing it against the symphysis) in anticipation of coughing, lifting, physical activity, or in response to urgency. This initiates a reflex that suppresses detrusor contractions.
  - A recent prospective randomized study comparing PFME with vaginal cones and vaginal electrical stimulation showed improved muscle strength in all three groups, but highest in PFME group (75%).
  - 78% of PFME group had significant decrease in urine leakage (compared to 30% for cone, 13% for electrical stimulation groups).
- Given the proposed mechanism for the development of POP, it can be theorized that PFME *may* improve mild to moderate POP and *may* slow its progression. Data are needed on this subject.

WEIGHTED VAGINAL CONES

- The vaginal cone is a form of simple biofeedback for PFME, as is the perineometer.

- Weighted vaginal cone regimen (Dacomed cones: cone #1 = 20 g → cone #5 = 70 g; other cone systems 20–100 g):
  ○ Vaginal cone of the least weight (20 g) is placed inside the vagina and prevented from slipping out by contracting the levator ani muscles.
  ○ This must be done two times a day for 15 minutes, while patient performs routine activities.
  ○ Once she is able to do it, a vaginal cone of greater weight is used.
- Vaginal cones may be helpful for some patients because they improve compliance.
- Is as effective as PFME if performed with the same regularity, intensity, and duration as PFME programs.
  ○ Which is better (PFME vs. vaginal cone-assisted PFME)? One study showed they are equivalent.

FORMAL BIOFEEDBACK

- Biofeedback is a form of intensive therapy that helps change one's behavior. Since detrusor control and contraction of the urethral sphincter are learned behaviors, one can reduce incontinence using biofeedback.
- Biofeedback is useful for urinary and fecal incontinence (EMG biofeedback may be useful in women with anal sphincter weakness without anatomic sphincter disruption).
- Rectal probes or vaginal perineometers can measure the pressure created by pelvic muscle contraction.
- Electromyographic (EMG) electrodes on the skin surface can help isolate the correct muscles that must be contracted.
- Feedback from the EMG can give immediate audio or visual feedback of pelvic muscle activity to the patient.
- Amplitude and duration of each contraction is recorded and can be reviewed later.
- Once the appropriate muscle has been isolated, patient can monitor and enhance those contractions.
- Five steps must be learned:
  ○ Learning to control abdominal pressure
  ○ Learning to isolate and contract PFM quickly without increasing abdominal pressure
  ○ Learning to contract PFM for 10 seconds without increasing abdominal pressure
  ○ Learning a *slow, deliberate* PFM contraction
  ○ Individualization: performing activities that ordinarily would provoke leakage at work or home (e.g., drink 400 mL fluid then cough) and practice control with PFM contraction while relaxing abdominal muscles
- Results from biofeedback are often seen in short amount of time (e.g., 2 weeks or after a few sessions).

- Biofeedback with a personal trainer is better than biofeedback using only electrodes or manometry for many patients.
- Biofeedback can be added to PFME or bladder retraining.
  ○ Which is better (PFME vs. biofeedback-assisted PFME)? Biofeedback-assisted PFME is equivalent to PFME alone.
- Main disadvantages of biofeedback: (1) cost and (2) time required for office programs.

FUNCTIONAL ELECTRICAL STIMULATION

Functional electrical stimulation is also known as FES, ES, E-stim, or external electrical stimulation (EES).
- Used for SUI, OAB, UUI, mixed urinary incontinence.
- FES ≠ sacral neuromodulation (Interstim), which is implanted for the treatment of detrusor overactivity not responsive to other therapies.
- FES is a battery-operated electrical device that produces low-level electrical current and delivers it to the patient through vaginal, anal, and intravesical plugs or catheters (which come in various shapes and sizes).
- The current is monophasic and rectangular.
  ○ The intensity of the current, frequency of pulse, duration of pulses (width), and the character (continuous vs. intermittent) can be controlled on the device.
  ○ In clinical use today: intermittent and alternating pulses; pulse frequency = 20–50 Hz (pelvic floor and striated urethral muscle contraction) and 10–12 Hz (low frequency for inhibition of involuntary detrusor contractions); pulse duration = 1–5 minutes (for SUI) and 10 minutes (for OAB).
- May be performed 15–30 minutes bid and a response may be seen in 6–8 weeks.
- Some women may experience temporary exacerbation of symptoms followed by improvement (patient should be warned about this).
- FES inhibits detrusor activity and activates PFM; although several theories exist, the mechanism of action is currently not understood.
- Theoretically, the path of electrical current is as follows:

Pudendal nerve afferent → sacral nerve root → efferent nerves → PFM contract *or*

Pudendal nerve afferent → spinal cord → pelvic nerves (parasympathetic) → detrusor inhibition

  ○ Example: mechanical dilation of anus leads to detrusor inhibition

- The goal of FES is to help the patient identify the PFM and to stimulate them enough so the patient can eventually achieve voluntary control.
- Indications for FES:
  - SUI
  - Detrusor overactivity (idiopathic or neurogenic)
  - Mixed incontinence
  - Sensory-urgency syndrome
  - Neuropathic voiding dysfunction
- Contraindications to FES:
  - UTI
  - Pregnancy
  - Vesicoureteral reflux (VUR) or dilated upper urinary tract
  - Urinary retention (elevated postvoid residual [PVR])
  - Cardiac pacemaker
  - History of cardiac arrhythmia
  - Vaginitis
  - Heavy vaginal bleeding (especially undiagnosed bleeding)
- Advantages of FES:
  - Is noninvasive
  - Some patients enjoy it
  - Has modest improvement rating
  - May be cost-effective for treatment of SUI
- Disadvantages of FES:
  - Is time consuming
  - May be painful
  - Requires commitment on part of patient and physician
  - Total cure rate is low
- More data are needed; however, the following are some outcome data:
  - Cure (or totally dry) is only 10–30%.
  - Improved: 60–70% decrease in incontinence episodes is possible.
  - Improved: increase in functional urethral length (FUL), increase in maximum cystometric capacity, and decrease in detrusor contractions.
- ES protocols are too variable to make proper comparisons to PFME.
  - Which is better (PFME vs. FES)? Several conflicting studies, but PFME *may* be better than FES.
  - Which is better (PFME vs. PFME + FES)? One study showed equivalent results.

MECHANICAL DEVICES

Urethral plugs, caps, and patches
- The above devices have been used successfully for SUI.
- They have been more popular in Europe than the United States.

- Urethral plugs are single-use, disposable, intraurethral devices which situates between bladder neck and external urethral sphincter. It is inserted by the patient and removed just before urination.
  - Example of plugs: Reliance Urinary Control Insert (Uromed Corp.) → approved by FDA
  - Leakage episodes decreased by 90%
  - Plugs need to be changed after each void (expense may be an issue)
  - Contraindicated in: history of recurrent UTIs or artificial heart valve
- Caps and patches are occlusive devices which block urinary leakage at the urethral meatus by using suction and adhesive, respectively.
  - Examples of *patch*: Impress Softpatch (Uromed Corp.), Miniguard (Advanced Surgical Innovations)
    - Minguard patch is effective for mild to moderate SUI but does not completely resolve symptoms because adhesive is weak.
    - Patch is safe in patients with detrusor contractions → not at risk for VUR as patch dislodges with contractions.
    - New patch has to be used after each void (expense may be an issue).
  - Examples of *cap*: FemAssist (Insight Medical) and Capsure (CR Bard)
    - FemAssist efficacy is limited.
    - Cap may be discontinued by many (≈40%) because of discomfort or dissatisfaction.
    - Caps may be reused for up to 1 week.
- These devices can cause discomfort, irritation, hematuria, and can lead to UTI.

PESSARIES

- Introduction:
  - Pessaries have been used for thousands of years.
  - Contraceptive diaphragms and short, large width tampons are self-prescribed by patients for mild incontinence and incontinence during exercise.
  - Although recently interest in the use of pessary has increased among graduating gynecologists, there had been a reluctance and discomfort in the use of pessaries by both the patient and the physician not long ago.
  - Pessaries are safe, cost-effective, minimally invasive, and may prevent patients from going to the operating room.
  - It is vital that the clinician ensures that appropriate care is provided to a patient wearing a pessary, regardless of the fact that she may have a nurse taking care of her at her own home or at a skilled nursing facility. Neglect of a patient wearing a pessary can

lead to problems that could have been easily avoided.

- Current uses of the pessary:
  - Pessaries are most helpful for managing POP.
  - Pessaries may be used to manage SUI; however, patients with SUI are likely to discontinue it.
    - Pessaries that provide support to the bladder neck include: Conveen Continence Guard (Johnson & Johnson), Introl (Uromed), incontinence dish (with or without support), incontinence ring pessary, Cook continence ring, even conventionally pessaries can be utilized to provide support.
    - In a study of the previously mentioned devices, large percentage of participants withdrew because of lack of efficacy and adverse events.
  - Although for most patients that use them, they are worn continuously, they can be used on a temporary basis in certain patients during times when symptoms may be at their highest.
    - Week before menses
    - Before anticipated long day of standing
    - With vigorous exercise (e.g., tennis match)
  - Pessaries can be helpful for alleviating symptoms related to POP, especially if the symptom is of much greater severity than the degree POP (e.g., severe back pain with mild POP).
  - They can be helpful in elucidating potential incontinence (aka occult or masked incontinence—see Chap. 5, Evaluation of Pelvic Organ Prolapse [POP]).
    - Some patients may benefit from injections with periurethral bulking agents for potential incontinence while continuing to use pessary.
    - Pessaries which provide support of the bladder neck may help in these patients.
  - Pessary *may* prevent progression of POP.
    - Although data are needed on this matter, the observation that some women with advanced POP need a smaller sized pessary over time is intriguing.
  - Pessaries may be used in pregnancy for POP or as an adjunct for cervical incompetence.
- Disadvantages of pessary:
  - Requires ongoing care
    - Therefore inability to comply with instructions (e.g., demented patient) or to follow-up with provider are both contraindications to pessary use.
  - Risk of vaginal discharge and odor
    - Noninflammatory leukorrhea is common.
    - More frequent pessary change (i.e., removal, cleaning with tap water, replacement) may help.
    - Douching with warm tap water may help.
    - Use of Trimo-San gel 1–2 times/week may reduce odors.
    - Antibacterial gel (Aci-Jel) may decrease amount of discharge.
  - Risk of vaginal infection
    - If symptomatic, can be treated with metronidazole gel (bacterial vaginosis [BV] is a common infection, especially among smokers).
    - Prophylactive metronidazole cream may be considered for recurrent BV.
    - Avoid broad-spectrum antibiotics or commercially available douches.
  - Risk of vaginal irritation, ulceration, and bleeding
    - Ulceration can develop in two ways: (1) advanced POP rubbed against underpants and exposed to outside environment can lead to ulcers, and (2) pessary used for POP if neglected for a long time can produce ulcerations.
    - In situation 1, pessary may help heal ulcers.
    - In situation 2, pessary should be discontinued temporarily.
    - In situation 2, if pessary is to be replaced after erosion has had time to heal, then sufficient local estrogen cream should be used each time pessary is inserted; also better follow-up and more frequent replacement of pessary is necessary.
    - In situation 2, if erosion does not go away then pessary must not be used and surgery should be contemplated.
    - If the ulceration is not healing with time, a biopsy of it should be taken to rule out cervical (if present) or vaginal cancer.
    - Evaluation of vaginal bleeding in a patient with pessary should include endometrial biopsy (EMB) and Pap smear, if uterus and cervix are present even if cause of bleeding appears to be from an ulceration.
  - If it is neglected, erosion and fistulas (rectovaginal or vesicovaginal) can occur
    - If erosions persist or fistula is present, then pessary must be discontinued.
    - Local estrogen is better at preventing erosions than water-based lubricants such as KY Jelly or Trimosan.
    - A neglected pessary that has caused a fistula may need to be taken out in the operating room because it may be embedded.
- A survey of American Urogynecologic Society (AUGS) members in 2000 showed the most common pessaries in use today are the (1) Ring (with or without support) (2), Gellhorn (3), doughnut, and cube.
  - Ring
    - Ring + support (or diaphragm)—is a ring with a filling disk which has four holes (two small holes facing each other and perpendicular to two large holes; the ring can be folded at the two large holes to form a half-moon)
    - Ring without support = a ring
    - May start with size 4 for most women

- Ring requires presence of some perineal support to stay in place
  - Easiest to insert and remove by the patient
  - Sexual intercourse is not a problem
- Gellhorn
  - From side-view, the Gellhorn looks like a pacifier
  - Rigid, semirigid, and flexible types are available
  - May start with size $2\frac{1}{2}$
  - Is used for advanced POP and uterine prolapse
  - Gellhorn must be removed to have sexual intercourse
  - It is more difficult to remove than the ring
- Doughnut
  - Is like a ring but occupies more space
  - May stay in place when ring fails
  - Preferred for apical prolapse
  - May be difficult to remove by the patient (try using Inflatoball or inflatable doughnut)
- Cube
  - Has six suction cups corresponding to six sides of a cube
  - Is pessary of last resort because of higher risk of erosion and fistula formation than any other pessary; therefore, if it is used, very regular follow-up must be ensured
  - Perineal support is not needed to keep cube in place
  - Sexual intercourse is not possible with cube in place
- Many other pessaries are available; these include but are not limited to: Lever, Gehrung, Inflatoball, Smith, Hodge, Risser, Shaatz, incontinence dish with support, incontinence ring, Introl.
- After the ring and Gellhorn have failed, the Gehrung pessary may be an option for anterior and posterior prolapses.
- All of the aforementioned pessaries are made of rubber, silicone, or latex (watch out for allergies).
- Double pessaries (ring + ring or doughnut + Gellhorn) are also used by some practitioners for patients with advanced POP. The use of estrogen releasing ring (Estring) in combination with a pessary also mimics this concept.
- Goals of pessary fitting:
  - Since the goal of pessary is to relieve the patient's symptom(s), even if a pessary that is deemed too small or in the wrong position works for the patient—leave it alone!
  - Try to use the smallest pessary that will reduce the POP and stay in place.
  - A well-supported pessary should not be visible at the introitus.
  - The patient should not feel a well-fitted pessary (pressure or discomfort may signify it is too big and sensation of pessary moving may signify it is too small).
  - A well-fitted pessary should not obstruct urinary flow.
- A pessary may be successfully fitted regardless of the degree of POP.

- A pessary may be successfully fitted regardless of presence or absence of a uterus.
- Highlights of pessary fitting:
  - The ring is folded in half (now it looks like a half-moon).
  - The ring can be inserted with straight edge facing the introitus (i.e., 90 degrees to the floor) or narrow end of the curved edge facing introitus (i.e., parallel to the floor).
  - Place lubrication on leading edge of the pessary (edge facing introitus) only, otherwise pessary may be too slippery to hold between the thumb and index.
  - Use ample estrogen cream as lubrication on pessary as well as vaginal introitus. Estring (Pharmacia & Upjohn) may also be used to provide longer local estrogen (3 months). Estring is placed inside vagina before (i.e., in front of) the pessary.
  - Pressure should always be directed inferiorly (or toward posterior wall) while inserting pessary to minimize discomfort.
  - The ring pessary should be parallel to the axis of the vagina (the Gellhorn is oblique with respect to the vaginal axis, in other words, its stem points toward the perineal body).
  - The ring pessary or the disk of the Gellhorn should be situated between the posterior fornix and the pubic symphysis.
  - If a patient has a cervix, it should rest on the flat of the pessary (on the diaphragm [ring] or on the disk [Gellhorn]).
  - One finger should fit between outer rim of pessary and vaginal wall after insertion and pessary should be able to slide up and down vaginal axis (if finger does not fit → use smaller pessary, if more than one finger fits → use larger pessary).
  - For the Gellhorn, if the stem protrudes or goes past introitus then a smaller size should be used.
  - Be sure to ask the patient to valsalva, cough, walk, and use the restroom before she goes home after initial pessary fitting.
  - If the patient is placing the pessary herself, it is best to do it while lying down or sitting so as to avoid gravity and intra-abdominal pressure.
- Although it can be left in place safely for months, it is ideal to remove it each night and replace it in the morning. However, since this is not practical, remove and replace it at least one to two times a week.
- Follow-up after pessary insertion:
  - Barring problems encountered by the patient after pessary insertion (e.g., inability to void, vaginal bleeding) the following follow-up schedule is adequate for proper pessary care:
    - Patient who self-inserts and removes pessary: 2–4 weeks (after initial insertion), then annually

- Patient who cannot or is not willing to change pessary: 2–4 weeks (after initial insertion), then every 3 months for the first year, then this interval may be increased to every 6 months
- Management of pessary problems:
  ○ Pessary falls out with straining
    ▪ Try larger pessary or a different type of pessary (ring → Gellhorn → Gehrung or cube).
    ▪ If pessary passes the tests in the office but falls out at home and usually during bowel movements (BM) then it may need to be removed prior to having BM. Also ensure that the patient has proper bowel care to avoid constipation and excessive straining.
  ○ She experiences pelvic pain
    ▪ Either pessary is too large or it may be too small and descended to the pain sensitive vaginal introitus.
  ○ Vaginal bleeding
    ▪ Pessary may be too large and need to be replaced.
    ▪ Use ample local estrogen and allow time to heal.
    ▪ EMB or Pap may be necessary.
  ○ Complains of vaginal discharge and odor (manage as stated earlier in this chapter)
  ○ Pessary becomes stiff → use new pessary
- After a pessary is successfully fitted, 50% will continue to use if for ≥1 year.
- Those who discontinue pessary do it within the first few days to weeks of fitting.

BIBLIOGRAPHY

Alling ML, Lose G, Jorgensen T. Risk factors for lower urinary tract symptoms in women 40 to 60 years of age. *Obstet Gynecol.* 2000;96(3):446–451.

Bergman A, Koonings PP, Ballard CA. Predicting postoperative urinary incontinence development in women undergoing operation for genitourinary prolapse. *Am J Obstet Gynecol.* 1988;158:1171–1175.

Bhatia N, Bergman A, Gunning J. Urodynamic effects of a vaginal pessary in women with stress urinary incontinence. *Am J Obstet Gynecol.* 1983;147:876–879.

Bourcier AP, Jras JC. Nonsurgical therapy for stress incontinence. *Urol Clin North Am.* 1995;22:613–627.

Bump RC, Sugerman JH, Fantl JA, et al. Obesity and the lower urinary tract function in women: effect of surgically induced weight loss. *Am J Obstet Gynecol.* 1992;167:392.

Burgio KL, Goode PS, Locher JL, et al. Behavioral training with and without biofeedback in the treatment of urge incontinence in older women: a randomized controlled trial. *JAMA.* 2002;288:2293–2299.

Burgio KL, Robinson JC, Engel BT. The role of biofeedback in Kegel exercise training for stress urinary incontinence. *Am J Obstet Gynecol.* 1986;154:58–64.

Elser Dm. Use of the vaginal pessary. In: Mann WJ Jr, Stovall TG, eds. *Gynecologic Surgery.* New York: Churchill Livingston; 1996:353–360.

Farrell SA. Nonsurgical management of pelvic organ prolapse. In: Bent AE, Ostergard DR, Cundiff GW, et al., eds. *Ostergard's Urogynecology and Pelvic Floor Dysfunction.* 5th ed. Philadelphia, PA: Lippincott Williams & Wilkins; 2003: 393–407.

Gormley EA. Biofeedback and behavioral therapy for the management of female urinary incontinence. *Urol Clin North Am.* 2002;29(3):551–557.

Greenhill JP. The nonsurgical management of vaginal relaxation. *Clin Obstet Gynecol.* 1972;15:1083–1097.

Iselin CE, Webster GD. Office management of female urinary incontinence. *Urol Clin North Am.* 1998;25(4):625–645.

Kegel AH. Progressive resistance exercise in the functional restoration of the perineal muscles. *Am J Obstet Gynecol.* 1948;56:238–248.

Meyer S, Lose G. Pelvic floor reeducation in urogynecology. In: Bourchier AP, McGuire EJ, Abrams P, eds. *Pelvic Floor Disorders.* Philadelphia, PA: Elsevier Saunders; 2004.

Miller DS. Contemporary use of the pessary. In: Sciarra JJ, ed. *Gynecology and Obstetrics.* Vol. 1. Philadelphia, PA: JB Lippincott; 1999:1–13.

Moore KH, Simons A, Dowell C, et al. Efficacy and user acceptability of the urethral occlusive device in women with urinary incontinence. *J Urol.* 1999;162:464–468.

Sand PK, Staskin D, Miller J, et al. Effect of a urinary control insert on quality of life in incontinent women. *Int Urogynecol J Pelvic Floor Dysfunct.* 1999;10:100–105.

Subak LL, Johnson C, Whitcomb E, et al. Does weight loss improve incontinence in moderately obese women? *Int Urogynecol J Pelvic Floor Dysfunct.* 2002;13:40–43.

Sulak PJ, Kuehl TJ, Shull BL. Vaginal pessaries and their use in pelvic relaxation. *J Reprod Med.* 1993;38:919–923.

Wyman JF, Fantl JA, McClish DK, et al. Comparative efficacy of behavioral interventions in the management of female urinary incontinence. Continence Program for Women Research Group. *Am J Obstet Gynecol.* 1998;179(4):999–1007.

QUESTIONS

QUESTIONS 1–3

Match the following statement with the word/phrase that best describes it. Each answer may be used once, more than once, or not at all.

    (A) Lifestyle modification
    (B) Bladder training
    (C) Pelvic floor exercises
    (D) Weighted vaginal cones
    (E) FES
    (F) Urethral plug
    (G) Urethral cap
    (H) Urethral patch
    (I) Ring pessary
    (J) Gellhorn pessary

1. In advanced POP, two of these may be used instead of just one
2. Is sometimes confused with sacral neuromodulation
3. Uses relaxation and distraction techniques to control impulses

QUESTIONS 4 AND 5

A 60-year-old gravida 3, para 3, presents to your office complaining of pelvic pressure and recurrent UTI. She has been placed on antibiotics six times over the last year. Her medical history is remarkable for hypertension, diabetes, and gastrointestinal reflux disease. She has had only one abdominal surgery in her life (an appendectomy 30 years ago). She just finished a course of ciprofloxacin. Her physical examination reveals an atrophic vagina and an anterior vaginal wall prolapse 2 cm past the hymen during valsalva. When her bladder is subjectively full, she does not leak urine in sitting position with and without reduction during valsalva. She is able to void 300 mL and has a catheterized PVR of 150 mL. Her urine dipstick is negative.

4. The best initial management of her problem is _____.

    (A) Ciprofloxacin
    (B) Ring pessary
    (C) Bladder retraining
    (D) FES
    (E) Behavioral modification

5. Addition of _____ would be helpful for prevention of UTI.

    (A) Doxycycline
    (B) Ampicillin
    (C) Metronidazole gel
    (D) Estrogen cream
    (E) Cranberry juice

ANSWERS

ANSWERS 1–3

1. *(I)*, 2. *(E)*, 3. *(B)*. Double pessaries (ring + ring or doughnut + Gellhorn) are used by some practitioners for patients with advanced POP. The use of estrogen releasing ring (Estring) in combination with a pessary also mimics this concept. FES and sacral neuromodulation (Interstim) are not the same thing. Sacral neuromodulation is an implanted lead attached to an electrical stimulator which is used for detrusor overactivity that is unresponsive to conservative management (see Chap. 24, Management of Detrusor Overactivity). During bladder retraining, urgency

control strategies such as relaxation and distraction techniques as well as a defensive posture (quick pelvic muscle contractions) are utilized.

ANSWERS 4 AND 5

4. *(B)*, 5. *(D)*. From the clinical scenario, it is apparent that the patient gets recurrent UTIs and has symptomatic POP. Patients with POP may retain urine in their bladders (stasis), which can predispose to lower UTIs. By reducing the prolapse with a pessary, she will reduce her PVR and may improve her bladder emptying capacity. Currently, she does not have symptoms of UTI; therefore ciprofloxacin would not be helpful. Bladder retraining is used for symptoms of detrusor overactivity. Behavioral modification would not be useful in this situation because there are no behaviors mentioned in this clinical scenario that need to be changed. FES is not helpful for POP or UTI. Patients who have urogenital atrophy will gain some protection against UTIs by using local estrogen cream. Metronidazole cream is used for BV. Cranberry juice, especially, that found in diluted proportions at the supermarket is not the best prophylaxis for UTIs. Cranberry extract has been shown to inhibit binding of *Escherichia coli* to urothelium. The other antibiotics, doxycycline and ampicillin, are not useful for prevention of UTI. In fact, there has been increasing resistance among uropathogens to ampicillin. A better choice would be nitrofurantoin, trimethoprim-sulfamethoxazole, or ciprofloxacin.

14 SURGICAL MANAGEMENT OF STRESS URINARY INCONTINENCE: VAGINAL PROCEDURES

Sujata Yavagal and Sam Siddighi

INTRODUCTION

- More than 150 surgical procedures have evolved for the management of stress urinary incontinence (SUI). The reasons for the existence of many procedures for one diagnosis are several: (1) technical innovation, (2) dissatisfaction with long-term results of existing treatments, (3) dissatisfaction with rate of complications of existing treatments, and (4) invasiveness of existing treatments.

- Continence is maintained because of (1) pelvic floor muscles (which are tonically contracted at rest and reflexively contracts with increases in intra-abdominal pressure), (2) suburethral endopelvic fascial hammock, (3) intrinsic urethral function which is determined by the intrinsic urethral smooth and striated muscles (and their intact innervation), supportive connective tissue, submucosal venous plexus, and urethral mucosa which aids in its sealing (coaptation).
- Integral theory: Successful surgeries which correct stress incontinence do so by reinforcing or repairing the connective tissue (via a support hammock underneath the urethra) or by improving urethral function so as to counteract intrinsic sphincteric deficiency (ISD). The urethra sits on top of and is invested by the fibromuscular layer of the anterior vaginal wall (known surgically as the pubocervical fascia or endopelvic fascia). In essence, the endopelvic fascia forms a hammock underneath the urethra. Additionally, the urethra is supported at its mid-portion by the pubourethral ligament. Normally, the urethra is compressed against this backboard during stress (e.g., cough) and becomes occluded. If the hammock is deficient, the urethra is not compressed and urine leaks during stress. Additionally, if the hammock is intact but the urethral function is poor (i.e., ISD), the urethra is unable to occlude completely (lack of coaptation) and thus leakage occurs.
- The integral theory gives a better explanation of the continence mechanism than historical explanations. Urethral hypermobility is a sign that the hammock is deficient (either broken or stretched). The retropubic location of the urethra and the idea of *zone of intra-abdominal pressure* is no longer the explanation for the mechanism of SUI. Studies have reported that hypermobility of the urethra persists following successful mid-urethral sling procedures. Therefore, when the hammock is deficient (thus rendering the urethra hypermobile), stress allows displacement of the urethrovesical junction, pressure transmission to the bladder, but not equally to the urethra. Since the urethra cannot be compressed against a stable backboard, urine loss occurs.
- Surgery for SUI is indicated when conservative management fails (pharmacologic, pelvic muscle exercises, pessaries, local electrical stimulation, and so forth) and the patient wants definitive surgical repair.
  1. Mild SUI should be approached nonsurgically first.
  2. Women who desire subsequent childbearing are not the best surgical candidates (we have little data on the effect of childbirth after surgical repair of incontinence).
  3. Poor surgical candidates (i.e., multiple medical conditions) should attempt medical management of SUI.

- Today, over 270,000 anti-incontinence surgeries are performed in the United States. Of these, 100,000 are retropubic procedures, 120,000 are slings. Of the slings, 80,000 are mid-urethral and 40,000 are proximal urethral slings.
- Patients with urodynamic stress incontinence, mixed incontinence with predominant stress symptoms, and ISD (formerly called Type III incontinence) are candidates for surgeries discussed in the following.
  ○ Currently, patients with SUI due to disruption of the hammock or hypermobile urethra (aka SUI with HMU) are candidates for retropubic urethropexy (e.g., Burch), traditional proximal urethral sling, or mid-urethral sling procedures.
  ○ On the other hand, patients with stress incontinence due to pure ISD are candidates for traditional proximal urethral slings, mid-urethral slings (although lower cure rate), bulking procedures, and artificial urinary sphincter. Additionally, patients with SUI with ISD have a low cure rates with Burch at 5 years ($\approx$50–60%).
  ○ Patients who have a combination of hypermobility *and* sphincteric deficiency may have a lower failure rate with sling procedures although retropubic urethropexy with or without modifications may be attempted.
- Ideally, the patient should be done with childbearing, as future pregnancies may negate the effectiveness of these procedures. Package insert for Gynecare tension-free vaginal tape (TVT) states, "it should not be performed in patients with future growth potential including women with plans for future pregnancy." This suggestion is based on theoretical risks rather than on long-term data.
- This chapter describes the chronologic evolution of vaginal surgeries for the treatment of SUI, discusses cure rates, and complications of incontinence surgery, especially the mid-urethral slings, and discusses the differences between TVT and trans-obturator sling (TOT).
- The mid-urethral tension-free sling has become the gold standard for the treatment of SUI because:
  1. It is minimally invasive (small incisions, vaginal route, estimated blood loss [EBL] $\leq$75 mL).
  2. It is rapidly performed (<30 min) and is done as outpatient (under local with conscious sedation [with caution!], regional, or general anesthesia).
  3. There is a short learning curve and it is highly reproducible.
  4. There exists long-term data (approximately 7.5 years for TVT).
  5. It promises a high cure rate.
  6. It promises faster recovery (can resume normal daily activity within 1–2 weeks).

7. It has less complications (such as de novo detrusor instability and voiding difficulties) than its predecessors.

ESSENTIAL PREOPERATIVE AND INTRAOPERATIVE STEPS

(See also Chap. 38, Preoperative Issues in Pelvic Surgery.)

- Must evaluate for pelvic organ prolapse (POP) prior to surgery for stress incontinence since symptomatic and significant prolapse should be corrected prior to or at the same time as incontinence surgery
- Simple or multichannel urodynamic testing (see Chap. 6, Evaluation of Urinary Incontinence in the Office and Indications for Referral to a Specialist)
- ± Fleets enema
- Perioperative antibiotics (e.g., cephalexin [Ancef], ampicillin/sulbactam [Unasyn])—give up to 1 hour before incision is made
- May use regional or general anesthesia
- Thromboprophylaxis
- ± Pubic hair shaving
- Properly position the patient in dorsal lithotomy with buttocks at level or just off the edge of table and legs in Allen Universal stirrups (Allen Medical systems). Legs should be slightly flexed and abducted. Care should be taken to avoid excessive extension or abduction of the thighs to avoid femoral nerve and peroneal nerve injury.
- Prepping and draping the abdomen, upper thighs, vulva, perineum, perianal areas, and vagina in sterile fashion
- Drain bladder with 18 Fr Foley catheter

PROCEDURES

KELLY PLICATION

Kelly plication is also known as Kelly-Kennedy, bladder buttress, anterior colporrhaphy with suburethral plication.

- Historically, anterior colporrhaphy with Kelly suburethral plication was the standard of treatment for patients with genuine SUI. It was first described by Howard Kelly in 1912.
- The goal is to restore the anatomic support of the bladder neck and the urethra. This is achieved by plicating the pubocervical fascia on both sides of the proximal urethra and bladder neck. Today, this procedure may be combined with anterior colporrhaphy.
- The success rates are operator dependent and the cure or improvement rate is in the range of 59–69%

at 1 year. The cure rate diminishes rapidly with time (i.e., at 5 years). Due to the poor long-term results in the cure rate, this procedure is no longer recommended in the treatment of SUI.

- However, the technique is occasionally combined with anterior colporrhaphy for the management of anterior POP.
- Kelly plication technique (modified):
  1. Anterior vaginal wall is injected with 0.25% Marcaine with Epi, dilute vasopressin, or lidocaine with Epi.
  2. Midline vaginal incision from bladder neck to cardinal ligament area is made.
  3. Lateral dissection (i.e., peeling the vaginal mucosa from underlying pubocervical fascia; care should be taken to leave the pubocervical fascia on the bladder rather than on the peeled vaginal mucosa).
  4. The urethrovesical junction is located by measuring 4.5–5.0 cm from the external urethral meatus or by palpating the balloon of the Foley catheter.
  5. Horizontal mattress sutures (permanent or delayed absorbable) are placed in two to three layers just below the urethrovesical in order to elevate and stabilize it. The goal is to create differential support between urethrovesical angle and the bladder base. Reapproximation and plication of rest of the pubocervical fascia with absorbable suture (e.g., 0 vicryl pop-offs).
  6. Excess vaginal mucosa is trimmed and edges reapproximated with continuous absorbable suture (e.g., 2.0 vicryl).

OPEN RETROPUBIC PROCEDURES

These have been described in detail in Chap. 15.

NEEDLE SUSPENSION PROCEDURES

- Pereyra was the first to describe needle urethropexy in 1959. Several modifications have been described since the original description. Stamey, Raz, and the bone fixation procedures are some of the other examples of needle suspensions.
- The goal of the procedure is to support the urethra and prevent descent during increase in intra-abdominal pressure. The main principle involves anchoring the perivesical fascia at the bladder neck to the abdominal fascia or the pubic bone. This is achieved by using a needle to carry the suture from the abdominal incision through the retropubic space to the vagina.
- The needle suspension procedures have also fallen into disfavor due to the low cure rates, especially as

compared to the retropubic procedures. The cure rates vary from 67 to 70% at 1 year in various studies, most of which are observational. The cure rates also diminish rapidly with time (i.e., at 5 years).

- These techniques are not described as they are rarely performed today.

THE PROXIMAL SUBURETHRAL SLINGS

The proximal suburethral slings are also known as traditional suburethral sling and urethrovesical junction slings.

- The suburethral sling procedures were traditionally used only to ISD and recurrent SUI because of their higher postoperative complications (voiding dysfunction/urinary retention, and sling erosion).
- The principle involves creating a hammock underneath the urethra and bladder neck to prevent descent and provide a backboard for compression of the urethra at the urethrovesical junction during increased intra-abdominal pressure.
- Traditional slings are done on an inpatient basis and are preferred by some female urologists.
- The first sling operation was described by Giordano in 1907 using gracilis muscle flap. In 1942, Aldridge developed the fascial suburethral sling, which after modifications, is in use today.
- Several biologic and synthetic materials have been used to make a sling (see Table 14-1). Theoretically, there is an increased risk of erosion, infection, and fistula formation with the synthetic materials. Cadaveric allograft fascia does not seem to carry a significant risk of infection, erosion, or fistula formation. (See Chap. 49, Female Sexual Dysfunction.)
- Bone-anchored slings were first introduced by GE Leach in 1988 in order to (1) decrease discomfort associated with tying sutures over rectus abdominis fascia and (2) minimize pull-through of suture from periurethral fascia.
- Modifications of the suburethral sling by anchoring it to the pubic bone does not increase the effectiveness, but does carry a risk of osteomyelitis, osteitis pubis, and erosion.

TABLE 14-1

BIOLOGIC SLINGS	SYNTHETIC SLINGS
Fascia lata	Mersilene
Rectus fascia	Nylon
Gracilis muscle flap	Marlex
Pectus or pyramidalis muscle flap	Gore-Tex
Round ligament	Silastic
ox dura mater	Polypropylene mesh
Porcine small intestine submucosa	
Cadaver fascia	

- Currently, many experts prefer autologous rectus fascia and soft polypropylene mesh. Allografts and xenografts are also used (see Chap. 50, Materials Used in Female Pelvic Reconstructive Surgery [FPRS]: Grafts, Meshes, and Sling Materials).
- Some experts will avoid use of synthetics for certain types of patients:
  ○ History of radiation
  ○ History of sling erosion
  ○ Having surgery on urethra as well as incontinence surgery (e.g., urethral diverticulectomy)
  ○ Having POP surgery at the same time as incontinence surgery (controversial)
  ○ Allergic reaction to synthetic materials
- The overall success rate for SUI with HMU is between 82 and 90% at 5 years and does not decrease much with time.
- The cure rate is better than once thought, since the majority of the studies of slings were on patients with severe ISD or recurrent incontinence (after previous incontinence surgery).
  ○ Cure rates for SUI with ISD at 5 years is ≈80–90% (higher than Burch and even mid-urethral slings).
  ○ Cure rates for primary incontinence are 80–95% and for recurrent incontinence 70–85%.
- Therefore, some experts will utilize proximal urethral slings (with subjective tension adjustments, [i.e., looser or tighter]) for all types of SUI (with primary or recurrent, and ISD, HMU, or both). It is better to error on the side of looser tensioning.
- The type of sling material probably does not significantly affect cure rates.
- Traditional sling technique using rectus fascia (helpful technical pearls in *italics*):
  1. A strip of rectus abdominus fascia is harvested as a strip or a patch (e.g., size ≈2 × 20 cm).
  2. Anterior vaginal wall is injected with dilute vasopressin, incised, and dissected as described for Kelly plication.
  3. Lateral dissection is carried to the inferior rami with the goal of opening the retropubic space on both sides of the bladder neck and proximal urethra. This space is finally entered and widened by a rotary motion of the index finger.
  4. Sling is put under bladder neck and proximal urethra (mostly under proximal urethra) then fixed in place with sutures.
  5. Stab incision is made at rectus fascia just above the symphysis pubis.
  6. Uterine packing forceps are passed through the stab incision posterior to the pubic bone (and under the guidance of index finger of the other hand) into the vaginal incision
  7. Sling material is pulled up into the abdominal incision and sutured to rectus fascia to anchor it.

Note: ends of the sling can be secured to rectus abdominis fascia, iliopectineal line, or pubic symphysis.

8. Cystoscopy is performed to rule out bladder injury and to confirm sling tension by observing closure of urethrovesical junction.

9. Sling is sutured to rectus abdominus fascia with nonabsorbable suture (e.g., Prolene). The tension placed on the sling is an art in itself. For example, experts will tie the sling with more tension in a patient with ISD and less tension for HMU. It is better to error on the side of less tension on the sling because urethral obstruction and urinary retention is a common complication of this procedure.

10. Abdominal and vaginal incisions are closed with absorbable suture.

- Effectiveness and complication rates (esp. urinary retention) are operator dependent. Although cure rates may be higher than other procedures, the complication rates (e.g., voiding dysfunction, prolonged catheterization, or permanent intermittent self catheterization [ISC]) are also higher.

MID-URETHRAL TENSION-FREE SLINGS

Mid-urethral tension-free slings are also known as minimally invasive mid-urethral sling (MIMUS), TVT, and trans-obturator sling (TOT).

TVT
- The TVT was first developed by Ulmsten in Sweden.
- It has been used extensively in Europe for the treatment of stress incontinence. It eventually caught on in the United States by gynecure and has now revolutionized the treatment of SUI.
- Indications for proximal and mid-urethral slings:
  ○ SUI with HMU
  ○ SUI with ISD
  ○ SUI with HMU/ISD spectrum
  ○ Mixed incontinence with stress predominance
  ○ Recurrent SUI
- Relative contraindications for proximal and mid-urethral slings:
  ○ Severe detrusor overactivity
  ○ Severe detrusor underactivity (acontractility)
  ○ High postvoid residuals (PVRs) without advanced POP
  ○ Valsalva voiding
  ○ Obstructive voiding on uroflow
  ○ Unwillingness to consider, perform, or learn intermittent self-catheterization
- Various mid-urethral slings are available for treatment of SUI. The success rates are initially high and durable (even at 7 years) for SUI and mixed incontinence;

success is lower for pure ISD. Mean objective cure rates for SUI with HMU are: 1 year ≥90% and 5–7 years ≈85%.
- However, TVT cure rates for SUI are lower in complicated patients at ≤4 years:
  ○ SUI with ISD ≈70–80%
  ○ Recurrent SUI ≈80–85%
  ○ Mixed incontinence ≈85%
  ○ Elderly ≈67%
- Additionally, patients with COPD, asthma, obesity, and so forth have higher risk for failure.
- TVT versus Burch (open and laparoscopic):
  ○ Compared to laparoscopic Burch, TVT is more cost effective, uses less operative time, and has higher objective cure rate (at <2 years)
  ○ Compared to pen Burch, TVT has similar cure rate for up to 2 years for treatment of primary incontinence (HMU-type)
- Three types of sling material are available (also see Chap. 50, Materials Used in Female Pelvic Reconstructive Surgery [FPRS]: Grafts, Meshes, and Sling Materials): synthetic (efficacious as per data but has risk of erosion), biological (theoretical decreased risk of erosion but efficacy remains to be seen), and combination or hybrid (theoretically retains adherent properties of synthetic with decreased risk of erosion).
- The various forms of TVT procedures are quickly and easily performed, minimally invasive, and have low complication rates.
- Possible mechanisms of cure:
  1. Formation of hammock (backboard) underneath urethra allowing its compression and thus occlusion
  2. Reformation of the pubourethral ligaments at mid-urethra which allows support at the normally high-pressure zone of the urethra
  3. Inflammation and metabolic changes induced by the procedure itself cause increase in collagen and stronger biomechanical properties of the endopelvic fascia (aka pubocervical fascia) supporting the urethra
- The procedures can be divided into categories depending on the route of insertion of the needle (or trocar). The TVT may be performed suprapubically (aka top-down approach) or vaginally (bottom-up approach). The TOT may be performed inside-out or outside-in.
- Currently available tension-free mid-urethral slings encountered commonly in the market are summarized in Table 50-2. The Gynecare TVT is the original TVT marketed in the United States. In the following we describe another type of mid-urethral sling called Uretex.
- Procedure (described in the text) and helpful technical pearls (in *italics*) and postoperative care—transvaginal (bottom-up) mid-urethral procedure using Uretex (CR Bard):

1. Quarter percent lidocaine with epinephrine is injected horizontally in the abdominal skin just above the symphysis pubis and downward along the back of the pubic bone in the space of Retzius. Lidocaine with Epi is also infiltrated suburethrally and paraurethrally into the vaginal wall.

2. Two small (5 mm) incisions are made about 1.5 cm from the midline on either side just above the symphysis pubis. Another 1–2 cm incision is made in the midline in the anterior vaginal wall (suburethral location) about a centimeter proximal to the external urethral meatus. *Note: (1) try to make a full-thickness vaginal dissection because it may help reduce erosions, (2) 1 cm is not exact distance, as long as the sling is placed in a mid-urethral location, it will be successful in curing stress incontinence.*

3. The paraurethral tissues are dissected bilaterally for about a centimeter.

4. The bladder is drained using a catheter. A rigid catheter guide is used to deflect the urethra to the patient's left (i.e., handle to the patient's right).

5. The trocar with a blue "guide wire" attached to its end is then introduced through the vaginal incision and advanced into the right paraurethral space and directed toward the patient's right shoulder. As soon as the trocar perforates the pubocervical fascia, it is redirected toward the patient's head. *Note: If the trocar is not redirected, it stays lateral and may migrate cranially and may risk injury to the bowel, nerves, and major vessels.* The trocar is then advanced slowly while in close contact with the posterior aspect of the pubic bone (in the space of Retzius and in front of the bladder and under constant tactile feedback) and is brought out through the right suprapubic incision. *Note: The trocar is kept in close contact to the pubic bone so as to avoid bladder perforation.* As the trocar is pulled out through the skin incision, the guide wire is left behind in the path that the trocar just created. This exact procedure is repeated on the opposite side while the urethra is held to the patient's right with the rigid catheter guide.

6. Cystoscopy is performed (+/- indigo carmine) to rule out injury to the urethra and the bladder. If the blue guide wire is seen inside the bladder, it is removed and the procedure is repeated with slightly more lateral aim of trocar while attempting to stay in apposition to the back of pubic bone. *Note: Bladder perforation is a common (5–10%) complication of this procedure and it heals spontaneously without catheterization beyond immediate postoperative period. Thus some experts recommend no catheter drainage after perforation,* *especially if a small caliber trocar is utilized for the TVT procedure. Others recommend indwelling catheterization overnight after bladder perforation. To reduce bladder perforation, hug the back of the pubic bone and empty bladder before inserting trocar.*

7. If the blue guide wire is not visible during cystoscopy, then polypropylene mesh tape and its plastic sheath is attached to the blue guide wire on both sides in the vaginal area, and the other end of the blue guide wire is pulled out though the skin in the abdominal end leaving behind the mesh and its plastic sheath. Just before the tape lies flat against the suburethal tissue at mid-urethral level, the tab in the middle part of the plastic sheath is cut.

8. A blunt instrument such as a Hegar dilator (size 8 or 9) or Mayo Scissors is left between the urethra and the mesh tape while the plastic sheath is pulled off completely so as to prevent any tension on the mesh. When the procedure is done, there should be a space (3–5 mm) between the urethra and the polypropylene mesh tape, hence tension-free sling (the cough stress test may be performed at this point if patient is awake). Additionally, some experts insert a dilator into the urethra after sling tensioning, and if narrowing or bumps are felt while sliding dilator through urethra, the sling is loosened. Some experts will leave less space between the urethral and the mesh tape in patients with ISD (esp. low LPP) and obese patients. *Note: Until the surgeon has sufficient experience with the technique to determine appropriate spacing between sling and urethra, it can be performed while the patient is awake so that the cough stress test can be performed. Alternatively, it can be performed under general or spinal anesthesia and the anesthesiologist can increase intra-abdominal pressure.*

9. Excess mesh ("sling arms") is cut just below the skin at the abdominal end. *Since the polypropylene weave grips onto tissue (like Velcro), and therefore* (we have little data on the effect of childbirth on surgical repair of incontinence) *does not need to be sutured onto any tissue. Friction between tissue and the mesh keeps it in place initially and later tissue ingrowth keeps it in permanently.*

10. The abdominal skin incisions and the vaginal incision are closed and a Foley catheter is left for less than 24 hours.

11. PVRs are checked by intermittent catheterization or bladder ultrasound and the patient is discharged home when bladder function is adequate.

12. Postoperative hemoglobin is recommended by some, since this is a blind procedure with risk of hemorrhage.
13. Patients are instructed to avoid heavy lifting (>12 lb), strenuous exercise, and to maintain pelvic rest for 4–6 weeks after the procedure. Patients may climb stairs the same day of surgery and may perform light activity (e.g., power walk) in 2 weeks.
14. Oral analgesics for 1 week are appropriate.
15. Postoperative antibiotics for 5–7 days are physician dependent.

- The suprapubic mid-urethral procedure (aka top-down) is similar in concept to the one described earlier. With this approach, the trocar is introduced through the suprapubic incision, pushed through the rectus fascia, passed behind the pubic bone, and pushed out from the vaginal incision. The sling is then attached and the trocar is brought out through the suprapubic incision. This is repeated on the contralateral side and cystoscopy is performed. The mesh is connected to the needle on the vaginal side and pulled out through the abdominal incisions.
- Both the suprapubic as well as transvaginal techniques of mid-urethral sling are acceptable and effective as long as the mesh is placed in a mid-urethral location.
- Experts who prefer the transvaginal approach claim that it has higher efficacy because there is more consistent placement of the mesh at the mid-urethra and there is a lower rate of bladder injury.
- On the other hand, experts who prefer the suprapubic approach claim that it has a lower rate of bowel and major vessel injury.

TOT

- The TOT is also a type of mid-urethral sling; however, it leaves the sling in a more horizontal ("hammocklike" orientation) or meniscuslike rather than a U created by TVT.
- It uses less operative time and is easier to learn than TVT. This may appeal to generalists and gynecologic surgeons who may not be as comfortable with the anatomy of the retropubic space.
- The TOT was designed to reduce complication rates of TVT. The TOT avoids the retropubic space and theoretically avoids injury to the bladder, bowel, and major vessels. In actuality, bladder perforation has been reported, though rarely.
- Anatomy review: Obturator foramen = oval window made of half ilium and half pubis. *Boundaries*: superior = superior pubic ramus + body of pubis, inferior = ischium, anterior = inferior pubic ramus + ischial ramus, posterior = ischium + pubis. Is sealed by the dense sheath, the obturator membrane, except at its most lateral, posterior, and superior border where the obturator vessels and nerve exit. This obturator canal is 4.4 cm lateral to the pubic rami. Originating from the obturator foramen edges and the obturator membrane lies the obturator internus muscle and obturator externus muscle inside and outside the pelvis, respectively. Both of these muscles attach to the femur.

- If performed correctly, the TOT sling is a safe distance from important structures:
  ○ Obturator canal = 2.4 cm
  ○ Obturator nerve (anterior division) = 3.4 cm
  ○ Obturator nerve (posterior division) = 2.7 cm
  ○ Obturator vessels (most medial, at risk branch) = 1.1 cm
- Procedure (described in the text) and helpful technical pearls (in *italics*): inside-out TOT procedure using TVT-O (Ethicon-Gynecare):
  1. Exit points on the skin are marked at a level 2 cm above the external urethral meatus and 2 cm lateral to the folds of the thigh, then two 5–10 mm stab incisions are made.
  2. The anterior vaginal wall mucosa is injected with a dilute vasopressin then a 1 cm incision is made about a centimeter proximal to the urethral opening.
  3. Lateral dissection by push-spread technique is achieved with the tips of the scissors pointed slightly upward (45 degrees to the horizontal). *Note: Anatomically, the track is above the perineal membrane and below the pubocervical fascia, therefore the space of Retzius is never entered.*
  4. Perforate the obturator membrane at the junction between the body of the pubic bone and the inferior pubic ramus (loss of resistance is felt).
  5. Insert winged guide into dissected track, insert the helical passer needle (with its plastic tube covering and attached tape and plastic sheath) through the guide just passing the obturator membrane. *Note: it is important to stay medial and superior on the obturator foramen because the origin of the vessels and nerve is at the most lateral-posterior, and superior position on the obturator foramen.*
  6. Then remove the winged guide and rotate the handle of the helical passer needle counterclockwise to the patient's right while moving the handle of the helical passer toward the midline.
  7. Exit the helical passer needle and plastic tube at exit points on the thigh. Note: the helical passer needle has passed through the following layers: obturator internus muscle (OI) → obturator membrane (OM) → obturator externus muscle (OE) → adductor magnus muscle → adductor brevis muscle → gracilis muscle → fascia lata → subcutaneous → skin exit. Three "pops" will be felt as you go through OI, OM, and OE.

8. When the tip of the plastic tube appears at the skin, grasp and clamp it then remove the helical passer needle by a reverse rotation of the handle (leaving behind the plastic tube and its attached tape and plastic sheath).

9. Pull the plastic tube completely through the skin until the tape appears.

10. Repeat the same steps on the other side, make sure the polypropylene mesh is not twisted in the mid-urethral area underneath the urethra.

11. When the tape is in position, pull the plastic sheath off while placing a blunt instrument as a spacer between the urethra and the polypropylene tape (therefore tension-free).

12. Cut the excess tape ends at the exit sites and close the thigh skin incision and the vaginal incision with absorbable suture or skin adhesive.

- Expert opinion:
  ○ Some experts believe that young, thin, and active women and patients with ISD are not the ideal candidates for the TOT procedure.
  ○ On the other hand, obese women and those with the following conditions may be better candidates for the TOT. Data are needed on this matter:
    ▪ Milder forms of SUI
    ▪ Occult incontinence
    ▪ Significant voiding dysfunction (valsalva voiding, poor detrusor contractility)
    ▪ Overactive bladder/mixed incontinence
    ▪ History of Burch procedure or other incontinence surgery
    ▪ History of some abdominal operation (anterior abdominal wall hernia repair with mesh, kidney transplant, or history of colovesical fistula repair)
- *TOT versus TVT* (all data are preliminary and data with longer follow-up are needed).
  ○ 12-month follow-up data show similar objective cure rates for the TOT; long-term data are needed especially in subgroups of SUI (e.g., pure ISD).
  ○ TOT seems to have less voiding difficulties than the TVT (esp. less urinary retention).
  ○ TOT seems to have lower infection, bladder perforation, and erosion rate, but 3% rate of obturator hematoma.
  ○ TOT has no bowel injury and lower nerve injury.
  ○ Cystoscopy is not required for TOT, therefore gynecologist may still perform this surgery in hospitals where they may not have cystoscopic privileges. However, some experts recommend performing a cystoscopy even after a TOT because bladder injury has been documented after a TOT and the true rate of bladder injury is presently unknown.
  ○ Less operating room time (15 min vs. 27 min).
  ○ Easy to learn and teach.

COMPLICATIONS OF VAGINAL PROCEDURES FOR THE CORRECTION OF STRESS INCONTINENCE

- Vaginal procedures for the management of SUI can have the following complications: *intraoperative* (injury to urinary tract, blood vessels or nerves, hemorrhage, injury to bowel), *early postoperative* (urinary retention with prolonged catheterization [≥4 weeks], urinary tract infection), and *late postoperative* (de novo detrusor overactivity, failure of treatment, recurrence of symptoms, graft erosion, infection, POP).
- Voiding difficulties in the form of urinary retention requiring prolonged catheterization or de novo OAB or urge incontinence are among the most common complications of these procedures. Generally, traditional slings have more severe and higher rate of complication than the mid-urethral slings. For example, the traditional sling procedures have the highest rate of urinary retention (2–37%) (traditional sling>Burch>TVT>TOT). The rate of urinary retention is operator dependent and also depends on how tight the sling is tied.
- The TVT has the following complication rates:
- *Voiding difficulties >UTI (up to 17%)>bladder perforation (5–10%)>erosions (3–5%)>vascular injuries>bowel injuries>hematoma>nerve injuries>death (6 women by Sept. 2002).*
- Vascular injuries are usually in the form of hematomas (retropubic>vaginal). Major vessel injuries are *uncommon,* but when it occurs, the external iliac vessels are the most commonly injured major vessels (external iliac>femoral>obturator>inferior epigastric).
- Other complications: erosions (vaginal (3%)> urethral>bladder); nerve injuries (esp. obturator nerve, ilioinguinal nerve), and enterocele, rectocele, and rarely necrotizing fasciitis.

MANAGEMENT OF COMMON COMPLICATIONS OF MID-URETHRAL SLINGS

The following suggestions are based on review of the literature and opinions of experts in the field.
- Voiding difficulties:
  ○ Postoperative urinary retention or incomplete bladder emptying usually resolves within 2 days of surgery. Chapter 23, Voiding Dysfunction and Urinary Retention, describes patients at higher risk for urinary retention in detail.
    1. An indwelling Foley catheter may be left in with removal 3–7 days (or more) postoperatively. Clean ISC or suprapubic catheterization is preferred for longer periods of retention as they are associated with lower incidence of UTI.

2. Tamsulosin (Flomax)—alpha-1 antagonist may relax smooth muscle in bladder neck enough to facilitate urine flow rate; this is expert opinion and lacks level 1–3 evidence.

3. Hegar dilator may be inserted in the urethra with downward traction.

4. Sling revision—the most common reason for retention is excess tension on the sling.

   ▪ Identification of the location of sling can be facilitated by placing cystoscope in urethra and placing tension on the sling.

   ▪ Vaginal midline transection or lysis of the mesh tape under intravenous (IV) sedation and local anesthetic. Additional retropubic and paraurethral dissection as needed, or,

   ▪ Rectus fascia slings may be released by cutting sutures which attach sling to the rectus fascia.

   ▪ Loosening of mesh tape—movement of mesh as a unit by downward traction on the loop underneath urethra with blunt instrument. However, this can only be done inslings with a built-in tensioning suture (e.g., SPARC[AMS]), otherwise the mesh will stretch. Ideally, loosening should be done within 2.5 weeks of surgery before capsule has formed around the mesh tape.

○ De novo detrusor overactivity may occur because of (1) worsening of preexisting symptoms after mesh placement; in a patient with mixed incontinence, conservative management should be done before attempting surgery for this reason. (2) Unmasking of OAB in patient with ISD. Since detrusor contractions cannot be appreciated on cystometry when there is no urethral resistance (i.e., ISD). De novo detrusor overactivity can be as high as 50% 1 week after surgery and may decrease to 10% by 10 weeks. Irritative symptoms should be evaluated and treated by bladder retraining and anticholinergics (see Chap. 13, Conservative Management of Incontinence and Pelvic Organ Prolapse).

○ UTI and wound infections—perioperative intravenous antibiotics, the plastic sheath covering the mesh, and the Prolene made up of the mesh (Prolene is a synthetic material with low risk of infection and rejection) reduce the risk of infection. However, postoperative antibiotics, vaginal estrogen cream, and pelvic rest may be required to treat infections.

• Bladder perforation:
   ○ If it occurs during surgery and 1–2 perforation(s) noted, trocar may be taken out and replaced. According to some experts, no prolonged catheterization is necessary if the patient is able to void prior to discharge. Others will leave a catheter in for a couple of days.
   ○ If it occurs during surgery and many perforations are noted, prolonged catheterization may be required.

Some experts suggest a cystogram after catheter is removed to evaluate bladder integrity.
   ○ If perforation is discovered long time after surgery (rare), it may be repaired with operative cystoscopic techniques.

• Excessive bleeding in the retropubic space or vagina may occur rarely and may resolve spontaneously. It may be diagnosed by suprapubic/pelvic discomfort, decreasing hemoglobin, bimanual examination fullness, and/or ultrasound confirmation: (1) avoid surgery on patients with bleeding disorder or those on anticoagulants, (2) suturing, manual compression, vaginal packing, or Gelfoam may be required, (3) Katske-Raz tamponade—place 30 mL Foley catheter into bleeding space and inflate, (4) fill the bladder with 400–500 mL of fluid for 5 minutes and apply suprapubic pressure.

• Mesh erosion:
   ○ *Vaginal* is the most common type. May have symptoms of new-onset vaginal discharge, bleeding, pelvic pain, and dyspareunia. Colposcopy may be helpful in visualization of erosion. May occur because of (1) technique—incorrect trocar application in patient with vaginal atrophy, (2) hematoma—bleeding underneath vaginal mucosa which drains through incision and leaves mesh exposed, (3) inadvertent button-hole during surgery. Vaginal mesh erosion may be ignored in a patient who is not sexually active. However, in a sexually active patient, experts suggest observation, pelvic rest, and antibiotics for 8 weeks to 3 months because growth may occur through the mesh pores and the mucosa may heal on its own. If after conservative management, mesh is still exposed, then cut excess mesh, free edges of vaginal mucosa, suture vaginal wall with absorbable suture, and give antibiotics. Cutting of mesh may not change effectiveness of sling in a patient who had hypermobile urethra type of SUI (it may, however, decrease effectiveness of sling in patient with ISD type of SUI).
   ○ *Bladder* is the least common type. May have symptoms of recurrent UTIs, hematuria, and irritative voiding symptoms. It is difficult to remove if discovered weeks after the procedure and depending on the type of mesh (e.g., Gore-Tex is easier to remove while Mersilene is tougher). It may be removed via operative cystoscopy (endoscopic scissors), vaporization by laser, or actual opening of bladder, removal, repair, and prolonged catheterization.

• Still has incontinence after mid-urethral sling placement:
   ○ If less than 2.5 weeks since surgery, patient may return for sling tightening (if sling has built-in tensioning-sutures [e.g., SPARC] that prevent stretching of mesh during tightening). Under IV sedation and

local anesthetic, the excess loop of mesh is reduced using Mayo scissors while the patient performs cough stress test. The loop of mesh is sequentially reduced and held in place with hemoclips until the space between the urethra and mesh is small enough to prevent leakage of urine during stress test. Then, the excess mesh is excised. The new ends of the mesh are sutured with several interrupted 4.0 Prolene sutures and the hemoclips are removed.

○ If it has been some time after surgery, the patient needs to be reevaluated objectively (urodynamics ± cystoscopy) to differentiate between urge, stress, mixed incontinence, or other reasons for incontinence.

○ A second sling is possible if >3 months have elapsed after first sling placement and the patient still has urodynamic stress incontinence. Experts prefer placement of the second sling in tandem fashion (next to the original sling) instead of on top of the original sling as it may increase surface area underneath the urethra. This is consistent with hammock theory.

• Bone anchoring complications (see Chap. 15, Surgical Management of Stress Urinary Incontinence: Open Retropubic Operations).

PREPUBIC MID-URETHRAL SLINGS

• Some physicians are experimenting with this technique. However, there are currently no data.
• The procedure involves placement of a synthetic sling underneath the mid-portion of the urethra in a tension-free fashion with the arms of the sling not anchored (as in TVT), and placed in front of the pubic bone instead of behind it (therefore, avoiding both retropubic space and obturator foramen).

RADIOFREQUENCY

• Radiofrequency is electromagnetic energy that induced thermal changes in tissues resulting in heating and shrinkage. This technique can be applied to the endopelvic fascia to shrink and stabilize the fascia to improve the support for the urethra and bladder neck.
• The SURx Transvaginal System (SURx, Inc., Livermore, California) is a device that is designed as a transvaginal treatment of urinary stress incontinence.
• The procedure can be performed under general anesthesia as an outpatient procedure.
• An incision is made in the vagina lateral to the urethra, exposing the endopelvic fascia. Radiofrequency energy is applied over the endopelvic fascia resulting in blanching and shrinkage of the tissue.

• Though long-term data are lacking, the 12-month overall cure rate is <73% according to studies.
• This method is used by some experts for occult or mild SUI.
• SURx may be better for treatment of paravaginal defect.

BIBLIOGRAPHY

Alcalay M, Monga A, Stanton SL. Burch colposuspension: a 10-20 year follow up. *Br J Obstet Gynaecol.* 1995;102: 740–745.

Biedmead J, Cardozo L. Sling techniques in the treatment of genuine stress incontinence. *Br J Obstet Gynaecol.* 2000;107: 147–156.

Blomquist J, Germain MM. Surgical correction of stress incontinence with hypermobility. In: Bent AE, Ostergard DR, et al., eds. *Ostergard's Urogynecology and Pelvic Floor Dysfunction.* 5th ed. Philadelphia, PA: Lippincott Williams & Wilkins; 2002:457–468.

Brubaker L. Suburethral sling release. *Obstet Gynecol.* 1995;86 (4 Pt 2):686–688.

Carr LK, Webster GD. Voiding dysfunction following incontinence surgery: diagnosis and treatment with retropubic or vaginal urethrolysi. *J Urol.* 1999;161(4):1268–1271.

Chaikin DC, Rosenthal J, Blaivas JG. Pubovaginal fascial sling for all types of stress urinary incontinence: long-term analysis. *J Urol.* 1998:160:1312–1316.

Clemens JQ, DeLancey Jo, Gaerber GJ, et al. Urinary tract erosions after synthetic pubovaginal slings: diagnosis and management strategy. *Urology.* 2000;56(4):589–594.

de Leval J. Novel surgical technique for the treatment of female stress urinary incontinence: transobturator vaginal tape inside-out. *Eur Urol.* 2003;44(6):724–730.

Delorme E, Droupy S, de Tayrac R, Delmas V. Transobturator tape (Uratape): a new minimally-invasic procedure to treat female urinary incontinence. *Eur Urol.* 2001;45(2): 203–207.

Klutke C, Siegel S, Carlin B, et al. Urinary retention after tension-free vaginal tape procedure: incidence and treatment. *Urology.* 2001;58:697–701.

Kohli N. Open compared with laparoscopic approach to Burch colposuspension: a cost analysis. *Obstet Gynecol.* 1997;90(3): 411–415.

Meschia M, Pifarotti P, Bernasconi F, et al. Tension-free vaginal tape (TVT) in women with recurrent stress urinary incontinence: a long-term follow-up. *Int Urogynecol J Suppl.* 2001;2:S24–S27.

Mohehrer B, Carey M, Wilson D. Laparoscopic colposuspension: a systematic review.*Br J Obstet Gynaecol.* 2003;110: 230–235.

Nilssonn CG, Kuuva N, Falconer C, et al. Long-term results of the tension-free vaginal tape (TVT) procedure for surgical treatment of female stress urinary incontinence. *Int Urogynecol J Suppl.* 2001;2:S5–S8.

Petros P, Ulmsten U. An integral theory of female urinary incontinence, experimental and clinical considerations. *Acta Obstet Gynecol Scand.* 1990;69(Suppl 153).

Pubic osteomyelitis and granuloma after bone anchor placement. *Int Urogynecol J Pelvic Floor Dysfunct.* 1999;10(5):346–348.

Rezapour M, Flaconer C, Ulmsten U. Tension-free vaginal tape (TVT) in stress incontinence women with intrinsic sphincteric deficiency: a long-term follow-up. *Int Urogynecol J Suppl.* 2001;2:S15–S18.

Ross JW, Galen DI, Abbott k, et al. A prospective multisite study of radiofrequency bipolar energy for treatment of genuine stress incontinence. *J Am Assoc Gynecol Laparosc.* 2002;9(4): 493–499.

Sand PK, Bowen LW, Panganiban R, et al. The low pressure urethra as a factor in failed retropubic urethropexy. *Obstet Gynecol.* 1987;69:399–402.

Schrepferman CG, Griebling Tl, Nygaard IE, et al. Resolution of urge symptoms following sling cystourethropexy. *J Urol.* 2000;164(5):1628–1631.Steel SA, Cox C, Stanton SL. Long-term follow-up of detrusor instability following the colposuspension operation. *Br J Urol.* 1986;58:138–142.

Tanagho EA. Colpocystourethropexy: the way we do it. *J Urol.* 1976;116:751–753.

Ulmsten U, Flaconer C, Johnson P, et al. A multicenter study of tension-free tape (TVT) for surgical treatment of stress urinary incontinence. *Int Urogynecol J.* 1998;9:210–213.

Ulmsten U, Henriksson L, Johnson P, et al. An ambulatory surgical procedure under local anesthesis for treatment of female urinary incontinence. *Int Urogynecol J.* 1996;7:81–86.

Ustun Y, Engin-Ustun Y, Gungor M, et al. Tension-free vaginal tape compared with laparoscopic Burch urethropexy. *J Am Assoc Gynecol Laparosc.* 2003;10(3):386–389.

Vierhout ME. Severe hemorrhage complicating tension-free vaginal tape (TVT): a case report. *Int Urogynecol J.* 2001;12: 139–140.

Walters MD, Daneshgari F. Surgical management of stress urinary incontinence. In: Weber A. *Clinical Obstetrics and Gynecology- Incontinence 2004.* Philadelphia, PA: Lippincott Williams & Wilkins; 2004: 93–103.

QUESTIONS

1. A 42-year-old, para 3, woman presents to you complaining of loss of urine during coughing, laughing, and exercise. This has had an impact on her quality of life. Review of symptoms is negative for symptoms of OAB. She has a history of a Burch colposuspension which was performed 7 years ago. She also had a splenectomy 3 years ago after a car accident. Upon pelvic examination, all three compartments are well supported. U_{dip} is negative and PVR = 10 mL after voiding 200 mL. During complex cystometry, she has a positive stress test in sitting position at 150 mL and she reveals maximum urethral closure pressure (MUCP) of 15 cm H_2O and valsalva leak point pressures (VLPP) at 50 cm H_2O. The best management of this patient is ____.

   (A) Duloxetine
   (B) TVT sling
   (C) Transobturator sling
   (D) Retropubic urethropexy
   (E) Radiofrequency procedure

2. The MOST common complication of mid-urethral slings is ____.

   (A) Excessive bleeding
   (B) Urinary retention
   (C) Bladder perforation
   (D) Major vessel injury
   (E) Vaginal erosion of tape

3. Currently, those who perform proximal urethral slings prefer using ____

   (A) Cadaveric fascia lata
   (B) Autologous rectus fascia
   (C) Mersilene tape
   (D) Porcine dermis

QUESTIONS 4–7

Any of the four answer choices may be used once, more than once, or not at all.

   (A) Comparable
   (B) Higher
   (C) Lower
   (D) Data not yet available

4. When compared to the TVT, the cure rates for open Burch at 3 years follow-up are

5. When compared to the TVT, the cure rates for laparoscopic Burch are

6. When compared to TVT, the cure rates for traditional slings at 5 years follow-up are

7. When compared to traditional sling, the cure rates for open Burch at 10 years are

ANSWERS

1. *(C).* Based on the symptoms, the patient has SUI. Based on urodynamic studies, the patient has a low-pressure urethra consistent with ISD. A sling procedure is preferable to a retropubic procedure when there is a low-pressure urethra. Additionally, many experts recommend performing a TOT rather than a TVT in patient who has had previous abdominal surgery or a previous anti-incontinence procedure. This patient has had both. Duloxetine is not yet approved by the Food and Drug Administration (FDA) for SUI.

It may not be effective in this patient. Currently, radiofrequency procedure may be used for occult or mild SUI. Long-term data are needed.

2. *(B)*. The TVT has the following complication rates: Voiding difficulties >UTI (up to 17%) >bladder perforation (5–10%) >erosions (3–5%) >vascular injuries >bowel injuries >hematoma >nerve injuries >death

3. *(B)*. Autologous rectus fascia is safe (no risk of erosion, minimal risk of surgery, no risk of rejection or autolysis), inexpensive, and easily harvested during surgery. Cadaveric fascia lata has a risk of autolysis and early failure (up to 20%).Mersilene tape is not preferred as it has higher risk of erosion and infection. Among synthetic materials, polypropylene is the most commonly utilized. Porcine dermis (e.g., Pelvilace) is not often used for traditional slings. See Chap. 50, Materials Used in Female Pelvic Reconstructive Surgery (FPRS): Grafts, Meshes, and Sling Materials.

ANSWERS 4–7

4. *(A)*, 5. *(C)*, 6. *(A)*, 7. *(C)*. Mean objective cure rates for SUI with HMU for the TVT are as follows: at 1 year ≥90% and 5–7 years ≈85%. The overall success rate for SUI with HMU for the traditional sling is between 82–90% at 5 years and does not decrease much with time. Compared to laparoscopic Burch, TVT is more cost-effective, uses less operative time, and has higher objective cure rate (at <2 years). Compared to open Burch, TVT has similar cure rate for up to 2 years. Based on long-term data, cure rate for SUI after Burch declines with time and plateaus by 10–12 years at ≈70%.

15 SURGICAL MANAGEMENT OF STRESS URINARY INCONTINENCE: OPEN RETROPUBIC OPERATIONS

Sam Siddighi

BACKGROUND

- More than 150 surgical procedures have evolved for the management of stress urinary incontinence (SUI). The reasons for the existence of many procedures for one diagnosis are several: (1) technical innovation, (2) dissatisfaction with long-term results of existing treatments, (3) dissatisfaction with rate of complications of existing treatments, and (4) invasiveness of existing treatments.

- Continence is maintained because of (1) pelvic floor muscles (which are tonically contracted at rest and reflexively contracts with increases in intra-abdominal pressure), (2) suburethral endopelvic fascial hammock, (3) intrinsic urethral function which is determined by the intrinsic urethral smooth and striated muscles (and their intact innervation), supportive connective tissue, submucosal venous plexus, and urethral mucosa which aids in its sealing (coaptation).

- Integral theory: Successful surgeries which correct stress incontinence do so by reinforcing or repairing the connective tissue (via a support hammock underneath the urethra) or by improving urethral function so as to counteract intrinsic sphincteric deficiency (ISD). The urethra sits on top of and is invested by the fibromuscular layer of the anterior vaginal wall (known surgically as the pubocervical fascia or endopelvic fascia). In essence, the endopelvic fascia forms a hammock underneath the urethra. Additionally, the urethra is supported at its midportion by the pubourethral ligament. Normally, the urethra is compressed against this backboard during stress (e.g., cough) and becomes occluded. If the hammock is deficient, the urethra is not compressed and urine leaks during stress. Additionally, if the hammock is intact but the urethral function is poor (i.e., ISD), the urethra is unable to occlude completely (lack of coaptation) and thus leakage occurs.

- The integral theory gives a better explanation of the continence mechanism than historical explanations. Urethral hypermobility is a sign that the hammock is deficient (either broken or stretched). The retropubic location of the urethra and the idea of "zone of intra-abdominal pressure" is no longer the explanation for the mechanism of SUI repair. Studies have reported that hypermobility of the urethra persists following successful midurethral sling procedures. Therefore, when the hammock is deficient (thus rendering the urethra hypermobile), stress allows displacement of the urethrovesical junction, pressure transmission to the bladder, but not equally to the urethra. Since the urethra cannot be compressed against a stable suburethral backboard, urine loss occurs.

- Surgery for SUI is indicated when conservative management fails (e.g., pharmacological treatments, pelvic muscle exercises, pessaries, and local electrical stimulation) and the patient wants definitive surgical repair.
  ○ Mild SUI should be approached nonsurgically first.
  ○ Women who desire subsequent childbearing are not the best surgical candidates (little data are available on the effect of childbirth after surgical repair of incontinence).

○ Poor surgical candidates (those with multiple medical conditions) should attempt medical management of SUI.

• Patients with urodynamic stress incontinence, mixed incontinence with predominant stress symptoms, and ISD (or formerly called Type III incontinence) are candidates for SUI surgery.

• Today, over 270,000 anti-incontinence surgeries are performed in the United States. Of these, 100,000 are retropubic procedures, 120,000 are slings. Of the slings, 80,000 are midurethral and 40,000 are proximal urethral slings.

• Currently, patients with SUI due to disruption of the hammock or hypermobile urethra (HMU) but intact intrinsic function of the urethra (aka formerly Type I and II incontinence or currently SUI with HMU) are candidates for retropubic urethropexy (e.g., Marshall-Marchetti-Krantz [MMK] and Burch), traditional proximal urethral sling, or midurethral sling procedures (e.g., tension-free vaginal tape [TVT] and transobturator tape [TOT]).

• On the other hand, patients with stress incontinence due to pure ISD are candidates for traditional proximal urethral slings, midurethral slings (although lower cure rate), bulking procedures, and artificial urinary sphincter.

• Patients with SUI with ISD have a much lower cure rates with Burch at 5 years (≈50–60%).

• Patients with mixed incontinence also have a 30% lower cure rate after Burch.

• Patients who have a combination of hypermobility and sphincteric deficiency (SUI with ISD + HMU) may have a lower failure rate with sling procedures although retropubic urethropexy with or without modifications may be attempted.

• Ideally, the patient should be done with childbearing, as future pregnancies may negate the effectiveness of these procedures. This suggestion is based on theoretical risk rather than long-term data.

• In this chapter, abdominal operations (retropubic operations: MMK, Burch, modification of Burch, and paravaginal repair) for correction of SUI will be discussed in detail.

ABDOMINAL OPERATIONS FOR SUI

INTRODUCTION

• The main goal of the retropubic operation is to reinforce, repair, and suspend the endopelvic fascial hammock which supports the urethra; incidentally, this operation places the bladder neck and proximal urethra in the retropubic position. As mentioned above, the relocation of the bladder neck and proximal urethra to the retropubic position currently is not the primary explanation for the mechanism of SUI repair.

• Unfortunately, since the retropubic urethropexies are not the fanciest and newest surgical technique, they have become less popular today.

• This is a shame since the Burch retropubic urethropexy is still the gold standard for the treatment of SUI. This is based on a large volume of well-designed and properly conducted studies showing its safety and efficacy.

• Most experts in female pelvic medicine and reconstructive surgery (FPMRS) believe that the Burch should remain among the top choices in the armamentarium of procedures for correction of SUI.

• Currently, experts will choose a Burch over other procedures for correction of SUI based on the following factors and indications:
  ○ Need for laparotomy for other pelvic diseases (e.g., concomitant hysterectomy, abdominal sacral colpopexy, and abdominal paravaginal repair)
    ▪ Prophylactic Burch for potential incontinence after an abdominal sacral colpopexy (this is controversial; data are pending)
  ○ Expertise of the surgeon in performing this procedure (since currently many graduating residents may not be comfortable with this procedure)
  ○ Preference of the patient
  ○ Need for concomitant pelvic organ prolapse (POP) surgery (e.g., if a surgeon feels more comfortable repairing POP vaginally or if a vaginal repair of POP is indicated, then the surgeon may also prefer a vaginal procedure to correct SUI after repair of the POP)
  ○ SUI with HMU only
  ○ SUI with HMU + ISD (may have higher failure rate)
  ○ Minimal number of factors which increase its failure rate:
    ▪ Pure ISD
    ▪ Abnormal perineal electromyography (EMG)
    ▪ Urodynamic bladder overactivity
    ▪ Chronic obstructive pulmonary disease (COPD), allergy, chronic cough
    ▪ Smoking
    ▪ Menopause (rather than advanced age)
    ▪ Prior hysterectomy
    ▪ Prior anti-incontinence surgery
    ▪ Intraoperative estimated blood loss (EBL) > 1000 mL
    ▪ Obesity
    ▪ Occupational or recreational repetitive heavy lifting or straining
    ▪ Short, small caliber, scarred, immobile vagina (since retropubic procedure elevates anterior vaginal wall,

and in essence, shortens the vagina; theoretically, the vaginal tissue should be pliable and the vaginal length adequate)
- ○ Prophylactic Burch after radical vulvectomy (radical surgery injures urethral sphincter mechanism and also may shorten urethral length)
- Patients with mixed incontinence should be managed by nonsurgical therapy first because (1) up to one-third may become dry with nonsurgical therapy and (2) they have lower cure rates after Burch.
  - ○ 30% of patients with SUI have coexistent detrusor overactivity. This is referred to as mixed urinary incontinence
  - ○ Mixed incontinence + Burch →
    - improved detrusor overactivity = 60%
    - worsened detrusor overactivity = 5–15%
    - continued detrusor overactivity = 20–30%

ESSENTIAL PREOPERATIVE AND INTRAOPERATIVE STEPS

For detailed review, see Chap. 38, Preoperative Issues in Pelvic Surgery.
- Must evaluate for POP prior to surgery for stress incontinence since symptomatic and significant prolapse should be corrected prior to or at the same time as incontinence surgery
- Simple or multichannel urodynamic testing (see Chap. 6, Evaluation of Urinary Incontinence in the Office and Indications for Referral to a Specialist)
- ±Fleets enema
- Perioperative antibiotics (e.g., cephalexin [Ancef])
- May use regional or general anesthesia
- Thromboprophylaxis
- ± Pubic hair shaving
- The patient should be properly placed in dorsal lithotomy position with buttocks at level or just off the edge of table and legs in Allen Universal stirrups (American Medical Systems). Legs should be slightly flexed and abducted. Care should be taken to avoid excessive extension or abduction of the thighs to avoid femoral nerve and peroneal nerve injury
- During the operation, you should have the ability to place two fingers of one hand inside the vagina to lift the endopelvic fascia into the surgeon's field of view (see description of technique below)
- Cleaning and draping the abdomen, upper thighs, vulva, perineum, perianal areas, and vagina in sterile fashion
- Insertion of a 16-20 Fr Foley catheter (±three-way for infusion of methylene blue) with large balloon (20–30 cc) into the bladder to help identify the location of the urethrovesical junction during the operation

ANATOMY OF THE RETROPUBIC SPACE (QUICK REVIEW PRIOR TO PROCEDURE)

- Anterior to bladder is the retropubic or space of Retzius (cave of Retzius). The boundaries are: anterior = symphysis pubis, lateral = pubic bone and obturator internus muscle, superior = superior ramus of pubic bone, inferior = pubocervical fascia, pubourethral ligaments, pubovesical ligaments, urethrovesical angle, proximal urethra, and the extraperitoneal part of the bladder.
- The space of Retzius also contains: (1) loose adipose tissue, (2) directly behind the pubic symphysis and in the midline are a symmetric network of vessels called the anterior vesical and retropubic vessels which are both branches of the internal pudendal artery, (3) veins of Santorini (rich venous plexus in the paravaginal fascia [endopelvic fascia] traveling parallel to each other and perpendicular to the arcus tendineus fascia pelvis [ATFP]; they arise from the vaginal and internal pudendal vessels), and (4) the obturator neurovascular bundle going into the obturator canal. An accessory obturator artery and vein (aka aberrant, anomalous) is usually also encountered leaving the obturator neurovascular bundle near the canal and traversing laterally and superiorly to connect with the inferior epigastric system near the top of the pubic bone. The inferior epigastric vessels connect to the external iliac vessels.
- The accessory obturator vessels are within 4–5 cm of the pubic tubercle and cross over Cooper's ligament. Therefore, they must be recognized before placing stitches during Burch retropubic urethropexy (see procedure described in the following text, while the technical pearls are given in italics).

PROCEDURE, HELPFUL TECHNICAL PEARLS, AND POSTOPERATIVE CARE

RECOMMENDED MODERN BURCH RETROPUBIC URETHROPEXY TECHNIQUE
1. Transverse skin incision (a low-midline incision), is made (either Pfannenstiel, Cherney, or Maylard).
2. Go through the layers as usual and enter the peritoneum.
3. If a concomitant procedure was planned (i.e., abdominal hysterectomy or abdominal sacral colpopexy), it should be performed first.
4. A prophylactic enterocele repair (obliteration of cul-de-sac of Douglas) via McCall's, Moschowitz, and Halban's culdoplasty should be performed before the Burch stitch is placed. *Note: Several studies have noted the development of enteroceles*

after the Burch procedure (5–13.6% depending on study and the number of years of follow-up).

5. The peritoneum may be closed at this point.

6. Patient is placed in reverse Trendelenburg position.

7. The rectus abdominis muscles are separated in the midline and retracted laterally with self-retaining retractors (e.g., Balfour and Bookwalter). *Note: A Maylard or Cherney may be performed to get more exposure if needed.*

8. Near the inferior end of the rectus abdominis, the transversalis and the parietal peritoneum are entered in the direction of the pubic bone.

9. The anterior bladder wall and back of pubic symphysis are separated by gentle blunt dissection with a moist sponge or sponge stick to expose the space of Retzius (see Chap. 2, Anatomy Relevant to Female Reconstructive Pelvic Surgery: Part II, for detailed description of this space). Try to stay close to back of the pubic symphysis. *Note: Use of lighted suction-irrigator or lighted retractor may help during this entire operation; dissection may be more difficult in someone who has had previous surgery in the space of Retzius, as there may be adhesions. (1) Infusion of methylene blue into the bladder through the three-way Foley and its spillage into the surgical field can help in recognizing incidental bladder injury during separation of the bladder from the pubic bone, (2) you may need to use sharp dissection, (3) a controlled, purposeful vertical incision (using scalpel or Metzenbaum scissors) in the dome of the bladder may be helpful in these patients with separation of bladder wall from pubic bone.*

10. Place the index and middle fingers of your non-dominant hand inside the vagina (palm-up). *Note: Make sure you remain sterile by using a sleeve, additional glove, and avoiding contamination while inserting your fingers into the vagina.*

11. Identify the area near the urethrovesical junction with the aid of the Foley balloon (i.e., junction of Foley balloon and Foley drainage tube) and partially fill the bladder to identify its lower margin. Stay lateral to the urethra (in the lateral vaginal fornix) and use your two fingers to gently rotate (laterally), then simultaneously push medially and elevate the anterior vaginal wall by flexing your fingers (toward the ceiling). This maneuver along with gentle small-sponge stick dissection (>2 cm lateral to urethra to avoid injury to high density of small veins and nerves around urethra) and clearing of fat in the retropubic space should expose the "glistening white" endopelvic fascia which will receive the Burch stitch. *Note: (1) The final stitch will be at the level of the urethrovesical junction and 4–5 cm proximal to the external urethral meatus and (2) this area is lined with very rich venous plexus.*

12. Full thickness of the anterior vaginal wall (where the elevated, glistening white endopelvic fascia was exposed) may be grasped with long Allis forceps (optional) to aid in placement of suture. *Note: (1) Be careful and stay 2 cm lateral to the urethra when grasping with the Allis forceps to prevent damage to the delicate urethral musculature and supplying nerves and vessels and (2) two stitches with two bites on each suture will be used.*

13. First stitch (i.e., distal stitch, close to midurethra): Use permanent (e.g., braided, treated, and coated polyester) or delayed absorbable 0 or 1 suture (on a Mayo #5 tapered needle; with ≈18 in. of suture), two passes are made (needle parallel to the urethra) through the entire thickness of the vaginal wall (without going through epithelium), 2 cm lateral to the urethra and the sutures tagged with a Kelly forceps. Do the same thing on the other side of the urethra. *Note: Permanent suture may have better results as it is long enough to allow scarring to reinforce the repair (approximately 6 months).*

14. Second stitch (i.e., proximal stitch, slightly proximal to urethrovesical junction): The same suture and needle are used with a double pass just cephalad or more proximal along the urethra with respect to the first pair of sutures and then tagged (again, be sure to remain 1.5–2 cm lateral to the urethra).

15. Each of the tagged sutures is untagged and made equal, then passed through the ipsilateral Cooper's ligament just above the location where the suture emerges from the anterior vaginal wall (i.e., ≈3 cm lateral to symphysis for midurethral stitch and 1 cm lateral to first for urethrovesical junction stitch). The Mayo needles are removed and the sutures tagged again.

16. Tensioning of sutures: The surgeon has his or her two fingers in the vagina at the urethrovesical junction where the sutures have been passed. Fingers are used to elevate the urethrovesical junction (i.e., causing a dimple in the anterior vaginal wall). At the same time, assistant surgeon ties the sutures (distal then proximal) to suspend the endopelvic fascia from Cooper's ligament at the appropriate tension. *Note: (1) Do not tie with such great tension as to directly juxtapose the endopelvic fascia to Cooper's ligament (especially if using permanent suture). Two fingers should fit between pubic bone and urethra after sutures are tied. (2) Error on the side of less tension (as too much tension will kink or obstruct the urethra) may cause pressure necrosis at the points of attachment. (3) Suturing in this vascular area may have caused excessive bleeding. If you are concerned about a hematoma, you may apply direct pressure, electrocautery, hemoclips, or suture*

as needed. Additionally, you can place a drain (e.g., Jackson-Pratt [JP] and Blake) in the space of Retzius with suction-end of tube out through a separate skin-stab incision. (4) Some experts will add Gelfoam just below Cooper's ligament over the obturator internus fascia to help with hemostasis and to promote scarring and healing-in of tissue.

17. Approximate but do not strangulate the rectus abdominis muscles in the midline with several sutures to prevent herniation of bladder or bowel.

18. Close the rest of the incision in routine fashion.

19. Cystoscopy may be done transurethrally to document lack of suture in the bladder and bilateral ureteral patency by extrusion of blue-colored indigo carmine (5 mL given IV). *Note: Alternatively, you may perform telescopy with purse string suturing and stab incision through the dome of the bladder (extraperitoneal) or you may perform a larger cystotomy if needed. The suprapubic catheter end should also be brought out through a separate skin incision. It is easy to check postvoid residual volume (PVR) with suprapubic catheters since at postoperative day (POD) 2 or 3 they can be clamped and the patient can attempt to void when she has urgency. The PVR is measured simply by unclamping.*

20. The bladder should be drained routinely for 1–2 days either via a transurethral or suprapubic catheter. *Note: This is important to prevent overdistention which (1) delays return to normal voiding, (2) may promote anoxia of the urothelium, and (3) may increase urinary tract infections (UTIs).*

21. Then PVR should be checked and catheter removed if the PVR is consistently low. If PVR is high an indwelling catheter may be left or intermittent self-catheterization performed.

POSSIBLE MECHANISMS OF CURE: MODERN RETROPUBIC URETHROPEXY

- Provide and repair endopelvic fascia which serves as a suburethral hammock against which the urethra is compressed and occluded during stress (e.g., cough).
- Preservation of intrinsic urethral function by avoiding damage to delicate urethral musculature and its nerve and vessel supply.
- Downward-displaced urethra may be funneled proximally (i.e., dilation of proximal urethra with urine inside) → Burch stitches can lift urethra and resolve funneling at rest by compression against the stable, lifted, suburethral backboard. This increases pressure transmission ratio (PTR).
- Placement of only two stitches (one at midurethral level and one at urethrovesical junction level) → allows posterior rotational descent of the bladder

during stress which helps in compression of proximal urethra against stable endopelvic hammock.

EVOLUTION OF RETROPUBIC PROCEDURES
- Original MMK
  ○ Is of historical significance (published in 1949) because it was not only a paradigm shift of treatment of SUI via an abdominal approach (both sling and Kelly are vaginal), but also was the first retropubic urethropexy operation.
  ○ Differences in MMK technique versus modern retropubic urethropexy
    ▪ Extensive dissection within 1 cm of external urethral meatus
    ▪ Chromic #0 suture with two bites × 3 (i.e., three stitches) on either side of and perpendicular to urethra (the goal as it was described originally, was to bring urethral and urethrovaginal [UV] junction in direct apposition to pubic symphysis)
    ▪ Fourth stitch on either side of urethrovesical junction
    ▪ ±Fifth stitch on either side of urethra if sagging of vagina observed among last four stitches
    ▪ With rounded-curved needle, these sutures *were passed through periosteum of symphysis pubis and into cartilage if possible* (this is the step that most people consider MMK). Note: Posterior aspect of rectus abdominis fascia sometimes was also an attachment point of these sutures
    ▪ Additional sutures through bladder muscle to suspend it to posterior rectus abdominis fascia
  ○ Even though cure rates are not different between Burch and MMK, most surgeons no longer perform the MMK due to the risk of osteitis pubis (see complications below).
- Original Burch
  ○ Is of historical significance (published by John Burch [JB] in 1961).
  ○ JB observed that MMK sutures pulled out of periosteum easily.
  ○ Differences in original Burch technique versus modern retropubic urethropexy
    ▪ Chromic catgut #2 × 3 stitches on either side of urethrovesical junction
    ▪ Sutures suspended to ipsilateral Cooper's ligament (instead of pubic periosteum in MMK) directly above (Note: Suspend means gentle tension rather than tight apposition.)
  ○ JB noticed that Burch also corrected associated cystocele (as opposed to MMK).
  ○ JB noticed that Burch predisposed to enterocele in patients with SUI + uterine prolapse; therefore, he recommended both hysterectomy and culdoplasty at same time as Burch.

- Paravaginal repair for treatment of SUI
  ○ Mentioned here for historical purposes only.
  ○ Cullen Richardson (CR) described paravaginal repair for correction of cystourethrocele.
  ○ Although it has a lower rate of voiding dysfunction than other retropubic procedures, its cure rate for SUI is much lower than other retropubic operations (61% at 3 years).
  ○ Technique: Endopelvic fascia of the anterior vaginal wall (full-thickness bites) is reattached to the ATFP (white line) or obturator internus fascia via five stitches of nonabsorbable suture.
  ○ Today this repair is used for the correction of anterior vaginal prolapse.
- Tanagho's modification of Burch
  ○ Emil Tanagho's (ET) modification in 1976 is basis of the modern retropubic urethropexy.
  ○ Differences between original Burch and Tanagho's modification
    ▪ Placement of each stitch should be achieved via a full-thickness bite through anterior vaginal wall (sparing mucosa) → allows good lift of urethrovesical junction and better support of the endopelvic fascial hammock
    ▪ Placement of each stitch lateral to the urethra → to prevent compression of urethral lumen + prevent damage to delicate urethral muscle
    ▪ Removal of retropubic fat after entry into space of Retzius
    ▪ Two stitches of delayed absorbable (polyglycolic acid #1) instead of 3 (chromic on both sides of the urethra. Distal stitch at level of midurethra and proximal stitch at level of urethrovesical junction (Note: One stitch-only procedures have a higher failure rate.)
  ○ ET warned to avoid direct apposition of periurethral tissue to Cooper's ligament as this would cause obstruction of the urethra.

CLINICAL RESULTS AND CURE RATES
- The objective cure rate for the open Burch at 1 year is ≈85–90% and is maintained at ≈5 years (≈77–86%). Satisfaction and subjective improvement rate is higher than objective cure rate at 5 years.
- Cure rates after Burch are lower for those who had a previous anti-incontinence procedure (80–85%).
- Based on long-term data, cure rate for SUI after Burch declines with time and plateaus by 10–12 years at ≈70%.
- As previously mentioned, cure rates after Burch are lower for those who have complicating factors (e.g., mixed incontinence, ISD, and previous anti-incontinence surgery).

- 1 of 10 patients will need at least one additional surgery for correction of SUI 10 years after Burch.
- Addition of abdominal hysterectomy to the Burch does not increase the efficacy (cure rate) of Burch retropubic urethropexy.
- The objective cure rates of Burch ≈ MMK; however, the MMK has risk of osteitis pubis and may have higher recurrence of SUI over time.
- Although theoretically, if a laparoscopic Burch (LB) is performed in the same manner as the open Burch (surgical technique, two stitches instead of one, suturing instead of stapling, nonabsorbable suture), then it should have the same cure rate. The success of LB is highly dependent on the skill of the surgeon. In practice, however, LB has somewhat lower cure rate (based on short-term data), higher complication rate (inferior epigastric vessel, bowel, bladder), and operating room cost than the open Burch; however, it has less postoperative pain, shorter hospital stay, shorter time to voiding, and less time to return to normal activity.
- Open Burch has a similar cure rate as proximal and midurethral sling procedures (at least for 2 years after the procedure). In addition, the TVT has a higher bladder injury rate than open Burch but less time is required in the operating room and less time is necessary to achieve normal voiding and for return to normal activity.
- Compared to LB, TVT is more cost-effective, uses less operative time, and has higher objective cure rate (at <2 years).

COMPLICATIONS OF OPEN RETROPUBIC URETHROPEXIES (MMK AND BURCH) AND SUGGESTED MANAGEMENT
- UTIs (most common)
  ○ The most common complication after retropubic urethropexy is UTI and wound complications.
  ○ During operation, try to avoid injury to the urinary tract.
  ○ During operation, try to minimize manipulation and injury to the nerves of the bladder which may delay return of bladder activity to normal.
  ○ After operation, ensure that the bladder is not overdistended as this may increase risk of infection (1) by causing anoxia of the transitional epithelium and (2) by prolonging catheterization.
  ○ Patients usually resume complete voiding by POD 7 after Burch.
  ○ Advantage of suprapubic catheter placement over transurethral placement is lower infection rate.
  ○ Intermittent self-catheterization has lower infection rate then indwelling catheter placement.
  ○ Management → prophylactic antibiotics, above cautions, and possible need for treatment with antibiotics.

- Voiding difficulties
  - Urinary retention (11–12.5%)
    - After Burch, patients usually void by POD 3 but on the average most patients will have voided by POD 12. It is uncommon to have urinary retention past POD 30.
    - Urinary retention mainly occurs as a result of tying the sutures too tight → apposition of endopelvic fascia and Cooper's ligament → kinking of urethra.
    - Urinary retention also occurs if sutures are placed too close to the urethra. The more lateral the sutures are placed in a Burch, the lower the rate of urinary retention.
    - Occasionally, bladder denervation may contribute to urinary retention.
    - Preoperative voiding studies (e.g., uroflowmetry and pressure flow) may help predict which patients are at risk for this (e.g., Valsalva voiding: low flow rates and high bladder pressures).
    - Other factors which may increase risk of voiding dysfunction: high first sensation to void on cystometry, high PVR, postoperative cystitis, advanced age, previous anti-incontinence surgery.
    - Overdistention of bladder delays the time to return to normal voiding (as described earlier in step 20, Note); therefore, catheterize bladder postoperatively until repeat PVR is low.
    - Management → catheterization of bladder longer, when tying sutures during retropubic operations → error on the looser side, diazepam (2–10 mg tid) as a striated muscle relaxant may help urinary retention. Rarely, release of sutures may be necessary for prolonged retention (>30 days) or alternatively, the patient may perform intermittent self-catheterization.
  - *De novo*, detrusor overactivity (≈16%)
    - 7–27% of patients who did not have bladder overactivity prior to Burch develop it by 5 years after surgery. Up to 40% of these patients are asymptomatic; ≈10% will develop *de novo* urge incontinence.
    - 25–45% of those with mixed incontinence prior to retropubic urethropexy have same or worse detrusor overactivity after surgery.
    - The mechanism of *de novo* detrusor overactivity is unknown, but few theories exist.
    - Management of symptomatic prolapse → anticholinergic medication, bladder retraining, behavioral modification.
- Bleeding and hematoma formation in space of Retzius
  - Injury of longitudinal venous plexus with needle → try to insert needle adjacent to rather than into veins if possible.
  - Bleeders → you may need to use direct pressure, hemoclips, or by just tying sutures bleeding may resolve.
  - Hematoma or urinoma risk → you may need to use JP drain as described above for potential hematomas or in cases of injury to urinary system (as urine may collect in retropubic space).
  - Additionally, you can prevent formation of infected hematomas or abscess in this space by: (1) placing a drain for at-risk patients, (2) ensuring that as your needle goes through the full thickness of the vaginal wall for the proximal and distal stitch placement, it does not penetrate the vaginal mucosa which contains bacteria, and (3) giving prophylactic antibiotics before skin incision is made.
- Enterocele formation (7–14%)
  - The retropubic urethropexy stitches cause anterior displacement of the vagina (thus change the angle of inclination or vaginal axis), this directs intra-abdominal pressure to posterior cul-de-sac thus predisposing to enterocele formation or vaginal vault prolapse within 5 years of surgery. However, some of these enteroceles may have been present at the time of the Burch but were not recognized or corrected.
  - Management → prophylactic culdoplasty (McCall's, Moschcowitz, or Halban's) at the time of retropubic urethropexy (as described above in step 4).
- Cystocele and rectocele formation
  - Discovery of cystocele and rectocele after retropubic urethropexy is most likely a result of not having diagnosed them before the surgery.
  - As described by JB in 1961, the Burch retropubic urethropexy can correct a cystocele.
  - In one study, 26% of patients at 10–20 years after Burch were observed to have undergone rectocele repair.
  - Rectoceles should only be repaired at the time of retropubic urethropexy, if they are large and symptomatic.
- Failure of retropubic urethropexy (≈15%) → "still wet"
  - Maybe because of wrong preoperative diagnosis of SUI and type (e.g., ISD is better treated with a sling procedure).
  - Maybe because of technical error while performing the surgery.
  - Maybe because of failure of suture material.
  - Maybe because of failure of tissue being suspended (paraurethral endopelvic fascia).
  - Presence of complicating factors which increase failure rate of retropubic urethropexies (see factors which increase failure rate in beginning of this chapter).
  - Failure rate of retropubic urethropexy increases with time and plateaus at 10–12 years.
- Postcolposuspension syndrome (12%)

○ Pain in low, midpelvis related to Burch suture tension.

○ Management → pain management (nonsteroidal anti-inflammatory drug [NSAID], narcotics, and so on) or takedown sutures.

• Osteitis pubis (2–3%)

○ The MMK has been studied the most when it comes to complication of retropubic urethropexies.

○ Osteitis is not unique to MMK; it also may occur after bone-anchored pubovaginal slings, artificial urinary sphincter, and radical pelvic surgery for cancer.

○ Is an aseptic (noninfectious) inflammation of the periosteum, bone, cartilage, and ligaments of the symphysis pubis.

○ May resolve spontaneously.

○ Not related to type of suture.

○ Cause is unknown.

○ Symptoms of severe, abrupt onset of lower pelvic pain and surprapubic swelling. Pain may radiate to thighs. It may present anytime up to 3 months after surgery. The pain is made worse with activity. There is also severe tenderness and swelling over the symphysis pubis.

○ X-ray may reveal loss of cortical bone and separation of two halves of pubic bone months after surgery.

○ Management of osteitis pubis → bedrest, physical therapy, NSAIDs, and steroid injections (200 mg/day × 1 week).

○ On the other hand, infectious osteitis is called osteomyelitis and may be suspected because of failure to resolution of what was thought to be osteitis pubis. Diagnosis is established by bone scans (tagged WBC or gallium), bone biopsy, and culture. This is treated with prolonged IV antibiotics. Surgical debridement or resection of bone may be necessary.

• Injury to lower urinary tract (1–3%)

○ Especially with history of previous operation in retropubic space.

○ Extraperitoneal, intentional cystotomy may help if visualization reduces inadvertent injury and certain sutures are not placed into bladder or around/through ureters.

○ Laceration or inadvertent suturing of lower urinary tract occurs in < 1% of patients and bladder is the most commonly injured (bladder > urethra> ureter).

○ Ureteral injury is rare but can be a serious complication because it can result in loss of ipsilateral kidney function.

▪ Burch stitches may indirectly cause injury, stretch, kink, or ligation of ureter (after they are tied).

▪ This is the reason why intraoperative assessment of bladder and ureter always should be done after retropubic urethropexy.

▪ Management → release of suture and stent ipsilateral ureter.

○ Rare events like genitourinary fistulas (slightly more with MMK), bladder stone formation (with bladder penetration of suture), and painful voiding may occur after retropubic urethropexy.

• Dyspareunia

○ Some women develop narrowing at level of the proximal Burch stitch. This may cause pain and tenderness for up to several months after surgery.

○ The retropubic urethropexy may also shorten the vagina by elevating the anterior vaginal wall (as described in the start of this chapter, under Factors that Increase Failure Rate). Thus, patients with short, small caliber, scarred, immobile vaginas may be more prone to dyspareunia.

○ Even higher rates of postoperative dyspareunia is observed when Burch is combined with posterior colporrhaphy.

BIBLIOGRAPHY

Alcalay M, Monga A, Stanton SL. Burch colposuspension: a 10-20 year follow up. *Br J Obstet Gynaecol.* 1995;102:740–745.

Burch JC. Urethrovaginal fixation to Cooper's ligament for correction of stress incontinence, cystocele, and prolapse. *Am J Obstet Gynecol.* 1961;81:281–290.

Columbo M, Milate R, Vitobello D, et al. A randomized comparison of Burch colposuspension and abdominal paravaginal defect repair for female stress urinary incontinence. *Am J Obstet Gynecol.* 1996;175(1):78–84.

Eriksen C, Hagen B, Eik-New SH, et al. Long-term effectiveness of the Burch colposuspension for female urinary stress incontinence. *Acta Obstet Gynecol Scand.* 1990;69:45–50.

Fine PM, Antonini TG, Appell RA. Clinical evaluation of women with lower urinary tract dysfunction. In: Weber A, ed. *Clinical Obstetrics and Gynecology, Incontinence.* Philadelphia, PA: Lippincott William & Wilkins; 2004:44–52.

Karram M, Culligan P, Fleischman SJ. The role of the ob/gyn in evaluating and managing urinary incontinence. *OBG Manage.* 2002;(Suppl):1–11.

Marshall VF, Marchetti AA, Krantz KE. The correction of stress incontinence by simple vesicourethral suspension. *Surg Gynecol Obstet.* 1949;88:509–518.

McDuffie RW Jr, Litin RB, Blundon KE. Urethrovesical suspension (Marshall-Marchetti-Krantz): experience with 204 cases. *Am J Surg.* 1981;141:297–298.

Persson J, Wolner-Hassan P. Laparoscopic Burch colposuspension for stress incontinence: a randomized comparison of one or two sutures on each side of the urethra. *Obstet Gynecol.* 2000;95:151–155.

Walters MD, Daneshgari FD. Surgical management of stress urinary incontinence. In: Weber A, ed. *Clinical Obstetrics and Gynecology—Incontinence.* Philadelphia, PA: Lippincott William & Wilkins; 2004:93–103.

Ward K, Hilton P. Prospective multicentre randomized trial of tension-free vaginal tape and colposuspension as primary treatment for stress incontinence. *BMJ.* 2002;325:1–7.

QUESTIONS

1. A 53-year-old, gravida 2, para 2 presents to your office because she leaks urine with exertion. She is 5 ft 6 in. tall and weighs 125 lbs. She has no significant past medical or surgical history. She works as an editor at an internationally renowned publishing company and does aerobic exercises five times per week. Her last menstrual period was 2 years ago and is on a daily estrogen/progesterone oral regimen. On physical examination, there is some laxity of the apical segment (cervix comes down to 1 cm proximal to the hymen) and points Aa = −1, Ba = −1. The posterior segment is well supported. Her PVR = 30 mL and U_{dip} is negative. During office cystometry, she leaks urine with Valsalva in sitting position with 200 mL inside the bladder. In the United States, the best management of her condition could be _____.

   (A) sling
   (B) Burch retropubic urethropexy
   (C) total vaginal hysterectomy (TVH), McCall's culdoplasty, uterosacral ligament vault suspension, anterior vaginal repair
   (D) total abdominal hysterectomy (TAH), Halban's culdoplasty, Burch retropubic urethropexy, paravaginal repair
   (E) TVH, McCall's culdoplasty, uterosacral ligament vault suspension, anterior repair, and sling

2. A 60-year-old, para 4 complains of leakage of urine during coughing, sneezing, laughing, and getting up from a chair. Occasionally, she also loses a large volume of urine on the way to the bathroom. She denies bedwetting. She has past medical history significant for asthma and diabetes mellitus. She had a vaginal hysterectomy 8 years ago because of POP. Currently, she is not taking any oral medications. On physical examination, the vaginal mucosa is moist and pink. Her pelvic muscles are 4/5 in strength. There is no significant POP. Her PVR = 10 mL after voiding 250 mL. Her U_{dip} is negative. Multichannel urodynamic testing reveals three detrusor pressure elevations > 30 cm H_2O during filling (at 200, 250, and 290 mL) and a leakage of urine with Valsalva at maximum bladder capacity = 310 mL. Her Valsalva leak point pressure (VLPP) = 130 cm H_2O. Initially, the best management of this patient is _____.

   (A) estrogen cream
   (B) bladder training
   (C) functional electrical stimulation
   (D) Burch
   (E) sling

QUESTIONS 3–5

Match the statement below with the percentage which is the closest approximation. Each answer choice may be used once, more than once, or not at all.

   (A) 10%
   (B) 20%
   (C) 30%
   (D) 40%
   (E) 50%
   (F) 60%
   (G) 70%
   (H) 80%
   (I) 90%

3. Cure rate of abdominal paravaginal repair for treatment of SUI.
4. Cure rate for Burch at 12 years follow-up.
5. Patients with mixed urinary incontinence have an approximately _____ lower cure rate after Burch.

ANSWERS

1. *(E).* A sling would resolve her symptoms of SUI; however, it would not address the asymptomatic POP which may become symptomatic in the future. In the European system, this patient would undergo a sling only. The choices with Burch retropubic urethropexy are not the best management options because the retropubic urethropexy causes anterior deviation of the vaginal axis which predisposes to apical prolapse and enteroceles. In a patient who already has significant yet asymptomatic apical prolapse, vaginal axis deviation may lead to symptomatic POP in the future. Choice C does not address SUI. Therefore, the best answer is E.

2. *(B).* This patient has symptoms of mixed urinary incontinence (leakage with exertion and large-volume leakage on way to bathroom). According to the complex cystometric analysis, she has significant detrusor contractions prior to the leakage of urine with Valsalva. Therefore, this patient cannot be considered "mixed incontinence with stress predominance."

Patients with mixed urinary incontinence have a 30% lower cure rate after Burch. Patients with mixed incontinence should be managed by nonsurgical therapy first because up to one-third may become dry with nonsurgical therapy. Similarly, a sling procedure would not be the best initial management. Estrogen cream is not helpful in someone without signs of urogenital atrophy. Functional electrical stimulation is useful for pelvic muscle strengthening and for inhibition of detrusor contractions. This patient has good pelvic muscle strength. Additionally, bladder retraining is usually tried first for patients with symptoms of detrusor overactivity.

ANSWERS 3–5

3. *(F)*, 4. *(G)*, 5. *(C)*. Based on long-term data, cure rates for SUI after Burch declines with time and plateaus at 70% by 10–12 years. Although abdominal paravaginal repair has a lower rate of voiding dysfunction than other retropubic procedures, its cure rate for SUI is much lower than other retropubic operations (61% at 3 years). Patients with mixed incontinence have a 30% lower cure rate after Burch.

16 URETHRAL AUGMENTATION FOR CORRECTION OF STRESS URINARY INCONTINENCE: BULKING PROCEDURES AND ARTIFICIAL URINARY SPHINCTER

Sam Siddighi and Sujata Yavagal

URETHRAL BULKING PROCEDURES (UBPS)

INTRODUCTION

- First described by Murless in 1938.
- Less invasive method to correct stress urinary incontinence (SUI) by strategically placing a semisolid implant underneath the mucosa at the urethrovesical junction (UVJ) (hence re-creating mucosal coaptation) using a needle and an urethrocystoscope.

- UBPs increase the ability of the internal urethral sphincter to resist abdominal pressure.
- Advantages of UBPs
  - Can be performed in the clinical office instead of operating room (OR).
    - Avoids OR and anesthesiology cost
    - Avoids OR turnover delays
    - Avoids regional or general anesthesia
    - Results can be appreciated at the completion of procedure (by doing provocative maneuvers)
  - The procedure is less invasive than surgery.
  - Can be used in SUI patients who have contraindications or do not desire surgery.
    - Medical condition(s) that precludes surgery
      • Elderly patients
      • Previous surgical failure
      • History of radiation therapy
      • Patient who has failed or cannot perform pelvic floor exercises
- Disadvantages of urethral bulking agents
  - Still invasive
  - Costly (multiple injections required)
  - Cure rate not optimal
  - Requires repeat injection
  - Ideal agent for injection not found
- Indication(s) for UBPs
  - SUI with pure intrinsic sphincteric deficiency (ISD)
    - Quick review of features suggestive of ISD
      • History: leaks while in bed
      • Physical examination: (1) empirical Bayesian significance test (EBST) positive and (2) Q-tip test negative
      • Urodynamics: (1) lack of detrusor contractions (P_{det}) and (2) leak point pressure (LPP) < 60 cm H_2O is consistent in ISD (<60 cm H_2O has 90% sensitivity but 64% specificity for diagnosing low pressure urethra; lower LPP cutoffs decrease sensitivity but increase specificity)
      • Videourodynamics: open bladder outlet at rest and lack of detrusor contractions
  - SUI with ISD + hypermobile urethra (HMU) (LPP 60–100 cm H_2O)
    - Controversial—although UBPs have been used for this purpose, some experts believe this is not the ideal indication; sling or artificial urinary sphincter (AUS) may be a better choice for these patients.
    - There is evidence that UBPs work equally well for ISD or ISD + HMU.
- Absolute contraindications to UBPs
  - Allergy or hypersensitivity to the injection agent (aka implant)
  - Severe overactive bladder (OAB) (considered absolute contraindication by some experts)
  - Active urinary tract infection (UTI)

INJECTABLE MATERIALS

- The ideal injection agent should have the following properties:
  - Can be injected using currently available cystoscopy equipment (i.e., not so viscous and dense that it cannot be injected easily thorough injection port using 20–22-gauge needle).
  - Does not cause severe inflammation and scarring, or a foreign body inflammatory reaction (i.e., formation of granuloma with giant cells).
  - It stays where it is injected. In other words, it does not migrate to other parts of the body (e.g., lymphatics, lungs, brain, kidney, and spleen) causing infarction and/or cardiopulmonary arrest.
  - Coaptation does not dramatically reduce in size either because of enzymatic degradation of agent, redistribution, diffusion, or absorption.
  - Promotes secretion of host's own collagen and remodeling of host's urethra at injection site (with incorporation and angiogenesis into injected implant).
  - Does not cause an allergic reaction.
  - It is not carcinogenic (i.e., it is safe for humans).
  - It is easily obtainable.
  - It is inexpensive.
- Historically, the following have been used but each has had associated problems:
  - Cod liver oil → severe inflammation; migration leading to death
  - Autologous blood → coaptation size reduces rapidly; does not promote host's own collagen secretion
  - Autologous fat → coaptation size reduces (absorption); severe inflammation
  - Silicone macroparticles (Macroplastique [Uroplasty]) → migration; extravasation of macroparticles; negative publicity
  - Polytetrafluoroethylene (PTFE [Mentor]) → migration; foreign body reaction; carcinogenic in rat/mice
- None of the currently available agents is ideal.
- Three injection agents will be discussed in detail. Other available agents are also mentioned.
- Cross-linked collagen (Contigen) and carbon-coated beads (Durasphere) are the two Food and Drug Administration (FDA) approved bulking agents (Table 16-1).

TABLE 16-1   Comparision of FDA Approved Bulking Agents

	CROSS-LINKED COLLAGEN	CARBON-COATED BEADS
Hypersensitivity	4%	None
Reinjection rate	Higher	Lower (more durable)
Migration	Rare	Low

Additionally, dimethyl sulfoxide (DMSO)/ethylene vinyl alcohol copolymers (EVOH [Tegress]) is a new agent that is currently available in the United States.

- Cross-linked collagen (Contigen [CR Bard])
  - Bovine collagen (>95% Type I collagen; remaining is Type II collagen). Processing decreases enzymatic digestion and inflammatory potential (hydrolysis of collagen terminals and glutaraldehyde to cross-link collagen fibers—aka glutaraldehyde cross-linked [GAX] bovine collagen).
  - Advantages: (1) coaptation size does not reduce rapidly, (2) does not form foreign body reaction, (3) does not migrate or if it does, it has not created any problems, (4) promotes host's collagen secretion.
  - Disadvantages: (1) expensive, (2) requires more treatment sessions (degradation begins in 3 months and is complete by ≈1.5 years), (3) allergy in 4% of patients; thus, skin testing for hypersensitivity is appropriate.
- Carbon-coated beads (Durasphere [Carbon Medical Technologies])
  - Pyrolytic zirconium oxide microbeads coated with carbon (200–500 µm).
  - Injected at bladder neck using 18-gauge needle.
  - Is more viscous → more difficult to inject than collagen.
  - Not absorbed with time like collagen.
  - Radiopaque thus can be seen on plain x-ray.
  - Migration has not been a problem.
  - More data are needed.
- EVOH/DMSO (Uryx [Genyx], Tegress [CR Bard])
  - It is a solution of EVOH in a DMSO carrier.
  - It has been used as an embolic agent.
  - After injection, the DMSO carrier diffuses and then the EVOH precipitates into a soft gel at the injection site.
  - Advertised advantages: (1) promotes host remodeling in area of injection, (2) coapt size does not change dramatically from degradation, absorption, or enzymatic digestion of implant.
  - $N = 174$, one to three injections in 3 months: 12 months after last procedure, 24% patients are dry, 59% are dry or improved after an average of 2.1 injections per patient.
  - More data are needed on safety and efficacy.
- Other agents being used in UBPs
  - Human collagen (Urologen [Collagenesis]) → cadaveric dermis processed and suspended in solution; high viscosity; good tissue in-growth; used in other fields of medicine; more data are needed.
  - Autologous ear chondrocytes → cells from patient's own pinna tissue cultured and added to suspension

gel for injection (issues of labeling error); more data are needed.
  ○ Cross-linked hyaluronic acid (HA, Hyagel [Biomatrix]) → is used in other medical fields; HA is insoluble glycosaminoglycan which is safe, soft, elastic, and biocompatible; more data are needed.
  ○ HA and dextranomer (Deflux [Q-med], Zuidex) →low viscosity; HA easily injects dextranomer microspheres into proper location; microspheres remain at site for 4 years; more data are needed.
  ○ Calcium hydroxyapatite spheres in carboxymethyl-cellulose carrier (coapatite) → same material found in bones and teeth; can be seen on x-ray; more data are needed.
• The future is here! Injection of myoblast itself or viral vectors which can deliver genes coding for proteins and connective tissue capable of producing muscle function have been successful in the rat urethra and bladder. The process is under investigation.

PROCEDURE AND TECHNIQUE

• The procedure can be performed as an office procedure under local anesthesia. The patient is placed in a dorsal lithotomy position. Topical 2% lidocaine jelly is applied in the periurethral region and 2–4 mL 1% lidocaine is injected at 3 and 9 o'clock positions, respectively. *Note: To aid with injection of 1% lidocaine, a urethral sound may be inserted to straighten the urethra which normally curves ventrally just at the level of the UVJ.* The aim of UBPs is to deliver the bulking material into the lamina propria at the UVJ and proximal urethra. This can be done either transurethrally or periurethrally (Table 16-2).
• Transurethral injection technique (The procedure is described in the text and helpful technical pearls are in *italics.*)
  (1) After application of local anesthetic, 0 degree urethrocystoscope with special needle attachment is inserted into the urethral, (2) the needle is inserted into the urothelium just past the midurethra and advanced to area before the internal urethral sphincter (i.e., in area of UVJ and proximal urethra). *Note: (1) Injection too far in (i.e., too close to bladder) will fail, (2) the purpose of needle bevel entry at a distance from UVJ where the injection material will be deposited → to minimize extravasation, (3) once the bevel of needle is out of view and just below the urothelium (i.e., in the lamina propria), injection is begun, (4) (A) inject at 4 and 8 o'clock positions, respectively. Note: Few authors describe multiple injections instead of just two and injections of urethra proximal to external urethral meatus to achieve coaptation of most of the urethral length, and (B) at each injection site, inject until coaptation of mucosa (i.e., bulging toward the urethral lumen) is one-half of total coaptation. Note: As needle is being withdrawn, continue to inject as this will fill the track created by the needle with bulking agent.*
• Periurethral injection technique (The procedure is described in the text and helpful technical pearls are in *italics.*)
  (1) After application of local anesthetic, a 0 or 30 degree urethrocystoscope is placed into the urethra. *Note: To facilitate accurate placement of injection material at UVJ with this technique, methylene blue mixed with lidocaine may be injected before bulking material is injected.* (2) A 20- or 22-gauge needle is introduced periurethrally at 4 or 8 o'clock positions with the bevel turned toward the urethral lumen. (3) While observing the mucosal bleb created by the needle tip through the cystoscope, the needle is advanced slowly and with little resistance if it is in the right plane (i.e., lamina propria). *Note: Only a mucosal bleb at tip of needle should be seen with advancement (i.e., bevel is properly positioned in the lamina propria) rather than movement of the entire urethra. If the latter is true, then the needle is too deep below the urethra (i.e., below lamina propria).* (4) At the level of the proximal urethra and UVJ, bulking material is injected. *Note: One-half mucosal coaptation created by 4 o'clock site and one-half coaptation by 8 o'clock site (achieving complete coaptation).*

TABLE 16-2   Comparison of Periurethral vs. Transurethral Injection of Bulking Agents

PERIURETHRAL INJECTION	TRANSURETHRAL INJECTION
Needle is inserted adjacent to external urethral meatus and mucosal protrusion by needle is observed	Needle is directly visualized with urethrocystoscope at all times
Requires a more experienced practitioner	Allows more accurate placement of needle
Preferred by many experts	Less operative time
No loss of injected material by extravasation from injection site	Injected material leaks out from urethral mucosa and urethral lumen
Minimal bleeding and does not hinder view of operative field	Bleeding at urethral mucosa puncture site into operative field

- Transvaginal ultrasound-guided injection technique has also been described in the literature. This method obviates urethral instrumentation.

AFTER THE PROCEDURE

- With either approaches, after the procedure the patient is instructed to perform various provocative maneuvers (Valsalva, cough) to check for SUI.
- A postvoid residual volume is measured and if abnormal, the patient is taught intermittent self-catheterization (ISC). Retention of urine or difficulty in voiding is usually temporary.
- Repeat injections may be necessary. Patients receiving Contigen implants will need more injections than patients receiving Durasphere or Tegress injections.

COMPLICATIONS

- Urinary retention (15–25%)
  - Usually transient if it occurs (1–2 days); teach ISC (see Chap. 40, Absorptive Products [Pantiliners, Pads, and Undergarments] and Bladder Catheters and Ureteral Stents in Use Today)
  - Avoid indwelling catheter as the injection material molds around catheter tube and leaves a hollow, open internal urethral meatus after removal of catheter
- UTI (5–30%) → most experts will give 3 days of prophylactic antibiotics to minimize this complication
- Transient urgency, frequency, or dysuria (<20%)
- Hematuria

RESULTS

- Long-term data and strong scientific data are few regarding UBPs.
- Cure rates vary in the literature because of how the terms "continence," "dry," or "success" are defined (e.g., social continence and Stamey grade dry).
- Cure rates also vary depending on the type of bulking agent injected used, quantity injected, and number of injections within a given period of time.
- A comparative study is needed.
- The following are some ranges quoted in the literature for collagen:
  - The actual ranges (cure)/(improve)/(fail) at 12 months are approximately 25-52/17-47/10-35.
- 25-50-25 Rule: At 12 months follow-up, 25% are almost completely dry (cured), 50% improve, 25% need repeat injections. Therefore, 25 + 50 = 75% are either dry or improved.

- Some literatures quote dry or improved rates as high as 80–95%.

ARTIFICIAL URINARY SPHINCTER

- Essentially, artificial urinary sphincter (AUS) is an inflatable cuff that surrounds the proximal urethra and bladder neck. It provides mechanical obstruction of the urethra when it is inflated and it allows voluntary relief of the obstruction when the patient is ready to void. The cuff is controlled by a pump which is placed underneath the skin of the labia majora.
- The first artificial sphincter was implanted by F. Brantley Scott in 1972.
- AUS has undergone several modifications since 1972. The current model in use is manufactured by American Medical Systems (AMS).
  - Model AS721(1972) → AS742 (1974) → AS791 (1979) → AS792 → AMS800 (1983, present model)
    - Inflation and deflation pumps not separate anymore
    - Fewer components
    - All controlling components incorporated into the accessible pump
    - Teflon-coated silicone cuff instead of Dacron
    - Automatic cuff closure
    - Kink resistant
    - Color-coded tubing
- Important concepts in AUS technology
  - The cuff should deflate and thus open completely when patient activates it.
  - The cuff should open partially when the bladder pressure is high.
  - The AUS should allow insertion of catheter (e.g., ISC) without difficulty.
  - Cuff should only cause urethral mucosal coaptation rather than tight closure leading to pressure necrosis. Therefore, the cuff pressure can never exceed the diastolic blood pressure.
- Candidates for AUS must satisfy all of the following criteria (proper patient selection is one of the most important factors contributing to a successful AUS operation):
  - ISD
  - Lack of the two absolute contraindications to AUS
    - Detrusor overactivity that is not amenable to therapy
    - High-grade vesicoureteral reflux
  - Must undergo the following testings:
    - Cystoscopy
    - Complex urodynamic testing (with LPP and maximal urethral closure pressure [MUCP]) or videourodynamic testing or both

- Must have three essential qualities to be able to operate the AUS on a daily basis
  - Manual dexterity
  - Mental capacity
  - Motivation
- Besides proper patient selection, the ability of the surgeon is crucial in rendering a successful AUS implantation. Hence, not many women have received AUS in the past 20 years. The obstacles to receiving implantation are the following:
  - Surgeons belief that implantation of AUS is an extremely difficult surgery.
  - Many candidates of this surgery have already undergone multiple incontinence surgeries (which may have caused the ISD); the operation is more difficult because of adhesions, scar tissue, and anatomic distortion.
  - In order to place the cuff around the proximal urethra and bladder neck, tunneling needs to be done between the urethra and the vaginal mucosa. Since this is not a true surgical plane, surgeons may fear injury to structures surrounding the urethra and the urethra itself.
- The AMS800 has four components
  - Cuff → surrounds urethra and bladder neck and occludes them; it is analogous to a blood pressure cuff except it is on a much smaller scale.
  - Pump → placed below labia majora; regulates inflation/deflation; contains control panel.
  - Tubing → one from pump to cuff and another from pump to balloon; special hemostats must be used during surgery in order to prevent damage or leaking of the tubes. Also care should be taken to not allow blood to enter tubing as this will cause malfunction of the entire system.
  - Balloon → placed next to the bladder; the thickness of the balloon wall determines how much pressure is created by the fluid-filled balloon; a detrusor contraction that is stronger than the pressure created by the balloon will push fluid out of the cuff and into the balloon (thus allowing deflation of the cuff).
- Before the operation
  - Very close attention should be paid to sterility and efforts to reduce infection because the device is a foreign body placed in a site with little access to the immune system or antibiotics.
    - Handle AUS as few times as possible.
    - Soak AUS in antimicrobial solution.
    - Achieve antibiotic levels before incision is made.
    - Preoperative shaving just before surgery instead of night before by patient reduces skin surface bacterial load.
    - Skin is prepared and draped in sterile fashion.
    - Ample irrigation throughout surgery.
  - Ask the patient whether she is right-handed or not before she is placed under anesthesia → it is easier

for a right-handed patient to operate the pump in her right labia majora.
- Abdominal approach for placement of AUS (The procedure is described in the text and the helpful technical pearls are in *italics*.)
  (1) After general or regional anesthesia is administered, patient is placed on Allen stirrups (AMS) with thighs abducted but only minimally flexed at the hips. *Note: This allows cystoscopy during the operation.* (2) After preparing and draping, a low transverse skin incision is made and then either Cherney or Maylard performed to give maximal exposure. (3) The retropubic space is entered. *Note: A cystotomy may need to be performed to aid with dissection of retropubic space. This can also help avoid the ureteral orifices when creating a tunnel between the bladder neck and anterior vaginal wall.* (4) The bladder neck is identified with the help of 30-mL Foley balloon and the endopelvic fascia investing the urethra and supporting the bladder is dissected and cleaned just lateral to the bladder neck and the proximal urethra. A Babcock clamp may be used to grasp the urethra and to visualize area between urethra and vaginal wall (the nonexistent anatomical plane → urethra–vaginal septum). (5) A special device (cutter clamp) is positioned just between the bladder neck/proximal urethra and the anterior vaginal wall; the clamp is used to create a tunnel within the urethra–vaginal septum with care to prevent injury to the proximal urethra and bladder neck. *Note: (1) The tunnel created by the clamp must be distal to the ureteral orifices, (2) the cutter clamp is a long, U-shaped clamp (when clamp is closed); it contains a blade which can be advanced within the device itself; once activated, the blade creates a tunnel in any tissue that is grasped between its jaws.* (6) Once the device is engaged and tunnel has been created, the clamp is dismantled, leaving a blade (in the urethra–vaginal septum) and an eye for receiving suture (at the tip of the blade). (7) The eye is threaded with suture and the blade is removed, leaving a suture in the tunnel created by the device. (8) The suture is used to guide a right-angle clamp through the tunnel; the clamp is spread to dilate this tunnel enough so the AMS800 cuff can fit (2 cm wide). (9) At this point two steps must be undertaken to ensure safety of urethra and bladder. (A) Cystoscopy to make sure urethra is clear and that the tunnel is away from the ureteral orifices inside the bladder and (B) bubble test → the bladder neck area is filled with bacteriostatic saline or antibiotic solution then air is put into the urethra and bladder. If bubbles are seen in the fluid, then the urethra or bladder integrity has been breached. The site must be identified and repaired. (10) Place cuff sizer around bladder neck and measure (usually it is 7–9 cm). (11) Then using the clamp, pull in to position

the AMS800 cuff. (12) Attach tubing to the cuff. (13) Create a space adjacent to the bladder in the retropubic space for placement of the balloon. *Note: (1) The balloon wall thickness chosen should provide adequate pressure to the cuff, but not excessive or else pressure necrosis of urethra can occur (the appropriate pressure is usually between 50 and 90 cm H_2O, (2) the balloon should be filled with 22 mL of temporary fluid and some radiopaque contrast material).* (14) The balloon is attached to the cuff (temporary connection; not found at the conclusion of the operation) allowing further tubing and cuff to fill with fluid (charging the system). (15) The balloon and cuff are now disconnected. (16) The balloon is emptied and refilled with 20 mL of the recommended fluid. (17) A tunnel is created using a Hegar dilator from the suprapubic area to the appropriate labia majus. (18) The tubing is directed away from the balloon and the cuff toward the labia making sure there is no tension, twisting, or kinking, along their path. (19) The pump is placed in a superficial and dependent position in the labia majus after the tubing from the cuff and balloon is separately attached to the pump. (20) System is activated/deactivated. When activated, the cuff squeezes around proximal urethra/bladder neck. Then the system is deactivated by squeezing pump and deflating the cuff (this fills the pump with fluid). *Note: The AMS800 is left deactivated for 6-12 weeks postoperatively.* (21) A Foley catheter is inserted and left in for 1–2 days. *Note: If the bladder or urethra were opened then the catheter should be left for 7–10 days.* (22) The wound is closed in standard manner. *Note: Be careful to avoid needle injury or blood contamination of tubing while closing abdomen.*

- Combined approach for placement of AUS
  ○ The combined or vaginal approach for insertion of the AMS800 was described by R. Appell in 1988 in order to reduce chance of injury to the proximal urethra and bladder neck during dissection.
  ○ Vaginal portion: An inverted U-shape incision is made in anterior vaginal wall and lateral dissection is performed. The retropubic space is entered and the proximal urethra and bladder neck are mobilized. Catheter is removed. Cuff sizer is passed around bladder neck. Cystoscopy is performed.
  ○ Abdominal portion: Small transverse incision just above pubic symphysis. Tonsil clamp is used to pull tubing from the cuff into the abdominal incision. Balloon and pump are placed through the abdominal wound. Tubing is connected and the system is filled as described before.
  ○ Abdominal and vaginal incisions are closed in standard fashion. Martius flap may be interposed if

necessary before closure. Gauze soaked in conjugated estrogen cream is packed inside the vagina until POD#1. Foley catheter is left inside the bladder for an appropriate amount of time. Cuff is activated 6 weeks later.

- Results and complications
  ○ In the past, mechanical complications (e.g., cuff leak and tubing kinks) outnumbered biological complications. Today the opposite is true (e.g., erosions and infections).
  ○ Largest drawback of AUS is the possibility of further surgery = 8.8–56%.
  ○ If patients are properly selected and the operator is experienced in placement of this device, then the AUS is extremely successful.
  ○ Abdominal procedure: 85–92% success for up to 9 years follow-up.
  ○ Vaginal procedure: 90–100% success with minimal complications.

BIBLIOGRAPHY

Abbassian A. A new operation for insertion of the artificial urinary sphincter. *J Urol*. 1988;140:512–513.

Appell RA. Techniques and results in the implantation of the artificial urinary sphincter in women with type III SUI by vaginal approach. *Neurourol Urodyn*. 1988;7:613–619.

Appell RA. Implantation of artificial urinary sphincters. In: Hurt GW, ed. *The Master's Techniques in Gynecologic Surgery*. 2nd ed. Philadelphia, PA: Lippincott William & Wilkins; 2000a: 159–166.

Appell RA. Periurethral injections. In: Hurt GW, ed. *The Master's Techniques in Gynecologic Surgery*. 2nd ed. Philadelphia, PA: Lippincott William & Wilkins; 2000b:149–158.

Bent AE, Tutrone RT, McLennan MT, et al. Treatment of intrinsic sphincter deficiency using autologous ear chondrocytes as a bulking agent. *Neurourol Urodyn*. 2001;20:157–165.

Chon JK, Leach GE. Surgical treatment in men. In: Bourcier AP, McGuire E, Abrams P, et al., eds. *Pelvic Floor Disorders*. Philadelphia, PA: Elsevier; 2004:424–431.

Elson ML. Adverse reaction to tretinoin and collagen injections. *J Am Acad Dermatol*. 1989a;20:861–862.

Elson ML. The role of skin testing in the use of collagen injectable materials. *J Dermatol Surg Oncol*. 1989b;15: 301–303.

Gross M, Appell RA. Periurethral injections. In: Bent AE, Ostergard DR, Swift JR, Cundiff MD, et al., eds. *Ostergard's Urogynecology and Pelvic Floor Dysfunction*. 5th ed. Philadelphia, PA: Lippincott William & Wilkins; 2003: 495–502.

Herschorn S, Radomski SB, Steele DY. Early experience with intraurethral collagen injections for urinary incontinence. *J Urol*. 1992;148:1797–1800.

Lightner D, Calvosa C, Andersen R, et al. A new injectable bulking agent for treatment of stress urinary incontinence: results of a multicenter, randomized, controlled, double-blind study of Durasphere. *Urology.* 2001;58:12–15.

Neal DE Jr, Lahaye ME, Lowe DC. Improved needle placement technique in periurethral collagen injection. *Urology.* 1995; 45:865–866.

O'Connell HE, McGuire EH, Aboseif S, et al. Transurethral collagen therapy in women. *J Urol.* 1995;154:1463–1465.

Politano VA, Small MP, Herper JM, et al. Periurethral Teflon injection for urinary incontinence. *J Urol.* 1974;111:180–183.

Swami S, Batista JE, Abrams P. Collagen for female genuine stress incontinence after a minimum 2-year follow-up. *Br J Urol.* 1997;80:757–761.

Webster GD, Perez LM, Khoury JM, et al. Management of type III stress urinary incontinence using the artificial urinary sphincter. *Urology.* 1992;39:499–501.

QUESTIONS

QUESTIONS 1 AND 2

Match the statement below with the injectable material(s) which best describe(s) it above. Each answer may be used once, more than once, or not at all

- (A) Calcium hydroxyapatite
- (B) Autologous ear chondrocytes
- (C) Silicone macroparticles
- (D) PTFE
- (E) EVOH/DMSO
- (F) Carbon-coated beads
- (G) Cross-linked collagen
- (H) liver oil

1. Injectable agent composed of salts found in bones and teeth.
2. Has shown to have carcinogenic potential in mice.
3. The cure rate (completely dry) of bulking agent is approximately __ at 1 year after injection.
   - (A) 15%
   - (B) 30%
   - (C) 60%
   - (D) 80%
   - (E) 90%
4. A 67-year-old woman is about to undergo placement of an AUS. It is particularly important for the surgeon to pay close attention to ___ before and during surgery.
   - (A) blood pressure
   - (B) heart rate

   - (C) sterility
   - (D) thromboprophylaxis
   - (E) antibiotic concentration
5. An 87-year-old, para 4 presents to your office 2 months after being fitted for an incontinence pessary with knob by her gynecologist for SUI. She has a history of pelvic radiation 6 years ago for cervical cancer. She also has diabetes mellitus, hypertension, arthritis, and coronary artery disease (2-vessel). Her past surgical history is remarkable for total abdominal hysterectomy with bilateral salpingoopherectomy (TAH-BSO) and lymph node sampling. As she positions herself on the stirrups, she involuntarily loses urine. On examination, she has Stage 2 pelvic organ prolapse. With a subjectively empty bladder (100 mL) and without reduction of her anterior prolapse, the patient demonstrates a positive stress test. The Q-tip angle changes 10 degrees on Valsalva. Cystometrogram (CMG) did not show any detrusor contractions throughout filling. Her Valsalva leak point pressure (VLPP) = 30 cm H_2O and MUCP = 10 cm H_2O. During cystoscopy, open UVJ was observed. The next best step in management of this patient is ____.
   - (A) duloxetine
   - (B) Introl (proximal urethral support)
   - (C) periurethral bulking agent
   - (D) midurethral sling
   - (E) Burch retropubic urethropexy

ANSWERS

ANSWERS 1 AND 2

1. *(A)*. Calcium is found in bones and teeth.
2. *(D)*. PTFE has been shown to provide cured in mice.
3. *(B)*. Remember the 25-50-25 rule. At 12 months follow-up, 25% are almost completely dry (cured), 50% improve, 25% need repeat injections. Therefore, 25 + 50 = 75% are either dry or improved.
4. *(C)*. Very close attention should be paid to sterility and efforts to reduce infection because the device is a foreign body placed in a site with little access to the immune system or antibiotics. Antibiotic concentration by itself is not the most important concept for AUS placement. Thromboprophylaxis is important for any major surgery not just for AUS placement. From the surgeon's perspective, during any elective surgery, vital signs are important considerations during acute hemorrhage and should be monitored

by the anesthesiologist administering medications which influence blood pressure and heart rate.

5. *(C)*. This patient is the prototype of "drain-pipe" urethra or ISD. Since ISD is a severe form of incontinence and duloxetine has not yet been approved for SUI, it is not the best answer. Introl is similar to the pessary that the patient already has, i.e., not effective. Burch is relatively contraindicated in a patient with pure ISD because of the high failure rate. Midurethral slings such as tension-free vaginal tape (TVT) may be attempted, though the cure rates would not be as high. Additionally, in an elderly patient with multiple medical problems, it may be better to try an in-office, less invasive procedure.

17 SURGICAL MANAGEMENT OF ANTERIOR VAGINAL WALL PROLAPSE

Sam Siddighi

SURGICAL MANAGEMENT OF PELVIC ORGAN PROLAPSE

- The majority of surgeries for pelvic organ prolapse (POP) are elective so the patient needs to understand the following before going to the operating room: (1) she may not have resolution of her symptoms, (2) she may have worsening of symptoms, (3) and there may be complications of surgery (e.g., prolonged catheterization and need for self-catheterization).
- If conservative management of POP is not desired or nonsurgical therapy has failed then the patient should be optimized for surgery with vaginal estrogen for 1–2 months prior to surgery.
- The management of anterior POP is controversial. In this chapter two theories for the etiology and management of cystoceles are discussed.

INTRODUCTION

- The following physicians have contributed greatly to our understanding of anterior wall prolapse and its management (also see Chap. 51, Essential Information About Female Pelvic Medicine and Reconstructive Surgery and Application to OB/GYN Subspecialty Fellowships in the United States):
  - George White (1909)
  - K.M. Fugurnov (1948)
  - B.R. Goff (1948)
  - Wayne Baden and Tom Walker (1968)
  - Cullen Richardson (1981)
  - Bob Shull (1989)

- Today there is debate among leading urogynecologists as to why anterior POPs result and what is the best way to manage them. There are two explanations
  - Anatomical defect: Majority of anterior wall prolapses occur because of detachment of fibromuscular layer of the vagina, which has been referred to by gynecologic surgeons as the "pubocervical fascia (PCF)," from the pelvic sidewall. These paravaginal defects have been observed on both MRI and ultrasound and can be seen during surgery.
  - Fibromuscularis attenuation: Attenuation and weakening of the fibromuscular layer of the vagina, or PCS, leads to anterior POP. Attenuated PCS is often found during surgery.
- There are no studies to compare the two explanations above because such a study would be difficult
  - Many patients would be necessary.
  - Long follow-up is necessary.
  - There is variability between surgeons and their techniques.
- Today, urogynecologists choose paravaginal defect repair versus anterior colporrhaphy based on their training and route of surgery undertaken.
- Apical, anterior, and posterior prolapses are associated with each other 67% of the time. Concomitant anterior prolapse occurs 7% of the time, posterior prolapse in 30%, and multiple compartment prolapse occurs up to 30% of the time.
- Therefore, an effort should be made to correct apical and posterior defects when anterior wall prolapse is being repaired.
- The reader should keep in mind that many of the percentages quoted in this chapter are based on expert experience and retrospective data rather than from prospective, randomized studies. Level I studies are in dire need.

VAGINAL SUPPORT ANATOMY (QUICK REVIEW)

For detailed review, see Chap., Anatomy Relevant to Female Reconstructive Pelvic Surgery: Part II.

- The vagina can be conceptualized as a fibromuscular, collapsed, cylindrical tube with three attachment systems. The anterior portion of this cylindrical tube is called the PCF, but pubocervical septum (PCS) is preferred since this structure is not true fascia. The posterior portion of this cylindrical tube is called "rectovaginal fascia (RVF)" or "rectovaginal septum (RVS)." The top portion of our conceptualized cylindrical tube is called the "pericervical ring." *Note: The RVS does not extend to the sacrum. Instead, RVS exists only in the distal, posterior vaginal wall and only folds of peritoneum extend to the sacrum.*
  - DeLancey's level I support (apical support)
    - Cardinal ligament: Attaches PCS of the anterior vaginal wall and the RVS of the posterior wall to the pelvic sidewall (e.g., obturator internus fascia) at the apex of vegina.
    - Uterosacral ligament: Attaches the PCS of the anterior vaginal wall and the RVS of the posterior vaginal wall to the back wall (sacrum) at apex of vagina.
    - Pericervical ring: Near the cervix, the cardinal ligaments concentrate, narrow, and attach to the capsule of the cervix forming the pericervical ring. Reconstruction of the pericervical ring structure is essential after a hysterectomy in order to provide support for the anterior (PCS) and posterior (RVS) vaginal walls and the vaginal apex.
  - DeLancey's level II support (midvaginal support)
    - Anterior: The middle segment of the anterior vaginal wall is attached by its PCS to the arcus tendineus fascia pelvis (ATFP).
    - Posterior: The middle segment of the posterior vaginal wall is attached by its RVS to the arcus tendineus fascia rectovaginalis (ATFRV).
  - DeLancey's level III support (distal-vaginal support)
    - The distal vagina is fused with the levator ani.
    - Distally, the PCS attaches to the perineal membrane and the RVS attaches to the perineal body.

ANATOMICAL DEFECT

- The areas where the anterior vaginal wall can become defective are represented by a hypothetical trapezoid. The long end of the trapezoid can be thought of as the pericervical ring. The sides represent attachment to the ATFP. The short end represents attachment to the perineal membrane.
- Detachment of trapezoid sides: Most anterior vaginal wall prolapses result from separation of the PCS from the ATFP. This is known as a lateral or paravaginal defect (≈80%) and may be observed during abdominal surgery.
  - This separation may occur in three ways
    - Detachment of the endopelvic fascia lateral to the ATFP (i.e., entire ATFP is detached from parietal

fascias of the obturator internus and levator ani)—most common situation. We will refer to this type of detachment as Type 1 for discussion purposes later in this chapter.
    - Detachment of endopelvic fascia through the middle of the ATFP—easiest to repair (Type 2).
    - Detachment of the endopelvic fascia medial to the ATFP (Type 3)—this leaves an irregular-edged endopelvic fascia thus making it the more difficult of the three to repair.
  - Diagnosis of paravaginal defect
    - Palpation: If there is a defect, then the index finger will have no resistance as it is swept up the pelvic sidewall in the direction of the top of the pubic ramus.
    - Observation: After the posterior vaginal wall is retracted (by Sims or weighted speculum), the lateral vaginal fornices are held at their normal positions with a pair of instruments (e.g., uterine forceps and Ayre spatulas). This maneuver will eliminate the vaginal bulge even after Valsalva if the defect is paravaginal. The maneuver can be repeated with just one lateral fornix supported with an instrument to determine if the paravaginal defect is unilateral (most of them are right-sided).
    - Mobility: Identify the vesical neck area and situate it between index and middle finger. The vesical neck should not have side-to-side mobility. If it does, then there is probably a break in the periurethral fascia (i.e., distal paravaginal defect).
    - Vaginal rugae are present over bulge (indicating that the PCS is intact underneath the bladder).
  - Patients with paravaginal defect may present with symptoms of POP and stress urinary incontinence (SUI).
  - Paravaginal defect is best repaired by paravaginal repair. Some experts claim that the abdominal route (vs. laparoscopic or vaginal) has the highest success rate.
  - Repair of a paravaginal defect will create an anterior vaginal fornix.
- Detachment within the trapezoid itself—less common (as a single defect), an anterior prolapse may result because of a central defect, which is a vertical tear of PCS down the midline or just lateral to the midline.
  - Diagnosis of a central defect
    - Loss of vaginal rugae over vaginal bulge.
    - Mobility of the vesical neck is possible.
    - Dilator placed into urethra will be easily palpated (i.e., very thin) at level of the bladder neck without intervening PCS.
    - When the maneuver described for diagnosis of paravaginal defect (described above) is performed,

Valsalva will cause bulging of the anterior vaginal wall.

- ◦ Patients with central defect may complain of SUI (especially if central defect of PCS is beneath the bladder neck and mobility exists).
- ◦ Patients who have undergone Burch retropubic urethropexy are at risk for a central defect because suturing of the PCS on either side of bladder neck to Cooper's ligament places tension which may lead to vertical breakage of this endopelvic fascia.
- ◦ Repair of central defect is achieved best by anterior colporrhaphy.
- Detachment of long end of the trapezoid—much less common is a transverse defect ($\approx$5%), or separation of the PCS from the cervix and base of the broad ligament.
  - ◦ Diagnosis of transverse defect
    - ▪ Bulge in the proximal anterior half of the vagina
    - ▪ Loss of anterior vaginal fornix
    - ▪ Loss of rugae over vaginal bulge (hence, absence of PCS beneath this area)
    - ▪ When the maneuver described above is performed, Valsalva will cause bulging of the anterior vaginal wall; therefore, either a transverse or central defect exists
  - ◦ Patients with transverse defect may present with increased postvoid residual (PVR) volume.
  - ◦ Occurs in patients with advanced uterine prolapse.
  - ◦ Transverse defect is repaired more easily by vaginal surgery
    - ▪ Nonhysterectomized patient → reattach PCS to pericervical ring with 0 Vicryl
    - ▪ Hysterectomized patient → reattach PCS to RVS with interrupted 0 Vicryl and resuspend the vaginal apex
- $\approx$15% of patients will have a combination defect, i.e., paravaginal + transverse.
- Detachment of small end of trapezoid—very rarely, a portion of the anterior prolapse may arise because of a distal defect. This results from detachment of the PCS from the perineal membrane and thus from the overlying pubic symphysis.
  - ◦ Patients with paravaginal defect may present with symptoms of outward protrusion or "telescoping" above the external urethral meatus during strain.
  - ◦ Only few complain of urethrocele or SUI.
  - ◦ Patients who have undergone radical vulvectomy are at risk for distal defect because of amputation of distal urethra.
- Most patients with advanced paravaginal defects will also complain of SUI. Proper correction of the paravaginal defect can correct the SUI in these patients. However, paravaginal repair is not the procedure of choice for SUI; the Burch and tension-free vaginal tape (TVT) are better choices for SUI.

ANATOMY OF THE RETROPUBIC SPACE (QUICK REVIEW)

- Anterior to bladder is the retropubic or space of Retzius (cave of Retzius). The boundaries are: anterior = symphysis pubis, lateral = pubic bone and obturator internus muscle, superior = superior ramus of pubic bone, inferior = PCS, pubourethral ligaments, pubovesical ligaments, urethrovesical angle, proximal urethra, and the extraperitoneal part of the bladder.
- The space of Retzius also contains (1) loose adipose tissue, (2) directly behind the pubic symphysis and in the midline are a symmetric network of vessels called the anterior vesical and retropubic vessels which are both branches of the internal pudendal artery, (3) veins of Santorini (rich venous plexus in the paravaginal fascia [endopelvic fascia] traveling parallel to each other and perpendicular to the ATFP; they arise from the vaginal and internal pudendal vessels), and (4) the obturator neurovascular bundle going into the obturator canal. An accessory obturator artery and vein (aka aberrant, anomalous) is usually also encountered leaving the obturator neurovascular bundle near the canal and traversing laterally and superiorly to connect with the inferior epigastric system near the top of the pubic bone. The inferior epigastric vessels connect to the external iliac vessels.
- The accessory obturator vessels are within 4–5 cm of the pubic tubercle and cross over Cooper's ligament. Therefore, they must be recognized before placing stitches during Burch retropubic urethropexy (see procedure described in the following and the helpful technical pearls in *italics*).
- The obturator neurovascular bundle is lateral and superior to the ATFP.

PROCEDURE AND HELPFUL TECHNICAL PEARLS

Abdominal paravaginal defect repair may be performed laparoscopically, abdominally, or vaginally. Many experts believe this repair is accomplished best abdominally.

1. Pfannenstiel skin incision is made.
2. All the layers are opened and the retropubic space is entered (as described in Chap. 14, Surgical Management of Stress Urinary Incontinence: Vaginal Procedures, for Burch procedure).
3. The bladder is pushed medially with sponge stick while the surgeon's nondominant hand elevates the anterolateral sulcus of the vagina.

4. Prominent veins can be seen in the retropubic space which follow the course of the superior, lateral sulcus. *Note: A paravaginal defect can be seen just lateral to these veins.*

5. The entire ATFP line should be dissected and exposed. *Note: (1) Expose from back of the pubic symphysis to the ischial spine, (2) the goal is to reattach the detached PCS to the ATFP, (3) the first stitch for reattachment is the most important because it determines where the vagina will be situated. This stitch is important regardless of whether it is placed near the pubic bone, between pubic bone and ischial spine, or near ischial spine, (4) permanent suture (e.g., Ethibond) on a SH-1 needle (or similar) may be used and six throws may be necessary to ensure a secure knot.*

6. The torn-away lateral, superior sulcus is elevated with the vaginal hand while the needle is placed underneath the prominent veins and through the PCS. *Note: Traction is held with the needle in the direction of the ischial spine to attempt alignment of PCS with its previous attachment located on the ATFP. During traction, the external urethral meatus is drawn inward and almost flush with the inferior pubic symphysis.*

7. The needle is then passed through the arcus tendineus levator ani (ATLA) (see Chap. 1, Anatomy Relevant to Female Reconstructive Pelvic Surgery: Part I) for Type 1 detachment, through remnant of the ATFP on pelvic sidewall for Type 2 detachment, or entire ATFP in Type 3 detachment.

8. Then a row of sutures is placed in a similar fashion at 1 cm intervals and tied. *Note: (1) The stitch near the pubic bone end of ATFP should be just adjacent to the bone while the stitch near the ischial spine end of ATFP can be 1 cm from ischial spine, (2) if bleeding occurs during needle passage, they usually resolve when the knot is tied. Warm water may also help visualization of bleeding vessels.*

9. The opposite side is sutured in a similar fashion even if there is no paravaginal defect for reinforcement.

10. The bladder is replaced and the abdomen is then closed in standard fashion.

11. An indwelling Foley catheter is not necessary after a paravaginal procedure alone because most patients will void in the immediate postoperative period.

RESULTS OF PARAVAGINAL REPAIR

- Success rate is 95% for abdominal route.
- Recurrence rate of anterior POP is 5% for abdominal route.

- Up to 98% success rate for vaginal route at 1 year, although many experts believe abdominal approach has a higher success rate than vaginal approach.
- More data are necessary.

COMPLICATIONS OF PARAVAGINAL REPAIR

- Recurrence of prolapse due to defect other than paravaginal + recurrence of prolapse due to breakdown of paravaginal repair ≈ 10%.
- Urinary retention is rare.
- Hemorrhage (usually in patients with previous retropubic operations) is rare.
- Vault prolapse or enterocele after paravaginal repair is very rare (in contrast to Burch—see Chap. 15, Surgical Management of Stress Urinary Incontinence: Open Retropubic Operations).
- More data are necessary.

PROCEDURE AND HELPFUL TECHNICAL PEARLS

The procedure is described in the following text and the technical pearls are in *italics*

- Anterior colporrhaphy for repair of anterior vaginal wall prolapse (due to fibromuscularis attenuation)

1. After prophylactic antibiotic has been given and the patient is prepared and draped in usual sterile fashion, a transurethral Foley catheter (or suprapubic catheter, see Chap. 40, Absorptive Products [Pantiliners, Pads, and Undergarments] and Bladder Catheters and Ureteral Stents in Use Today) is placed for continuous drainage of the bladder. *Note: Many experts begin an anterior repair after the total abdominal hysterectomy with bilateral salpingoopherectomy (TAH-BSO), culdoplasty (e.g., McCall's), and vaginal vault suspension if these procedures must also be done in the same operation. Other experts repair prolapses in a hysterectomized patient beginning with the most prominent compartment prolapse.*

2. The vaginal mucosa is grasped with three Allis clamps in the midline, vertical anterior vaginal wall.

3. The potential space along the vertical line grasped by the three Allis clamps is injected with 0.25% Marcaine with epinephrine (or dilute vasopressin [20 U vasopressin in 30 cc normal saline, NS], or 1% lidocaine with epinephrine). *Note: Injection accomplishes two things: (1) hydrodissection of the potential space and (2) vasoconstriction to minimize bleeding when the mucosa is dissected. Also an attempt must be made to inject without formation of a wheal so that one is injecting into the potential space rather than into the fibromuscular layer or PCS.*

4. An incision is made along the Allis clamps from 1 to 2 cm proximal to external urethral meatus to the cervix or vaginal cuff.

5. Cut edges of the vaginal mucosa are grasped with a series of Allis clamps or other type of tissue retraction device.

6. The vaginal mucosa is sharply dissected away from the PCS laterally to the inferior pubic ramus. *Note: (1) If the correct tissue plane is found, this dissection is very easy and there is minimal bleeding. The detrusor muscle bleeds, the PCS does not, (2) the defect in the PCS is identified by contrast in color between tissues. Irrigate at this point. The PCS is glistening white while the prolapsed, muscular detrusor wall is reddish in hue.*

7. If necessary, at this point the Kelly plication stitch can be done as described in Chap. 15. *Note: If Kelly plication is performed, it is important to avoid truncation of more layers of tissue plication underneath the bladder in comparison to the urethra (i.e., normally there is an angle between the urethra and the bladder). Plication of the PCS beneath the bladder more than the tissue beneath the urethrovesical junction flattens or eliminates this angle and predisposes to SUI.*

8. One to two layers of interrupted, 2-0 Vicryl (some experts will use 2-0 Ethibond for the second layer) may be placed laterally on the PCS in a mattress fashion. This will plicate the tissue underneath the bladder forming a shelf. *Note: (1) Be careful to avoid plication of tissue directly underneath the urethra as this may injure its blood supply and its delicate musculature. If any repair is necessary near the urethra, fine suture and small needle should be used. (2) Avoid inclusion of urethral tissue or urethrovesical junction tissue in the plication stitches. (3) The "good" fibromuscular tissue is found laterally, close to the inferior pubic ramus.*

9. Prior to closure of the vaginal mucosa, some experts will eliminate the space between the repaired PCS and the vaginal mucosa by placing stitches between these tissues.

10. Excess vaginal mucosa flaps are trimmed of excess tissue.

11. The resulting vaginal mucosa flaps are closed with 2.0 Vicryl (or other absorbable suture) with a running or interrupted suture(s).

12. Other prolapses are then repaired (see also Chap. 18, Surgical Management of Apical and Posterior Wall Prolapse).

13. Vagina is packed with dry gauze for 12–24 h. *Note: Packing accomplishes two things: (1) minimizes bleeding beneath vaginal mucosa and (2) keeps anterior and posterior vaginal walls separated during initial healing.*

14. Indwelling catheter (or suprapubic catheter) is placed and removed when patient is able to void adequately. *Note: Indwelling catheterization minimizes overdistention of the bladder, which can prolong return to normal voiding and predispose to urinary tract infection (UTI).*

15. Ensure that excessive or heavy lifting, constipation, and pelvic trauma (tampons, douching, intercourse) are minimized for the first few weeks after surgery for proper healing.

INDICATIONS FOR ANTERIOR COLPORRHAPY (AKA ANTERIOR REPAIR)

- Anterior vaginal wall prolapse (especially fibromuscular attenuation or central defect)
- SUI with anterior vaginal wall prolapse is best addressed by adding an incontinence procedure (e.g., midurethral sling) to the prolapse repair. However, for mild or occult SUI the following has been done:
  - Mild SUI (must use anterior colporrhaphy with Kelly plication stitches)
  - Occult or potential SUI (must use anterior colporrhaphy with Kelly plication stitches)
- Anterior repair should be performed in conjunction with other POP repairs (if present) and prior to sling procedures (if necessary)

RESULTS OF ANTERIOR REPAIR

- The success rates for SUI are operator dependent and the cure or improvement rate is in the range of 59–69% at 1 year. The cure rate diminishes rapidly with time (i.e., at 5 years).
- Success rate with anterior colporrhaphy for recurrent anterior POP ≈ 66%.
- Success rate with anterior colporrhaphy + synthetic mesh is higher than 75% but there may be complications associated with use of a synthetic material (e.g., erosion and infection).
- ≈10–30% of women will fail primary prolapse repair (i.e., recurrent POP).
- Failure rate of anterior wall repair may be greater than that of posterior repair (≈30% vs. ≈20%).

COMPLICATIONS OF ANTERIOR REPAIR

- Direct injury to bladder > urethra > ureter; Therefore it is a good idea to perform cystoscopy even after an anterior repair
- Indirect injury from hematoma or denervation

- Injury to bladder neck or urethra leading to intrinsic sphincteric deficiency (ISD)
- Urinary retention (see Chap. 23, Voiding Dysfunction and Urinary Retention)
- Persistence of SUI (i.e., *still wet*, failure of surgery—see Chap. 14)
- Vaginal narrowing
- Female sexual dysfunction (see Chap. 49, Female Sexual Dysfunction)

PROCEDURE AND HELPFUL TECHNICAL PEARLS

VAGINAL–PARAVAGINAL DEFECT REPAIR FOR ANTERIOR VAGINAL WALL PROLAPSE

1. Steps 1–6 described for anterior colporrhaphy technique are performed (as described earlier).
2. The paravaginal space (aka retropubic space) is entered by continuing the dissection of PCS laterally past inferior pubic ramus along the vaginal sidewall.
3. Once retropubic space is entered, it is widened by a rotary motion of the index finger.
4. The index finger of the right hand is inserted into this space and the patient's right ischial spine is palpated. The ATFP runs along the medial aspect of the index finger and attaches to the back of the pubic bone (1 cm above inferior margin of pubic bone and 1 cm lateral to middle of pubic symphysis [i.e., 1 cm lateral to arcuate ligament]).
5. Place permanent interrupted sutures from the ischial spine to the pubic bone in same manner as done abdominally and hold each of them with a Kelly clamp in a fan-like configuration. Do not pop off or cut the needle yet. Stitches should be 1 cm apart. *Note: Placement of sutures can be difficult as there is a small space to operate and there may not be adequate lighting. Use of a lighted suction-irrigation device (or light attachment device to suction, or a headlight) may help visualization of the location where stitches must be placed. Placement of a suture with one needle holder and while grasping of needle near the tip with another needle holder is helpful. Some physicians may use the Capio needle to place sutures into the ATFP.*
6. Once all sutures have been placed, connect each one to the corresponding location on the PCS (lateral to midline) and then tie all of them. *Note: (1) While tying sutures make sure the knot is pushed toward the tissue rather than pulling them apart. (2) When all the sutures are tied, the PCS is reattached to the ATFP, and the paravaginal defect is eliminated.*
7. Do the same thing on the patient's left side.
8. The postoperative recovery period should be shorter than that of an abdominal paravaginal defect repair.

OTHER METHODS OF ANTERIOR VAGINAL WALL PROLAPSE REPAIR

- Laparoscopic paravaginal defect repair if performed exactly the same way as an abdominal repair (usually by a skilled laparoscopist) has the same success rate (see Chap. 19, Laparoscopic Surgery for Pelvic Organ Prolapse and Stress Urinary Incontinence).
- Repair of anterior vaginal wall prolapse, central defect type, via an abdominal route is as efficacious as the traditional anterior colporrhaphy; however, there is an increased risk of bleeding and denervation of the bladder.
- Patients with weak, attenuated tissue or those with recurrent prolapse are candidates of anterior repair using mesh or graft (see Chap. 50, Materials Used in Female Pelvic Reconstructive Surgery [FPRS]: Grafts, Meshes, and Sling Materials). The procedure is achieved in the same way as described for vaginal–paravaginal repair with a few caveats
  - ° Defects in the PCS are still repaired prior to placement of graft material.
  - ° Lateral attachment: The sutures, which have been placed through the ATFP, are secured to the graft sequentially from most proximal to most distal.
  - ° Proximal attachment: The graft must be attached to the pericervical ring (if uterus is present) or apical support network (if hysterectomized), i.e., cardinal–uterosacral–PCS–RVS.
  - ° Distal attachment: The graft may be attached to the PCS with two laterally placed (to avoid urethra) 0 Vicryl stitches if distal connection of PCS to perineal membrane is adequate.

BIBLIOGRAPHY

Benson JT, Lucente V, McClellan E. Vaginal versus abdominal reconstructive surgery for the treatment of pelvic support defects: a prospective randomized study with long-term outcome evaluation. *Am J Obstet Gynecol.* 1996;175:1418–1422.

Huddleston HT, Dunninhoo DR, Huddleston PM III, et al. Magnetic resonance imaging of defects in DeLancey's vagina support levels I, II, and III. *Am J Obstet Gynecol.* 1995; 172:1778–1784.

Sand PK, Kodure S, Lobel RW, et al. Prospective randomized trial of polyglactin 910 mesh to prevent recurrence of cystoceles and rectoceles. *Am J Obstet Gynecol.* 2001;184: 1357–1364.

Shull BL, Bachofen C, Coates KW, et al. A transvaginal approach to repair of apical and other associated sites of pelvic organ prolapse with uterosacral ligaments. *Am J Obstet Gynecol.* 2000;183:1365–1374.

Shull BL, Baden WF. A six year experience with paravaginal defect repair for stress urinary incontinence. *Am J Obstet Gynecol.* 1989;160:1432–1440.

Van Rooyen JV, Cundiff GW. Surgical management of pelvic organ prolapse. In: Bent AE, Ostergard DR, et al., eds. *Ostergard's Urogynecology and Pelvic Floor Dysfunction.* 5th ed. Philadelphia, PA: Lippincott William and Wilkins; 2003.

Weber Am, Wlaters MD. Anterior vaginal prolapse: review of anatomy and techniques of surgical repair. *Obstet Gynecol.* 1997;89:311–318.

White GR. Cystocele, a radical cure by suturing lateral sulci of vagina to white line of pelvic fascia. *JAMA.* 1909;53: 1707–1711.

Young SB, Daman JJ, Bony LG. Vaginal paravaginal repair: one-year outcome. *Am J Obstet Gynecol.* 2001:185(6):1360–1366.

Youngblood JP. Paravaginal fascial defect repair for SUI. *Contemp Ob Gyn.* 1990;35:28–38.

QUESTIONS

1. The term pubocervical fascia is a surgical term which is often used in dictations of anterior colporrhaphy and is also used commonly because of ease of communication between surgeons. However, based on histology, this layer is actually _____.
   (A) fibrous tissue
   (B) adventitia tissue
   (C) smooth muscle
   (D) fibromuscularis + adventitia tissue
   (E) endopelvic fascia

2. A 70-year-old patient who had undergone radical vulvectomy for vulvar carcinoma presents to you because of an uncomfortable bulge "down there." Upon straining you notice the urethra protruding outward like a radio antenna. You suspect ____ defect in the fibromuscular layer of the anterior vaginal wall.
   (A) proximal
   (B) distal
   (C) paravaginal
   (D) central
   (E) transverse

3. During surgical repair of the anterior compartment, one of the most important concepts to remember to achieve a strong repair _____.
   (A) type of suture
   (B) meticulous hemostasis
   (C) sterile technique
   (D) elimination of dead space
   (E) sufficient lateral dissection

QUESTIONS 4 AND 5

Match the statement below with the word(s) which best describe(s) it above. Each answer may be used once, more than once, or not at all.
   (A) Paravaginal defect
   (B) Distal defect
   (C) Central defect
   (D) Transverse defect
   (E) Cardinal ligament
   (F) Round ligament
   (G) Uterosacral ligament
   (H) Ovarian ligament

4. Arcus tendineus fascia pelvis
5. Attaches the uterus to the labia majora

ANSWERS

1. *(D)*. The layers of the vagina are in sequence: nonkeratinizing stratified squamous epithelium → loose connective tissue (lamina propria) → fibromuscular layer → adventitia. Note that the outer part of the histologic fibromuscular layer and adventitia is referred to during surgery as the PCS. However, this is not true fascia. Therefore, endopelvic or PCS are not the best terms.

2. *(B)*. Distal defects results from detachment of the PCS from the perineal membrane and thus from the overlying pubic symphysis. Patients with paravaginal defect may present with symptoms of outward protrusion or "telescoping" above the external urethral meatus during strain. Only few complain of urethrocele or SUI. Patients who have undergone radical vulvectomy are at risk for distal defect because of amputation of distal urethra.

3. *(E)*. Sharp lateral dissection to the underplane of the inferior pubic ramus is important in this repair because of two reasons: (1) it allows identification and mobilization of "good tissue" (i.e., the more lateral you go, the more glistening white strong tissue you will be able to pick-up for placation) and (2) it allows identification of a paravaginal defect which must be addressed as described in this chapter. Type of suture is not necessarily the most important concept as any absorbable suture should be fine. Studies are needed on this. Meticulous hemostasis is important for any surgery (especially fistula repairs) but not particularly in this surgery. Sterile technique although important for any surgery (especially for placement of an artificial urethral

sphincter) are not the key point of an anterior repair. Elimination of dead space is important in abdominal wall surgery and may reduce fluid collection and subsequent infection.

ANSWERS 4 AND 5

4. *(A)*, 5. *(F)*. The round ligament is attached to the dermis of the labia majora through the inguinal canal and connected to the uterus. It does not provide much support to the uterus. Detachment of the ATFP or the white line is responsible for a paravaginal defect.

18 SURGICAL MANAGEMENT OF APICAL AND POSTERIOR WALL PROLAPSE

Rajiv B. Gala, Sujata Yavagal, and Sam Siddighi

INTRODUCTION

- Pelvic floor prolapse can severely affect a woman's quality of life. Not only will women complain about pelvic pressure and an unsightly bulge, but bowel and sexual function can also become seriously compromised (see Chap. 5, Evaluation of Pelvic Organ Prolapse [POP]).
- Vaginal vault prolapse or apical prolapse occurs when the dome of the vagina loses its support and bulges into the vagina or outside. This may be accompanied by anterior prolapse (cystocele), posterior prolapse (rectocele), and/or enterocele.
- The incidence varies between 0.1 and 18.2% after a vaginal or abdominal hysterectomy. It is seen to occur more commonly if a patient received a hysterectomy for POP.
- The preoperative plan should include
  ○ Approach of surgery: abdominal, vaginal, or laparoscopic
  ○ Coexistent multiorgan prolapse and repair
  ○ Presence of stress urinary incontinence and correction
  ○ Preservation of functional vagina (e.g., length)
- The approach of surgery chosen will depend largely on the surgeon's training and to some extent on the patient's characteristics.
- The abdominal sacral colpopexy (ASCP) has a >90% cure rate. The "high" uterosacral ligament suspension (HUSLS) may have up to 90% cure rate. Prospective

randomized comparisons of ASCP versus HUSLS are needed.
- The sacrospinous ligament suspension (SSLS) has a variable cure rate (60–97%) and may have higher POP recurrence and deviation of the vaginal axis.
- Newer techniques are also discussed in this chapter.
- Prior to deciding on surgical management of apical prolapse one must have an understanding of the anatomy.

BASIC ANATOMY REVIEW

For detailed review of anatomy, see Chap. 2, Anatomy Relevant to Female Reconstructive Pelvic Surgery: Part II.
- To ensure long-term success of apical and posterior wall defects, vaginal support must be reestablished.
- DeLancey describes three types of support around the vaginal tube
  ○ DeLancey's level 1: suspension of the upper quarter of the vagina by the cardinal–uterosacral ligament complex
  ○ DeLancey's level 2: lateral attachment of the middle half of the vagina to the arcus tendineus fascia pelvis (ATFP)
  ○ DeLancey's level 3: fusion of the lower quarter of the vagina to the perineal membrane (anteriorly) and perineal body (posteriorly)
- Primary support of the posterior wall is the rectovaginal fascia (or Denonvilliers' fascia), which is the endopelvic fascia that normally attenuates before attaching to the cardinal–uterosacral ligament complex superiorly. Laterally, the rectovaginal fascia is attached to the arcus tendineus fascia rectovaginalis (ATFRV).
- One must always remember the ureter while performing pelvic surgery, which courses along the pelvic sidewall and is 1–1.5 cm lateral to the uterosacral ligament as the ureter passes underneath the uterine artery.

OBJECTIVE OF TREATMENT

- The ultimate goal of surgical therapy is to relieve symptoms, restore anatomy, and improve or maintain sexual and visceral functions.
- Nichols classified enteroceles into four groups based on etiologies: congenital, pulsion, traction, and iatrogenic. A clear understanding of each aid in the anatomical considerations necessary for surgical correction (see Chap. 5).
- Proposed mechanism of POP development: damage to levator ani muscle and pelvic nerves → decrease muscle tone and strength (Type I, slow-twitch) →

muscle disuse atrophy → muscle descent and widened levator hiatus → now intra-abdominal pressure is unopposed thus places added forces on tissue → connective tissue stretches and tears over time → prolapse results depending on where defects or attenuation have occurred.

- Thus, not only is the surgical repair of the fascial defect/attenuation crucial in the correction of enteroceles, but the pelvic muscles must be reconditioned as well.
- Finally, in the select patient with multiple medical problems who is not interested in preservation of sexual function, choose the safest and quickest procedure.

PRINCIPLES OF REPAIR

PROPHYLACTIC SURGICAL TECHNIQUES

- Prior to discussing specific surgical techniques used in repairing pelvic floor dysfunction, it is worth mentioning some common techniques used to prevent future enterocele development at the time of hysterectomy.
  - After hysterectomy: After removing the uterus, the apex of the vagina should be sutured to the uterosacral ligaments (distal or low on the uterosacral ligament) or if they are attenuated, the cuff may be attached to either one or both sacrospinous ligaments.
  - Enterocele prevention: Perform a culdoplasty (Moschowitz, Halban's, or McCall's [see below]) → try to include the bladder peritoneum to prevent anterior enterocele.
- Supracervical versus total hysterectomy → Is there any benefit to retaining the cervix and its uterosacral ligament and simply shortening the USL? Little data exist at this point to make such recommendations. Most urogynecologists will remove the cervix when correcting POP.
- Transabdominal culdoplasty
  - Marion-Moschowitz
    - Number 0 permanent suture is stitched in the peritoneum around the cul-de-sac in a purse string fashion. Careful examination of the ureters after the procedure is necessary to ensure their integrity. Cystoscopy may also be performed to check for efflux of indigo carmine.
    - Additional sutures may be placed if the cul-de-sac is still not obliterated.
  - Halban's
    - Number 0 permanent suture is stitched starting at the posterior vagina and proceeding longitudinally over the cul-de-sac peritoneum and then over the inferior sigmoid serosa.

- Multiple sutures are placed about 1 cm apart and then tied in the end.
- Compared to the Moschowitz procedure, there is less chance of involving the ureters, but careful examination with cystoscopy is still recommended, if needed.
- Transvaginal culdoplasty
  - McCall's
    - Purse string sutures concentrically in the peritoneal surface of the redundant cul-de-sac incorporated into the uterosacral ligaments bilaterally.
    - Two to three nonabsorbable sutures (e.g., 0 Prolene) are used.
    - Tying the sutures leads to obliteration of the cul-de-sac. (internal McCall's)
    - If sutures are used to suspend open ends of vagina by being brought into the vaginal mucosa, this is called a modified McCall's culdeplasty.

APICAL REPAIRS

- Vaginal approach: One prospective study showed there is a higher recurrence rate (mostly anterior compartment) of POP if corrected by vaginal approach. However, SSLS was the procedure used by vaginal route. As discussed in the following, SSLS predisposes to anterior POP.
  - SSLS: Vaginal procedure with randomized controlled trials showing lower success rates as compared to ASCP and higher recurrence rates (12% vs. 2.5%, respectively). SSLS shifts the vaginal axis posteriorly, which leaves the patient susceptible to future anterior compartment prolapse. Either unilateral or bilateral SSLS can be performed. Unilateral suspension deviates the vagina laterally while bilateral creates a trapezoid-shaped vaginal apex. Nevertheless, this procedure is useful in those patients who wish to preserve coital function where a vaginal approach is undertaken.
    - The procedure involves anchoring apex of the vagina to the sacrospinous ligament. This ligament lies on the posterior aspect of coccygeus and extends from the lateral aspect of the sacrum and coccyx to the ischial spine. The pudendal nerve with its accompanying vessels lies just lateral to the ligament at its attachment to the ischial spine.
    - Preoperative treatment with vaginal estrogen may be warranted in some patients. Prophylactic antibiotic is given to all patients.
    - The procedure is usually performed on one side though bilateral sacrospinous ligament fixation has been described.
    - With the patient under anesthesia in dorsal lithotomy position pelvic examination is done to confirm the

findings. In a patient with a uterus and multicompartment prolapse, the hysterectomy is done first and the apex can be addressed next. In a hysterectomized patient, the compartment with the largest prolapse should be addressed first.

- In one method, one can open the posterior vaginal mucosa and dissect out the rectovaginal space.
- Lateral blunt dissection is carried to reach the pararectal space. The sacrospinous ligament can be reached through the pararectal space.
- Rectal examination is done to make sure there has been no injury to the rectum during the dissection.
- The ischial spine and the attached sacrospinous ligament are then palpated.
- Various techniques can be used to pass the suture through the ligament. Deschamps ligature carrier and nerve hook, Miya hook ligature carrier and Capio suture-capturing device (Boston Scientific) are some of the examples.
- With the rectum displaced to the patient's left, the operator's left index and middle fingers are placed at the medial aspect of the patient's right ischial spine. The Deschamps ligature carrier with the nonabsorbable or delayed absorbable suture is then used to penetrate the sacrospinous ligament 2–3 cm medial to the ischial spine. Considerable resistance must be encountered during this step.
- The ligature is then grasped with a nerve hook and pulled. Another similar suture is placed about a centimeter medial to the first one.
- The Capio suture-capturing device from Boston Scientific is designed to make the technique safer and easier. Placement and retrieval of the suture are both accomplished in one step. The proposed advantage includes decrease in risk of injury to the surrounding vessels and nerves.
- The free end of each suture is then threaded to a free needle and placed through the fibromuscular layer and epithelium of the undersurface of the vaginal vault. These sutures are held on hemostats and tied after the upper half of the posterior wall of vagina is closed. If nonabsorbable suture is being used, the sutures are placed including only the fibromuscular layer of the vagina and tied. This knot is not exposed through the vagina.
- When the suspension sutures are tied the vaginal apex is pulled up to the sacrospinous ligament and suspended. A rectal examination is performed.
○ High uterosacral ligament suspension (HUSLS): Easier to perform than a sacrospinous vault suspension with more anatomical results and preservation of coital function. There is a higher risk of ureteral injury and theoretically may not have as much tensile strength as the sacrospinous ligaments. Sutures have to be placed at or higher than the level of the ischial spine, as the uterosacral ligaments can be attenuated or detached distal to this landmark. Currently, this procedure is preferred by experts in the field of female pelvic medicine and reconstructive surgery (FPMRS) when performing apical repairs by the vaginal route. HUSLS also leaves the vagina with greater depth (10.8 cm vs. 8.3 cm) when compared to SSLS. No randomized controlled trials have been performed comparing the two vaginal procedures.

- The principle is to suspend the prolapsed vaginal vault to the uterosacral ligaments. Once a vaginal incision is made to open the apex, the enterocele sac is dissected, enterocele is reduced, and the redundant sac is excised (see below).
- The bowels are packed away with several moist Kerlexes and the uterosacral ligaments are identified. A lighted headlamp or a lighted suction-irrigator may help identification of USL. The middle of the entire USL is the optimal location for suture placement because it is a compromise between safety and strength. A safe area of the uterosacral ligament is its posterior border at the level of ischial spine. There is minimal risk of injury to the vessels, nerves, and ureter at this level. *Note: The ureter is closest to USL at the level of the cervix and farthest to USL at level of sacrum. The ureter lies 1–1.5 cm lateral to the anterior border of the USL at its closest point. Sometime the ureter is attached to the USL by a fibrous band* which is not easily palpated or dissected in the operating room.
- Two to three permanent suture is then placed through the uterosacral ligament remnant (in a figure-of-eight fashion) at the level of ischial spine toward its posterior border (i.e., 1 cm posterior to the anterior border). One of the free ends of the suture is brought out through the dissected rectovaginal septum and the other through the dissected pubocervical septum. *Note: (1) Some experts attach both of these sutures to the rectovaginal septum only and close the cuff mucosa at the end of the procedure. There is no data on which method is better. (2) Some experts use absorbable sutures and suture through to the vaginal mucosa. This obviates dissection at PCS and RVS at the apex.*
- Similar suture is placed through the uterosacral ligament on the other side and attached to the rectovaginal and pubocervical septi.
- The vaginal vault with its underlying fascia is closed medial to these uterosacral sutures. The uterosacral sutures are then tied to close and suspend the angles of the vaginal vault.
- Several variations of this procedure have been described. Some authors plicate the uterosacral ligament in the midline and suspend the vaginal apex to the plicated firm uterosacral ligament complex.

Others have described placing few more sutures (usually two to three) in the uterosacral ligaments, each successive suture more cephalad (higher) to the previous and anchoring them to the vaginal vault more medially. In other words, the highest suture on the HUSL anchors medially on the cuff.

- Some experts would perform an internal McCall's culdoplasty prior to closure of the cuff.
- Cystoscopy is performed to rule out obstruction of either ureter which is up to 10%. The obstruction may be reversed by releasing the uterosacral sutures. If more extensive damage has occurred reimplantation may be necessary.

○ Iliococcygeus suspension (ICS)

- Iliococcygeus muscle arises from the arcus tendineus levator ani (ATLA), a thickening of obturator internus parietal fascia from pubic bone (posterior, lateral, and superior on the pubic bone) to ischial spine from which the levator ani originates.
- The iliococcygeus passes behind the rectum and inserts into the anococcygeal raphe and the coccyx.
- The iliococcygeus fascia can be used to suspend the vaginal vault in cases where the uterosacral ligament is attenuated.
- The procedure is similar to that described for USLS. Once the posterior vaginal wall is opened the pararectal spaces are dissected and the ischial spines are identified.
- The suture is placed into the iliococcygeus fascia anterior to the ischial spine and is brought out through the rectovaginal and the pubocervical fascia. This is then repeated on the other side. When these sutures are tied the vault is elevated and suspended to the iliococcygeus fascia.

○ Newer vaginal techniques: IVS tunneler, Apogee, and others (these are described in Chap. 50, Materials Used in Female Pelvic Reconstructive Surgery [FPRS]: Grafts, Meshes, and Sling Materials; here we briefly describe the IVS tunneler). More data are needed on long-term efficacy and safety of these procedures.

- IVS tunneler (aka posterior intravaginal slingplasty or infracoccygeal sacropexy)
  - The first IVS procedure was performed in Australia by Dr. P.E. Petros in 1997. It has been widely used in Europe and Australia since then. The procedure was approved by Food and Drug Administration (FDA) in March 2003.
  - The IVS tunneler manufactured by Tyco healthcare employs an 8-mm polypropylene tape to suspend the vaginal vault. It is composed of a stainless outer sheath, a blue polypropylene stylet with an eyelet to thread the tape and a tension-free multifilament polypropylene mesh.

- The patient is positioned in a dorsal lithotomy position with the buttocks slightly off the table. An incision is made in the posterior vaginal wall about 2 cm below the vaginal vault. Lateral dissection is carried out in the pararectal spaces bilaterally till the ischial spines can be identified. This exposes the underside of the sacrospinous ligament on both sides.
- Two 5-mm skin incisions are made one on each side: 2 cm lateral and 2 cm posterior to the anal verge
- The stainless steel outer sheath is then introduced through the skin incision. It is advanced forward into the ischiorectal fossa lateral to the puborectalis. Two fingers of the other hand are placed through the vaginal incision at the level of ischial spine palpating the margin of the levator ani muscle.
- The outer sheath is further advanced through the levator ani using the vaginal fingers as a guide. It is then brought out through the vaginal incision. The outer sheath is left in this position and the blue stylet is removed and reversed. The tape is threaded through the eyelet and the stylet is reinserted in the sheath. The entire instrument is then removed while holding the tape in place. The procedure is then repeated on the contralateral side.
- The U-shaped loop of the tape lies in the vaginal incision. It is sutured to the underlying vaginal submucosa using three absorbable interrupted sutures. Gentle traction is applied to the ends to position the vagina in the normal horizontal axis.
- The ends of the tape are cut just below the surface of the skin and the vaginal and skin incisions are closed.

○ LeFort colpocleisis (aka partial colpocleisis): In a patient who is at high surgical risk and is not sexually active, a colpocleisis may be performed under local + IV sedation or regional anesthesia. It requires minimal dissection and has less and more gradual blood loss than the restorative procedures described above. The traditional LeFort is performed in someone with a uterus. If this procedure is planned, a Pap smear, ultrasound, and endometrial biopsy should be done prior to the procedure to exclude cancer. Urodynamics evaluation also should be performed to evaluate for urinary incontinence. The LeFort leaves lateral channels in the vagina through which uterine bleeding can be detected.

- Two straps of vaginal mucosa, one anteriorly and one posteriorly, are excised and carried down to the pubocervical septum and rectovaginal septum, respectively.
- Down the lateral sides of uterus, approximate the pubocervical septum anteriorly to the rectovaginal septum posteriorly using Lembert inverting sutures.

- Then, approximate the anterior and posterior segments over the opening of the cervix.
- Embrocate the remnant of the cervix in an anterior/posterior fashion.
- The anterior and posterior walls are not attached to each other all the way to the hymenal ring because this flattens the vesical neck angle and predisposes to stress urinary incontinence.
- Finally, close the vaginal mucosa.

○ Total colpectomy and colpocleisis: In the absence of a uterus, a complete colpocleisis or total colpectomy can be performed. It has a reported success rate of 90–100%. Most common complication is *de novo* stress urinary incontinence (<10%).

- The procedure involves making a circumferential incision in the vaginal mucosa after holding and pulling the vaginal apex. Four quadrants are marked on the vagina and each is dissected from the underlying tissue. A series of purse string sutures is placed to approximate the anterior pubocervical and posterior rectovaginal septum. As the purse string sutures are tied the soft tissue is reduced and the prolapse corrected.
- Levator ani plication and posterior colporrhaphy are also performed. Both stress and urge urinary incontinence can occur after this procedure. With preexisting stress urinary incontinence an anti-incontinence procedure (e.g., tension-free vaginal tape [TVT]) may be performed before closing the vagina. Alternatively, a kelly plication may be performed.

• Abdominal approach: The abdominal approach allows repair of the apex (discussed below) and also the anterior compartment by way of an abdominal paravaginal repair. However, the posterior compartment is difficult to address abdominally and therefore the patient must be repositioned or prepositioned in Allen stirrups for a vaginal repair of the posterior compartment. This can add extra time and morbidity to the surgery.

○ ASCP: Selection of patients is very important for this procedure. It provides a strong and long-lasting support to the vault, thereby making it the procedure of choice in younger patients. Some of the other indications include pelvic pathology, poor vaginal tissues, and medical conditions such as chronic cough or constipation. Some reserve this procedure for patients who have recurrent prolapse.

○ This procedure has higher morbidity and requires a longer hospital stay and recovery. However, the results are better.

○ The first attempt at ASCP was done by Arthure, Savage, and Falk who attached the vaginal vault to the sacrum. The use of a suspension tissue between the vault and the sacrum was first introduced by Embrey. This prevented undue tension on the vault.

Several synthetic and autologous grafts are available and can be used for the suspension. The various allografts include fascia lata, cadaveric fascia, and rectus fascia. The synthetic materials that can be used to suspend the vagina are polypropylene, polytetrafluroethylene, or Dacron mesh.

- With the patient in Allen stirrups, a sponge stick is placed in the vagina for elevating it during the procedure. Laparotomy is performed via a Pfannenstiel or a vertical midline incision. Small bowel and sigmoid colon are packed away from the site of surgery. While elevating the vagina with an end to end anastomosis (EEA) sizer, an incision is made in the peritoneum over the vaginal vault and the bladder and the rectum are dissected off the anterior and the posterior vaginal walls, respectively. Any defects in the pubocervical and the rectovaginal fascia are repaired and they are attached to each other at the apex of vagina if separated.
- The two strips of grafts are then attached anteriorly and posteriorly using permanent sutures (e.g., Ethibond) to the muscular wall of the vagina avoiding the vaginal epithelium. The graft extends about halfway down the posterior vaginal wall.
- It is preferable to perform a culdoplasty at this time to prevent future enterocele formation behind the posterior mesh.
- The presacral space is opened by incising the peritoneum over the sacrum. It is important to identify the aortic bifurcation, the iliac vessels and nerves, middle sacral vessels, and the ureter. The presacral space is then gently dissected to expose the anterior sacral ligament.
- Two permanent sutures are placed through the ligament at the level of S2-S3 and then through both the anterior and the posterior mesh. The sutures are tied down avoiding unnecessary tension on the mesh. The peritoneum over the sacrum and bladder flap are closed.

○ Abdominal SSLS is possible but is rarely undertaken because of difficulty of the procedure by this route and less optimal surgical results obtained by its vaginal counterpart.

• Laparoscopic technique (see Chap. 19, Laparoscopic Surgery for Pelvic Organ Prolapse and Stress Urinary Incontinence)

○ Laparoscopic uterosacral ligament suspension: Abdominal or laparoscopic USLS have the advantage of allowing uterine preservation in patients who do not want a hysterectomy. Here we describe the Richardson-Saye technique.

- The most important consideration after proper patient selection is appropriate port placement and technique

- Four ports: 1st umbilicus (10/12 mm), 2nd a 10/12-mm midway between umbilicus and pubic bone but fingerbreadth left of midline, 3rd and 4th left and right midlower abdomen.
- Use nonabsorbable 2-0 suture on a 5/8 circle curved needle.
  - Invert the vaginal vault using a rectal sizer.
  - Identify the uterosacral ligaments while paying special attention to the anterolateral relationship of the ureters.
  - Tag the unbroken portions of uterosacral ligament with 2-0 permanent suture as they enter into the sacrum.
  - Identify the pubocervical and rectovaginal septum after separation of the peritoneum.
  - Stitch the apical corner and lateral edges of the vaginal vault and incorporate into the ipsilateral uterosacral ligament thus, reapproximating the rectovaginal and pubocervical septum overlying the vaginal mucosa.
  - Repeat the same process on the contralateral side.
  - Use interrupted sutures to reapproximate the rectovaginal and pubocervical septum across the center of the vaginal vault.
  - Place reinforcing sutures from the ipsilateral uterosacral ligament to posterior rectovaginal fascia bilaterally, avoiding to cross the midline in an effort to re-create the natural anatomical planes.

ENTEROCELE REPAIR

- Bear in mind that correction of the herniation starts with adequate attention to the apical fascia and suspension of the vaginal vault.
- Classic transvaginal technique
  - At the posterior hymenal ring, make a vertical incision with a scalpel through the vaginal epithelium after injection with 1% lidocaine with epinephrine (or similar).
  - Use several Allis clamps to hold the edge of the cut vaginal mucosa and Metzenbaum scissors to dissect the vaginal epithelium from the rectovaginal fascia.
  - Staying in the midline, continue the dissection toward the vaginal apex until loss of the rectovaginal fascia is noted and the enterocele sac is visible.
  - Carefully enter the enterocele sac and excise the excess peritoneum.
  - Demarcation of the sac by the rectovaginal septum posteriorly and the pubocervical septum anteriorly is noted. This demarcation can be better observed by placing nondominant index finger in the rectum and lifting anteriorly.

- The anterior vaginal mucosa is dissected off the pubocervical septum.
- The uterosacral ligaments are reattached to the vaginal apex.
- Use 2-0 permanent suture to reapproximate the pubocervical septum anteriorly and the rectovaginal septum posteriorly in an interrupted fashion.
- Finally, tie the uterosacral suspension sutures down thus resuspending the new apex.
- Perform transurethral cystoscopy to confirm bilateral ureteral patency.

POSTERIOR REPAIR (AKA POSTERIOR COLPORRHAPY)

- Transvaginal approach: traditional posterior colpoperineorrhaphy with levator ani plication
  - The rectovaginal fascia is typically over sewn or plicated in the midline (the attenuated rectovaginal fascia is repaired without identification of defect(s)).
  - The vaginal bulge is eliminated and excess vaginal mucosa is removed.
  - The levator ani muscles and connective tissue are identified, mobilized, and brought together in the midline by a series of interrupted sutures.
  - Aggressive plication of the levator ani high in vagina (i.e., proximal) can result in a transverse ridge, narrowing, and can lead to dyspareunia (see Chap. 49, Female Sexual Dysfunction).
- Defect-specific repair
  - The "site-specific" defect or well-defined defect in the rectovaginal septum is uncommon. Instead, the rectovaginal fascia or the posterior fibromuscular layer of the vagina must be plicated in the midline while a finger is placed in the rectum to identify areas of deficiency.
  - Many urogynecologists are moving toward this type of repair as the literature continues to validate its superiority to traditional posterior colporrhaphy (i.e., less pain and decreased incidence of sexual dysfunction). The repair has proven to provide durable anatomical support along with restoration of bowel function. The success rate is ≈80–90% at 1-year follow-up.
    - Inject the posterior vaginal wall and perineum with 1% lidocaine with epinephrine (or similar).
    - With the nondominant finger in the anus, make a vertical incision in the posterior vaginal mucosa (a transverse incision technique may also be performed).
    - Use Mayo scissors to make a plane in the rectovaginal space. The goal is to leave as much of the fascia on the rectum as possible.

- Carry the dissection superiorly to the vaginal apex, laterally to the tendinous arch of the levator ani (ATFRV), and inferiorly to the perineal body.
- With the nondominant finger lifting anteriorly, inspect the rectovaginal septum for attenuation or discrete breaks.
- Identify uncovered muscularis in areas of fascial defects and perform the repair (in placating fashion) using interrupted, absorbable 2-0 suture (e.g., 2-0 Vicryl).
- Trim the vaginal epithelium as needed.
- A perineorrhaphy is not routinely performed unless the patient has a gaping genital hiatus or separation of the superficial transverse perineal muscles and bulbocavernosus requires perineal body reconstruction. The goal is to achieve a vaginal diameter of 2–3 finger's width.
- Be sure to attach the plicated tissue of posterior fibromuscular vaginal wall (i.e., rectovaginal septum) to the perineal body before closing the vaginal mucosa.
- Posterior repair with augmentation (see Chap. 50, Materials Used in Female Pelvic Reconstructive Surgery: Grafts, Meshes, and Sling Materials)
- Transanal repair
  - This is the preferred route of the colorectal surgeon.
    - In patients with thinning of the rectal submucosa and increased reservoir size, use endorectal plication to reduce the luminal size.
    - Two obliterative layers starting at the mucocutaneous junction incorporating the full-thickness of the rectal wall.
  - No difference has been found in dyspareunia, constipation, or fecal incontinence when compared to the traditional posterior colporrhaphy.

COMPLICATIONS

SEXUAL DYSFUNCTION AND PAIN

- Posterior colporrhaphy will usually correct the anatomical defects, but multiple retrospective studies show an association with increased sexual and bowel dysfunction. The fundamental portion of the procedure, the levator plication, is felt to be the leading source of pain and dyspareunia in 19–33% of women because of muscle atrophy due to pressure and subsequent scarring.
- Some postulate that the selected cohorts of elderly women who are postmenopausal and suffer from vaginal atrophy predispose them to difficulties with intercourse. Nevertheless, sexual dysfunction is more

common with posterior repairs than any other vaginal procedure (see Chap. 49, Female Sexual Dysfunction).

BOWEL DYSFUNCTION

- Symptoms of pelvic heaviness and difficulty with rectal emptying are relieved in as many as 91% of women undergoing rectocele repair. Caution should be exercised and a thorough workup, including defecography, may be undertaken in women with a primary complaint of rectal emptying difficulties. Patients with pathological transit studies may benefit from maximization of conservative therapy prior to surgical intervention.

SUTURE EROSION AND WOUND DEHISCENCE

- The types of suture materials used in all of the procedure above are surgeon dependent and based on their personal experiences. A common maxim in surgical repairs of hernias is to use permanent suture materials. Some feel like vaginal surgery is unique in that the connective tissue and vaginal epithelium tend to be thinner and less vascular after obstetric injuries thus impairing wound healing at baseline.
- One retrospective analysis suggests that absorbable suture material decreases the incidence of both wound dehiscence and suture erosion. A randomized prospective trial would strengthen this argument.

MESH EROSION AFTER SACRAL COLPOPEXY

- To reduce the risk of mesh erosion after ASCP the following is suggested:
  - Local vaginal estrogen cream prior to surgery and after surgery to strengthen tissue
  - Sterile technique during attachment of mesh
  - If using synthetic material → use soft, pliable material and only a single-thickness to attach to the cuff (instead of doubling or folding which increase amount of foreign body)
  - Use biological material (e.g., derma graft and rectus fascia)
  - Monofilament suture to attach mesh instead of braided suture
  - Avoid full-thickness stitches into the vagina
- Erosion may occur a few weeks to years after surgery. The sooner the erosion occurs, the higher the likelihood of recurrence of POP.
- When erosion occurs, there are a few options for management:

○ Conservative (vaginal estrogen and expectant management) → wait 2 months, but this may a lengthy process and may not be successful.

○ Mobilization of vaginal mucosa and closure → is not successful.

○ Vaginal excision of all visible mesh then closure → is successful, less invasive, and has low chance of POP recurrence.

○ Abdominal excision of distal mesh then closure → is successful and low chance or POP recurrence. Be sure to not remove mesh at sacrum (proximally) because this can lead to life-threatening hemorrhage.

CONCLUSIONS

IMPROVING LONG-TERM SUCCESS IN PELVIC FLOOR RECONSTRUCTION

- Multiple studies demonstrate that cadaveric fascia lata and dermis, despite significant increases in cost, do not improve long-term success rates. As technology continues to integrate stronger surgical materials into the operating theater, one must consider the future of synthetic absorbable meshes to decrease failure rates in pelvic surgery (see Chap. 50, Materials Used in Female Pelvic Reconstructive Surgery: Grafts, Meshes, and Sling Materials).

- One series demonstrated that polyglactin 910 mesh reinforcement did prevent the recurrence of cystoceles. The literature must still address numerous questions like should we overlay or reinforce natural fascia with synthetic materials, which is the best absorbable material, can growth factors help in healing, and what is the exact role of nerves and muscles of the pelvic floor in future success rates?

BIBLIOGRAPHY

Carter JE. Enterocele repair and vaginal vault suspension. *Curr Opin Obstet Gynecol.* 2000;12:321–330.

DeLancey JO. Anatomic aspects of vaginal eversion after hysterectomy. *Am J Obstet Gynecol.* 1992;166:1717–1724; discussion 1724–1728.

DeLancey JO, Morley GW. Total colpocleisis for vaginal eversion. *Am J Obstet Gynecol.* 1997;176:1228–1232; discussion 1232–1235.

Holley RL. Enterocele: a review. *Obstet Gynecol Surv.* 1994; 49:284–293.

Kahn MA, Stanton SL. Posterior colporrhaphy: its effects on bowel and sexual function. *Br J Obstet Gynaecol.* 1997;104: 82–86.

Lopez A, Anzen B, Bremmer S, et al. Durability of success after rectocele repair. *Int Urogynecol J Pelvic Floor Dysfunct.* 2001;12:97–103.

Lovatsis D, Drutz HP. Vaginal surgical approach to vaginal vault prolapse: considerations of anatomic correction and safety. *Curr Opin Obstet Gynecol.* 2003;15:435–437.

Luck AM, Galvin SL, Theofrastous JP. Suture erosion and wound dehiscence with permanent versus absorbable suture in reconstructive posterior vaginal surgery. *Am J Obstet Gynecol.* 2005;192:1626–1629.

Nichols DH. Types of enterocele and principles underlying choice of operation for repair. *Obstet Gynecol.* 1972;40:257–263.

Paraiso MF, Falcone T, Walters MD. Laparoscopic surgery for enterocele, vaginal apex prolapse and rectocele. *Int Urogynecol J Pelvic Floor Dysfunct.* 1999;10:223–229.

Porter WE, Steele A, Walsh P, et al. The anatomic and functional outcomes of defect-specific rectocele repairs. *Am J Obstet Gynecol.* 1999;181:1353–1358; discussion 1358–1359.

Sand PK, Koduri S, Lobel RW, et al. Prospective randomized trial of polyglactin 910 mesh to prevent recurrence of cystoceles and rectoceles. *Am J Obstet Gynecol.* 2001;184:1357–1362; discussion 1362–1364.

Segal JL, Karram MM. Evaluation and management of rectoceles. *Curr Opin Urol.* 2002;12:345–352.

Waters E. A diagnostic technique for the detection of enterocele. *Am J Obstet Gynecol.* 1946;52:810.

Wheeless C. Atlas of pelvic surgery. In: Mitchell CW, ed. Baltimore, MD: Williams & Wilkins; 1997.

QUESTIONS

1. A 57-year-old woman presents to her gynecologist with complaints of pelvic pressure and is noted to have a significant vaginal vault prolapse. The decision was made to proceed with a transvaginal sacrospinous colpopexy. The procedure was uneventful and the patient was discharged on postoperative day 1. At her 6-week postoperative follow up, the patient notes that she has numbness on her perineum and has started having fecal incontinence. The most likely etiology is

   (A) normal postoperative course
   (B) damage to the pudendal nerve
   (C) side effects from anesthesia
   (D) damage to the obturator nerve

2. A healthy 43-year-old woman with two prior cesarean sections and an appendectomy secondary to rupture was having severe menorrhagia secondary to fibroids. Her gynecologist decided to perform an abdominal hysterectomy. The patient had extensive pelvic scarring from her prior surgeries and her gynecologist wanted to decrease her chances of requiring another procedure and performed

a prophylactic Moschowitz procedure. On postoperative day 3, the patient began complaining of fevers, chills, nausea, and nonspecific flank/abdominal pain, and clear leakage from her vagina. Her white blood cell (WBC) count was 21,000, packed cell volume (PCV) was 32, and blood urea nitrogen/creatinine (BUN/Cr) was 40/2.1. Which of the following is the most likely cause of her symptoms?

(A) vaginal cuff cellulitis

(B) urinary tract infection (UTI)

(C) ureteral obstruction

(D) ileus

3. A 64-year-old woman, postmenopausal since her total abdominal hysterectomy with bilateral salpingoopherectomy (TAH-BSO) 20 years ago, complains of feeling a bulge in her vagina. She does not have any problem with urination but is having to use a finger in her vagina to help with defecation. She also notes that it is worse when she is up on her feet. Moreover, it has been interfering with sexual activity and she wants definitive treatment. On examination, you can see the bulge immediately and when you use a Sims speculum, the bulge is mostly posteriorly. When you perform a rectovaginal examination, your finger can palpate part of the bulge but not all of it. The most likely diagnosis is

(A) cystocele

(B) enterocele

(C) rectocele

(D) rectocele + enterocele

(E) complete procidentia

ANSWERS

1. *(B)*. During the sacrospinous colpopexy, knowledge of the coccygeus muscle-sacrospinous ligament is critical. The pudendal artery and nerve pass about 2 cm medial and beneath the ischial spine. An improperly placed suture can damage the nerve and lead to a significant hematoma if the vessel is disrupted as well. The obturator nerve is more likely damaged during retroperitoneal surgery and is associated with inability to adduct the thighs.

2. *(C)*. When a culdoplasty is performed at the time of an abdominal hysterectomy, the two most common techniques are the Moschowitz procedure and the Halban's technique. Of the two techniques, the Moschowitz is more likely to injure the ureter. Nevertheless, this patient had multiple risk factors for having ureteral damage (prior surgery, scar

tissue, and performing a hysterectomy). All of her symptoms are explained by a ureteral injury and treatment is based on when the injury is first recognized. Since her injury was noted on postoperative day 3, immediate repair could be performed.

3. *(D)*. Her examination is classic of a combined lesion, especially with the findings of an apical bulge above her rectal finger. Cystocele is an anterior lesion and procidentia refers to uterine prolapse.

19 LAPAROSCOPIC SURGERY FOR PELVIC ORGAN PROLAPSE AND STRESS URINARY INCONTINENCE

Justin Thien Lee

INTRODUCTION

- Over the past 30 years, Laparoscopic surgery has been evolving from a simple diagnostic tool to a broader major surgical technique to treat a variety of disease processes.
- Laparoscopy was first used in Gynecology in an effort to replicate procedures that were performed by laparotomy.
- Like any other surgical procedure, plenty of practice is necessary to become a skilled laparoscopist. There is an initial steep curve while learning to perform laporoscopic procedures.
- This essential diagnostic and therapeutic operative tool will be reviewed in this chapter.

INDICATIONS FOR LAPAROSCOPIC PROCEDURES IN GYNECOLOGIC SURGERY—BASIC REVIEW

- *Diagnostic laparoscopy*: Gynecologic surgeons often need to assess the etiology of chronic and acute pelvic pain, such as endometriosis, ectopic pregnancy, and adnexal torsion. In addition, the physician may need to perform chromopertubation for evaluation of tubal patency in infertility work-up. In this procedure, the camera lens is often introduced into the abdomen via the infraumbilical trocar port. A second trocar port is usually placed at suprapubic region or at the lower abdomen where an atraumatic probe is used to systematically evaluate the pelvic organs.

- *Permanent tubal sterilization*: Different instruments and devices have been used to occlude the tubes at the isthmic portion which is approximately 3 cm lateral to the cornua. The bipolar electrocautery, Silastic bands, and Filsche clips have been used depending on the physicians' preferences. The failure rate using these devices to achieve the permanent sterilization is about 1–3% in 10 years prospective follow-up. The trocar placements are also at the infraumbilical and suprapubic region of the abdomen.
- *Ovarian cystectomy and oophorectomy*: The ovarian simple cyst can be removed laparoscopically. Signs of malignancy such as ascites, tumor implants on the peritoneum, liver, or excrescences on the ovary can be diagnosed when a complex ovarian cystectomy procedure is attempted. A good effort should be made to remove the cyst intact at all times. An endobag may be used to assist in removal of the cyst out of the abdomen via a 10-mm trocar. However, if cyst is too large then drainage of the cyst prior to removal of the endobag is possible. Specimens should be sent for permanent section and pathological diagnosis. If there are any signs of malignancy, the cyst must be sent for frozen section to rule out malignancy or potential for malignancy. Laparotomy should be performed immediately after confirming malignancy by frozen section. The peritoneal cavity should be rinsed copiously with Ringer's lactate solution in event of ruptured cyst during removal. When a dermoid cyst is ruptured, great effort should be made to remove all sebaceous content of the dermoid cyst. The contamination of peritoneal cavity with dermoid cyst material can cause a severe chemical peritonitis.
- *Laparoscopic oophorectomy* can be performed safely. There are many different laparoscopic instruments, such as bipolar, staplers, prettied loops, and vibrating devices used to hemostatically occlude the infundibulopelvic (IP) ligament in order to remove the ovary. An endobag is needed to remove ovarian tissue. The ovary is often removed via a 10- or 12-mm trocar port site. The physician must pay attention to any signs of malignancy as mentioned before. An intraoperative consult or an immediate laparotomy for staging is needed if malignancy is found on frozen section of ovarian tissue.
- *Treatment for endometriosis*: Fulguration of endometriosis can be performed by using laparoscopic instruments, where endometriotic lesions may be resected or ablated. This procedure may improve fertility and reduce pelvic pain.
- *Treatment of ectopic pregnancy*: Linear salpingostomy or salpingectomy can be performed with laparoscopic instruments to remove a tubal embryo and gestational sac. Stapling devices and prettied loops are used for salpingectomy. On the other hand, the monopolar and bipolar devices are often used for salpingostomy. The endobag usually is suited for removal of the ectopic conception.
- *Myomectomy*: For women who have desire for preservation of the uterus and fertility, laparoscopic myomectomy is an option for a symptomatic fibroid uterus. An injection of vasopressin into the uterus is often used to reduce heavy bleeding, especially with intramural leiomyomas. After removal of the fibroid, the defect on the uterus must be sutured laparoscopically. This task may be difficult and time-consuming for an inexperienced surgeon. A morcellator may be used to expedite the removal of the fibroid. A barrier material is often used to reduce the risk of adhesion formation at the end of laparoscopic myomectomy procedure.
- *Hysterectomy*: There are several approaches for hysterectomy—laparoscopic-assisted vaginal hysterectomy (LAVH), laparoscopic supracervical hysterectomy (LSH), and total laparoscopic hysterectomy (TLH). Radical laparoscopic-assisted vaginal hysterectomy and radical total laparoscopic hysterectomy are also being attempted by some gynecologic oncologists.
  - LAVH is often performed by using 3- to 4-port sites. The intra-abdominal peritoneal cavity is inspected, and lysis of adhesion and washing sampling may be performed if necessary. The IP ligaments or the utero-ovarian ligaments are clamped and transected, depending on the indication of removal of the ovaries. The round ligaments are cut in a similar fashion. The uterovesical peritoneum is opened and cut. The gynecologic surgeon can choose to occlude the proximal uterine blood supply and uterine arteries. The physician may then reposition vaginally. The rest of the hysterectomy can be performed vaginally, including closure of the vaginal cuff.
  - LSH procedure preserves the cervix and is technically easier to perform. The LSH procedure is performed with a similar technique as LAVH. However, the entire fundus is removed from the cervix after the pedicles, uterine vessels, and dissection of the bladder from the uterus. The entire fundus is transected from the cervix with a cautery device, and removed from the abdomen by a laparoscopic morcellator through a 12-mm port.
  - TLH procedure is performed similar to an LAVH. However, the entire hysterectomy procedure is done laparoscopically. The gynecologic surgeon would prefer TLH approach for patients whose uteri do not descend or vaginal access is limited (narrow) which make the LAVH impossible. After occlusion and transection of the pedicles, IP, utero-ovarian, and round ligaments, the bladder is dissected off of the uterus. The uterine vessels and uterosacral ligaments are occluded and transected. The posterior

and anterior cul-de-sac is incised and the specimen is then removed vaginally. The vaginal cuff is closed laparoscopically with intracorporeal or extracorporeal knot-tying techniques. It is important to identify the ureters throughout laparoscopic hysterectomy procedure.

- Radical LAVH and radical total laparoscopic hysterectomy are experimental at this point. Currently, gynecologic oncologists at several academic centers are involved in research involving radical LAVH and lymph node dissection. Some believe that laparotomy can be replaced by laparoscopy for staging and treatment of early stage endometrial carcinoma.

INDICATIONS FOR LAPAROSCOPIC SURGERY IN FEMALE PELVIC RECONSTRUCTIVE SURGERY

- *Female pelvic reconstructive surgery*: Traditionally, pelvic organ prolapse and incontinence have been corrected by vaginal or abdominal reconstructive surgery. Laparoscopy has been used with varying success to perform following reconstructive operations: paravaginal repair, Burch, enterocele repair, and vaginal vault suspension (e.g., uterosacral ligament suspension and sacral colpopexy).
  - Laparoscopic paravaginal repair has been performed for anterior compartment prolapse with a paravaginal or lateral type of defect in the supportive tissue. According to certain experts in the field of female pelvic medicine and reconstructive surgery (FPMRS), most cystoceles are a result of lateral defects. The paravaginal defect is repaired by suturing the lateral aspect of the vaginal wall to arcus tendineus fascia pelvis (ATFP) or "white line" (see Chap. 1, Anatomy Relevant to Female Reconstructive Pelvic Surgery: Part I and Chap. 2, Anatomy Relevant to Female Reconstructive Pelvic Surgery: Part II). Paravaginal repair can be performed concomitantly with other prolapse and/or incontinence procedures (e.g., sacralcolpopexy and Burch). If the paravaginal repair is performed in exactly the same manner as the open procedure, then the cure and complication rates should be similar. More data is needed on this.
  - Open Burch retropubic urethropexy is a highly effective procedure for the treatment of stress urinary incontinence (see Chap. 15, Surgical Management of Stress Urinary Incontinence: Open Retropubic Operations). Laparoscopic Burch procedure can be accomplished by placement of permanent sutures at the level of the midurethra and bladder neck to the Cooper's ligament. The complication of this procedure includes bladder or ureter injury, voiding dysfunction,

hemorrhage, incomplete bladder emptying, and urinary retention. Theoretically, if the laparoscopic Burch is performed in exactly the same way as the open Burch then the cure rates would be comparable. According to recent studies, laparoscopic Burch has lower subjective and objective cure rates than the open Burch. Additionally, compared to tension-free vaginal tape (TVT), the laparoscopic Burch is less cost-effective, uses more operative time, and has a lower objective cure rate (at < 2 years).

  - *Laparoscopic culdoplasty*: Enterocele repair can be performed laparoscopically. An enterocele is defined as a protruding peritoneal sac with or without intestinal content in direct contact with the vaginal epithelium (see Chap. 6, Evaluation of Urinary Incontinence in the Office and Indications for Referral to a Specialist). In order to repair the enterocele, continuity in the supporting tissue is reestablished by suturing the pubocervical septum to the rectovaginal septum.
  - Vaginal vault prolapse often occurs when there is a defect or attenuation of the uterosacral ligaments. This usually occurs distal to the ischial spine. The vaginal apex can lose its support following a hysterectomy or even in the intact uterus because of attenuation or breaking of the uterosacral ligament. There are several ways to support the vaginal apex (see Chap. 18, Surgical Management of Apical and Posterior Wall Prolapse).
    - Laparoscopic uterosacral ligament suspension can be performed by placing sutures high on the uterosacral ligaments (HUSLs) and connecting this to the vaginal apex (see Chap. 18 for a full description).
    - Laparoscopic sacral colpopexy is another reconstructive surgery for the correction of vaginal vault prolapse. It is technically challenging and only few surgeons report good results. The sacral colpopexy is performed by suturing a synthetic mesh that connects the proximal anterior, apical, and posterior vaginal walls to the sacrum. In sacral colpopexy, the peritoneum which is incised and opened for attachment of the mesh to the sacrum should be closed to reduce the risk of adhesion formation and of the possibility for bowel strangulation. The results of the laparoscopic sacral colpopexy are comparable to the open sacral colpopexy if the laparoscopic procedure is performed in the same way as the open procedure.

LAPAROSCOPIC TECHNIQUES

- There are approximately four common ways of placing a laparoscopic port into the abdomen and creating pneumoperitoneum: (1) Veress needle followed by a primary trocar, (2) open laparoscopy, (3) direct trocar insertion, and (4) optical trocar placement. Each approach offers its own advantages. Gynecologic surgeon choice of technique varies due to individual experiences. There are also two types of instruments: (1) reusable (metallic trocar) and (2) disposable (plastic trocar).

○ Veress needle followed by a primary trocar technique
  ▪ Veress needle is introduced into the abdomen through the umbilicus.
  ▪ The patient's position should be completely horizontal.
  ▪ The abdominal wall is grasped manually or with towel clips at the base of the umbilicus, and elevated to create a pocket of space in the peritoneum just below the umbilicus. This maneuver may lessen the likelihood of the intestinal tract and retroperitoneal vessels injury.
  ▪ It is important to assess patient's body habitus prior to placing the primary trocar. For an average weight patient, the Veress needle is inserted at a 45-degree angle and pointed toward the hollow of the sacrum. For an obese patient, the Veress needle is placed at 70–80 degree because the thickness of the abdominal wall is increased. Extreme care must be taken when introducing the Veress needle into the abdomen in a thin patient. Because the vital structures such as retroperitoneal vessels are much closer to the abdominal wall, the margin of error is reduced when inserting the Veress needle at 45-degree angle.
  ▪ After placing the Veress needle, confirmation of correct placement can be performed by different methods, such as hanging drop test, measurement of intra-abdominal pressure with carbon dioxide insufflation, or injection and aspiration of fluid through the Veress needle.
  ▪ The primary trocar is placed with similar angle to the Veress needle after pneumoperitoneum has been accomplished.
○ Open laparoscopy is performed with an incision of infraumbilical skin and rectus abdominis fascia.
  ▪ The peritoneal cavity is then entered with a Crile or a Kelly clamp.
  ▪ The trocar with sleeve is now introduced into the peritoneal cavity.
  ▪ Pneumoperitoneum is then achieved.
  ▪ For the Hasson open laparoscopy, the sutures are placed on the fascia to hold, anchor the sleeve, and maintain pneumoperitoneum. General Surgeons believe that open laparoscopy reduces the risk of bowel injury and avoids injury to retroperitoneal vessels. For these reasons, many laparoscopists choose this method for placing the primary trocar.
○ Direct trocar insertion is the technique in which the primary trocar is introduced into the peritoneal cavity without having inserted the Veress needle and established pneumoperitoneum.
  ▪ After the trocar has been inserted into the cavity, the pneumoperitoneum is achieved.
  ▪ Rate of complications such as vessel and bowel injury between this technique and the Veress technique are unknown. However, most laparoscopists believe that the incidence of injury is higher with direct trocar insertion technique.
○ Optical trocar insertion is performed in a similar manner as direct trocar insertion.
  ▪ A clear, hollow trocar sleeve is used with the laparoscope inside to visualize the layers of abdominal wall while penetrating into the peritoneal cavity. The risk of retroperitoneal vessel and bowel injury has not been established with this technique. However, some laparoscopists believe that optical trocar insertion may help in recognizing the complications as vessel and bowel injury.
• Secondary trocar insertion is often required to proceed with operative gynecologic procedures. The secondary trocars are introduced with direct visualization via laparoscope and after identification of inferior epigastric vessels. The secondary trocars are usually placed either at approximately 5 cm lateral to the midline and 8 cm above the pubic symphysis or at midline 3 cm above the pubic symphysis. It is important to close the fascia when a greater than 5 mm trocar is used in order to reduce the risk of incisional hernia.

POWERHOUSE INSTRUMENTS

• Technology in laparoscopic surgery has been advancing rapidly in the past 20 years. The monopolar electrosurgery was developed for the gynecologic surgeon to maintain hemostasis during laparoscopic procedure. Due to electrical current, monopolar devices carry a higher risk of injury to the adjacent tissue than the bipolar electrosurgery in which injury is limited by thermal spread.
• New instruments have been developed to minimize the risk of injury and maximize the safety margin. These include the stapling devices, the tripolar, and the vibrating device which uses high frequency ultrasonic waves to cut and coagulate.
• Additionally, laser provides a precise and rapid method of using thermal energy to destroy tissue. Other accessories are hooks, scissors, ball, atraumatic graspers, prettied suture loop, and so on.
• These newly developed instruments have also offered surgeons an efficient method to occlude and to cut large vessels in gynecology surgery.

COMPLICATIONS

- Some of the risks of laparoscopic surgery are: vascular injury, bowel injury, urinary tract injury, gas embolism, incisional hernia, neuropathy, and port site metastasis.
- Major vascular injury is one of the most life-threatening complications in laparoscopic surgery. It occurs seldom and usually occurs during introduction of the Veress needle or the primary trocar.
  - Due to the proximity of the umbilicus to the bifurcation of the aorta and the inferior vena cava, the laparoscopist should be careful when inserting the Veress needle or primary trocar.
  - Additionally, retroperitoneal vessel trauma can occur when the Veress needle or trocar is introduced into the abdomen in a thin patient because the proximity of the umbilicus and major intra-abdominal vessel could be less than 3–4 cm.
  - The abdominal wall vessels such as the inferior epigastric, superficial epigastric, and the superficial circumflex iliac vessels can be injured during laparoscopic surgery when multiple trocars are inserted. Knowing the anatomy and origins of these vessels is very important to avoid this complication or to be able to deal with it before there is significant blood loss.
- Bowel injury during laparoscopy can be life threatening if it is not recognized.
  - The risk of bowel injury during introduction of the Veress needle or the primary trocar is higher in patient who has history of multiple abdominal surgeries or intraperitoneal infection (e.g., pelvic inflammatory disease [PID] and ruptured appendix) because the small and large intestines are likely to be adhered to abdominal wall.
  - Thermal injury to the intestines is also a major complication during laparoscopy, especially when monopolar electrocautery is used. Thermal injuries to the intestines are often unrecognized and life-threatening situations. Patients usually present with acute peritonitis during the postoperative period (i.e., 3–4 days after discharge from hospital).
- Urinary tract system including bladder and ureters can be injured during laparoscopy at time of introducing the trocar and during use of powerhouse instruments.
  - Bladder injury can cause significant morbidity if it is not recognized. Patients may present with low urine output, hematuria, suprapubic pain, acute renal failure, and postoperative ileus.
  - With ureteral injuries, patients present with similar symptoms and often are unrecognized. It can occur during laparoscopic procedures involving powerhouse instrumentation in proximity to the ureters, thermal injury from laser or cautery pointed lateral to the uterosacral ligaments, ligation with suture, or transection.
- Gas embolism is a rare complication. However, it could be fatal if it occurs.
  - Gas embolism often occurs by inadvertent placement of the Veress needle into the intra-abdominal vessels, such as aorta and inferior vena cava, prior to obtaining the pneumoperitoneum with carbon dioxide gas.
  - Carbon dioxide gas can occlude the aorta and produce an ischemic event. Luckily, the carbon dioxide gas is rapidly absorbed from the arterial vessels.
  - However, if it is introduced into the inferior vena cava, carbon dioxide can produce the complete occlusion of pulmonary artery, an acute fatal event.
  - The signs of carbon dioxide gas embolism in the pulmonary system include severe hypotension, decreased oxygenation saturation, tachycardia, and cardiac arrest.
- Incisional hernia can occur when larger than 5-mm trocars are used and the fascia is left open. The abdominal fascia defects allow the bowel to trap, which can lead to bowel obstruction. Therefore, any abdominal fascia defect larger than 5 mm should be closed to reduce the risk of incisional hernia.
- Peripheral neuropathy can occur with laparoscopic surgery. Nerve compressions are often the complication resulting from the wrong patient positioning. Brachial plexus, peroneal nerve, and obturator nerve injury are the few examples.

TIPS FOR COMPLICATION PREVENTION

- Just as for open surgery, the patient must be evaluated. History and physical examination, risk factors, and alternative options must be discussed. Laparoscopic surgery is not an exception. The most important thing to remember about a laparoscopic complication is to recognize the injury and immediately repair or obtain appropriate intraoperative consultation for it.
  - *Major intra-abdominal vessels injury*: (1) During introduction of the Veress needle or primary trocar, patient should be in complete horizontal position (not Trendelenburg), (2) 45-degree angle toward the hollow of the sacrum for an average body habitus patient, 70- to 80-degree angle (vertical) for an obese patient, (3) injection and aspiration of fluid, (4) hanging drop test, (5) measurement of intra-abdominal pressure, (6) open laparoscopy
  - *Bowel injury*: (1) Preoperative bowel preparation, (2) open laparoscopy, (3) conical-tip trocars, (4) bipolar preferred rather than monopolar electrocautery

○ *Urinary tract injury*: (1) Foley catheter prior to trocar placement, (2) intravenous indigo carmine and cystoscopic evaluation

○ *Gas embolism*: (1) Open Veress needle valve, (2) aspirate with syringe through the Veress needle, (3) hanging drop test

○ *Incisional hernia*: Facial closure for a larger than 5-mm trocar

BIBLIOGRAPHY

A consensus document concerning laparoscopic entry techniques. Middleborough, March 19–20, 1999. *Gynecol Endosc.* 1999;8:403.

Chandler JG, Corson SL, Way LW. Three spectra of laparoscopic entry access injuries. *J Am Coll Surg.* 2001;192:478.

Garry R, Reich H. *Basic Techniques for Advanced Laparoscopic Surgery.* Oxford: Blackwell Scientific; 1992:46.

Hasson HM, Rotman C, Rana N, et al. Open laparoscopy. *Obstet Gynecol.* 2000;96(5):763–766.

Hay-Smith EJC, Bø K, Berghmans LCM. *Ostergard's Urogynecology and Pelvic Floor Dysfunction.* 5th ed. Philadelphia, PA: Lippincott Williams & Wilkins; 2003.

Hurd WW, Bude RO, DeLancey JO, et al. The relationship of the umbilicus to the aortic bifurcation: implications for laparoscopic technique. *Obstet Gynecol.* 1992;80(1):48–51.

Marcovich R, Del Terzo MA, Wolf JS. Comparison of transperitoneal laparoscopic access techniques: Optiview visualizing trocar and Veress needle. *J Endourol.* 2000;14(2):175–179.

Miklos JR, Kohli N, Moore R. Laparoscopic surgery for pelvic support defects. Curr Opin Obstet Gynecol. 2002;14(4):387–395.

Miklos JR, Kohli N. Paravaginal plus burch procedure: a laparoscopic approach. *J Pelvic Surg.* 1998;4(6):297–302.

Philosophe R. Avoiding complications of laparoscopic surgery. *Fertil Steril.* 2003;80(Suppl 4):30.

Poindexter AN, Ritter M, Fahim A, et al. Trocar introduction performed during laparoscopy of the obese patient. *Surg Gynecol Obstet.* 1987;165:57.

Saini J, Kohli N, Miklos JR, et al. Nonsurgical and minimally invasive outpatient treatments for stress urinary incontinence and pelvic organ prolapse. *Female Patient.* 2004;29:45–54.

Westhoff C, Davis A. Tubal sterilization: focus on the U.S. experience. *Fertil Steril.* 2000;73(5):913–922.

Yuzpe AA. Pneumoperitoneum needle and trocar injuries in laparoscopy. *J Reprod Med.* 1990;35(5): 485–490.

QUESTIONS

1. A 35-year-old white female who has undergone a laparoscopic cystectomy for a 6-cm persistent right ovarian cyst presents to your office. She also has prior surgical history of appendectomy for ruptured appendicitis, a remote history of PID in the past, and no other medical conditions. An extensive lysis of adhesion was performed to complete the cystectomy. Patient presented at emergency room on the fourth day after the outpatient surgery with complaints of nausea, vomiting, abdominal distention, minimal urination, and feeling sick. Patient is afebrile, tachycardia at 105 heart beat per minute, blood pressure 120/80 mmHg, respiratory rate at 18. Laboratory findings include serum blood urea nitrogen (BUN) 25, creatinine 2.1, no other electrolytes abnormality. CT-scan of abdomen shows dilated loop of small bowel, moderate fluid in abdomen. No free air in the abdomen by abdominal x-ray. The next step in management for this patient is

    (A) an MRI

    (B) small bowel follow through to rule out bowel obstruction

    (C) paracentesis and send fluid for analysis of its chemistry

    (D) gastrointestinal service consultation

    (E) continue to observe

2. After a presacral neurectomy with laparoscopic laser, patient presented to emergency room on fourth day after outpatient surgery with abdominal distention, guarding, nausea, vomiting, fever, tachycardia, severe abdominal pain, and increased white blood cell count. Abdominal x-ray shows free air under the diaphragm. The most likely diagnosis is

    (A) acute peritonitis

    (B) acute bowel obstruction

    (C) acute appendicitis

    (D) acute PID

    (E) acute postoperative ileus

3. After an extensive laparoscopic treatment for endometriosis, a 28-year-old white female complaints of weakness on her left leg, and diminished control of her left foot. The most likely diagnosis is

    (A) deep vein thrombosis (DVT)

    (B) tibial artery thrombosis

    (C) foot drop

    (D) posttraumatic syndrome

    E) femoral nerve compression

4. After introducing the second trocar into the lower quadrant of abdomen for operative laparoscopy, surgeon noticed a hematoma formation at his second trocar site. The most likely vessel that he has just severed is

    (A) internal iliac vessel

    (B) superior vesicle vessel

(C) inferior epigastric vessel

(D) inferior vesicle vessel

(E) external iliac vessel

5. During the laparoscopic paravaginal repair for cystourethrocele, the surgeon tries to attach the following structures:

(A) Cooper's ligament to "white line"

(B) pubocervical tissue to arcus tendineus

(C) arcus tendineus to "white line"

(D) pubocervical tissue to pubic symphysis

(E) pubocervical tissue to rectus muscle

ANSWERS

1. *(C)*. Urinary tract injury is well known in gynecologic surgery complication. Ureter and bladder injury may not be recognized. In this particular case, the most likely ureter injury has occurred at the site of extensive lysis of adhesion for cystectomy. The leakage of urine in the peritoneal cavity can cause postoperative ileus and increased BUN/creatinine.

2. *(A)*. Acute peritonitis is the most likely complication. Laser energy used in presacral neurectomy can damage the bowel integrity, especially in unrecognized complication of bowel injury. The bowel can be ischemic and complicated as bowel perforation. Bowel contents then subsequently cause acute peritonitis.

3. *(C)*. The most likely diagnosis of this patient is foot drop. This complication is resulted from the peroneal nerve compression due to incorrect positioning of patient's lower extremity for a long extensive surgical procedure.

4. *(C)*. The most likely cause of anterior abdominal hematoma is an injury to the inferior epigastric artery which is a branch of the external iliac artery. This complication often occurs at the site of secondary trocar placement.

5. *(B)*. The paravaginal repair for cystourethrocele is performed by attaching the pubocervical tissue to the ATFP which is also known as "white line."

20 FECAL INCONTINENCE

Jessica Bracken

FECAL INCONTINENCE

- The loss of anal sphincter control leading to unwanted release of feces or gas is called fecal and flatal incontinence, respectively.

EPIDEMIOLOGY

- Estimation of the prevalence of fecal incontinence in the general population is challenging due to several factors.
  - More than one definition for fecal incontinence is used.
  - Methods of inquiry vary.
  - Patients are often embarrassed by their incontinence and are unwilling to inform their primary care physician of their problem.
  - Physicians are reluctant to inquire about it.
- Fecal incontinence is more prevalent in the elderly particularly those in hospitals, psychiatric wards, and in nursing homes. It is the second leading cause for admission to nursing homes. Approximately, half a billion dollars per year are spent on adult diapers.

ANATOMY AND PHYSIOLOGY OF CONTINENCE AND DEFECATION

- The anal canal is the distal outlet of the intestinal tract and is approximately 3–4 cm long. Closure of this outlet is controlled by various muscles. The *puborectalis* muscle attaches to the symphysis pubis and wraps around the posterior aspect of the anorectal junction. Normally this U-shaped muscle is contracted and acts as a sling, creating an angle of about 80 degrees between the rectum and anal canal. This angle provides a barrier to the passage of stool. The *internal anal sphincter* (IAS) is a smooth muscle and is continuous with the distal portion of the circular muscle of the rectum. It is contracted a greater part of the time and accounts for 75–80% of the anal canal resting pressure. When the rectum is distended with advancing feces, the IAS reflexively relaxes allowing the stool to reach the sensitive anal canal mucosa. The *external anal sphincter* (EAS), a striated muscle that surrounds the IAS, contracts enough to keep stool from exiting the gut and allows the rectum to fill. When the volume in the rectum exceeds 300 mL, the intraluminal pressure increases and this causes a feeling of urgency. When defecation is desired, the pelvic floor relaxes, (increasing the angle of the puborectalic sling). IAS automatically relaxes, the EAS is voluntarily inhibited, and the bolus is expelled.

ETIOLOGY

- Normal continence relies on multiple factors including mental function, stool volume and consistency, bowel motility, rectal distensibility, anal sphincter function, anorectal sensation, and anorectal reflexes. Incontinence usually occurs when abnormalities present with one or more of the above factors.

CAUSES OF FECAL INCONTINENCE
- Trauma
  - Surgical: Damage can occur to the anal sphincter or surrounding structures when repairing anal fistulas, hemorrhoids, after injection of botulinum toxin for anal fissures.
  - Obstetrical: Vaginal delivery can result in fecal incontinence immediately or after several years resulting from mechanical trauma to the anal sphincter or injury to the pudendal nerve. Risk factors for nerve damage during childbirth include use of forceps, high-birth-weight infant, prolonged second stage of labor, and occiput-posterior presentation of the fetus. Vacuum-assisted deliveries are associated with less trauma than forceps to the perineum.

○ Accidental: Impalement on a spike or pole may cause a sphincter injury. Sepsis can ensue and cause scar formation that may result in a patulous anal canal and an incompetent sphincter.

• Colorectal disease: Rectal prolapse or hemorrhoids can interfere with closure of the anal canal. Stretching of the sphincter by the mass may lead to incontinence. Attenuation of the pudendal nerve from the rectal prolapse can lead to sphincter atrophy. Other conditions such as inflammatory bowel disease, malignancy, infection, and parasitic diseases can also cause incontinence.

• Congenital anomaly: Neural tube defects such as spina bifida, meningocele, and myelomeningocele can lead to congenital incontinence.

• Neurological disease: It can cause fecal incontinence by damage to the central nervous system (CNS) or to the peripheral nervous system (PNS).
  ○ CNS: includes dementia, neoplasm, stroke, trauma, multiple sclerosis, and so on
  ○ PNS: includes diabetic peripheral neuropathy

• Miscellaneous
  ○ Laxative abuse: Leads to stools that are greasy. It slides through the sphincter without causing pressure to dilate the sphincter. It leads to atrophy of the muscle.
  ○ Diarrheal condition: Large volumes of stool can overwhelm a normal sphincter. Consider infectious causes, inflammatory bowel disease, short-gut syndrome, and radiation enteritis.
  ○ Fecal impaction: Impaction leads to inhibition of IAS tone which allows leakage of stool around the impaction. Decreased mobility, inadequate fluid intake, a low fiber diet, rectal hyposensitivity, and impaired mental function can lead to impaction.
  ○ Encopresis: The repeated, generally involuntary, passage of feces in inappropriate places is considered to be a mental disorder if it occurs in a child over 4 years. It occurs more often in boys than girls. Behavioral factors that may lead to the problem include
    ▪ Family or personal stress
    ▪ Fear of the toilet
    ▪ Desire for attention
    ▪ Laxative abuse
    ▪ Excessive, harsh, or lax toilet training methods by the parents
  ○ Excessive retention of stools leads to change in rectal wall. Sphincter contractility becomes more lenient and leads to constipation, intestinal obstruction, and fecal impaction. Treatment includes stress reduction, psychological counseling, and bowel management training.
  ○ Idiopathic: The denervation of the sphincter muscles by an unknown cause is considered idiopathic.

EVALUATION OF FECAL INCONTINENCE

• History: True incontinence must be defined. The diagnosis must be established separate from urgency and frequency but without loss of bowel function.
  ○ Onset, duration, frequency, severity of problems, precipitating events, history of vaginal delivery if female, anorectal surgery, pelvic irradiation, diabetes, neurological disease, and whether symptoms occur with diarrhea are all important components to a good history.
  ○ A symptom diary is helpful for diagnosis and for evaluating efficacy of treatments.

• Physical examination
  ○ Inspection: Visualizing the anus may demonstrate a patulous anus (loss of sphincter tone or neurological impairment), rectal prolapse, fistulas, hemorrhoids, or a perineal tear, scar, or deformity.
  ○ Palpation: Performing a digital rectal examination allows assessment of resting sphincter tone and increase in tone when the patient is asked to contract the muscle. A defect in the sphincter muscle can be perceived. It can also determine if there is a mass, fecal impaction, or presence of a rectocele. Sensory function can also be determined by evoking the anocutaneous reflex. This reflex should be elicited bilaterally. Absence suggests nerve damage and interruption of the spinal arc.
  ○ Anoscopy and sigmoidoscopy: Visualizing the rectal cavity is important to rule out tumors, inflammatory causes, or impaction as cause for incontinence.
  ○ Anal ultrasonography: This highly sensitive and minimally invasive sonogram allows visualization of the internal and external sphincters, the puborectalis sling, and the anococcygeal ligament. Ultrasound can localize defects, muscular thickness, and asymmetry in the two sphincters. It is well tolerated by patients. Many obstetric-related defects in the IAS and EAS are anterior (12 o'clock) in location.
  ○ Anal manometry: Manometry is the most useful method to analyze anal sphincter function. It measures resting and maximal contraction pressures of the anal canal using balloons, solid-state microtransducers, or water perfused multichannel catheters. It can record the sphincter response to stress and determine if the rectoanal inhibitory reflex is present. Manometry also assesses rectal compliance and sensation. It can determine spatial sphincter defects by cross-sectional mapping of the whole sphincter. It helps to perform and predict response to biofeedback training.
  ○ Electromyography (EMG): It determines the functional activity of the anal sphincter and pelvic floor muscles and the neuromuscular integrity of the anal canal. It measures action potentials generated by the external sphincter and puborectalis muscle while at rest, during contraction, and in response to a variety

of reflexes. This method involves inserting needle electrodes into the sphincter muscle, which can measure the activity of individual muscle fibers within a motor unit. This particular technique is uncomfortable for the patient and has a risk of infection. To improve the patient's comfort, an anal plug electrode was designed that is inserted into the rectum. It consists of two longitudinal wires mounted on its surface. It is less invasive than the needle electrodes and has been found to be equally accurate. It is important to note that EMG cannot differentiate myopathic and neurogenic disorders when analyzing abnormal electrical activity. Used in conjunction with endoanal ultrasound, the two studies compliment each other with a morphological and neurological assessment of the muscles.

○ Evacuation proctography/cinedefecography: Barium solution is inserted into the rectum and a patient can be radiographed using fluoroscopy while at rest, during muscular contraction of pelvic floor muscles, and while defecating. This method allows measurement of the anal canal, visualization of the perianal descent, the anorectal angle, how well the patient can empty the rectum, and any anatomical abnormalities. The radiation exposure is high and this study is only recommended when other studies have failed to demonstrate a cause of functional obstruction to the passage of stool.

○ Endoluminal MRI: An MRI study of the anal canal anatomy using endoanal coils can be done to assess the sphincter muscles. Lesions such as defects and scars can be identified with an accuracy of greater than 90%. In comparison to anal ultrasonography, the sonography can image the IAS better than the MRI. The two are equal in determining EAS defects. However, MRI has better detection of atrophy of the EAS.

NONSURGICAL TREATMENT

• It is important to treat the underlying medical and surgical problems first, such as cancer resection, treatment of inflammatory bowel disease, repair of rectal prolapse, and removal of impactions.

○ Medical treatment

■ Bulking agents (Metamucil, Citracel) make stool well-formed and easier to control. Begin with one teaspoon and gradually increase the dose to one tablespoon three times a day to avoid side effects. Restricting fluid intake will help increase stool bulk.

■ Anti-motility agents (loperamide hydrochloride, Lomotil) decrease the motility of the bowel allowing greater resorption of fluid and more time for the bulk density to increase. Rectal compliance will increase while decreasing urgency. Recommended dose of loperamide is 2–4 mg before meals with a maximum dose of 16 mg. Lomotil is a schedule V drug with a minimal potential for physical dependence. The recommended dose is 2.5–5 mg once daily to four times a day. Side effects include abdominal distention, dizziness, depression, nausea, headache, blurred vision, dry mouth, and drowsiness.

○ Biofeedback: For patients who are alert and motivated, pelvic floor exercises with a therapist are successful. Biofeedback involves placing two balloons, one in the rectum and one in the anal canal. The balloon in the rectum is dilated until the patient senses the expansion and contracts the anal sphincter. The second balloon measures this contraction. The therapist can offer visual feedback regarding the contraction of the EAS and encourages the patient when the correct sphincter response is made. Gradually, the rectal balloon volume is decreased and the patient learns to recognize smaller volumes in the rectum; 63–90% of patients experience improvement with this method.

○ Kegel exercise: Pelvic floor exercises have shown no proven benefit but are not harmful and are free. A physical therapist can measure the contractions and have the patient hold the contraction for 10 seconds. The patient can watch a screen that shows when the contraction is decreasing.

○ Daily enemas and suppositories are preferred by some patients.

SURGICAL TREATMENT

The following preoperative and postoperative pearls are helpful:

• Bowel prep is given to cleanse the bowel (e.g., polyethylene glycol [Golytely], Magnesium citrate, Fleets phosphosoda).

• Prophylactic antibiotics should be given during the preoperative period. Intravenous metronidazole and a third generation cephalosporin are recommended. Antibiotics should be continued postoperatively as well.

• If the surgery is correcting an injury, the injury should be allowed to heal for 3–6 months. Inflammation will impair the healing of reparative surgery.

• Foley is placed.

• After surgery the following steps should be considered:

○ Intravenous antibiotics should be given for 2–3 days.

○ Patient should be NPO for at least a day. Low residue (low fiber) diet for a short period of time is recommended by colorectal surgeons especially after hemorrhoidectomy.

○ Foley should be discontinued for postoperative day 2 (if possible).

○ 1 oz. of mineral oil should be given daily with the diet.

○ If no bowel movement by postoperative day 7, 1 oz of milk of magnesia should be given twice a day until a motion occurs. It is common to not stool for several days.

- Sphincteroplasty: When a defect is found in the sphincters, reapproximation of the two ends is attempted. It is important to remember that the pudendal nerve branches innervate the EAS from the posterolateral position. The patient is placed in jackknife prone position. Dissect down the rectovaginal septum. Dissect laterally to the ischiorectal fat. If you tear into the anal mucosa, use 4.0 chromic suture in interrupted fashion for repair. The injury to the rectal sphincter usually has scar tissue. Divide the scar tissue in the midline and leave it attached to the sphincter end for added strength. You may need to use a needle-point on your electrocautery device to distinguish contractile tissue (muscle) from scar tissue. If the IAS/EAS are both injured, they can be repaired as one unit. If the IAS is intact and the EAS is disrupted, then repair only the EAS. If the IAS is not disrupted but is redundant, it can be plicated before repairing the EAS. The ends of the sphincter should be overlapped and mattress sutures are placed (three on each side) with 2.0 polyglycan suture. *Thus, a secondary repair of the anal sphincter should be by overlapping sphincteroplasty.* The repair should be tightened enough to only allow the index finger to pass. Antibiotic solution should be used to irrigate the wound. The skin is closed in a V-Y fashion. The center can be left open for drainage. If there is a large amount of dead space then a Penrose drain should be placed for 2 days.
- Postanal pelvic floor repair: For patients whose sphincter has no defects but still suffer from fecal incontinence, a postanal pelvic floor repair may be the appropriate surgery for them. It is also recommended for those with neuropathic incontinence. Optimal results are seen in patients with anal sphincter stretch and loss of the anorectal angle. This procedure reestablishes the anorectal angle while increasing the length and tightening of the anal canal. An inverted V incision is made 5–6 cm from the anal verge posteriorly. The intersphincteric plane is identified and dissection is directed cephalad to Waldeyer's fascia. The fascia is dissected to expose mesorectal fat. The two sides of the ileococcygeus muscle are brought together with figure-of-eight 2.0 polypropylene sutures. They do not approximate because they are too distal from each other. The pubococcygeus muscle is identified next. A lattice of figure-of-eight sutures is placed in a similar fashion and the anterior ends should be approximated. The puborectalis and EAS are then plicated. Skin is closed in a V-Y fashion. Improvement is seen in approximately 28% in the long term. The procedure may lead to worsening of the neurogenic damage to the pelvic floor.
- Muscle transposition procedure: For some patients, repair of the sphincter muscle is impossible or efforts of repair have failed. Another option for them is transposition of the gracilis or gluteus muscle to create a neoanal sphincter. It is contraindicated in neurological disease such as multiple sclerosis. The gracilis muscle contains Type II fibers which are unable to maintain sustained contraction. Success rates were improved with implantation of a pacemaker that releases a chronic low-frequency electrical stimulation which maintains muscle contraction. When a patient desires defecation, they can turn off the pacemaker and the muscle can relax. Success of this procedure has lead to less anxiety and improved quality of life. There is high morbidity associated with this procedure, including infections and complications with the pacemaker, and a steep learning curve for the surgeon. Success rate ranges from 23 to 65% of patients. It is important to consider the normal function of the gluteus muscle in normal daily activities such as running, rising from a seated position, and climbing stairs. After muscle transposition the patient may have new problems to overcome.
- Artificial anal sphincter: An artificial anal sphincter is an implantable device that is inflated to occlude the anus. Only a few centers perform this procedure. Up to a third of patients experience infection or complications. However, approximately 75% of patients obtained improvement in their incontinence even if not regaining full continence.
- Colostomy or ileostomy: Diverting the bowel in the form of a colostomy or ileostomy is sometimes the best option for some patients particularly when other surgical attempts have failed. It gives them control over their incontinence, allowing them to go out into public places without fear of having an episode.

BIBLIOGRAPHY

Barnett JL. Anorectal diseases. In: Yamada T, ed. *Textbook of Gastroenterology.* 1st ed. Philadelphia, PA: Lippincott Williams & Wilkins; 1999:2094–2098.

Corman ML. Anal incontinence. In: Corman ML, ed. *Colon and Rectal Surgery.* 4th ed. Philadelphia, PA: Lippincott-Raven; 1998:285–343.

Furner S, Cautley E, Norton N, et al. Community-based prevalence of anal incontinence. *JAMA.* 1995;274:559–561.

Giordano P, Wexner S. The assessment of fecal incontinence in women. *J Am Coll Surg.* 2001;193(4):397–406.

Hinninghofen H, Enck P. Fecal incontinence: evaluation and treatment. *Gastroenterol Clin North Am.* 2003;32:685–706.

Hull TL. Fecal incontinence. In: Walters MD, Karram MM, eds. *Urogynecology and Reconstructive Pelvic Surgery.* 2nd ed. St. Louis, MO: Mosby; 1999:259–268.

Johanson JF, Lafferty J. Epidemiology of fecal incontinence: the silent affliction. *Am J Gastroenterol.* 1996;91:33–36.

Ludwig KA. Urogynecology and pelvic floor dysfunction. *Obstet Gynecol Clin.* 1998;25(4):923–944.

Madoff RD, Williams JG, Caushaj PF. Fecal incontinence. *N Engl J Med.* 1992;326:1002–1007.

Sultan AH, Kamm MA, Hudson CN, et al. Anal-sphincter disruption during vaginal delivery. *N Engl J Med.* 1993;329: 1905–1911.

QUESTIONS

1. _____ has superiority for the visualization of the IAS.
   (A) Plain x-ray
   (B) Ultrasound
   (C) MRI
   (D) Defecography
   (E) Anoscopy

2. A 45-year-old, para 4 had her last vaginal delivery 2 years ago. She recently underwent testing. It is apparent that the EAS is defective at 2 o'clock position and the pudendal nerve function is intact. If she was to undergo repair of the EAS, the appropriate term to describe the repair is _____.
   (A) primary end-to-end sphincteroplasty
   (B) primary overlapping sphincteroplasty
   (C) secondary end-to-end sphincteroplasty
   (D) secondary overlapping sphincteroplasty
   (E) EAS placation

3. Flatal and fecal incontinence occurs in someone who has fecal impaction because ___.
   (A) large bulk of stool can overwhelm a normal sphincter
   (B) sliding occurs through the sphincter without causing pressure to dilate it
   (C) inhibition of IAS tone
   (D) reflexive inhibition of perirectal autonomic nerves

ANSWERS

1. *(B).* Ultrasound can image the IAS better than the MRI. The other modalities are not as good as MRI or ultrasound. Anoscopy cannot see the full depth of the sphincter.

2. *(B).* As some time has passed since the primary obstetrical trauma which resulted in defect of the EAS, the repair is secondary. Immediate repair of a fourth degree obstetrical trauma is usually by primary end-to-end sphincteroplasty. Overlapping sphincteroplasty has better results than end-to-end for secondary type of repairs. However, for primary repairs, results are comparable. Since end-to-end is easier to perform and requires less dissection, this type of repair is preferred for primary obstetrical repairs.

3. *(C).* Choice A is the mechanism of fecal incontinence due to diarrhea. Choice B is the mechanism of fecal incontinence due to laxative abuse. Impaction leads to inhibition of IAS tone which allows leakage of stool around the impaction. Choice D is also incorrect.

21 RECTOVAGINAL FISTULA

Bogdan A. Grigorescu

DEFINITION

- A rectovaginal fistula is an epithelium-lined communication between the rectum and vagina. The lower rectovaginal fistulas (<3 cm from the anal orifice) are in fact anovaginal fistulas, but are still referred to by most clinicians as rectovaginal fistulas.

INCIDENCE

- There is a lack of reliable data on the prevalence of obstetric fistulas. Based on women who sought treatment, the WHO estimated that there are >2 million women worldwide with obstetric fistulas and there are 50,000–100,000 new cases per year. The incidence in some countries is as high as 350 per 100,000 live births with >1 million unrepaired cases in Nigeria alone.

- It has been reported that third-degree perineal tears follow 0.6% of vaginal deliveries, and 6% of these may result in a rectovaginal fistula (1 in 3000 deliveries overall).

- The incidence of anal sphincter lacerations has been reported to be between 0.5% and 2.5% in cases where mediolateral episiotomy was performed, and 11% in cases where midline episiotomy was performed.

ETIOLOGY

- Most rectovaginal fistulas are acquired although congenital abnormalities have been reported.

- Obstetric injury accounts for the occurrence of most rectovaginal fistulas. Thus, vaginal delivery, and in particular, instrumental delivery is the most frequent cause associated with perineal and anal sphincter injury.
- Among the most common causes responsible for rectovaginal fistula formation are the breakdown of repair of third- and fourth-degree perineal lacerations, unrecognized injury during forceps, or precipitous vaginal delivery. Perineal and vaginal lacerations have been classified as follows according to the tissues involved:
  - First-degree laceration involves the vaginal epithelium or perineal skin only
  - Second-degree tear involves the vaginal epithelium, perineal skin, perineal muscles + fascia
  - Third-degree laceration is a defect of the vaginal epithelium, perineal skin, perineal body, and external anal sphincter muscle and it can be subdivided into
    - Partial laceration of the external sphincter (less than 50% thickness)
    - Complete tear of the external anal sphincter (EAS)
    - Disruption of the internal anal sphincter (IAS)
  - Fourth-degree tear is a third-degree laceration plus involvement of the anal epithelium.
- In developing countries, necrosis of the vaginal septum from ↑ compression by the fetal presenting part is a main causative factor in the → of rectovaginal fistulas.
  - During normal labor, in the anterior pelvis, the bladder base and urethra are compressed between the posterior surface of the pubis and the fetal head. This may result in vesicovaginal or urethrovaginal fistulas.
  - In the posterior pelvis, ↑ compression of the soft tissues between the sacral promontory and the presenting part → necrosis and ischemia of the posterior vaginal wall and underlying rectum, → in a rectovaginal fistula.
- Inflammatory bowel disease (IBD): While both ulcerative colitis (UC) and Crohn's disease can cause a recto-vaginal fistula, it is more commonly seen in Crohn's disease. In a study of 886 female patients with Crohn's disease, 90 (9.8%) developed a rectovaginal fistula. A study on UC showed a 3.6% incidence in women.
- Diverticular disease may cause colovaginal fistulas and colouterine fistulas.
- Carcinoma, whether it is primary, recurrent, or metastatic → rectovaginal fistula. The most common cancers that lead to rectovaginal fistulas are rectal, cervical, vaginal, and uterine. If a patient with a rectovaginal fistula has a history of any of these cancers or other perineal cancers, a biopsy of the fistula is necessary.

- Patients whose cul-de-sac is obliterated with endometriosis, chronic inflammation, or pelvic abscess and who undergo surgery are at risk of rectal injury and high rectovaginal fistulas.
- In patients with pelvic malignancy, high rectovaginal fistulas may be caused directly by radiation injury to the rectum adjacent to the posterior vaginal fornix; any such fistula tract should be biopsied to exclude a cancer recurrence.
- Other causes of rectovaginal fistulas include infections (tuberculosis, schistosomiasis, and lymphogranuloma venereum), trauma, and foreign bodies (e.g., neglected pessary).

CLASSIFICATION

- Most authorities classify rectovaginal fistulas depending on their location in the rectovaginal septum into low, middle, or high.
- Low fistulas enter the vagina at the posterior fourchette.
- High fistulas enter the vagina at the vaginal apex.
- Middle fistulas are located between the low and high fistulas.
- Rectovaginal fistulas >2.5 cm in size are considered large in size and may require a diverting colostomy (see below).
- Simple fistulas are rectovaginal fistulas located in the distal half of the vagina and complex fistulas enter into the proximal half of the vagina.

CLINICAL PRESENTATION

- The majority of women with perineal and anal sphincter disruption present a few years after the injury. Some present during the perimenopausal years because of embarrassing leakage of liquid or solid stool from the vagina. Still others see their physician for estrogen deficiency or pelvic neuropathy and are diagnosed with rectovaginal fistula.
- If the defect is small enough, it may be asymptomatic, especially with a small amount of gas and feces passing through to the vagina. Moreover, rectovaginal fistulas may become asymptomatic because of the scarring and contracture of the vagina, which occurs after tissue sloughing.
- When the fistula is larger, the patient complains of escape of gas and liquid stool per vagina and an offensive odor in the vaginal discharge.
- When the fistula is large, the entire bowel movement is evacuated through the vagina. These patients awaiting surgical repair have voluntary constipation.

- Tenderness of the fistula orifice on palpation is likely caused by Crohn's disease until proven otherwise. In cases with active Crohn's disease, multiple fistulas may occur between ileum, colon, rectum, and the vagina; the patients present with mucous or bloody diarrhea and discharge per vagina, abdominal tenderness, sepsis, and weight ↓. A single rectovaginal orifice may be connected by several circuitous tracts with microabscesses to multiple anorectal orifices.
- Patients with colovesical and colovaginal fistulas present with urinary tract infections (UTIs) and pneumaturia (air in urine).

DIAGNOSIS

- Most rectovaginal fistulas of obstetric origin are located in the lower one-third of the vagina.
- Vaginal examination and examination under anesthesia (EUA) with a bivalve speculum is essential for the detection of rectovaginal fistulas. The vulva and perineum may be wet, if a genitourinary fistula is also present and accompanied by urine, fecal odor, or skin excoriation. A small, high posterior horseshoe-shaped rectovaginal fistula may only be diagnosed during the repair of a vesicovaginal fistula.
- For patients with colovesical fistulas, urine culture and sensitivity (C&S) should be done and UTIs must be treated with appropriate antibiotics.
- Dye tests are not as useful as for genitourinary fistulas (see Chap. 27, Bypass Mechanisms: Vesicovaginal, Uretherovaginal, and Ureterovaginal Fistulas). However, multiple sinuses in the perineum may be traced in the office with methylene blue injections and a carmine marker taken PO may confirm the presence of intestinal fistulas.
- Methylene blue test may be done if the fistulous tract is not visible on EUA. A solution of diluted methylene blue is instilled in the rectum after placement of a vaginal tampon. After 15–20 minutes, staining of the tampon confirms the presence of a rectovaginal fistula.
- Contrast studies—contrast enemas and cystography—are important for diagnosis of fistulous tracts, and for detecting underlying colonic disease, such as diverticular disease, Crohn's disease, and colon carcinoma. Contrast enemas using barium (BE), Gastrografin, or ionic contrast have a sensitivity of 70% for the diagnosis of colonic fistulas. Cystography demonstrates air in the bladder in about 30% of colovesical fistulas.
- In patients with suspected enterovaginal fistulas, a BE, colonoscopy, gastrointestinal (GI) series with small bowel follow-through (SBFT). GI series excludes bowel obstruction. Excretory urography (intravenous pyelogram [IVP]) images the distal genitourinary tract and rules out concurrent ureterovaginal fistulas.
- Sigmoidoscopy and proctoscopy are essential for the diagnosis of IBD. Rectal distension with air through a sigmoidoscope may show bubbling of air in a vagina filled with saline in the presence of a low fistula. Biopsy of the fistula edge is important to rule out malignancy.
- Sinography (fistulography)—a ureteric or a Foley catheter may be used to deliver radiopaque dye into vaginal fistulas which have an intervening abscess cavity. If the vaginal aperture communicates with a loop of bowel, its nature may become apparent from the radiological appearance of haustrations.
- Computed tomography (CT) and magnetic resonance imaging (MRI) are used for the assessment of complex fistulas and for evaluation of renal function and the distal genitourinary tract.
- Anal endosonography and endoluminal MRIs are useful diagnostic tools because they identify anatomical defects in the anterior portion of the anal sphincter prior to repair of rectovaginal fistulas. If a rectovaginal fistula develops after a vaginal delivery, an occult anal sphincter defect may be present, even after proper surgical repair, *thus anal endosonography is indicated prior to repair of a rectovaginal fistula.*

MANAGEMENT

- The best management is to prevent the occurrence of rectovaginal fistulas.
- In the developing world, better education of girls, women, and community leaders and ↑ economic opportunities may delay childbearing and ↑ awareness of obstetric fistulas. Fistula prevention programs in sub-Saharan Africa can provide access to emergency obstetric care, including safe cesarean sections for women with obstructed labor. It has been shown that >5% of deliveries must be done by cesarean section to ↓ maternal morbidity and mortality. In the majority of countries in sub-Saharan Africa, the cesarean section rates were <5% (<2% in half of them).
- In the developed countries, it is important to ensure that anal sphincter injuries associated with vaginal instrumental deliveries are recognized immediately and repaired properly at the time of the primary repair. Moreover, there is new evidence that with restrictive episiotomy, the anal sphincter laceration rate and the risk of anal sphincter laceration attributable to episiotomy were ↓ by about 50%.
- Although mediolateral episiotomies do not prevent sphincter ruptures, they may be protective against severe sphincter lacerations compared to midline episiotomies.

TIMING OF REPAIR AND PREOPERATIVE MANAGEMENT OF RECTOVAGINAL FISTULAS

- For most fistulas, the timing of the surgical repair is the most contentious issue. However, most authorities agree that surgical repair of rectovaginal fistulas should be delayed until the tissues are free of edema, induration, and infection.
- Postirradiation rectovaginal fistulas may require more than 3 months, and often 12 months before the tissues are suitable for repair.
- Preoperative broad-spectrum prophylactic antibiotics (to cover both aerobic and anaerobic bacteria) are recommended by most surgeons prior to secondary anal sphincter repair and rectovaginal fistula repair.
- In some cases, a temporary sigmoid or transverse colostomy may be performed to divert the fecal stream from the operative field, especially if the fistula is large (>2.5 cm), is located high in the vagina, or is a result of irradiation treatment for pelvic malignancy. Indications for colostomy in the treatment of rectovaginal fistulas include
  ○ A large fistula (>2.5 cm)
  ○ Location near the vaginal apex
  ○ Distal bowel obstruction
  ○ IBD
  ○ Presence of an intra-abdominal or pelvic abscess
- However, in most cases, colostomy is not necessary before the surgical repair of a simple rectovaginal fistula in the lower vagina
- Mechanical bowel preparation is given to all patients prior to rectovaginal fistula repair to ↓ the bacterial number in the colon and anal canal. First, the patient is given clear liquids for 24–72 hours before surgery, and then a PO bowel slush preparation (GoLytely) is started at noon, the day before the surgery.
- Erythromycin 500 mg and neomycin 1 g are given PO at 1, 2, and 10 PM the day prior to surgery and rectal irrigation is performed in the morning of the surgery until the fluid returns clear. Patients who underwent a colostomy prior to rectovaginal fistula repair should use a neomycin solution to irrigate the lower colon and the rectum, and a PO bowel preparation is not necessary.

SURGICAL TREATMENT OF RECTOVAGINAL FISTULAS

- It is important to recognize that some low rectovaginal fistulas may cause only minor symptoms and may not require surgical repair. Close to one in four small rectovaginal fistulas heal spontaneously before epithelialization of the fistulous tract in patients treated with a low-residue diet and diphenoxylate hydrochloride (Lomotil). In another series comprising 52 patients with rectovaginal fistulas, 12.2% (5 patients) achieved cure with conservative management only.
- In general, the management of rectovaginal fistulas depends on the origin, size, location, and the number of fistulas.
- The basic principles of rectovaginal fistula repair are
  ○ Wide mobilization of tissues around the vaginal and rectal orifice
  ○ Removal of the scar tissue and excision of the entire fistulous tract
  ○ Closure of tissue layers without tension on the suture lines
  ○ Precise closure of the rectal fistulous orifice with approximation of broad tissue surface to broad tissue surface ensures adequate closure of the high-pressure end of the fistula
- The choice of suture used in rectovaginal fistula repair is another important factor. Delayed absorbable suture (e.g., polyglactin –[Vicryl]) is preferred to chromic or to permanent suture and it ensures that tissue reaction is ↓, the knot is more secure, and the tensile strength is maintained for a ↑ time.

METHODS FOR SURGICAL REPAIR OF RECTOVAGINAL FISTULAS

- Most of the lower vaginal fistulas can be repaired by a transvaginal or a transrectal approach, and many high rectovaginal and sigmoidovaginal fistulas may be repaired transvaginally using the Latzko's technique.
- Transabdominal repair is indicated for patients with high rectovaginal fistulas associated with primary bowel pathology (e.g., IBD, diverticulitis) when bowel resection and reanastomosis may be performed.
- The main methods used by gynecologists for repairing rectovaginal fistulas in the lower vagina are the transvaginal pursestring method, perineoproctotomy followed by a layered closure (sphincteroplasty), and transverse transperineal repair.
  ○ In general, the transvaginal pursestring method is the procedure of choice for small (<1.5 cm) rectovaginal fistulas situated within 5 cm of the vaginal furchette.
  ○ In patients with larger fistulas (>1.5 cm) lying just above the external anal sphincter and with evidence of anal incompetence, the preferred method of repair is perineoproctotomy followed by a layered closure (sphincteroplasty). A Martius bulbocavernosus muscle or labial fat pad is used in patients exposed to radiation treatment and provide tissue support and an additional blood supply.

○ *Latzko's closure* is an effective method for closing a high rectovaginal fistula at the vaginal apex (see Chap. 27, Bypass Mechanisms: Vesicovaginal, Uretherovaginal, and Ureterovaginal Fistulas).

○ Occasionally, high rectovaginal or sigmoidovaginal fistulas require a transabdominal repair, especially in patients with fistulas associated with IBD and diverticulitis when bowel resection and reanastomosis may need to be performed.

○ The segment of involved rectum is isolated from the vagina and resected. Bowel continuity is reestablished with an end-to-end circularly stapled anastomosis or hand-sewn anastomosis. The anastomosis site is separated from the vagina with an omentum or a fat pad. If bowel continuity cannot be reestablished → Hartmann's procedure or → a double-barrel or loop colostomy.

• A vascular graft of omentum or nonirradiated bowel may be used to provide additional blood supply in patients with rectal fistulas induced by radiation treatment.

THE TECHNIQUE OF TRANSVAGINAL REPAIR OF RECTOVAGINAL FISTULAS

• The " purse string" technique is as follows:
  ○ A vaginal incision is made to encircle the fistulous opening.
  ○ Dissection of vaginal mucosa circumferentially for 2 cm from the margin of the fistula orifice to allow mobility of the bowel wall. Injection of sterile NS or lidocaine with Epi into the vaginal mucosa may facilitate dissection and access to the proper plane, and hemostacis (if Epi used).
  ○ A suture of 3-0 polyglactin (Vicryl) is placed in the vaginal submucosal opening in a purse-string fashion, a few millimeters from the mucosal edge. Placement of sutures must avoid perforation of bowel mucosa. The purse-string suture is tied while the edges of the fistula are inverted into the bowel lumen.
  ○ A second and possibly a third purse-string suture is placed around the first suture in the muscularis tissues.
  ○ Rectovaginal septum (RVS) is approximated in the midline with interrupted sutures of 2-0 delayed absorbable suture (e.g., polyglactin [Vicryl]).
  ○ Excess vaginal mucosa is excised and the mucosa is closed with a continuous locking suture (e.g., 3-0 polyglactin [Vicryl]).
• Complications include
  ○ Vaginal constriction
  ○ Injury to the external anal sphincter
• In *perineoproctotomy with layered closure*, the fistula is converted into a fourth-degree laceration by excising the perineal bridge between the vaginal fourchette and the fistula orifice. The defect is then closed in a standard layered fashion identical to the repair of a fourth-degree perineal tear.
• Complications include
  ○ Narrowing of the vagina
  ○ Dyspareunia
• The disadvantage of this procedure is that it may → improper healing and scarring of a prior intact anal sphincter.

THE TECHNIQUE OF TRANSVERSE TRANSPERINEAL REPAIR OF LOW RECTOVAGINAL FISTULAS

• The technique is as follows:
  ○ The patient is prepped and draped in the dorsal lithotomy position and the perineal tissues are injected with NS solution or lidocaine with Epi to ease dissection.
  ○ A transverse incision is made with the scalpel across the perineal body above the anal sphincter.
  ○ Dissection is carried between the anterior rectal wall and posterior vaginal wall around the fistula and it is continued superiorly several centimeters above the fistula.
  ○ The fistulous tract is transected by sharp dissection and the scar tissue from the vaginal orifice of the fistula is removed and the vaginal mucosa is approximated with one or two layers of interrupted 3-0 delayed absorbable sutures (e.g., polyglactin [Vicryl] suture).
  ○ Scar tissue from the anterior rectal wall is removed sharply and the anterior rectal wall defect is closed with interrupted 3-0 delayed absorbable sutures. A second layer of interrupted sutures is placed in the anterior rectal wall to imbricate and reinforce the first line of sutures.
  ○ Perineal body muscles are approximated in the midline with 2-0 delayed absorbable sutures (e.g., polyglactin [Vicryl] suture) to reinforce the fistula closure.
  ○ The perineal subcutaneous tissue is approximated with interrupted 3-0 delayed absorbable sutures and the skin is closed transversely with 4-0 delayed absorbable suture.
• This approach has several advantages over other methods of rectovaginal fistula repair:
  ○ Wider mobilization of tissues, adequate dissection of the posterior vaginal wall, and transection of the fistula tract
  ○ The margins of the rectal orifice are visible for a precise tension-free closure
  ○ A bulbocavernosus flap can be used for an additional layer of protection and blood supply in patients with poor tissue vascularization caused by irradiation or IBD

○ This technique may be used in patients with Crohn's disease without creating a diverting colostomy

○ In cases where the anal sphincter is weak or torn, it may be repaired through the same incision

• *Alternative procedures* may be used for patients who failed previous repairs, with a denervated anal sphincter, or for patients who are unsuitable to undergo a major operation.

○ Autologous fibrin glue, a mixture of autologous fibrinogen and cryoprecipitate with reconstituted bovine thrombin, creates a fibrin seal and subsequent scar formation. It has been used successfully in one study in four out of five patients with rectovaginal fistulas.

○ Neoanal sphincter created from transposed gracilis muscle with an electrical pulse generator has been implanted in patients with severe sphincter damage or whose sphincter was removed as a result of surgery for pelvic malignancy. In a series of 20 patients, 12 had a functioning neonatal sphincter and complications include sepsis and muscle ischemia.

○ An artificial sphincter may be placed around the anal canal in patients with severe fecal incontinence.

POSTOPERATIVE MANAGEMENT

• Patients are given liquid diet for 3 days followed by a low-residue diet and stool softeners for 2–3 weeks.

• Postoperatively, broad-spectrum antibiotics may be continued for 5–7 days.

• Continuous bladder drainage via a Foley catheter is recommended for 48 hours.

• For added comfort, ice to the perineum may be used three times/day for the first ten days.

PROGNOSIS AND CONCLUSIONS

• The cure rate for rectovaginal fistulas ranges from 70% to 100%.

• The type of procedure used for repair is not as important as following the basic principles of rectovaginal fistula repair.

• The best prospect for cure of the fistula is the first intervention, and it should be undertaken by surgeons experienced in these operations.

• Since rectovaginal fistulas are most commonly caused by unsuccessful repairs of third- and fourth-degree perineal tears, the focus should be directed toward preventive obstetrical practice and adequate surgical technique when perineal injury occurs.

BIBLIOGRAPHY

Abel ME, Chiu YS, Russell TR, et al. Autologous fibrin glue in the treatment of rectovaginal and complex fistulas. *Dis Colon Rectum.* 1993;36(5):447–449.

Cardozo L, Staskin D. *Textbook of Female Urology and Urogynecology.* London: ISIS Medical Media; 2001:286–297, 692–719.

Clemons JL, Towers GD, McClure GB, et al. Decreased anal sphincter lacerations associated with restrictive episiotomy use. *Am J Obstet Gynecol.* 2005;192(5):1620–1625.

DeDombal FT, Watts JM, Watkinson G, et al. Incidence and management of anorectal abscess, fistula and fissure in patients with ulcerative colitis. *Dis Colon Rectum.* 1966;9:201–206.

Donnay F, Weil L. Obstetric fistula: the international response. *Lancet.* 2004;363:71–72.

Goldaber KG, Wendel PJ, McIntire DD, et al.. Postpartum perineal morbidity after fourth-degree perineal repair. *Am J Obstet Gynecol.* 1993;168(2):489–493.

Hallan RI, George B, Williams NS. Anal sphincter function: fecal incontinence and its treatment. *Surg Annu.* 1993;25(Pt 2):85–115.

Hartmann K, Viswanathan M, Palmieri R, et al. Outcomes of routine episiotomy: a systematic review. *JAMA.* 2005;293(17): 2141–2148.

Hilton P. Fistulae. In: Shaw RW, Soutter WP, Stanton SL, eds. *Gynecology.* 2nd ed. Edinburgh: Churchill Livingstone; 1997:792–801.

Hueston WJ. Factors associated with the use of episiotomy during vaginal delivery. *Obstet Gynecol.* 1996;87(6):1001–1005.

Poen AC, Felt-Bersma RJ, Strijers RL, et al. Third-degree obstetric perineal tear: long-term clinical and functional results after primary repair. *Br J Surg.* 1998;85(10):1433–1438.

PROLOG. *Gynecology and Surgery*, 5th ed.Washington, DC: The American College of Obstetricians and Gynecologists; 2004:136.

Radcliff AG, Ritchie JK, Hawley PR, et al. Anovaginal and rectovaginal fistulas in Crohn's disease. *Dis Colon Rectum.* 1988;31:94–99.

Rahman MS, Al-Suleiman SA, El-Yahia AR, et al. Surgical treatment of rectovaginal fistula of obstetric origin: a review of 15 years' experience in a teaching hospital. *J Obstet Gynaecol.* 2003;23(6):607–610.

Snooks SJ, Swash M, Mathers SE, et al. Effect of vaginal delivery on the pelvic floor: a 5-year follow-up. *Br J Surg.* 1990;77(12):1358–1360.

Sorensen SM, Bondersen H, Istre O, et al. Perineal rupture following vaginal delivery. *Acta Obstet Gynecol Scand.* 1988; 67:315–318.

Stoker J, Rociu E, Schouten WR, et al. Anovaginal and rectovaginal fistulas: endoluminal sonography versus endoluminal MR imaging. *AJR Am J Roentgenol.* 2002;178(3):737–741.

Sultan AH, Johanson RB, Carter JE. Occult anal sphincter trauma following randomized forceps and vacuum delivery. *Int J Gynaecol Obstet.* 1998;61(2):113–119.

Sultan AH, Kamm MA, Hudson CN, et al. Anal-sphincter disruption during vaginal delivery. *N Engl J Med.* 1993;329(26): 1905–1911.

Sultan AH, Kamm MA, Hudson CN, et al. Third degree obstetric anal sphincter tears: risk factors and outcome of primary repair. *BMJ.* 1994;308(6933):887–891.

Wiskind AK, Thompson JD. Transverse transperineal repair of rectovaginal fistulas in the lower vagina. *Am J Obstet Gynecol.* 1992;167(3):694–699.

Wiskind AK, Thompson JD. Fecal incontinence and rectovaginal fistulas. In: Rock JA, Thompson JD, eds. *Operative Gynecology.* 8th ed. Philadelphia, PA: Lippincott Williams & Wilkins; 1997:1223–1236.

QUESTIONS

1. A 42-year-old G8P5A3 is status post- total abdominal hysterectomy with bilateral salpingo-oopherectomy (TAH/BSO) and drainage for a ruptured tuboovarian cyst. Surgery was difficult and patient lost 4 units of blood. Postoperative day, no. 4 patient did not pass flatus and she is still unable to take PO regular diet and she is passing stool and purulent discharge per vagina. She has a temperature of 38°C (100.4°F). Rectovaginal examination reveals a 3-cm rectovaginal fistula at the vaginal cuff. The most appropriate next step in management is
   (A) Vaginal rectovaginal fistula repair
   (B) Abdominal rectovaginal fistula repair
   (C) Expectant management
   (D) Somatostatin therapy
   (E) Diverting colostomy

2. A 32-year-old G1P1 presents with a foul vaginal discharge 10 days after a vaginal delivery complicated by a third-degree perineal laceration. Vaginal examination and EUA with a bivalve speculum shows a 3-mm rectovaginal fistula 1 cm from the vaginal introitus. Vaginal epithelium is pink and there are no signs of infection. The proper initial management of this patient is
   (A) Diverting colostomy followed by a layered closure
   (B) Perineoproctotomy with layered closure
   (C) Transvaginal pursestring
   (D) Conservative management (observation, a low-residue diet, and stool softeners)
   (E) Closure with a Martius bulbocavernosus muscle fat pad

3. A 35-year-old G2P2 presents to the office with complains of a 2-month history of a foul-smelling vaginal discharge and passage of gas per vagina. She underwent her last vaginal delivery 6 months ago and she delivered a healthy male baby weighing

4350 g. Her obstetrician performed an episiotomy and perineal repair at that time. Pelvic examination reveals a fistulous tract in the posterior vaginal wall, 1 cm size, 2 cm from the vaginal introitus and the vaginal mucosa looks pink, soft with no signs of infection. Rectovaginal examination demonstrates an attenuated perineal body and confirms the rectovaginal fistula. The most appropriate next step in the management of this patient is
   (A) Barium enema
   (B) Methylene blue test
   (C) Surgical repair
   (D) Conservative management (observation, a low-residue diet and stool softeners)
   (E) Anal endosonography

4. A 32-year-old G2P2 presents with a foul vaginal discharge 3 months after a vaginal delivery complicated by a fourth-degree perineal laceration repaired at that time by her obstetrician. Vaginal examination and EUA with a bivalve speculum shows a 1.2 cm rectovaginal fistula 2 cm from the vaginal introitus. Vaginal epithelium is pink and there are no signs of infection. The best surgical repair for this patient is
   (A) Transvaginal pursestring method
   (B) Perineoproctotomy followed by a layered closure
   (C) Conservative management (observation, a low-residue diet and stool softeners)
   (D) Rectovaginal fistula repair with a Martius bulbocavernosus muscle or labial fat pad
   (E) Latzko's closure of rectovaginal fistula

5. A 48-year-old G4P4 comes to the office complaining of offensive, brownish colored vaginal discharge. She is status postradiation therapy for stage IIb cervical cancer that she completed 5 months ago. She has no dysuria and urinalysis shows no leukocytes, nitrates, or bacteria. IVP shows no periureteric flare and no extravasation of contrast. Pelvic examination shows an obliterated, erythematous vaginal cuff with a moderate amount of fluid, and well-supported vaginal walls. A 2 cm high rectovaginal fistula is seen on examination and confirmed by a contrast enema using BE and colonoscopy. Patient underwent diverting colonoscopy and biopsy of fistula edge rule out a cancer recurrence. Patient desires bowel reanastomosis and surgical repair of the rectovaginal fistula. The most appropriate surgical management of this patient's rectovaginal fistula is
   (A) Transvaginal pursestring method with a Martius bulbocavernosus muscle graft in 12 months
   (B) Perineoproctotomy followed by a layered closure (sphincteroplasty) in 12 months

(C) Abdominal repair with an omental pedicle graft in 1 week

(D) Abdominal repair with an omental pedicle graft in 12 months

(E) Latzko's repair of rectovaginal fistula

ANSWERS

1. *(E)*. A colostomy is rarely indicated in the treatment of rectovaginal fistula. Indications for colostomy include prior pelvic radiation, IBD, the presence of an intra-abdominal or pelvic abscess, distal bowel obstruction, and a large (>2.5 cm) fistula near the vaginal apex. This patient has a large rectovaginal fistula at the vaginal cuff and she has a pelvic abscess, therefore a diverting colostomy is indicated. Before the colostomy is performed, it is necessary to perform a BE enema, GI series with SBFT, colonoscopy +/− injection of contrast to identify the colon segment that communicates with vagina.

2. *(D)*. It is important to recognize that some low rectovaginal fistulas may cause only minor symptoms and may not require surgical repair. Close to one in four small rectovaginal fistulas heal spontaneously before epithelialization of the fistulous tract in patients treated with a low-residue diet and diphenoxylate hydrochloride (Lomotil). In another series comprising 52 patients with rectovaginal fistulas, 12.2% (5 patients) achieved cure with conservative management only.

3. *(E)*. Anal endosonography imaging is a useful diagnostic tool because it identifies anatomical defects in the anterior portion of the anal sphincter prior to repair of rectovaginal fistulas. If a rectovaginal fistula develops after a vaginal delivery, an occult anal sphincter defect may lead to fecal incontinence, even after proper surgical repair, thus anal endosonography is indicated prior to repair of a rectovaginal fistula. Methylene blue dye and BE enema may detect the presence of a rectovaginal fistula but they do not detect anal sphincter disruption.

4. *(A)*. The transvaginal pursestring method is the procedure of choice for small (<1.5 cm) rectovaginal fistulas situated within 5 cm of the vaginal furchette.

   In patients with larger fistulas (>1.5 cm) lying just above the external anal sphincter and with evidence of anal incompetence, the preferred method of repair is perineoproctotomy followed by a layered closure (sphincteroplasty). Latzko's closure is an effective method for closing a high rectovaginal fistula at the vaginal apex.

5. *(D)*. This patient desires to undergo a laparotomy procedure for bowel reanastomosis, so it is easiest to perform an abdominal repair of the rectovaginal fistula. Omental pedicle grafts are used mostly for repair of postradiation fistulas. They are dissected from the grater curvature of the stomach and are rotated and brought into the pelvis along with the gastroepiploic artery to provide an additional blood supply to the tissues undergoing surgical repair. In radiation fistulas, there is ↑ tissue sloughing and it is necessary to wait at least 12 months before attempting surgical repair. Biopsy of the fistula edge is necessary to *rule out* cancer recurrence. The transvaginal pursestring method and the perineoproctotomy followed by a layered closure are transvaginal procedures.

22 RECTAL PROLAPSE AND HEMORRHOIDS: A BASIC OVERVIEW
Mayank Pandya

RECTAL PROLAPSE

- Full thickness intussusceptions of the rectum through the anal canal
- Associated with
  ◦ Straining
  ◦ Poor tone of pelvic muscles
  ◦ Tenesmus
  ◦ Neurological disease
  ◦ Multiparous women, 3–10 times
  ◦ Child (approximately 3 years)
  ◦ Those over 50 years (a 6:1 ratio, women > men)

ETIOLOGY

- Protrusion of the rectum beyond the anus
- Occult (internal)—when the rectum has prolapsed but not beyond the anus (aka intussusception), or external
- Rectal prolapse is a sliding hernia that protrudes through a defect in the pelvic fascia at the level of the anterior rectal wall

ASSOCIATED SYMPTOMS

- Constipation
- Solitary rectal ulcers

SOME ANATOMOMIC DISORDERS THAT PREDISPOSE TO PROLAPSE

- Deep peritoneal cul-de-sac (pouch of Douglas) loss of posterior rectal fixation
- Diastases of the levator ani
- Redundant rectum and sigmoid colon
- Presence of abnormal uterine and vaginal support— due to lax lateral ligaments or mobile mesorectum is associated
- Weakness of the internal and external sphincters may be associated with pudendal neuropathy

CLINICAL FEATURES OF EXTERNAL RECTAL PROLAPSE

The following are the clinical features of external rectal prolapse
- Soilage
- Prolapse
- Mucous discharge
- Itching
- Bleeding facilitated by venous congestion

CLINICAL FEATURES OF OCCULT RECTAL PROLAPSE

The following are the clinical features of occult rectal prolapse
- Incomplete evacuation
- Tenesmus—trauma, irritation, and bleeding
- Rectal pain

EVALUATION

- History and physical examination (H&P) (focus on good gynecological history, like a hysterectomy and vaginal prolapse repair, along with a history of rectocele, enterocele, and cystocele)
- Neurological examinations
- Symptoms of urinary and fecal incontinence, and or constipation
- Physical (helpful tips)
  - It is helpful to show an occult prolapse with straining in standing position
  - Inspect perianal skin (look for excoriation secondary to soiling and itching)

- Test anocutaneous reflex
- Prolapsed segment on digital segment can often be felt
- Look for associated rectocele, enteroceles, and cystocele (pelvic floor defects)
- Flex sigmoidoscopy may be used for biopsies and localizing inflammations if necessary
- Defecography may show a sigmoid that prolapses into the anal canal
- Also do a flex sigmoidoscopy to rule out other issues like malignancy or solitary rectal ulcer syndromes

SURGICAL REPAIRS

- The goal of treatment is to
  - Control the prolapse
  - Stop constipation
  - Restore continence
- There are two ways of doing that
  - Remove the redundant bowel
  - Fix the rectum to the sacral ligaments
- Two categories of repair
  - Abdominal
    - Suture rectopexy: The rectum is mobilized onto the pre sacral fascia. With healing and fibrosis, it becomes fixed in its new location
    - Prosthetic (mesh) rectopexy; placement of a foreign body with the above procedure in the hopes that the foreign body will elicit more of a reaction leading to stronger fixation
      - Posterior mesh rectopexy: When there is a synthetic material positioned between the rectum and the sacrum (sutured into the rectum and the periosteum of the sacral promontory). Using absorbable versus nonabsorbable materials has similar effects. Risk of sepsis is 2–16% with the main risk factor being a pelvic hematoma (drain all blood). If a pelvic sepsis occurs, then it will be necessary to remove the foreign material
      - Ripstein procedure (anterior sling rectopexy). This is done by first mobilizing the rectum completely, then an artificial anterior sling is placed synthetic or fascia lata) and attached to the sacral promontory. This goal is to restore the posterior curve decreasing the effect of the intra-abdominal pressure and restoring the anatomical position of the rectum
    - Resection: By itself it is not used much today. Usually used in combination with other procedures like a suture rectopexy. This is known as the Frykman-Golberg procedure

- Laparoscopic rectopexy: Less pain and shorter hospital stay, and involves a postmesh rectopexy with or without resection. It is as effective as the open procedure, but due to the longer surgery times, the overall cost may be more
  - Perineal, well suited to the high-risk patient or elderly
    - Delorme operation: Dilate the anus, separate the mucosa from the sphincter and plicate the muscularis propria. This is a surgical alternative for patients with a prolapse who may not be able to tolerate a more extensive operation
    - Perineal rectosigmoidectomy, a resection and repair of a full thickness rectum and part of the sigmoid colon, but more suited for the male patient
- The best surgery? Early and late complications were shorter for the perineal approach, but abdominal procedures have lower recurrence rates but higher complication rates

HEMORRHOIDS

- Hemorrhoids (haima = blood; rhoos = flowing)
- This condition has been reported since the beginning of history. It is estimated that about 10 million people suffer from this condition in the United States (about 4% of the population)
- One-third seek medical treatment
- This occurs in people who are 45–65 years old
- Often a chronic problem that gets worse with time
- The term hemorrhoids is commonly misused by patients and many times refers to any anal problem experienced by the patient; so it is important to consider other etiologies
- Ninety percent need no surgery
- Common symptoms are bleeding, pain, protrusion, and itching
- Remember all patients who say they have bleeding need a colposcopy
- Bleeding is bright red, not dark or mixed with feces. Those situations are more worrisome

DIFFERENTIAL DIAGNOSIS

- Fissures
- Abscesses
- Fistulas
- Pruritus ani
- Condylomatas
- Viral and bacterial skin infections
- Colorectal cancer (important to rule out!)
- Rectal prolapse
- Polyps
- Carcinoma
- Hypertrophies of anal papilla

ANATOMY

- It is important to realize that these entities are not actually *varicose*-like. They are a collection of a vascular type tissue, containing venules and arterioles with elements of smooth muscle and connective tissue
- There are two types of hemorrhoids, which are anatomically separated by the dentate (pectinate) line

INTERNAL HEMORRHOIDS

- These contain three vascular beds (described earlier) that get their blood supply from the superior hemorrhoid, middle and inferior arteries. They are located in the left lateral, right anterior, and right posterior positions (at 3, 6, and 9 o'clock) in the anus. Fed by the terminal branches of the superior rectal arteries, their drainage is by the inferior, middle, and superior rectal veins. Anal subepithelial smooth muscle arises from the conjoined longitudinal muscle layer, passes through the internal anal sphincter and inserts into the subepithelial vascular space. There the smooth muscle suspends and contributes to the bulk of the hemorrhoidal cushions. These cushions also supply important sensory information that let the patients know when and what they may be passing (i.e., stool, liquid, and even flatus). These are not supplied by somatic sensory nerves and therefore cannot cause pain. These vascular beds also assist with continence because they occlude the anus in part as they protrude into the lumen and are subjected to the downward pressure of any Valsalva maneuver. As people age, the fibers that attach these vascular beds to their normal anatomical positions begin to deteriorate, this can lead to bleeding, prolapse, and congestion. When bleeding occurs, it is arterial not venous. Vascular cushions are anchored to the underlying muscle by the mucosal suspensory ligament.

EXTERNAL HEMORRHOIDS

- They are hemorrhoids covered by squamous epithelium. They form from venous thrombosis, or bleed from eroded blood clots. The cutaneous nerves that supply the perianal area innervate external hemorrhoids. These nerves include the pudendal nerve and branches of the sacral plexus. *Many times, external skin tags may be confused with external hemorrhoids.* No classification system for these. These tend to be more painful because the pain fibers that are lacking in the internal hemorrhoids are present here. A patient generally gets symptoms when there is inflammation, enlargement, a thrombus formation, or prolapse. Acute pain is caused by the occlusion of the external hemorrhoidal vein, which leads to distention of the overlying tissue. This distention (caused by edema) usually starts to resolve around the 7–14th day as the thrombus resolves. These usually do not bleed unless you have a patient who has a thrombosis which is resolving. Thrombus formation is often preceded by an acute event, like physical exertion, lifting, constipation with associated straining, or a change in the diet. The distention that occurs can sometimes leave skin tags. Hygiene often becomes a problem.

SYMPTOMS BASED ON LOCATION

INTERNAL HEMORRHOIDS
- Bleeding (usually painless, on toilet paper, dripping into the toilet bowl at the end of defecation)
- Usually bright
- In itself do not cause pain, but may illicit spasms of the sphincter
- Strangulation with or without necrosis (causing a deep discomfort)
- Pruritus ani
- Deposition of mucous on the perianal tissue (due to the prolapse)
- Localized dermatitis
- Soiling
- Most problems arise from these hemorrhoids, not external

EXTERNAL HEMORRHOIDS
- Asymptomatic usually unless there is a thrombosis, which expands the overlying skin
- When they heal they may leave a skin tag that may cause hygiene problems with secondary irritation
- Pain with a palpable lump is a hallmark of a thrombosed external hemorrhoid

CLASSIFICATION OF INTERNAL HEMORRHOIDS (BASED ON DEGREE OF PROLAPSE)

- First degree—vascular cushions that do not descend, only bleed
- Second degree—vascular cushions protrude below the pectinate line on straining but then return to normal when that straining stops
- Third degree—vascular cushions protrude to the exterior of the canal during straining often may need reduction
- Fourth degree—vascular cushions that are irreducible and stay prolapsed even without straining

DIAGNOSIS

- The key to diagnosing is with a thorough history
- Ask about symptoms mentioned previously
- Physical examination
  - It is usually a good idea to warn the patient before you decide to poke or probe them
  - Digital examination—make sure patient is on left (or right) lateral decubitus position, permitting optimal visualization of the anal region
  - Feel for rectal masses or tender points
  - If you get extreme pain, then you may be feeling external hemorrhoids, thrombosis, or an anal fissure
  - Anal fissures and perianal dermatitis (pruritus ani) are easily visible without internal probing
  - Internal hemorrhoids are soft vascular structures (the cushions). They are usually not palpable
  - Make a note of any skin tags and the presence of any thrombosis
  - *Anal wink* with stimulation confirms *intact sensation*
- For viewing internal hemorrhoids, *anoscopy* is the key, while the patient performs a Valsalva
- Anoscopy detects more lesions in the anorectal region than flex sigmoidoscopy, especially the slotted anoscope (it is sometimes helpful to have the patient strain to improve visualization)
  - Perform Valsalva without the anoscope, to see if there is any prolapse
- Consider a proctosigmoidoscopy to rule out the ever important specter of colon cancer, and to check for polyps

LAB

- Hematocrit/Hemoglobin
  - Barium enema to rule out colon disease

HISTOLOGIC FINDINGS

- Generally noncontributory but send anything suspicious to pathology

TREATMENT

- Only symptomatic hemorrhoids need any treatment. Most cases can be handled in the primary care setting
- External hemorrhoids
  - Minimize straining
  - Fiber (good for internal grades I and II internal hemorrhoids and can also help prevent future episodes)

- Exercise
- Limiting time on the toilet, little evidence but does not do any harm
- Anything that would decrease the downward force of defecation
- Analgesic and hydrocortisone—use the two no longer than 7–10 days due to side effects of contact dermatitis and mucosal atrophy
- Warm sitz two to three times a day works by relaxing the internal sphincter
- Best is excision with a local
- Internal hemorrhoids
  - Remove excess hemorrhoidal tissue, subsequent process of healing/scarring will attach the residual tissue to the anorectal muscular ring
  - Rubber band ligation: The best treatment for grades I–III that fail conservative therapy is rubber band ligation. This is a safe method, important to warn the patient that the tissue will slough off in 4–7 days. In the meantime, give them sitz bath instructions and fiber. The band is placed 5 mm above dentate line. Often there is a complaint of "tightness." A possible complication may be infection, abscess, sepsis, but overall risk is low. Rubber band ligation has become one of the most frequently applied methods for the treatment of internal hemorrhoids—applied on an insensitive area just above the dentate line (anesthesia is unnecessary). Give instructions for high-fiber diet following the procedure
  - Sclerotherapy: The injection of sclerosants causes an intense inflammatory reaction. Sclerosing agents cause fibrosis of the vascular cushions—obliterating hemorrhoids. Used for first- and second-degree hemorrhoids but not for external hemorrhoids, thrombosed, or ulcerated internal hemorrhoids. Some sclerosing therapy agents used are phenol 5% in vegetable oil, quinine, and urea hydrochloride. This technique is good for those with coagulation disorders. However, with this therapy there is a high relapse rate
  - Diathermy coagulation—nonoperative technique for second and third degrees and when medical therapy for first degree has failed—can be repeated if necessary
  - Bipolar coagulation—nonoperative technique for second and third degrees and when medical therapy for first degree has failed—can be repeated if necessary
  - Infrared coagulation—nonoperative technique for second and third degrees and when medical therapy for first degree has failed—can be repeated if necessary
  - Cryotherapy—not used any longer—for second and third degrees and when medical therapy for first degree has failed—can be repeated if necessary
  - Sphincter dilation—daily dilation for several weeks—it is painful and you may need may need general anesthesia. Possible side effect may be incontinence

- Surgery—indicated for those who fail medical and nonoperative therapy, symptomatic third or fourth degree, or mixed internal and external hemorrhoids. Use operative treatment if there are external components, ulceration, gangrene, extensive thrombosis, hypertrophies papillae, fissure, or failure of rubber band ligation to alleviate symptoms. Most are outpatient procedures. Closed hemorrhoidectomy—where an elliptical incision is made on the external hemorrhoidal tissue and extended proximally to the superior extent of the hemorrhoidal column. Usually three hemorrhoidal columns are treated at a time and the defect is closed with a continuous absorbable suture with a 95% success rate. Open hemorrhoidectomy—not commonly used due to complication rate. Involves excision and ligation without closure. Used to decrease the rate of infection, however, there is a slower healing rate
- Medical therapy for first degree (cornerstone being fiber and water), topical steroids, analgesics for the skin irritation
- Summary of medical and surgical treatments of hemorrhoids

TREATMENT	INDICATION
Analgesics/anti-inflammatories	Grades I–IV and thrombosed external hemorrhoids
Topical analgesics	Grades I–III
Corticosteroids	
Fiber	Grades I–II
Office procedures	Rubber band ligation
Phlebotonics	Grades I–II
Hemorrhoidectomy	Grades II–IV

REFERENCES

1. Mediba TE, Baig MK, Wecner SD. Surgical management of rectal prolapse. *Arch Surg.* 2005;140(1):63–73.
2. Walters MA, Karram MM. *Urogynecology and Reconstructive Pelvic Surgery.* St. Louis, MO: Mosby; 1999:285–294.
3. Gopal DV. Diseases of the rectum and anus: a clinical approach to common disorders. *Clin Cornerstone.* 2002; 44(4):34–48.
4. Khawaja Azimuddin MD, et al. Rectal prolapse: a search for the best operation. *Am Surg.* 2001;67:622–627.
5. Sardinaha TC, et al. Hemorrhoids. *Surg Clin N Am.* 2002;82:1153–1167.
6. Alonso-Coello P, Castillejo MM. Office evaluation and treatment of hemorrhoids. *J Fam Pract.* 2003;52I(5):366.
7. American Gastroenterological Association Medical Position Statement. Diagnosis and treatment of hemorrhoids. *Gastroenterology.* 2004;126:1061–1146.
8. American Gastroenterological Association. American Gastroenterological Association technical review on the diagnosis and treatment of hemorrhoids. *Gastroenterology.* 2004; 126:1463–1473.

QUESTIONS

1. A 50-year-old White female G_3P_3 comes in because sudden pain in the anus. It started when she went to the bathroom to have a bowel movement two nights ago. She states that the pain is intense—a 7/10. When questioned further, she states that she has been suffering from chronic constipation since she has been on the Atkins diet which she started 1 year ago. Her diet consists of red meats and chicken. She has lost about 30 lb since she has been on the diet. The correct diagnosis is
   (A) Internal hemorrhoid
   (B) External hemorrhoid
   (C) Occluded rectal prolapse
   (D) Pruritus ani

2. A 3-year-old girl has been having multiple bowel movements in a span of a few hours. This has been distressing for her mother. There are no signs of bleeding. The baby is afebrile and is not showing any signs of distress. She is active and playful. The mother when wiping notices a small piece of *tissue* from the anus that often disappears. The correct diagnosis is
   (A) Internal prolapsed hemorrhoids
   (B) Rectal prolapse
   (C) Healed external thrombosis
   (D) Fissure

3. A 50-year-old male has been having some rectal bleeding. The bleeding is not mixed with the feces, and usually comes at the end of the bowel movement. He has not been bothered by it until recently when he began to worry that something more serious may be going on. He had a father who died of colon cancer. Patient's diet has been low in fiber. He has a bowel movement every two days. Patient feels as if his BMs are complete, and does not suffer from any rectal pain. Correct diagnosis is
   (A) Internal hemorrhoid
   (B) External hemorrhoid
   (C) Occluded prolapse
   (D) Complete prolapse
   (E) Suspected colon cancer

4. A man whose internal hemorrhoids have vascular cushions that are irreducible without straining. This is a _____ degree hemorrhoid
   (A) First
   (B) Second
   (C) Third
   (D) Fourth

ANSWERS

1. *(B)*. Notice the sudden onset associated with straining. Pain can be intense, and often preceded by prolonged straining. Remember to check for associated pathology, like internal hemorrhoids, which can coexist with external hemorrhoids. Occluded rectal prolapse would not present with a sudden onset of pain. Pruritus ani is associated with fecal soilage that often accompanies rectal prolapse.

2. *(B)*. Internal prolapsed hemorrhoids usually are in the elderly, not the young. Also there is an associated bleeding. The same goes with healed external hemorrhoids. Also one should be suspicious of some pain. If there is no pain, then thrombosed hemorrhoid is unlikely. Fissures often are found in the young, but in this case there are no signs of this event occurring. A rectal prolapse is commonly discovered in this age group. The tissue described could be from a healed thrombi but again no sign of distress in the baby.

3. *(A)*. Patient's description of rectal bleeding is classic for internal hemorrhoids. The bleeding is not mixed with the feces, which is more worrisome with colon cancer or upper gastrointestinal (GI) bleed. However, this painless bleeding seems benign enough. However, due to the patient's age and history, it would be prudent to have colon cancer screening. External hemorrhoids are painful. There is no prolapsed tissue eliminating a complete prolapse.

4. Classification of internal hemorrhoids (based on degree of prolapse):
   (A) First degree: Vascular cushions that do not descend, only bleed.
   (B) Second degree: Vascular cushions protrude below the pectinate line on straining but then return to normal when that straining stops.
   (C) Third degree: Vascular cushions protrude to the exterior of the canal during straining often may need reduction.
   (D) Fourth degree: Vascular cushions that are irreducible and stay prolapsed even without straining.
   The answer is (D).

23 VOIDING DYSFUNCTION AND URINARY RETENTION

J. Linn Daudel and Sam Siddighi

INTRODUCTION

- Voiding dysfunction—any difficulty or discomfort with the process of emptying the bladder
- Urinary retention—total inability to empty the bladder when there is an urge to void
- Voiding dysfunction and urinary retention are on a spectrum. Voiding dysfunction can progress to urinary retention (end-stage on the spectrum)
- In this chapter, we will look at voiding dysfunction from several different viewpoints (nerve pathway mechanism, acute vs. chronic, neurogenic vs. nonneurogenic, and common presentations in gynecologic and elderly female patients)
- Normal micturition involves neural input/output from four different areas in central nervous system (CNS) and peripheral nervous system (PNS). Any lesion of one of these areas can result in voiding dysfunction and possible urinary retention:
  - ○ Cerebral cortex—receives neural input from brain stem and spinal cord and releases inhibition on micturition reflex when it is socially acceptable to void
    - ▪ Lesion of cortex → (1) urinary retention secondary to urethral sphincter spasticity, (2) detrusor overactivity, urge incontinence, enuresis, (3) incontinence in public raises no social concern
    - ▪ Causes of cortical lesions: stroke, tumor, Parkinson's, multiple sclerosis (MS), trauma, normal pressure hydrocephalus (NPH)
  - ○ Pontine reticular formation (PRF)—micturition reflex is controlled by the PRF; it integrates all signals from above (cortex) and below (sacral spinal cord and peripheral nerves), then coordinates detrusor contraction and simultaneous urethral sphincter relaxation (or the opposite)
    - ▪ Lesion above PRF → spontaneous involuntary voiding (i.e., involuntary bladder contraction with simultaneous urethral relaxation)
  - ○ Sacral spinal cord (S2-S4)—contains upper motor neurons that innervate the detrusor muscle
    - ▪ Lesion above S2,S3,S4 → (1) detrusor overactivity, (2) detrusor-sphincter dyssynergia (DSD) → *voiding dysfunction*
    - ▪ Causes of sacral lesions: herpes zoster radiculitis, trauma, spinal stenosis, protruding vertebral disk, MS, tumor
  - ○ Peripheral nerves—sympathetic and parasympathetic nerves whose lower motor neurons synapse on ganglia, detrusor muscle, or urethral sphincter. Also important in voiding is the pudendal nerve which not only receives sensory information from the striated urethral sphincter (SUS), it also activates SUS as well as the pelvic floor muscles
    - ▪ Parasympathetic (pelvic nerves: most important for detrusor contraction): presynaptic neurons of S2-S4 (intermediolateral column of spinal cord) → ganglia near bladder → postsynaptic neurons release acetylcholine (Ach) onto muscarinic receptors on the detrusor muscle which leads to bladder contraction
    - ▪ Sympathetic (hypogastric and pelvic nerves)→ presynaptic neurons of T10-L2 pass through paravertebral chain (to pelvic nerves) or go to inferior mesenteric and hypogastric ganglia (through hypogastric nerves) → (1) detrusor wall relaxation and urethral sphincter contraction and (2) synapse with parasympathetic fibers at the spinal or ganglion level to inhibit them by releasing norepinephrine (NE)
    - ▪ Lesion pelvic nerves → detrusor muscle areflexia and lack of bladder sensation (thus *urinary retention*)
    - ▪ Causes of pelvic nerve lesions: trauma, radical pelvic surgery, diabetes mellitus (DM), alcoholism, herpes zoster, tabes dorsalis of syphilis
- Normal micturition mechanism: bladder fills with urine and stretches bladder wall with little risk in pressure (i.e., compliance) → afferent input to S2-S4

spinal cord, pons, then cortex → if socially acceptable, inhibition on micturition reflex is released by cortex → PRF mediates micturition → relaxation of SUS and pelvic floor muscles which are normally tonically contracted → bladder and upper two-thirds of urethra are mobile, therefore they descend and urethrovesical junction dilates → detrusor muscle contracts with sufficient pressure and coordination to produce urine flow

SIGNS AND SYMPTOMS

- Common symptoms: hesitancy (difficulty in initiating urinary stream), weak urinary stream, prolonged voiding time, use of suprapubic pressure to void, straining to void, a weak or interrupted voiding stream, and/or feeling of incomplete emptying
- Other symptoms: urinary frequency, nocturia, and overflow incontinence (intermittent dribbling or continuous wetness)
- Most patients with acute urinary retention feel pain in the lower, midpelvis; however, chronic urinary retention is usually painless
- Back pain, fever, and painful urination may indicate a urinary tract infection (UTI) (with or without a kidney infection) secondary to large residual urine volumes. Recurrent UTIs despite antibiotic therapy are also common
- Incidental discovery of large bladder volume on computed tomography (CT) scan for other indication

ETIOLOGY

- Urinary retention can result in only three ways:
  - Proper bladder function depends on normal detrusor muscle function. This muscle may be unable to generate adequate strength or duration of contractions to produce efficient bladder emptying or it may become completely acontractile
  - The urethra may become obstructed via overactivity or mechanical occlusion
  - The levator ani muscles of the pelvic floor may not be able to relax adequately
- Acute urinary retention
  - When voiding dysfunction presents acutely, urinary retention may occur transiently for a period of days to weeks
  - The most common causes for acute retention are surgery and childbirth
  - Herpes simplex is a common cause of transient, acute urinary retention in reproductive-aged women

- This is due to a combination of vulvovaginal pain, edema, levator spasm, and autonomic dysfunction of the detrusor muscle
- Urinary retention is managed by analgesia, antiviral therapy, and possibly transurethral catheterization for 2–3 days
  - Other common causes are new medication, severe constipation, UTI, endocrine abnormalities (hypothyroidism), and psychological problems
  - Finally, acute retention often results following pelvic/abdominal surgery or vaginal delivery
  - Treatment of the underlying cause, along with facilitating bladder emptying for a few days to weeks via intermittent catheterization or indwelling catheter, tends to alleviate the retention without the need for any involved work-up
- Chronic urinary retention
  - Sometimes voiding difficulties develop gradually over many months and are not detected until a patient presents with a variety of symptoms
  - Chronic urinary retention usually results from another disease process or neurologic problem, but occasionally, it may also result following surgery
- Another important classification system of urinary retention is neurogenic versus nonneurogenic causes. See Table 23-1
- Causes of voiding dysfunction in obstetric, gynecologic, and elderly female patients
  - Childbirth can cause urinary retention because of the following:
    - Trauma, edema, and hematomas caused by descent of the baby
    - Pain due to laceration or episiotomy → levator ani spasm → inhibits detrusor contraction and levator ani muscle relaxation
    - Overdistention episodes during labor should be avoided (intermittent catheterization) as they increase the likelihood of urinary retention
  - Anti-incontinence surgery-induced voiding dysfunction
    - Surgical correction of SUI is the most common cause of bladder outlet obstruction in women
    - Usually patients will return to normal voiding between 3 and 12 days after sling or Burch
    - It is uncommon to have urinary retention beyond 4–6 weeks. If this is the case, then pressure-flow studies should be done and more aggressive management contemplated (see section on Treatment)
    - The incidence of postoperative urinary retention depends on the type of anti-incontinence operation
      - The traditional sling procedures have the highest rate of urinary retention (2–37%)
      - For a traditional sling, the rate of urinary retention is operator dependent and depends on how tight the sling is tied

TABLE 23-1 Causes of Urinary Retention in Females

ACUTE	CHRONIC
Infectious	**Obstructive**
Urethritis/cystitis/vulvovaginitis	Neurogenic
Herpes simplex	Detrusor sphincter dyssynergia
Iatrogenic	Brain/spinal cord lesions (*upper motor neurons*)
Pharmacologic (*decreased bladder contractility*)	MS
Postpartum/postoperative (*localized edema and pain*)	Myelitis
Obstructive	Parkinson's disease
Fecal impaction	Nonneurogenic
Endocrine	Anatomic obstruction
Hypothyroidism	Primary bladder neck obstruction
Psychiatric Disorder (Diagnosed by Specific Pattern on EMG)	Inflammatory processes
Schizophrenia	• Bladder neck fibrosis
Depression	• Urethral stricture
	• Meatal stenosis
	• Urethral diverticulum
	• Skene's gland cyst/abscess
	Pelvic organ prolapse
	• Uterine prolapse
	• Cystocele
	• Enterocele
	• Rectocele
	Neoplastic
	• Urethral carcinoma
	Gynecologic (*extrinsic compression*)
	• Retroverted uterus
	• Vaginal carcinoma
	• Cervical carcinoma
	• Ovarian mass
	Iatrogenic obstruction (*elevation/obstruction of bladder neck*)
	• Anti-incontinence procedures
	• Multiple urethral dilatations
	• Urethral excision or reconstruction
	Other
	• Bladder calculi
	• Atrophic vaginitis/urethritis
	Functional obstruction
	External sphincter spasticity
	Dysfunctional voiding
	Decreased Bladder Contractility
	Neurogenic
	Lower motor neuron lesion
	Cauda equina injury
	Pelvic plexus injury
	• Postoperative denervation of bladder
	Peripheral neuropathy
	• DM
	• Alcoholic neuropathy
	• Pernicious anemia
	• Herpes zoster
	• Guillain-Barre syndrome
	• Tabes dorsalis
	MS
	Autonomic dysfunction
	Nonneurogenic
	Atony/hypotonia
	Chronic obstruction secondary to disease process (i.e., scleroderma)
	Radiation cystitis
	Tuberculosis
	Psychogenic retention
	Infrequent voiders syndrome

ABBREVIATION: EMG, electromyogram.

- Relative rates of urinary retention are as follows: traditional sling > Burch > TVT > TOT
- Early, transient voiding dysfunction is related to edema, inflammation, and pain
- Alteration of the anatomy of the bladder, neck, and proximal urethra can cause voiding dysfunction and urinary retention for a longer period
  - Sutures placed too close to the urethra can cause urethral deviation
  - Sutures not placed lateral enough (away from urethra) in Burch have higher risk for urinary retention
  - Sutures tied too tightly can overcorrect, kink, and shut the neck of the bladder
  - Sutures piercing the urethral lumen can lead to fibrosis and periurethral scarring
  - Even the surgical dissection itself may generate scarring which results in obstructive anatomy
- The patient history and the type of procedure may help predict the risk of postoperative urinary retention
  - Age > 65
  - Consistently elevated postvoid residual (PVR) on routine visits
  - History of voiding dysfunction for whatever reason
  - History of urinary retention after surgery or childbirth
  - Underlying chronic or permanent condition (e.g., MS, DM, hypothyroid, stroke, and so forth)
  - Undergoing other concomitant surgical procedure (e.g., anterior repair + sling)
  - Type of procedure: for example, a radical hysterectomy can result in pelvic nerve injury and subsequent bladder hypocontractility
- Additionally, pressure-flow studies may also help predict which patients will have postoperative urinary retention (this is controversial)
  - *Normal* and *abnormal* values for pressure-flow studies are
    - Normal $\rightarrow Q_{max} > 15$–20 mL/s and $P_{det} < 20$ cm H_2O
    - Outlet obstruction pattern $\rightarrow$ low flow rates and high detrusor pressure (P_{det}). $Q_{max} < 12$ mL/s and $P_{det} > 35$ cm H_2O (range: 20–50 cm H_2O) at Q_{max}
  - Pressure-flow study before surgical correction for SUI may help predict which patients are at risk for prolonged bladder catheterization (i.e., >7 days). Patients with low flow rate ($Q_{max} < 15$–20 mL/s) and those using Valsalva (high P_{det} at Q_{max} [>50 cm H_2O] $\rightarrow$i.e., detrusor peak flow pressure [PFP]) to void may be at risk for prolonged catheterization. These patients should be counseled preoperatively that clean intermittent self-catheterization is a possibility
  - After pelvic surgery in patients with consistently elevated PVRs: e.g., after a Burch urethropexy or suburethral sling (either from denervation injury during surgery or because of increased urethral resistance from suture or sling after SUI surgery). The outlet obstruction pattern may indicate need to takedown repair (urethrolysis)
- Reconstructive pelvic surgery-induced voiding dysfunction (temporary)
  - General anesthetic agents and analgesic agents contribute to voiding and bowel dysfunction after surgery
  - Anterior colporrhaphy
    - The surgical dissection can cause periurethral tissue inflammation and edema
    - Aggressive plication of endopelvic fascia may result in partial anatomical obstruction
    - Postoperative pain can prevent levator ani relaxation
  - Posterior colporrhaphy
    - Needle and suture stimulation of levator ani muscles during posterior repair can cause muscle spasm
    - In addition, stimulation and postoperative pain $\rightarrow$ (1) inhibits detrusor contraction and (2) prevents levator ani relaxation
  - Sacrospinous ligament suspension (SSLS)
    - Suspension sutures may cause levator ani muscle spasm
- Physical urethral obstruction
  - Advanced pelvic organ prolapse (POP) can cause kinking, compression, and occlusion of the urethra (especially anterior wall prolapse)
  - Extrinsic masses may obstruct the urethra: vaginal myoma, hematocolpos, Skene's gland cyst
  - Intrinsic disorders can occlude the urethra from inside: condyloma, cancer, edema, fibrosis
- Pelvic nerve injury
  - Injury to the pelvic, hypogastric, and pudendal nerves or to the pelvic plexus can cause voiding dysfunction because of denervation of the bladder and urethral sphincter
  - This injury can be the result of major surgeries (e.g., radical hysterectomy or colorectal resection), trauma, or cancer. The usual result is an areflexive bladder and other forms of voiding dysfunction
    - Parasympathetic nerve injury $\rightarrow$ hypocontractility and decreased sensation
    - Sympathetic nerve injury $\rightarrow$ decreased compliance and high storage pressure or as bladder neck incompetence and incontinence

- Some cases of nerve injury will resolve after several months, but for some patients, the injury will be permanent
- This is the reason why a suprapubic catheter is always placed just after a radical hysterectomy
  ○ Pharmacologic
  - Oral or intravenous (IV) medications from the following drug classes affect bladder function by affecting different areas in the nervous system or the bladder itself: anticholinergics, narcotics, Ca²⁺ channel antagonists, muscle relaxants, antihistamines, tricyclic antidepressants, α-adrenergic agonists, amphetamines, ganglion-blocking agents, theophylline, phenothiazines, and L-dopa
  - The desired effect or side effect of these drugs may cause a decrease in bladder contractility and/or increase in urethral sphincter tone. Here are three examples:
    • Diphenhydramine (antihistamine) → decreases bladder contractility
    • Ephedrine α-adrenergic agonist) → increases urethral sphincter tone
    • Imipramine (tricyclic antidepressant) → causes both the above
  - To know the effect of a particular drug on voiding, check a physician's desk reference (PDR) or drug information sheet for adverse effects and mechanism of drug action
  - Epidurals and spinals also result in urinary retention by blocking most nerve input/output at the level of the spinal cord
  ○ DSD
  - DSD results following neurologic damage to either the spinal cord above the sacral region or to the CNS
  - These patients have both hyperreflexic detrusor muscle activity and an increase in external sphincter activity
  - EMG diagnosis → increase in EMG electrode activity before and during the start of detrusor contraction
  - Therefore, a detrusor contraction against a closed sphincter occurs with subsequent urinary retention
  - MS, stroke, and spinal cord injury patients is systemic may have DSD. Additionally, MS can also lead to bladder acontractility as the cause of urinary retention
  - Pharmacologic therapy for DSD patients is aimed at reducing urethral sphincter tone (prazosin or phenoxybenzamine), relaxing the pelvic floor muscles (dantrolene, baclofen, or diazepam), and by reducing detrusor muscle hyperreflexia (oxybutynin, tolterodine)
  - Dysfunctional voiding in neurologically intact children may have a similar EMG electrode activity as

DSD. It results in an intermittent, interrupted urinary stream pattern on uroflowmetry (i.e., low peak flow rate, prolonged flow times) and a high PVR
  ○ Detrusor hyperactivity with impaired contractility (DHIC)
  - In some elderly, the detrusor muscle may have slow, weak overactivity but these contractions do not produce enough force to allow the bladder to empty
  - This may be due to replacement of bladder smooth muscle by collagen because of the process of aging or it may be because of dysfunction of the smooth muscle
  ○ Diabetic cystopathy
  - Since DM is such a prevalent disease, a brief mention of the disease's effect on the urologic function of women is warranted. Around the time that a diabetic begins to experience peripheral neuropathy, urologic manifestations of DM may begin to appear as well
  - The onset of dysfunction is characterized by a decrease in bladder sensation. This is followed by an increase in bladder capacity and high PVRs. Finally, detrusor hypocontractility will occur
  - Also, independently of these, diabetics tend to demonstrate detrusor overactivity that can produce urge symptoms in these patients
  ○ Chronic or permanent condition(s)
  - Chronic diseases affecting the nervous system can also result in functional abnormalities of voiding. These include but are not limited to the following: Parkinson's disease, dementia, stroke, MS, myelitis, alcoholic neuropathy, tabes dorsalis, pernicious anemia, and hypothyroidism

EVALUATION

- The complete evaluation of urinary incontinence and related issues is discussed in detail in Chap. 6, Evaluation of Urinary Incontinence in the Office and Indications for Referral to a Specialist
- History and physical examination key points (relevant to this chapter)
  ○ Did she just have anti-incontinence surgery, pelvic reconstructive surgery, or childbirth?
  ○ Does she have symptoms reminiscent of voiding dysfunction? Look at her urinary diary.
  ○ Does she have any of the risk factors for postoperative voiding dysfunction?
  ○ Does she have any contributing chronic or permanent medical condition?
  ○ Is she chronically constipated?
  ○ Does she take any over-the-counter medications or supplements which may cause urinary retention?

○ Inspect the vagina (rule out condylomas) and urethra, palpate the urethra (rule out urethral or suburethral mass), perform a speculum examination (rule out POP), bimanual examination (rule out pelvic mass, palpate bladder distention), rectal examination (fecal impaction).

○ Perform a complete neurologic examination (flexion and extension of knee against resistance [tests L2-L5], eversion/inversion of foot [tests S1-S2], deep tendon reflexes [DTRs] hyperreflexive and Babinski is present in upper motor neuron lesions, sensory function, and pelvic floor reflexes—anal wink, clitoral-anal, and cough reflexes indicate spinal cord below L4 is intact; see Chap. 6, Evaluation of Urinary Incontinence in the Office and Indications for Referral to a Specialist).

• Perform urinalysis (± urine culture and sensitivity [UC&S] and PVR (by catheterization or ultrasound)

○ PVR is usually <60 mL (60–100 mL can be normal; >200 mL is always considered abnormal)

○ Nevertheless, it is more useful to indicate PVR as a percentage of total volume voided (i.e., PVR/total voided volume). This value should be <20%

• Noninvasive uroflowmetry (NIF) and pressure-flow studies may be useful in objectively assessing obstructive versus underactive voiding patterns:

○ Bladder must contain at least 150–200 mL of urine because this influences test results (see Chap. 8, Urodynamics II: Tests that Evaluate Bladder Emptying)

○ A *normal* woman can void 200 mL in 30 second with a $Q_{max} > 15$–20 mL/s

○ Low flow rates and high detrusor pressures indicate obstruction → $Q_{max} < 12$ mL/s and PFP > 50 cm H_2O (i.e., $P_{det} > 50$ cm H_2O at Q_{max})

○ Said another way, an obstructed urethra has a high urethral resistance = PFP/$(Q_{max})^2 > 0.2$

○ Underactive detrusor pattern → low flow rate ($Q_{max} < 12$ mL/s) and low detrusor pressures PFP < 50 cm H_2O

• Urethral needle EMG may be useful in someone you suspect has DSD

• Cystoscopy can be used to rule out bladder or urethral masses, strictures, or foreign bodies which may contribute to voiding dysfunction

• Voiding cystourethrogram (imaging during urination) may also be helpful

• Renal ultrasound or IVP is useful for someone with long-standing urinary retention with symptoms of flank pain or recurrent pyelonephritis → rule out renal hydronephrosis or stone

• Routine screening of patients with voiding dysfunction and urinary retention with renal ultrasound or IVP is not appropriate

TREATMENT

• Urinary retention should be treated in a timely fashion in order to relieve the patient's symptoms, prevent bladder overdistention, and to avoid long-term damage to the kidney

• Treat pain but do not use excessive amounts of narcotics for postoperative patients as this may delay return of not only bowel but also bladder function

• Adequate analgesia is important, especially for patients with excessive pain and pelvic floor spasm

• Prevent and treat constipation as fecal impaction can contribute to voiding dysfunction (fluids, fiber, stool softeners, laxatives)

• Mild voiding dysfunction can be managed by special techniques/maneuvers

○ Frequent, scheduled voiding → void every 2 hours while awake

○ Double voiding → wait a few minutes after initial void then void again

○ Credé maneuver → take hand and press down on suprapubic region while simultaneously attempting to void

○ Valsalva voiding → use intra-abdominal pressure to void

○ Position changes such as bending forward

• Pharmacologic management of urinary retention

○ Bethanechol only → oral or subcutaneous doses do not help

○ Phenoxybenzamine + bethanechol → significant improvement in voiding

○ Local estrogen cream → important for postmenopausal women with atrophic and stenotic urethra

○ α-Adrenergic antagonists (e.g., prazosin, terazosin tamsulosin [Flomax]) → $α_1$ antagonist may relax smooth muscle in bladder neck enough to facilitate urine flow

○ Muscle relaxants (diazepam, baclofen, dantrolene) → can relieve levator ani muscle spasticity

○ Adequate pain control with non-steroidal anti-inflammatory drugs (NSAIDs) and narcotics (as necessary) → pain not only can aggravate levator ani muscle spasms, it can also create an anticipatory response which will prevent the patient from even attempting to void

○ Acyclovir, famcyclovir, or valacyclovir may be needed for acute urinary retention from herpes simplex

• The gold-standard treatment of severe or chronic urinary retention is regular clean intermittent self-catheterization (ISC) until urinary retention is resolved or for entire duration of life

○ Transurethral Foley catheter may be left in for a few days, but ISC is always preferred (see Chap. 40)

○ If the patient cannot perform ISC because of morbid obesity or disability then a suprapubic catheter should be placed (see Chap. 40)

• Voiding dysfunction and urinary dysfunction after anti-incontinence surgery can be managed with one or more of the aforementioned methods or by the following more aggressive methods if voiding dysfunction exceeds 4–6 weeks:

- Midurethral sling stretching → Hegar dilator may be inserted in the urethra with downward traction
- Midurethral sling revision:
  - Transection, takedown, or lysis of the mesh tape under IV sedation and local anesthetic or in operating room (OR)
  - Loosening of mesh tape—movement of mesh as a unit by downward traction on the loop underneath urethra with blunt instrument. However, this only can be done with slings with a built-in tension suture (e.g., SPARC), otherwise the mesh will stretch. Ideally, loosening should be done within 2.5 weeks of surgery before capsule has formed around the mesh tape
- Retropubic takedown of Burch or Marshall-Marchetti-Krantz (MMK) stitches
- Transvaginal urethrolysis → Foley with 30 mL balloon inserted to help identify bladder neck → midline vaginal mucosa injected, incised, and dissected to inferior pubic ramus as if performing a traditional sling (Chap. 15, Surgical Management of Stress Urinary Incontinence: Open Retropubic Operations) → retropubic space is entered digitally to allow some degree of urethrovesical junction and proximal urethral mobility
- Retropubic urethrolysis → the retropubic space is entered as for Burch procedure (Chap. 14, Surgical Management of Stress Urinary Incontinence: Vaginal Procedures), then the bladder neck and proximal urethral are mobilized with similar goal as transvaginal technique
- Other therapies for urinary retention based on cause:
  - Sacral nerve stimulation → has been helpful for some patients with nonobstructive urinary retention. Mechanism is unknown: it may decrease pelvic floor muscle spasticity and it may modulate detrusor muscle contractions
  - Patients with intrinsic urethral mass or stenosis → cystoscopy + urethral dilation using a 36 Fr dilator, then subsequent local estrogen cream
  - Neurologically-mediated spastic urethral sphincter muscle → sphincterotomy + urethrotomy
  - Urinary diversion may be indicated if urinary retention has caused renal deterioration (see Chap. 41)

BIBLIOGRAPHY

Germain MM. Urinary retention and overflow incontinence. In: Bent AE, Ostergard DR, et al., eds. *Ostergard's Urogynecology and Pelvic Floor Dysfunction*. 5th ed. Philadelphia, PA: Lippincott Williams & Wilkins; 2003.

Kobak WH, Walters MD, Piedmonte MR. Determinants of voiding after three types of incontinence surgery: a multivariable analysis. *Obstet Gynecol*. 2001:97:86–91.

Nitti VM, Raz S. Urinary retention. In: Raz S, ed. *Female Urology*. 2nd ed. Philadelphia, PA: W.B. Saunders; 1996.

Partoll LM. Voiding dysfunction and retention. In: Walters MD, Karram MM, eds. *Urogynecology and Reconstructive Pelvic Surgery*. 2nd ed. St. Louis, MO: C.V. Mosley; 1999.

Stanton SL, Ozsoy C, Hilton P. Voiding difficulties in the female: prevalence, clinical and urodynamic review. *Obstet Gynecol*. 1983:61:144–147.

Toglia MR. Voiding dysfunction and urinary retention. In: Weber AM, Brubaker L, et al., eds. *Office Urogynecology*. New York: McGraw-Hill; 2004.

Wall LL, Norton PA, DeLancey JOL. Bladder emptying problems. In: Wall LL, Norton PA, DeLancey JOL, eds. *Practical Urogynecology*. Baltimore, MD: Lippincott Williams & Wilkins; 1993.

Wein AJ. Neuromuscular dysfunction of the lower urinary tract and its treatment. In: Walsh PC, Retik AB, et al., eds. *Campbell's Urology*. 8th ed. Philadelphia, PA: W.B. Saunders; 2002.

QUESTIONS

1. A 58-year-old woman comes to your office for incomplete voiding. She is currently experiencing symptoms of difficulty in initiating urination, a weak urinary stream, and vague abdominal pain. She has been having symptoms for 5 months. These symptoms started after she had surgery for anterior vaginal prolapse. As part of your work-up, you decide to perform a PVR urine analysis. Which of the following results is most consistent with a diagnosis of urinary retention:

   (A) A total voided volume of 600 mL and a PVR volume of 100 mL
   (B) A total voided volume of 60 mL and a PVR volume of 60 mL
   (C) A total voided volume of 100 mL and a PVR volume of 40 mL
   (D) All of the above would be suggestive of urinary retention
   (E) None of the above would be suggestive of urinary retention

2. A 48-year-old woman comes to your office for difficulty with voiding. She has been experiencing painful urination with abdominal and back pain, and occasional leakage of urine. She has had these symptoms for the past month. The patient has no other medical problems and is not taking any medications. There has been no recent illness or trauma. The patient has had two prior cesarean sections, the last one was 22 years

ago. Which of the following is the most important test in determining the cause of her urinary difficulties:

(A) Multichannel urodynamic testing

(B) PVR urine analysis

(C) A urinalysis with cultures

(D) A neurologic examination

(E) A 24-hour voiding diary

3. A 72-year-old woman comes to your office for follow-up after having an anti-incontinence procedure. In your preoperative work-up, the patient denied having urinary symptoms. She is at postoperative day 14 and has had a Foley catheter in place since surgery for an inability to void. She reports having normal postoperative pain. There are no abnormal findings on physical examination. A voiding trial is performed: 400 mL of water is placed into the bladder and the catheter is removed. The patient is able to void 150 mL, but states she had strain and had poor flow. What is the next step of management:

(A) Multichannel urodynamic testing

(B) Surgical correction

(C) A urinalysis with cultures

(D) Intermittent self-catheterization and follow-up in 2 weeks

(E) Leave the Foley catheter in place and follow-up in 2 weeks

4. A 55-year-old woman with urinary retention for over 1 year has just completed a full evaluation. Her history is significant for MS diagnosed 7 years ago. The patient has a surgical history which includes a cholecystectomy and several knee surgeries. Her PVR urine volumes are constantly > 200 mL. A urodynamic study showed a peak urine flow of 25 mL/s with a detrusor pressure of 75 cm water. A cystourethroscopy did not reveal any abnormalities. An EMG was positive for an increase in ureteral external sphincter activity. What is the most likely diagnosis?

(A) Bladder outlet obstruction

(B) Dysfunctional voiding

(C) DSD

(D) Detrusor acontractility

(E) Pelvic nerve injury

5. A 70-year-old woman has just been diagnosed with detrusor areflexia secondary to long-term diabetes. What is the best treatment for her condition?

(A) Behavior modification—timed voiding, fluid restriction, and so forth

(B) Biofeedback/nerve stimulation device

(C) An anticholinergic medication (Urecholine)

(D) Surgical correction

(E) Intermittent self-catheterization

6. A 53-year-old woman with difficulty in initiating urination must use suprapubic pressure to generate a weak and interrupting urinary stream. She has had these symptoms for the past 8 months. Her PVR represents 75% of her total voided urine volume. A urodynamic study showed a peak urine flow of 10 mL/s with a detrusor pressure of 85 cm H_2O. Based on these findings, the next step for making a diagnosis should be

(A) A voiding cystourethrogram

(B) Have the patient keep a 24-hour voiding diary

(C) An intravenous pyelogram (IVP)

(D) An electromyography of the pelvic floor and external sphincter

(E) All of the above tests should be done for a thorough work-up

ANSWERS

1. *(B)*. The correct answer is B, because it demonstrates a larger PVR volume of urine versus voided urine. The PVR represents 100% of the voided total. These values definitely indicate urinary retention. Answer A is incorrect, because although the PVR volume of 100 mL could be considered high by some (100 mL is in the debate zone), the PVR represents only 17% of the voided total; thus, it is less likely that urinary retention is present. Answer C is incorrect, because although the PVR represents 40% of the voided total PVR volume, a PVR volume of less than 50 mL is always considered normal. Answers D and E are incorrect based on the explanations given.

2. *(C)*. The correct answer is C, because of the nature of the patient's symptoms of painful urination with accompanying back/abdominal pain and the shorter duration of symptoms. This patient is most likely experiencing short-term urinary retention secondary to a UTI, an acute and treatable form of urinary retention. Answer A is incorrect, because this form of testing is usually reserved until after the basic work-up studies have completed and a cause for chronic urinary retention is being sought. Answer B is incorrect, because although this test is often performed at the first visit and may help in diagnosing urinary retention, it will not help in determining the cause of urinary retention. Answer D is incorrect, because although a thorough physical examination should be performed at the first visit and may help in determining a cause of urinary retention, the patient's history is not suggestive of a neurologic problem. Answer E is incorrect, because a 24-hour voiding diary is useful for evaluating and treating

chronic urinary retention. This patient has only had symptoms for a month.

3. *(D)*. The correct answer is D**,** because the patient is able to void, but not completely. It is expected that her urinary retention will continue to resolve over the next few weeks. Answers A and B are incorrect, because it is premature to assume that this patient's urinary retention symptoms will not continue to resolve. Answer C is incorrect, because although it may be reasonable to perform this test at this visit, it is not the most appropriate step for managing the patient's current problem. Answer E is incorrect, because the patient now has some voiding capability. Leaving the Foley in place has a higher risk of infection, which would only complicate this patient's case. Furthermore, urinary function is more likely to return to normal with attempts at normal voiding, with support via intermittent catheterization as needed.

4. *(C)*. The correct answer is C, because the patient has both hyperreflexic detrusor muscle activity and an increase in external sphincter activity; therefore, a detrusor contraction against a closed sphincter occurs with subsequent urinary retention. MS is systemic neurologic disease that can cause detrusor-sphincter dyssynergia in women. Answer A is incorrect, because the patient has a normal cystourethroscopy and no other predisposing factors for obstruction are present (i.e., history of anti-incontinence surgery). Answer B is incorrect, because although these findings may occur with this diagnosis, the diagnosis requires a neurologically intact individual. This patient has MS. Answer D is incorrect, because although this is the more common finding for urinary retention in a patient with MS, the test results do not support this diagnosis. Answer E is incorrect, because this patient has no history of trauma or major pelvic/abdominal surgery.

5. *(E)*. The correct answer is E, because detrusor hypoactivity or areflexia is difficult to treat and intermittent catheterization is the only reliable treatment option. Answers A and B are incorrect, because while these treatments may be appropriate in diabetics treated early, this diagnosis, although new for the patient, implies extensive nerve degeneration has already occurred. Answers C and D are incorrect, because neither surgical nor pharmacologic therapies are effective treatments for total detrusor acontractility (areflexia).

6. *(A)*. The correct answer is A, because the patient is showings signs of an obstructive etiology; thus an imaging study is the next diagnostic test to perform. A radiographic/ultrasound evaluation or cystourethroscopy would also be reasonable diagnostic tests at this time. Answer B is incorrect, because it is clear that the patient is suffering from obstructive symptoms. A diary of symptoms at this time would not further the diagnosis. Answer C is incorrect, because although an IVP is an imaging studying, this test should be reserved for the evaluation of kidney function and is not the best test in determining the cause of this patient's obstruction. Answer D is incorrect, because although an electromyography of the pelvic floor and external sphincter could provide information about a possible cause for functional obstruction, causes of anatomic obstruction should be evaluated first with imaging studies. Answer E is incorrect, based on the explanations given.

24 MANAGEMENT OF DETRUSOR OVERACTIVITY
Tricia L. Fynewever and Sam Siddighi

INTRODUCTION

- Detrusor overactivity can be a distressing medical condition.
- The symptoms associated with urinary incontinence have implications on the activities of daily living, social relationships, sexual life, and self-esteem (see Chap. 46, Psychological Issues Related to Incontinence and Pelvic Organ Prolapse).
- Some women remain at home to be near the bathroom and to avoid loss of urine in public.
- When planning even a short trip, women with detrusor overactivity will "toilet map," or research the location of bathrooms along the way from home to final destination.
- Several aspects of detrusor overactivity have been discussed in previous chapters and others will be discussed in the following chapters. In this chapter, the reader will be prompted to also see Chap. 37 for a more detailed discussion of the pharmacologic management.
- Here, we will summarize current knowledge of detrusor overactivity and will give a detailed explanation of current therapies, especially sacral neuromodulation.

DEFINITIONS

- In recent years, the International Continence Society (ICS) has sought to standardize and clarify terminology related to the dysfunction of the lower urinary tract.
- The term *detrusor* refers specifically to the smooth muscle structure of the bladder, while bladder refers to the entire structure of the bladder.

- *Detrusor overactivity* refers to the involuntary contractions of the detrusor muscle during the filling phase of the bladder during urodynamic studies. Detrusor overactivity can be divided into phasic and terminal.
  - *Phasic detrusor overactivity* refers to a specific waveform, which may or may not be associated with sensation and or urinary incontinence.
  - *Terminal* means a single involuntary detrusor contraction at cystometric capacity, which cannot be suppressed or results in incontinence. This is often found with decreased bladder sensation.
- *Detrusor overactivity incontinence* is defined as an involuntary detrusor contraction resulting in incontinence. Also known as urinary urgency incontinence (UUI)
- *Idiopathic detrusor overactivity* replaces the former term *detrusor instability*. This describes a bladder, which contracts during the filling phase, documented on cystometrogram. Further conditions require either (1) a detrusor pressure rise of at least 15 cm H_2O or (2) a rise less than 15 cm of H_2O, but in the presence of urgency or urge incontinence.
- *Neurogenic detrusor overactivity* replaces the term *detrusor hyperreflexia* and refers to overactivity associated with a known neurological disorder.
- *Overactive bladder (OAB)*—a term coined by industry for purpose of coding and medication prescription; it includes any or all of the following: urgency, frequency, nocturia, and urge incontinence. The more types of OAB symptoms a patient has, the greater the chance that she has detrusor overactivity on complex cystometry.

SYMPTOMS

- OAB usually presents with some combination of these symptoms: urgency, frequency, urge incontinence, and nocturia.
- Frequency is defined as greater than 10 micturitions in 24 hours.
- These symptoms sometimes coexist with symptoms of stress incontinence in which case a person is said to have *mixed urinary incontinence.*

CAUSES

- *Neurogenic detrusor overactivity* formerly called detrusor hyperreflexia is associated with known neurological disorders of the brain and spinal cord.
  - Multiple sclerosis is a well-known disease affecting women between the ages of 20 and 40 years old. Although the etiology is unknown, pathologically

demyelinating plaques form in different areas of the nervous system producing varying symptoms depending on their location.
  - Parkinson's disease usually occurs after age 50 and involves the extrapyramidal system of the brain. This system is thought to inhibit the micturition center of the brain and with loss of control in this area urge incontinence occurs.
  - Cerebrovascular disease can produce bladder dysfunction by infarcting areas of the brain, which control micturition.
  - Dementia, including Alzheimer's disease, often involves diffuse areas of neurological function. Urge incontinence can occur either by pathologic involvement of areas that control micturition or merely by lack of attention to continence signals.
  - Spinal cord injury superior to the sacral spinal cord can cause upper motor neuron injury resulting in neurogenic detrusor overactivity.
- *Idiopathic detrusor overactivity* is the most common etiology of OAB, and 90% of women present with it.
  - These women seem to have a higher sensitivity to nervous system and acetylcholine stimulation.
  - Also vasoactive intestinal polypeptide (VIP), known to relax smooth muscle including the bladder, seems to be found in reduced concentrations in the bladders of these women.
- Bladder outflow obstruction (more common in men with enlarged prostates) can cause OAB in women who have severe pelvic organ prolapse. Also poor detrusor function can mimic obstruction with poor emptying during micturition.
- Bladder inflammation caused by urinary tract infection (UTI) can cause symptoms of OAB which resolve after treatment. This is why it is always important to perform urinalysis ± culture during evaluation.

BLADDER CONTROL AND OAB PATHOGENESIS

- The bladder is controlled by peripheral and central micturition reflex arcs.
- Parasympathetic nerves, which originate from S2–S4, have a stimulatory effect through acetylcholine on the bladder.
- Vasoactive intestinal peptide, which is abundant in normal bladders, relaxes smooth muscle and seems to have an inhibitory affect on the parasympathetic pathway.
- The bladder also appears to have its own pacemaker cells. It has been shown to be continuously active, undergoing rhythmic contractions, which can be seen on urodynamic studies. These contractions may be due to intrinsic bladder pacemaker cells.

- Sensory nerves also infiltrate the bladder, which gives rise to the sensations of bladder filling and the urge to void.
- In women with idiopathic OAB, there seems to be an increased sensitivity to acetylcholine causing a hyper-reflexive sympathetic response. Infiltration of the sacral spine with local anesthetic relieves this OAB.
- Additionally, VIP is found in decreased concentrations in the bladder possibly leading to decreased inhibition.
- Researchers have found greater density of sensory nerves than normal in these women, which could cause oversensation to otherwise normal filling.
- Also, there may be abnormal junctions between bladder muscle cells causing dysfunction of the pacemaker cells of the bladder.
- Other processes may be involved in the pathology of OAB. Positron emission tomography (PET) studies of women with OAB show reduced cerebral perfusion of the frontal lobes. The cause is unknown.

DIFFERENTIAL DIAGNOSIS OF OAB

- Severe stress urinary incontinence (SUI)
- Cystitis or urethritis
- Urethral diverticulum
- Foreign body in bladder
- Bladder carcinoma
- Vesicovaginal fistula

DIAGNOSIS

- When women come into the office with complaints of bladder dysfunction, it is important to delineate whether the symptoms are characteristic of OAB, stress incontinence, mixed incontinence, or overflow incontinence.
- A detailed history should be taken first. Include a detailed history of the onset, course, and current symptoms including frequency of leaking, timing, associated factors (such as urge and stress maneuvers), precipitants, and volume leaked.
- A focused past medical, obstetrical, gynecological, and neurological history is equally important.
- The physician should also ask how these symptoms have affected her quality of life.
- Assessment should be made of the patient's living environment and other social factors that may contribute to or exacerbate incontinence.
- The physician should perform a thorough physical examination.
  - General examination includes heart, lungs, and abdomen with special attention paid to a neurological

examination evaluating sacral nerve intactness: anal sphincter tone, anal wink, and bulbocavernous reflex, as well as motor strength and tone, vibration, and peripheral sensation.
  - Pelvic examination could be significant for signs of hypoestrogenism (vaginal atrophy) or decreased pelvic support (pelvic organ prolapse [POP] or urethral hypermobility). Bimanual examination assesses for masses. Rectal examination looks at rectal tone, mass, or impaction. (see Chap. 5, Evaluation of Pelvic Organ Prolapse)
  - In addition, a cough stress test should look for presence of SUI indicating either genuine SUI or mixed incontinence (see Chap. 6, Evaluation of Urinary Incontinence in the Office and Indications for Referral to a Specialist)
  - A postvoid residual (PVR) should be obtained which could indicate overflow incontinence. PVR less than 50 cc equals adequate emptying while greater than 200 is inadequate (see Chap. 8, Urodynamics II: Tests that Evaluate Bladder Emptying)
- The physician should ask the patient to keep a voiding or bladder diary indicating both times and amount of voiding and fluid intake (timing, amount, and type of fluid). The patient should also record the times and amount of leakage and timing of nocturia (see Chap. 6, Evaluation of Urinary Incontinence in the Office and Indications for Referral to a Specialist)
- Urinalysis and culture is necessary to assess for infection, white blood cells, glucose, or blood—all indicators of possible causes or contributing factors to OAB.
- More advanced testing using urodynamic studies can be used to evaluate both the structure and function of the lower urinary tract.
  - Cystometry is used to assess for the storing ability of the bladder. Previously it was thought that a pressure rise of greater than 15 cm of H_2O was needed to produce symptoms; however, now it is known that even contraction of the detrusor less than 15 cm of H_2O can be symptomatic. These rises in pressure must not be due to bladder compliance issues (see Chap. 7, Urodynamics Part I: Evaluation of Bladder Filling and Storage)
  - Provoking stimuli such as coughing, straining, jogging, or running water should be introduced to induce bladder contraction.
  - During cystometry, bethanechol chloride, a cholinergic agonist, which acts on postganglionic parasympathetic neural cells, can be used to evoke detrusor muscle contractions. While bethanechol has little effect on normal bladders, it will evoke contractions in unstable bladders.
  - Urethral pressure studies are not needed to diagnose OAB, however, the results can aid in choosing

treatment options. These studies, if positive, signal urethral instability. If concomitant urethral instability is found, these patients may respond better to treatment with alpha-sympathomimetic drugs, while patient without urethral instability may be treated better with anticholinergic medications (see Chap. 9, Urodynamics Part III: Evaluation of Urethral Function)

○ Electromyography assesses the function of the striated urethral sphincter muscles. It is useful to document that the detrusor muscle and the sphincter operate in a synchronized order. Also the control of the patient over the urethral sphincter can be documented (see Chap. 10, Electrophysiologic Testing)

MANAGEMENT

• Various methods and combinations of pharmacological and nonpharmacological treatment exist.
• Treatment should be tailored to the needs and desires of the patient, and also to the severity of her problem.
• Minimize foods with high acidity content (from anecdotal evidence). The following are foods with a high acid content (adapted from Food "Ash" pH Chart) listed in order of decreasing acidity. Note: A<<B means A has much lower pH than B (i.e., A is much more acidic than B):
  ○ Vinegar ——————→ pure acid
  ○ Alcohol (hard liquor < beer < wine)
  ○ Meats (pork<beef << chicken < fish)
  ○ Soy sauce
  ○ Fruit juice sweetened with white sugar
  ○ Artificial sweeteners (aspartame)
  ○ Tea < coffee
  ○ Chocolate
  ○ Mustard
  ○ Nuts
  ○ Honey
  ○ Milk ——————→ ≈ neutral
• Gradual elimination of other foods may also improve bladder control (mechanism not clear):
  ○ Soft drinks and carbonated beverages
  ○ Even decaffeinated tea or coffee
  ○ Corn syrup
  ○ Even milk and milk products (despite low acidity rating)
  ○ Highly spiced foods
• *Bladder retraining*, also known as timed voiding, should be integrated into the treatment of the patient. The patient should be educated on the anatomy of the urinary tract system, how it works, and the nature of her bladder dysfunction. She should then receive instruction as to how to "teach" her bladder to function according to the patient's schedule and not to the

bladder's schedule. She learns how to resist the sensation of urgency, postponing voiding until scheduled times. She should keep a daily diary, recording times of voiding and leaking. Timed voiding intervals can vary from 15 minutes to 1 hour, starting out with short intervals and then increasing in length as treatment progresses. The patient should be followed up every 1–2 weeks with total treatment time lasting 6–12 weeks (also see Chap. 13, Conservative Management of Incontinence and Pelvic Organ Prolapse).

• *Biofeedback* trains the patient to recognize otherwise unconscious signals from the bladder. Cystometry is used to show the patient visually what is occurring in the bladder as it fills. As the pressure in the bladder rises, the patient can see this on the graph; she can also see the increased pressure as the detrusor begins to contract. She attempts to inhibit these contractions when they occur. The bladder is filled multiple times during each session (which lasts ≈1 hour). Sessions should be repeated weekly for as many as 8 weeks (also see Chap. 13, Conservative Management of Incontinence and Pelvic Organ Prolapse)

• *Functional electrical stimulation* (FES) is a useful modality for retraining the bladders of patients with both neurogenic and idiopathic detrusor overactivity. During FES, the contractility of the pelvic floor and urethral striated muscles is increased while inhibiting the detrusor. This is done through the pudendal nerve reflex arc. The treatment is limited by the tolerance of the patient for stimulation, either transrectal or intravaginally. Researchers have now found that women are better able to tolerate a shorter period of stimulation (approximately 30 minutes) at the maximal tolerable intensity. This treatment should be performed daily and continued over several weeks. Despite drawbacks, patients have reported significant reduction in symptoms as well as some cures (see Chap. 13, Conservative Management of Incontinence and Pelvic Organ Prolapse)

• *Pharmacologic therapy* is the most commonly used treatment for OAB. Various classes of drugs are effective in treating OAB, although the extent to which they are effective for an individual patient as well as the severity of the side effects are variable. Classes of drugs include anticholinergic agents, tricyclic antidepressants, calcium channel blockers, and others. The major stimulus for bladder contraction is acetylcholine. Anticholinergics agents seek to block this resulting in increased bladder capacity and an increased volume of urine before an involuntary bladder contraction is stimulated. However, because of the lack of selectivity of these drugs for the acetylcholine receptors found primarily in the bladder (M2 and M3), the drugs are associated with many side effects. These include dry mouth and eyes, inhibition of gastrointestinal motility (constipation), gastroesophageal reflux, drowsiness, and cognitive dysfunction. See Chap. 37, Medicines Used in Urogynecology, for a detailed discussion of the following medications used to treat OAB: Oxybutynin, Tolterodine, Trospium, Darifenacin, Solefenacin, Propiverine, Atropine, Propantheline, Imipramine, and Botulinum Toxin.

- Although, *estrogen therapy* for the treatment of OAB has never been investigated in a placebo-controlled trial, it has been shown to improve sensory urgency. This probably occurs by raising the bladder's sensory threshold. However, estrogen therapy does not decrease the number of incontinence episodes (see Chap. 34, The Effect of Estrogen and SERMs on the Lower Urinary Tract and Pelvic Floor)
- *Subtrigonal phenol injection:* Phenol (6%) is injected cystoscopically into the pelvic plexus underneath the bladder trigone. Success rates vary.
- *Hyperbaric bladder distension:* Bladder is distended with water under high pressure to damage sensory nerves by causing ischemia.
- *Sacral neuromodulation* is reserved for those patients who fail first-line therapies described earlier. Patients must meet Medicare criteria in order to be *eligible* for the treatment. These include the following:
  - Failed conservative therapy: There must be documentation of failure of at least two medications and behavioral therapy
  - Symptoms must have been present for at least 12 months and have limited ability to participate in activities or work
  - Test stimulation must be successful
    - Office procedure with patient in prone position
      - Marking the skin → (1) S3 is 3 finger-widths superior and 1 finger-width lateral to tip/end of coccyx, or (2) level of the greater sciatic notch, 1 finger-width lateral to vertical midline (i.e., spinous processes)
      - At skin marking, if spinal needle is held at 60° angle, it will go into S3. However, if needle is held at 90° (perpendicular to skin), it will go into S4 instead
      - Anesthetize skin with 1% lidocaine (you may add bicarb to reduce stinging from acidic lidocaine)
      - Spinal needle is pushed into skin onto sacrum and then slight sliding movement drops needle tip into the third sacral foramen (this is done unilaterally or bilaterally)
      - Needle is connected to a temporary stimulator (10 Hz, 210 ms, 0.5–20 mA)
        - Appropriate response (S3): (1) bellows sign—contraction of levator ani results in deepening of groove between buttocks and inward perineal movement (majority will have this), (2) big

toe-plantar flexion (many do not have this), (3) sensation in vagina or rectum (some do not have this), (4) use of a Foley catheter ring electrode to sense striated urethral sphincter contraction during stimulation may improve ability to detect a proper S3 response.
        - Inappropriate response: S4 = similar to S3 response without motor activity (i.e.. absence of 2); S2 = anal sphincter contraction, calf contraction, foot plantar flexion, foot eversion
      - After S3 response is obtained, thin wire is threaded through spinal needle
      - Wire is secured to the skin with tape
      - An x-ray may be taken to document wire location
      - Patient is instructed to avoid bending, excessive movements, or strenuous activity during testing period (to prevent dislodging wire)
      - Wire is attached to stimulator and it is turned on to an intensity that is sensed but is not painful
    - Successful test stimulation is defined by at least 50% improvement of symptoms in UUI/frequency/urgency patients or PVR < 50 mL in urinary retention patients.
    - Improvement of symptoms is demonstrated by comparing a 3-day voiding diary during the test phase and comparing it to one performed before test stimulation. In the future, longer periods of time (2–4 weeks), minimally invasive techniques, and staged implantation will be done to improve identification of individuals who will respond to sacral neuromodulation.
  - Mechanism of neuromodulation: Not understood but may involve modulation of sacral reflex. Sacral neuromodulation may interfere with afferent nerve activity of bladder, urethra, vulvar structures, or anus. For example, afferent stimulation of the pelvic nerve by anal dilation will block efferent stimulation of the detrusor muscle.
  - Why is S3 important? (1) Is main autonomic innervation of detrusor and (2) Is main somatic innervation of levator ani.
  - Patients with an increased bladder-anal or clitoral-anal reflex have improved outcome with sacral neuromodulation.
  - Indications (disease that is refractory to standard therapy):
    - Urge urinary incontinence (OAB-wet)
    - Frequency-urgency
    - Urinary retention
    - Chronic pelvic pain
    - Interstitial cystitis (IC) (may help)
  - The currently available device is the InterStim Continence Control System which was first introduced in 1981 (Medtronic).

○ Permanent implantation is performed in the prone position in the operating room after successful test stimulation.
  ▪ After administration of prophylactic antibiotics, administration of general anesthesia (without muscle relaxants), proper positioning with pillow and rolls, skin marking, and sterile preparation of skin, a spinal needle is placed to confirm test stimulation then S3 location is marked and needle is removed
  ▪ A 10 cm midline incision (S4 → S1) is made down to lumbodorsal fascia and adequate exposure is developed by undermining the fatty layer
  ▪ Medial insertion of gluteus maximus is incised 1–1.5 cm, the sacrum is reached by sharp and blunt dissection, and the tissue is retracted
  ▪ Foramen is identified and the fascial covering is dilated with a probe
  ▪ The lead is placed as medial as possible. The lead contains four electrode stimulation sites (0, 1, 2, 3). At least two out of four sites must show appropriate S3 response with 0.5–2 mA of current only then lead stylet is removed. If not, lead is slightly tweaked/adjusted
  ▪ When lead is in perfect position, it is fixed to periosteum with permanent sutures distally
  ▪ A transverse buttock incision is made from the implantable pulse generator (IPG). Create a pocket for the IPG by leaving enough fat over muscle and under skin
  ▪ The lead is tunneled to the IPG site
  ▪ A plastic covering is placed over the lead and it is connected to IPG
  ▪ Fascia over the lead is closed; fatty layer over both lead and IPG is closed with absorbable suture; and the skin is closed with subcuticular stitch
  ▪ Patient may go home the same day after prolonged observation ·
  ▪ Device is turned "on" with remote control device on POD# 1 and stimulation intensity may be adjusted by patient
○ Multiple studies have shown successful treatment of urge incontinence, frequency, and urgency with neuromodulation. After successful test stimulation, >50% of patients are dry at 6 months follow-up and another large percentage (15–80%) of patients have shown more than 50% improvement in symptoms (reduced number of voids each day, volume of void, and urgency) and improved quality of life.
○ Treatment of urinary retention also has high cure rates at 6 months (69%).
○ Although sacral neuromodulation is not approved for IC, case series demonstrate improvement in pain and voiding in these patients.

○ Several important caveats: (1) The cure and improvement rates may be falsely elevated because of drop out of patients from the studies which tend to bias toward improvement, (2) some studies show a low cure rate, (3) there is a 15% complication rate, (4) despite these facts, the response rates are impressive and worthwhile to patients who are unhappy and have tried everything else in the book. Most ((70%) patients are satisfied with the procedure. Some achieve dramatic improvements.
○ Complications:
  ▪ Number one complication rate is return to operating room for revision (10–30%)
  ▪ Lead migration
  ▪ Pain at IPG site (less pain if placed in buttock vs. lower abdomen)
  ▪ Decreased efficacy with time. Note: Revision with late failures in patients with good S3 response has poor response
  ▪ Other complications: Change in bowel function, vaginal cramps, anal pain, new pain, leg stimulation, infection, herpes zoster, device failure
• *Surgery* tends to remain a last resort for treatment of OAB.
○ Permanent denervation can be obtained by a selective blockade of the sacral pelvic nerves of S3 using aqueous phenol.
○ Another procedure involves sacral laminectomy followed by a *selective sacral neurectomy* (bilateral transection of S3 root) using electrical stimulation to identify which nerves to transect.
○ Transvaginal partial denervation of the bladder by resection of the inferior hypogastric pelvic nerve plexus is known as the *Ingelman-Sundberg procedure*.
○ *Augmentation cystoplasty* creates a urinary reservoir which the patient must self-catheterize to empty. This is accomplished by bivalving the bladder and then using either a portion of the ileum (ileocystoplasty) or the cecum (ileocecocystoplasty) to create the pouch [see Chap. 41, Urinary Diversion (Reservoirs, Pouches, and Conduits)]

BIBLIOGRAPHY

Abrams P, et al. The standardisation of terminology of lower urinary tract function: report from the standardisation sub-committee of the International Continence Society. *Am J Obstet Gynecol.* 2002;187:1.

Amundsen C, Webster G. Sacral neuromodulation in an older, urge-incontinent population. *Am J Obstet Gynecol.* 2002; 187:6.

Chai TC, Zhang C, Warren JW, et al. Percutaneous sacral third nerve neurostimulation improves symptoms and normalizes urinary BB-EGF levels and antiproliferative activity in patients with interstitial cystitis. *Urology*. 2000;55:643–646.

DuBeau C. *Clinical Presentation and Diagnosis of Urinary Incontinence*. UpToDate. www.uptodate.com.

Fantl JA. Urinary incontinence due to detrusor instability. *Clin Obstet Gynecol*. 1984;27:474–489.

Flesh G. *Detrusor Overactivity in Women*. UpToDate. www.uptodate.com.

Groen J, Bsoch JLHR. Neuromodulation techniques in the treatment of the overactive bladder. *Br J Urol Int*. 2001;87: 723–731.

Hadley EC. Bladder training and related therapies for urinary incontinence in older people. *JAMA*. 1986;256:372–379.

Karram M. Detrusor instability and hyperreflexia. In: Karram M, Walter M. *Urogynecology and Reconstructive Pelvic Surgery*. 2nd ed. St Louis, MO: Mosby 1999 :297–314.

Klausner AP, Steers WD. Research frontiers in the treatment of urinary incontinence. In: Weber A, ed. *Clinical Obstetrics and Gynecology—Incontinence 2004*. Philadelphia, PA: Lippincott William & Wilkins; 2004:104–113.

McLennan MT. Sacral neuromodulation. In: Bent AE, Ostergard DR, et al. *Ostergard's Urogynecology and Pelvic Floor Dysfunction*. 5th ed. Philadelphia, PA: Lippincott William & Wilkins; 2003:325–337.

Montella JM. Management of overactive bladder. In: Bent AE, Ostergard DR, et al. *Ostergard's Urogynecology and Pelvic Floor Dysfunction*. 5th ed. Philadelphia, PA: Lippincott William & Wilkins; 2003:293–306.

Natarajan V, Singh G. Urinary diversion for incontinence in women. *Int Urogynecol J*. 2000;11:180–187.

Opsomer RJ, Klarskov P, Holm-Bentzen M, et al. Long-term results of superselective sacral nerve resection for motor urge incontinence. *Scand J Urol Nephrol*. 1984;18:101–105.

Schmidt RA, Jonas U, Oleson KA, et al. Sacral nerve stimulation or treatment of refractory urinary urge incontinence. *J Urol*. 1999;162:352–357.

Wein A, Rovner E. Pharmacologic management of urinary incontinence in women. *Urol Clin North Am*. 2002;29:3.

Zermann D-H, Weirich T, Wunderlich H, et al. Sacral nerve stimulation for pain relief in interstitial cystitis. *Urol Int*. 2000;65:120–121.

QUESTIONS

Match the statement below with the word that best describes it. Each answer may be used once, more than once, or not at all.

QUESTIONS 1–3

(A) Neurogenic detrusor overactivity
(B) Idiopathic detrusor overactivity
(C) OAB
(D) Sacral neuromodulation
(E) Functional electrical stimulation
(F) Ingelman-Sundberg procedure
(G) S2 response
(H) S3 response
(I) S4 response
(J) Pacemaker cells

1. Formerly referred to as detrusor hyperreflexia
2. A "sucking in" of the perineum and sensation in the vagina
3. Electrical stimulation inside the vagina leads to activation of pudendal reflex arc which inhibit detrusor contractions.
4. A 50-year-old patient presents to you in the office because of symptoms of urgency, frequency, and nocturia. She is healthy but relates two episodes of documented UTI this past year. She applies estrogen cream (Premarin) twice per week to the vagina. She is also taking Detrol LA 4 mg every day. She drinks one cup of coffee each day, a glass of wine at dinner, and eight glasses of cranberry juice each day to prevent bladder infections. Of the following, one of the simplest approaches to reduce her OAB symptoms is by _____
   (A) Discontinuation of coffee
   (B) Discontinuation of wine
   (C) Discontinuation of cranberry juice
   (D) Change to Ditropan XL
   (E) Discontinuation of estrogen cream
5. The *most* common complication of sacral neuromodulation is _____.
   (A) Vaginal cramps
   (B) Rectal pressure
   (C) Infection
   (D) Lead migration
   (E) Device malfunction

ANSWERS

ANSWERS 1–3

1. *(A)*, 2. *(H)*, 3. *(E)*. Neurogenic detrusor overactivity used to be called detrusor hyperreflexia. The inward movement of the perineum, sensations in the rectum or vagina, and plantar flexion of big toe are all S3 responses during testing for sacral neuromodulation. FES involves application of electrical current to the vagina, rectum, or bladder. FES has

produced improvement of symptoms in patients with detrusor overactivity.

4. *(C)*. Cranberry extract has been shown to reduce adherence of *Escherichia coli* to the urothelium and thus effective for UTI prophylaxis. However, cranberry juice purchased at the supermarket is highly acidic and may exacerbate symptoms of OAB (especially when taken in such high quantities). Discontinuation of coffee and wine may help, but neither is as acidic or consumed in as large a quantity as cranberry juice. Local estrogen is helpful for irritative symptoms. Changing to another medication (Detropan XL) is not the simplest of the listed approaches.

5. *(D)*. The three most common complications of sacral neuromodulation are return to OR for revision, lead migration, and pain at implantation site. Rectal pressure is not a complication. It may be experienced when the appropriate S3 response is attained. Vaginal cramps, infection, and device malfunction are less common complications.

25 LOWER URINARY TRACT INFECTIONS AND ASYMPTOMATIC BACTERIURIA

Sam Siddighi

INTRODUCTION

- Urinary tract infections (UTIs) account for 7 million visits to the doctor annually
- UTIs cost to society >$1.5 billion annually
- Fifty percent of women have at least one UTI in their lifetime
- Prevalence of asymptomatic bacteriuria increases with age:
  - 1 year = 1–2%
  - 15–24 years = 2–3% (increase because of sexual activity and pregnancy)
  - 60 years = 15%
  - 80 years = 25–50% (sharp increase because of pelvic organ prolapse, [POP], chronic illness, e.g., diabetes mellitus [DM], hospitalization)
- UTI is the no. 1 infection in hospitalized patients (catheterization or instrumentation is no. 1 contributing factor)
- Commonly confused terms:

- Asymptomatic bacteriuria: Growth of ≥100,000 CFU/mL on urine culture without symptoms
- Bacteriuria: Growth of bacteria in urine regardless of count; even low counts such as 100 CFU/mL may be symptomatic
- Urethritis: Symptoms are indistinguishable from cystitis in women and is uncommon in women
- Chronic UTI: do not use this term
- Reinfection: Most recurrent infections are due to reinfection with a different bacterial strain (although it may be the same species, like *Escherichia coli*), which is usually derived from gastrointestinal (GI) tract bacterial strain (bacterial species)
- Relapse: Repeat infection by same bacterial strain usually within 2 weeks of original UTI; this may occur because of a focus in the upper urinary tract such as a stone or a foreign body (e.g., after anti-incontinence procedure)
- Persistent: Continued presence of same bacteria that was present when she was first diagnosed; bacteria may persist because of (1) inadequate drug dosage, (2) resistance, (3) poor compliance, or (4) some underlying structural or functional problem in the urinary tract (congenital anomaly, stone, foreign body, and so forth) → computed tomography (CT) scan or cystoscopy may need to be done if this is suspected
- Complicated UTI: A UTI that has a higher chance of failing standard therapy. The presence of any of the following conditions makes a UTI complicated:
  - Pregnancy
  - Elderly patient
  - Structural or functional abnormality in urinary tract
  - Multidrug-resistant infection
  - Indwelling catheter present
  - Recent urinary tract instrumentation
  - Hospital-acquired infection
  - Childhood UTI history
  - DM
  - Immunosuppression
  - Patient presenting to urban emergency department (ED)
  - Recent antibiotic use
- The following are risk factors for development of UTI (Table 25-1).
- The following have not been shown to be risk factors for UTI in scientific studies: toilet-paper wiping patterns, delayed voiding, body mass index (BMI), restrictive, nonbreathable underpants, douching, voiding pattern after intercourse (although many women claim this works for them)
- Most UTIs are a result of ascending infections rather than from hematogenous or lymphatic seeding

TABLE 25-1. Risk Factors for Development of UTI

NONMODIFIABLE RISK FACTORS	MODIFIABLE RISK FACTORS
↓ bladder GAGs	Inadequate vaginal pH (acidic) → lactobacilli
↓ bladder mucosa secretory IgAs	Inadequate hydration and regular voiding pattern
↓ Tamm-Horsfall protein (secreted by loop of Henle; prevents bacterial adherence)	Diaphragm use
Blood group B and AB (+Lewis) (are nonsecretors of blood group antigens which may be protective)	High PVR (POP, DM, MS, SC injury, recent anti-incontinence surgery, and so forth)
HLA-A3 phenotype	↓ functional status (dementia, stroke, MIs, CNS disorders)
Bacterial adhesions (P-fimbriae [attachment to cells in kidney], X-adhesin, Type 1 pili [attachment to urethral and bladder cells])	Sexual intercourse (1) frequency, (2) new partner within last year, (3) use of nonoxynol-9 spermicide alters vaginal flora
Bacterial resistance mechanisms (plasmid transfer)	Nosocomial (catheterization or hospitalization)
Proteus enzyme urease	Pregnancy
Enterobactericeae virulence factors (hemolysin, colicin V)	Concomitant fecal incontinence
↓ distance from anus to urethral meatus	Anticholinergic medications

ABBREVIATIONS: CNS, central nervous system; GAGs, glycosaminoglycans; HLA, human leukocyte antigens; IgA, immunoglobulin A; MI, myocardial infarction; MS, multiple sclerosis; PVR, postvoid residual; SC, spinal cord.

- Although the majority (>80%) of uncomplicated UTIs are caused by *E. coli* and other gram-negative bacilli, knowledge of patterns of infection may be useful:
  - *Staphylococcus saprophyticus* is no. 2 most common cause of uncomplicated UTI (10%)
  - *Staphylococcus aureus* (if this is cultured → rule out hematogenous seeding/spread)
  - The most common species found in complicated UTIs are *Proteus, Klebsiella, Pseudomonas, Serratia, Staphylococcus,* and *Enterococcus fecalis* (accounts for 15% of nosocomial infections)
  - *Streptococcus agalactiae* (is associated with DM, immunosuppressed, and catheter use)
  - *Pseudomonas aeruginosa* UTI usually occurs because of instrumentation
  - Anaerobic bacteria do not cause UTIs
  - *Chlamydia trachomatis, Neisseria gonorrhoea, Mycoplasma hominis,* and *Ureaplasma urelyticum* may cause UTI-like symptoms, be misdiagnosed, and go untreated
  - UTI can be caused by other microorganisms besides bacteria (i.e., fungi and viruses)
    - *Candida albicans* (DM, immunosuppressed, catheter use) and *Torulopsis glabrata* (no. 2 most common cause of fungal UTI)
    - Viral UTIs are associated with acute infections and viremia (e.g., mumps and cytomegalovirus [CMV])

ASSESSMENT OF UTI

HISTORY AND PHYSICAL EXAMINATION

- Common symptoms of lower UTI: dysuria, frequency, urgency, hematuria, suprapubic discomfort
  - Frequency + urgency (but lack of dysuria) → maybe OAB
  - Recurrent symptoms of UTI (especially dysuria) but always negative cultures → maybe IC, urethral syndrome, or sensory-urgency syndrome
- Other UTI symptoms which are not usually thought of as UTI but should be incontinence and nocturia
- Common symptoms and signs of upper UTI (pyelonephritis): flank pain, fever, chills, malaise, nausea, vomiting, and costovertebral angle tenderness
- Symptoms of UTI are acute, more severe, and discovered earlier in younger women versus the elderly, who have milder or atypical symptoms and are diagnosed later (several days may elapse)
- Ask patient about the modifiable risk factors listed previously
- Ask patient about vulvovaginal itching, discharge, or recent use of antibiotics as vaginitis or sexually transmitted diseases (STDs) may mimic UTIs
  - If hematuria is a symptom or sign → vulvovaginitis and STD are unlikely (i.e., UTI is more likely)
- If the patient was recently treated for UTI ask her if (1) she completed antibiotic course, (2) urine culture was obtained, and (3) which antibiotic was she prescribed
- During the physical examination make sure to assess the following:
  - Costovertebral angle tenderness → to rule out upper UTI
  - Vaginal discharge → to rule out vaginitis (*Candida, trichomonas*)
  - Vulvovaginal atrophy → increases risk for UTI due to changed vaginal pH and microflora
  - Herpes simplex virus (HSV) lesions (multiple dewdrop on erythematous base) → HSV can cause UTI symptoms; also patient may feel pain when urine contacts lesions during voiding

○ Cervical culture for chlamydia and gonorrhea (maybe even mycoplasma and ureaplasma if symptoms are refractory to treatment) → both may cause dysuria and urethritis or can be asymptomatic

○ ↑ PVR → someone who is postsurgery for stress urinary incontinence (SUI), or who has advanced POP, or who has neurogenic bladder and cannot empty the bladder adequately

TESTING

- Office, dipstick urinalysis
  ○ Is a quick, convenient, and cheap screening test
  ○ Is best when performed in the morning on the first voiding attempt
  ○ Dipstick results are affected by medications/dyes that alter urine color (phenazopyridine, nitrofurantoin, metronidazole, bilirubin, methylene blue, and vitamin B complex)
  ○ Dipstick is falsely positive if the specimen is contaminated
  ○ Although sterile catheterization is the best way to obtain an uncontaminated sample, clean catch of midstream urine may be adequate if the patient has been properly instructed on how to obtain the sample
    ▪ Midstream clean-catch is contraindicated for obese, demented, and patients with physical disabilities
    ▪ Instruction should emphasize finger spreading of labia, proper front to back cleaning of periurethral area with water-moistened gauze, and collection of midstream rather than initial-stream urine while labia are still spread
  ○ Nitrite + → for gram-negative bacteria which convert nitrate to nitrite; high sensitivity (92–100%), low specificity; false negative (1) UTI with bacteria that do not reduce nitrate, e.g., (1) enter, (2) dilute urine, (3) excess dietary vitamin C intake, and (4) patient does not eat foods that contain nitrate therefore bacteria do not have substrate to convert into nitrite
  ○ Leukocyte esterase + → indicates presence of pyuria (white blood cell [WBC]) since leukocytes produced this enzyme; high specificity (94–98%), moderate-high sensitivity (75–95%)
- Laboratory, microscopic urinalysis
  ○ This test is unnecessary in a patient with uncomplicated UTI (empiric treatment is sufficient)
  ○ To avoid contamination of urine specimen with vaginal cells (and thus contamination with vaginal microflora), obtain a carefully catheterized specimen for laboratory, microscopic urinalysis

▪ Presence of ≥10 epithelial cells/hpf may suggest contamination

▪ Since epithelial cells are also found in the urethra and trigone of the bladder, it is possible that contamination with these cells rather than vaginal cells accounted for ≥10 epithelial cell/hpf on microscopic urinalysis

○ If microscopic urinalysis was obtained (for complicated or recurrent patient), then pyuria (≥10 WBC/mL) + microscopic hematuria (≥2–3 red blood cell [RBC]/hpf) + UTI symptoms → empiric therapy

○ Forty to sixty percent of UTIs have microscopic hematuria
  ▪ Presence of microscopic hematuria may rule out vaginitis (as mentioned previously)

○ Presence of casts → upper urinary tract disease

○ Most patients with UTIs have pyuria and at least some bacteriuria

○ Presence of pyuria without any bacteria (aka sterile pyuria) → rule out one of the following:
  ▪ Tuberculosis
  ▪ Interstitial cystitis (IC)
  ▪ Chlamydia
  ▪ Kidney problem (stone or glomerulonephritis)

- Urine culture and antibiotic sensitivity (aka UC&S)
  ○ Indications for urine culture are the following:
    ▪ Diagnosis of lower UTI is questionable
    ▪ Recurrent UTIs (to differentiate persistent vs. reinfection vs. relapse)
    ▪ Complicated UTI (see the criteria mentioned previously)
    ▪ Suspect treatment failure for any reason (e.g., noncompliant patient)
  ○ As seen from the indications, urine culture is not indicated for most UTIs
  ○ The traditional definition of UTI is no longer used (i.e., ≥100,000 CFU/mL)
    ▪ Up to 50% of patients with symptoms of UTI have<100,000 CFU/mL on culture of midstream urine
    ▪ Even a low count of only 100 CFU/mL may present as symptomatic UTI
  ○ Culture of a single organism + symptoms means UTI regardless of CFU/mL
  ○ Currently there are two methods available for urine culture (1) split agar → high accuracy and (2) dip-slides → quicker
  ○ Best way to report a UC&S is to (1) mention organisms besides the predominant organism (i.e., in mixed infections), (2) report bacterial count (CFU/mL) regardless of how low it is, and (3) to perform and report antibiotic sensitivities (since patients with complicated UTIs have resistant bacteria)

○ Patients who do not respond to antibiotic therapy after culture should undergo a (1) CT scan and/or renal ultrasound (U/S) to rule out structural anomalies and/or (2) cystoscopy (especially if risk factors such as smoking, old age, persistent hematuria, risky occupation are present) to rule out bladder cancer

TREATMENT OF UTI

- Adequate hydration is important in treatment; on the other hand, excessive hydration should be avoided as it may dilute antibiotic concentrations. Elderly may restrict their own fluid intake because of incontinence
- Three-day treatment is preferred for uncomplicated, community-acquired UTIs
- Seven-day treatment for uncomplicated UTI has no added benefit
- Single-dose treatment may be less effective and requires that the patient is aware that further treatment may be necessary if the infection persists. However, single dose may be (1) more cost effective, (2) circumvents problem of patient compliance, and (3) fewer adverse effects of antibiotic
- When in doubt about antibiotic dosage and when you are sure about her drug allergies, treat with higher doses because concentrations less than the minimum inhibitory concentration (MIC) can produce resistant organisms
- It is best to take antibiotics before bedtime (so as to minimize experience of adverse effects) and on an empty bladder (so that the maximum amount of excreted drug can accumulate within the bladder mucosa)
- Antibiotics can also be taken every other night or every third night in patients who cannot tolerate its toxicity (renal, hepatic d/o) and still be effective
- Complicated UTIs should be treated for 7–14 days using a fluoroquinolone as initial broad spectrum therapy until culture results return
  ○ Complicated UTI with multidrug-resistant bacteria may require intravenous (IV) antibiotic therapy (e.g., gentamicin)
  ○ If indwelling catheter is present → remove or change it
  ○ UTI with fungus can be treated with oral antifungal + bladder irrigation. It may be necessary to do a blood culture because fungemia has high mortality rate and requires aggressive IV therapy
- The first-line agent for uncomplicated, community-acquired UTI is trimethoprim-sulfamethoxazole (TMP-SMZ) except in high bacterial-resistant states

○ Twenty to forty percent of *E. coli* in California, Minnesota, and Michigan are resistant to TMP-SMZ
○ Ciprofloxacin is a better first-line agent in these states (fluoroquinolones have the highest efficacy, but are more expensive)
- Other common effective agents used for treatment of UTIs include the following:
  ○ Nitrofurantoin monohydrate macrocrystals (Macrobid) → 100 mg bid × 7 days
  ○ TMP-SMZ (Bactrim DS) → (160/800) mg bid
  ○ Ciprofloxacin (Cipro) → 250 mg bid
  ○ Levofloxacin (Levaquin) → 250 mg qd
  ○ Trimethoprim → 100 mg bid (useful for sulfa allergic patients; maintains efficacy)
  ○ Second- or third-generation cephalosporins → for complicated UTIs with contraindications (pregnancy, renal failure [use cephalexin 125 mg or cefixime<400 mg qd])
- The following agents should be avoided for certain types of UTIs:
  ○ Ampicillin and amoxicillin → *E. coli* resistant and high rate of *Candida* vaginitis
  ○ Nitrofurantoin → *Proteus* and *Pseudomonas* resistant
  ○ Cephalosporins → *Enterococcus* resistant
  ○ TMP-SMZ in California, Michigan, Minnesota → *E. coli* resistant
- The most common adverse effect of the most commonly used antibiotics for UTI
  ○ TMP-SMX (Bactrim DS or Septra) → allergic skin reaction from sulfa component
  ○ Nitrofurantoin (Macrobid) → GI problems (abdominal pain, diarrhea, nausea and vomiting)
  ○ Ciprofloxacin (Cipro) → GI problems (abdominal pain, diarrhea, GI bleed, N/V)
- Uncomplicated UTI symptoms usually resolve in 1–2 days after initiation of therapy
- Test-of-cure (TOC) is unnecessary with uncomplicated UTIs (because it is not cost effective, time effective, or prevent pyelonephritis)
- Treatment of recurrent infection
  ○ Recurrent means ≥3 per year or 2 or more in 6 months
  ○ The source for the majority of recurrent infections is fecal flora
  ○ Recurrent infections may have three patterns as defined previously: reinfection, relapse, and persistence
  ○ UC&S is important as many of these bacteria may be drug resistant
  ○ The same antibiotic agents that have been discussed are used, but with a UC&S to guide therapy and for longer duration (7–14 days)
  ○ Prophylaxis or self-treatment regimens (discussed further) may also be tried for recurrent infections

○ Vaginal estrogen cream or estrogen ring is helpful for postmenopausal women; oral estrogen is not helpful

○ Many women use postcoital voiding to prevent recurrence of UTI (however, the literature shows no association between voiding patterns before and after sexual intercourse)

○ Diaphragm users with UTI: (1) use of smaller diaphragm, (2) removal of diaphragm, or (3) change to another type of birth control method

• Phenazopyridine (Pyridium) × 2 days may be given with antibiotic therapy to relieve symptoms of UTI within hours

○ It is a urinary analgesic found over the counter as well as by prescription

○ Warn the patient that it will turn her urine bright orange

UTI PROPHYLAXIS

• Pure cranberry juice may be effective for prophylaxis as it can prevent adherence of bacteria to the urothelium

○ Cranberry juice or extract must be concentrated to be effective (i.e., dilute or cranberry mixtures may not be effective)

• Vaginal estrogen decreases recurrence of UTI in postmenopausal women but

○ Vaginal estrogen works but not as effectively as nitrofurantoin prophylaxis

○ Oral estrogens are not effective in reducing UTIs in postmenopausal women

• Continuous prophylaxis × 6–12 months

○ Use one of the following: Macrobid 100 mg qd, TMP-SMZ 240 mg, trimethoprim 100 mg, norfloxacin 200 mg

○ Use this prophylactic regimen only after treatment regimen is completed and the infection has resolved

○ One may try continuous prophylaxis for 6 months, then follow the patient with regular urine cultures

• Postcoital prophylaxis

○ Is cost effective when compared to continuous prophylaxis

○ Macrobid 100 mg or Septra after each episode of sexual intercourse

• Precoital prophylaxis

○ Application of cetrimide (0.5%) antiseptic cream to periurethral areas before intercourse may help

• Self-start therapy

○ Ciprofloxacin or norfloxacin are the best for this regimen

○ For a patient who refuses continuous prophylaxis

○ The patient must be reliable, compliant, motivated, and have good relationship with the physician

○ Adequate quantity of antibiotics and refills are prescribed

○ Some physicians will also give the patient a dipslide so she may culture her own urine just before starting antibiotics

○ The patient is instructed to start antibiotics and take them for 3 days as soon as she has symptoms of a UTI

○ She must also contact her physician if symptoms do not resolve after 2 days

• Prophylaxis against bacterial endocarditis should only be provided for the following patients 30 minutes before undergoing lower urinary tract procedure (e.g., cystoscopy, urethral dilation, any genitourinary [GU] procedure in presence of a UTI)

○ Conditions requiring prophylaxis (first in the list is high risk and last in the list is moderate risk)

▪ Prosthetic heart valves

▪ History of bacterial endocarditis

▪ Heart has been surgically reconstructed with shunts and conduits

▪ Cyanotic heart diseases (e.g., transposition great arteries [TGA] and tetralogy of Fallot [TOF])

▪ Rheumatic heart disease (i.e., heart valves dysfunctional)

▪ Mitral valve prolapse (MVP) with regurgitation

○ Antibiotic prophylaxis is *not* recommended for

▪ Urethral catheterization (if no UTI is present)

▪ Vaginal hysterectomy

○ Antibiotic regimen for moderate and high risk is as follows:

▪ High risk: Ampicillin 2 g IV + gentamicin 1.5 mg/kd or vancomycin 1 g IV over 2 hours + gentamicin 1.5 mg/kg (for penicillin allergic patients)

▪ Moderate risk: Ampicillin, amoxicillin, or vancomycin only (by mouth [PO] or IV)

ASYMPTOMATIC BACTERIURIA

• Definition: ≥100,000 CFU/mL of a single bacterial species on two consecutive clean-catch urine specimens, but without any symptoms of UTI

• Groups who are at high risk for asymptomatic bacteriuria include

○ ≈50% of institutionalized elderly

○ ≈50% of women performing clean intermittent self-catheterization

○ 100% of patients with long-term indwelling catheters

• Asymptomatic bacteriuria should not be treated with antibiotics except in the following situations:

○ Pregnancy

○ Diabetes (severe and long standing)

- ○ Immunosuppression
- ○ Proteus species found on urine culture
- ○ Those undergoing invasive GU procedures
- Why should asymptomatic bacteriuria not be treated?
  - ○ It is futile because the bacteria will recolonize
  - ○ Treatment may cause replacement of nonadhering, nonvirulent bacteria with virulent strains
  - ○ Treatment may promote development of antibiotic-resistant strains
  - ○ Treatment with antibiotics always has risk of allergic reaction and anaphylaxis
  - ○ Asymptomatic bacteriuria does not lead to renal disease (except in the above situations where it is possible)
- Therefore, do not treat elderly institutionalized patients with asymptomatic bacteriuria with antibiotics because it may by harmful

BIBLIOGRAPHY

Droegemueller W. Infections of the lower genital tract. In: Herbst AL, Mishell DR Jr, Stenchever MA, Droegemueller W, eds. *Comprehensive Gynecology*. 2nd ed. St Louis, MO: Mosby-Year Book; 1992:633–689.

Hoeprich PD, Jordan MC, Ronald AR. *Infectious diseases; a treatise of infectious processes*. 5th ed. Philadelphia, PA: J.B. Lippincott; 1994.

Karram MM, Mallipeddi PK. Anatomy of the lower urinary tract, rectum, and pelvic floor. In: Walters MD, Karram MM. *Urogynecology and Reconstructive Pelvic Surgery*. 2nd ed. St Louis, MO: Mosby; 1999:341–353.

Mayer TR. UTI in the elderly: how to select treatment. *Geriatrics*. 1980;35:67.

Platt R, Polk BF, Murdock B, et al. Mortality associated with nosocomial urinary tract infection. *N Engl J Med.* 1982;307:736.

Powers RD. New directions in the diagnosis and therapy of urinary tract infections. *Am J Obstet Gynecol.* 1991;164:1387–1389.

Raz R, Stamm WE. A controlled trial of intravaginal estriol in postmenopausal women with recurrent urinary tract infections. *N Engl J Med.* 1993;329:753.

Schaeffer AJ. Recurrent urinary tract infections in women. Pathogenesis and management. *Postgrad Med.* 1987;81:51.

Stamey TA, Condy M, Mihara G. Prophylactive efficacy of nitrofurantoin macrocrystals and trimethoprim-sulfamethoxazole in urinary tract infections: biologic effects on the vaginal and rectal flora. *N Engl J Med.* 1977;296:780.

Stamm WE, Counts GW, McKevitt M, et al. Urinary prophylaxis with trimethoprim and trimethoprim-sulfamethoxazole: efficacy, influence on the natural history of recurrent bacteriuria, and cost control. *Rev Infect Dis.* 1982;4:450.

Stamm WE, Counts GW, Running KR, et al. Diagnosis of coliform infection in acutely dysuric women. *N Engl J Med.* 1982;307:463.

Wallmark G, Arremark I, Telander B. *Staphylococcus saprophyticus*: a frequent cause of acute urinary tract infection among female outpatients. *J Infect Dis.* 1978;138:791.

QUESTIONS

QUESTIONS 1–3

For each of the clinical scenarios described below, choose the best diagnosis above. Each answer choice may be used once, more than once, or not at all.

- (A) Asymptomatic bacteriuria
- (B) Cystitis
- (C) Acute urethritis
- (D) Chronic urethritis
- (E) Pyelonephritis

1. A 25-year-old sexually active woman who continues to have urgency and frequency after antibiotic therapy. She has pyuria on dipstick urinalysis and a clean-catch culture shows more than 10^2 CFU/mL

2. A 20-year-old with symptoms of UTI and whose urine culture shows <10^2 CFU/mL

3. A 23-year-old woman who is discovered to have 10^5 CFU/mL on a clean-catch midstream urine during her first prenatal visit.

4. In Alabama, a 20-year-old sexually active, nulligravid college student is seen for symptoms of UTI. The most cost-effective treatment is _____.

- (A) Ciprofloxacin
- (B) Ampicillin
- (C) Cephalexin
- (D) Macrodantin
- (E) Trimethoprim-sulfamethoxazole

ANSWERS

ANSWERS 1–3

1. *(B)*, 2. *(C)*, 3. *(A)*. In symptomatic patients, 10^2 CFU/mL is the threshold for diagnosing cystitis. A culture showing less than the above with symptoms is considered acute urethritis. Chronic urethritis or urethral syndrome is diagnosed after 3 months of symptoms.

In question 3 there is no mention of symptoms yet the urine culture shows 10^5 CFU/mL. This is asymptomatic bacteriuria.

4. *(E)*. TMP-SMZ is the best choice because it has low resistance, is inexpensive, and has minimal side effects. In certain states such as California, 20–40% of *E. coli* are resistant to TMP-SMZ, so there ciprofloxacin is

preferred. However, Cipro is expensive. *E. coli* has high resistance to ampicillin. Cephalexin and Macrodantin may be effective but they require 7 days of treatment, which increases the cost.

26 INTERSTITIAL CYSTITIS, URETHRAL SYNDROME, AND SENSORY URGENCY-FREQUENCY SYNDROME

Dean E. Dagermangy

INTERSTITIAL CYSTITIS

INTRODUCTION

- The term interstitial cystitis (IC) was first used by Skene in 1887 to describe an inflammatory pattern within the bladder mucosa. In 1918, Hunner described what he saw on cystoscopy as red, bleeding areas of the bladder wall, eventually termed Hunner's ulcers. As cystoscopy advanced, these ulcer-like regions were later described as petechial hemorrhages by Hand in 1949 and given the term glomerulations by Walsh in 1978. It was not until Messing and Stamey, however, that the diagnosis shifted away from cystoscopic findings (secondary to low specificity) and toward symptom-based criteria.
- Also known as painful bladder syndrome, IC is a clinical diagnosis characterized by the triad of urinary frequency and urgency, pelvic pain, and sterile urine cultures. The exact etiology is unclear but it is believed to be multifactorial.
- Despite extensive research, little clinician uniformity exists on diagnostic criteria and treatment modalities. As such, diagnosis is often based on eliminating other possible disorders and treatment is usually empiric in nature.
- Overall, considered by many to be underdiagnosed, undertreated, and poorly understood. There is essentially no cure for the condition and the disease is considered to be chronic.

EPIDEMIOLOGY

- Believed to have a diagnostic female:male ratio of about 10:1.
- Studies of prevalence rates in the United States range from 60 to 865 per 100,000.

- Europe and Japan report prevalence rates of 18/100,000 and 4/100,000, respectively.
- It is estimated that between 700,000 and 1,000,000 people in the United States currently have IC.
- The median age of onset of IC is in the early 40s with an age range of between 30 to 70.
- Cases in children as young as 2 years old have been reported.
- Greater than 90% of patients are believed to be Caucasian.
- Patients with IC have been found to have a higher prevalence of first-degree relatives with IC than compared to the general population. Some studies have suggested a higher occurrence in twins.
- Some researchers have reported that patients with IC have a higher incidence of inflammatory bowel disease, Sjögren's syndrome, systemic lupus erythematosus (SLE), irritable bowel syndrome, fibromyalgia, and skin allergy diseases.
- There is a significant socioeconomic burden on patients diagnosed with IC. Depressive and anxiety symptoms are common and the medical costs associated with IC in the United States are believed to be more than $100 million annually.

ETIOLOGY AND PATHOGENESIS

- Several causes have been suggested, such as infection (because of symptoms and female predominance), an allergic reaction (because of often abrupt onset and probable mast cell involvement), an autoimmune response (based on the higher incidence of coexistent disorders such as SLE, Sjögren's syndrome, and fibromyalgia), epithelial dysfunction (as seen on cystoscopic evaluation), and inherited susceptibility (sighting associations among first-degree relatives and twins).
- The most recent theory centers on the idea that IC stems from a deficiency in the glycosaminoglycan (GAG) layer of the bladder epithelium. Such a defect is postulated to allow certain substances in the urine (e.g., chemicals, toxins, and bacteria) to cause irritation of the bladder wall and the subsequent symptoms. Many treatment modalities center on this belief.
- Several researchers have proposed that this irritation leads to an increase in activation of mast cells. Once mast cells are activated, a variety of substances are released (e.g., histamine, serotonin, substance P, proteases, tumor necrosis factor-alpha [TNF-alpha], and a host of cytokines). Sensory nerves subsequently become more sensitive, an inflammatory process is initiated, and immune tissue damage can initiate.
- Patients with IC have been found to have an increased number of submucosal mast cells. This increase in number has been proposed to be due to a

progesterone/estrogen imbalance, which some argue is why the disease is more prevalent in women.

DIAGNOSIS AND CLINICAL PRESENTATION

- *IC is a diagnosis of exclusion and is primarily based on a constellation of symptoms* rather than cystoscopic or histological-pathological findings. There is no pathognomonic microscopic picture consistent with IC and there is great histological variation of bladder wall tissue among patients and even among different samples taken from the same patient over time. Further, the severity of clinical symptoms does not correlate with the severity of pathological findings.
- Nevertheless, patients may present with symptoms of low pelvic pain, urgency, frequency, nocturia, and bladder pressure which is relieved by voiding.
- Some of the major inconsistent findings include mast cell infiltration, lymphocytic and perineural infiltrates, submucosal ulcerations and hemorrhage (Hunner's ulcers), thinning epithelium, granulation tissue, hypervascular mucosa, linear scarring, and even normal epithelial tissue.
- Urinalysis and urine culture and antibiotic sensitivity test to exclude urinary tract infection (UTI) and hematuria.
- Urodynamic testing reveals no detrusor overactivity, low bladder capacity (maximum bladder capacity <350 mL), and compliance (<130 mL/cm H_2O).
- Whether *cystoscopy with hydrostatic bladder dilation* is required for diagnosis (Hunner's ulcers in 10% of patients and pinpoint petechial hemorrhages [glomerulations] in three-fourth of bladder) is controversial, as negative findings do not rule out the diagnosis; *its use is to primarily rule out other differential diagnoses.* Several authors have suggested that hydrodistention of the bladder can be temporarily therapeutic in nature.
- Bladder biopsy during cystoscopy is useful to rule out other causes such as cancer, tuberculosis, and eosinophilic cystitis.
- Another diagnostic tool is the potassium sensitivity test, which measures the bladder wall's epithelial permeability. The test is performed by comparing the sensation response of intravesical instillation of water (no discomfort) to that of a potassium chloride solution (causing pain in IC patients). The test is positive in 75–80% of patients who actually have IC. A potassium solution of 40 mEq in 100 cc is instilled from or height of 80–100 cm above the symphysis and is kept for 5 minutes.
- Pelvic examination usually reveals a tender bladder base, although there are no pathognomonic physical examination findings.

- National Institute of Diabetes and Digestive and Kidney Diseases (NIDDK) criteria for diagnosis of IC:
  - Inclusion criteria
    1) Glomerulations in 3 quadrants of bladder and ≥10 glomerulations per quadrant or Humen ulcer
    2) Symptoms of pain associated with bladder or urgency
  - Exclusion criteria
    1) Bladder capacity >350 mL
    2) Intense urgency wrt >150 mL in bladder
    3) Bladder contractors on cystometry
    4) Duration of symptoms <9 months
    5) Nocturia
    6) Symptoms relieved by antibiotics, anticholinergics, or antispasmodics
    7) Void <8 times per day
    8) Cystitis diagnosed within 3 months
    9) Bladder stones
- The pain is classically relieved by voiding, but returns as the bladder refills. A persistent urge to void after the bladder is emptied is also characteristic, and patients commonly void repetitively throughout the day.
- The onset of symptoms is often acute and the syndrome can go through periods of exacerbation and remission.
- Many studies have remarked that symptoms are often worse immediately before menses.
- Symptoms can frequently be made worse after consuming acidic foods such as caffeine, alcohol, carbonated drinks, citrus fruits or fruit drinks, tomatoes and tomato products, and chocolate. (See Chap. 24 list of acidic foods)
- Dyspareunia is often present, although incontinence of urine is not.
- Urinalysis may indicate signs of slight hematuria; however, urine culture is always negative for infection.
- As a careful history is crucial to diagnosis, a variety of symptom indices have been developed: the O'Leary-Sant questionnaire and problem index, the University of Wisconsin IC scale, and the pain urgency and frequency questionnaire.
- A voiding diary is also imperative.

TREATMENT

- The goal is not cure but rather improvement of symptoms.
- Currently there is not one standard, accepted therapy for the treatment of IC. The only two Food and Drug Administration (FDA)-approved treatments are oral pentosan polysulfate sodium (PPS or Elmiron) and bladder instillation with dimethyl sulfoxide (DMSO).
- The most widely accepted management is to use a multimodal approach of supportive social measures, oral medications, intravesical pharmacological treatment, and interventional therapy.

- Nonpharmacological, conservative therapy
  - Supportive therapy includes aspects such as patient education, diet, behavioral therapy, stress and anxiety reduction, and exercise.
  - Diet restrictions include caloric reductions as well as limitations of smoking, alcoholic beverages, carbonated drinks, caffeine, citrus fruits, citrus drinks, tomatoes and tomato products, vinegar, and foods high in arylalkylamines (e.g., bananas, cheese, chocolate, aspartame, nuts, raisins, onions, sour cream, and yogurt). Tryptophan is an arylalkylamine, and two of its metabolites—3-hydroxykynurenine and hydroxyanthranilic acid—have been found to cause disruption of the GAG layer in the bladder.
  - Behavioral therapy centers on urge inhibition in order to lengthen voiding intervals (i.e., timed voiding, bladder retraining), and has been found to provide some relief in at least 50% of patients.
- Oral medications
  - Tricyclic antidepressants (e.g., *amitriptyline*, doxepin, and imipramine) are believed to improve pain symptoms through their anticholinergic, antihistamine, and serotonin/noradrenaline inhibitory reuptake mechanisms.
  - Antihistamines such as *hydroxyzine*, an H_1-receptor antagonist, are believed to exert their effect through the inhibition of mast cell activation by substance P and thereby block both the nerve sensitization and proinflammatory processes. It also has sedative and anxiolytic effects which may help.
  - PPS (Elmiron) functions by replacing the GAG layer that is often disrupted in patients with IC, thereby forming a barrier to irritating elements. Current recommendations are to treat patients with PPS for a minimum of 6 months. Adverse effects (4%) are diarrhea, nausea, headache, and alopecia.
  - Many clinicians prescribe a cocktail of medicines (e.g. amitriptyline, hydroxyzine, and PPS)
  - Both gabapentin and opiates are used intermittently for analgesic control and should only be considered as adjuvant therapy for severe pelvic pain.
  - Immunomodulators (e.g., cyclosporine, etanercept, infliximab, interleukin [IL]-10, imatinib, and methotrexate) have been proposed as treatments, but little widespread data exist on their utility.
- Intravesical therapy
  - DMSO infusion is believed to exert its effect through anti-inflammatory, muscle relaxant, and analgesic properties. It may desensitize nerves as well as increase bladder capacity. It is effective in 90% of patients.
  - Intravesical treatment with Bacille Calmette Guérin (BCG, an attenuated strain of *Mycobacterium bovis*) is thought to work by immunomodulation, although its exact mechanism of action is unknown.
  - Similarly, the exact mechanism of hyaluronic acid (and other infused GAGs such as heparin and chondroitin sulfate) is also unknown, but has been suggested to work in a similar fashion as oral PPS (i.e., proteoglycan layer replacement).
  - Resiniferatoxin is an extremely potent vanilloid receptor agonist that elicits relief through bladder afferent nerve desensitization.
  - Many clinicians have supported the idea of infusing a cocktail of the various substances (described earlier) in order to achieve maximum benefit to the patient for the greatest length of time.
- Interventional therapies
  - Hydrodistention, considered one of the mainstays of treatment in children, is believed to provide relief through both ischemia of the submucosal nerve plexus and by extensive mast cell degranulation (thereby exhausting inflammatory mediators). Relief of symptoms, however, is usually transient and only lasting several months.
  - The efficacy of sacral neuromodulation and nerve stimulation modalities has only recently been evaluated in a handful of small studies, and has shown some benefit.
  - Concerning surgical measures, it is widely accepted that such a therapeutic tool should only be used as a last resort. Options include removing Hunner's ulcers (if present) with a laser (fulguration), resection of bladder trigone with augmentation cystoplasty (bladder augmentation using bowel), or complete cystectomy with urinary diversion. Surgical success rates vary widely from 25 to 100%.

CONCLUSION

- Although researchers have been studying IC since it was first termed by Skene in 1887, little progress has essentially been made, primarily because its etiology and pathogenesis still remain a mystery.
- Although many theories have been postulated, clinicians are still uncertain as to how many of the pharmacological treatments work and why the pathological and histological findings do not correlate with symptom severity.
- Both clinicians and patients need to understand that, as of now, this condition is considered chronic by most authorities and requires patience and a willingness to most often explore several different treatment modalities.

URETHRAL SYNDROME

INTRODUCTION

- Urethral syndrome was initially described by Powell in 1949. In 1965, a group of physicians in New Zealand led by Gallagher used the term to classify a group of women with urinary symptoms that could not be attributed to an infection.

- There is great discrepancy in the literature, both amongst urogynecologists and between urologists and urogynecologists, of how to define urethral syndrome and even if such a condition exists. Recent authors have suggested that the condition is one of exclusion and that it should more appropriately be categorized under IC rather than hold its own domain.
- Often referred to as other entities (e.g., frequency dysuria syndrome and female prostatitis), urethral syndrome is most commonly described as urinary urgency, frequency, and dysuria; although many other urinary symptoms may be present.

EPIDEMIOLOGY AND ETIOLOGY

- The incidence of urethral syndrome is unknown due to a lack of epidemiological data. It is thought to occur most commonly in Caucasian women of reproductive age.
- Similar to IC, many patients have a coexistent depression or anxiety disorder believed to be secondary to the chronic discomfort.
- Numerous theories have been suggested concerning the etiology of the syndrome, including acute or chronic urethritis, hypoestrogenic (senile) urethritis, urethral stenosis or obstruction, urethral spasm, psychogenic factors, allergies, neurological disorder sequela, trauma, and noxious agents (e.g., environmental chemicals such as soaps and contraceptive gels), hormonal imbalances, and anatomical abnormalities. As with IC, there is usually no evidence of active bacterial infection.

DIAGNOSIS AND CLINICAL PRESENTATION

- Similar to IC, urethral syndrome is a diagnosis of exclusion. It is imperative to rule out diagnoses such as urethral stones, bladder cancer, urethral diverticula, urethral prolapse, cystocele, condyloma, and herpes.
- The most common presenting symptoms are frequency, urgency, and dysuria. Other complaints, however, may also be present including suprapubic pain, dyspareunia, urge or stress incontinence, urinary hesitancy and significant postvoid residual, malaise, and back pain. Nocturia, however, is classically absent with urethral syndrome (but normally present with IC).
- A urinalysis with a urine culture is invariably negative, and the physical assessment should include an adnexal examination, a pelvic and rectal examination, a neurological examination, urethral calibration, urethroscopy, and a cystometrogram.

TREATMENT

- Effective treatment is a function of likely etiology, and the goal of treatment should be aimed at symptom relief. Where appropriate, most authors suggest a conservative approach rather than invasive procedures secondary to the fact that urethral syndrome has a very high rate of spontaneous remission.
- Examples of some of the many proposed treatment possibilities include urethral massage, steroids or even fulguration for chronic urethritis, estrogen creams in the case of hypoestrogenic urethritis, the breaking of a constrictive ring and dilation for urethral stenosis, diazepam, skeletal muscle relaxants, tricyclic antidepressants, anticholinergics and alpha-adrenergic antagonists to treat urethral spasm or pain symptoms, electrical stimulation to counter neurogenic causes, diet modification, and psychotherapy and biofeedback to help with psychogenic causes or in instances where an etiological agent cannot be blamed.

CONCLUSION

- Because of the discrepancy around both the existence of urethral syndrome and what the proper definition is, there remain many unanswered questions pertaining to almost all aspects of the condition. To add to the dilemma, few articles have even been published on urethral syndrome since the late 1990s.
- As with IC, clinicians and patients must be willing to use numerous, varying and occasionally simultaneous treatment modalities. Although the problem may be chronic in nature, patients can be encouraged by the fact that cure rates appear to be high.

SENSORY URGENCY-FREQUENCY SYNDROME

OVERVIEW

- Many authors have suggested that the sensory urgency-frequency syndrome is either synonymous with or a component of IC and should therefore be categorized as such. As with the urethral syndrome, however, there exist historical differences between IC and the sensory urgency-frequency syndrome.
- The syndrome is an urodynamic diagnosis that can be defined as one of the two broad types of dysfunctional voiding, in which *voiding urgency occurs at low bladder filling volumes in the absence of detrusor overactivity.* Although the bladder has become hypersensitive, these patients technically do not have a fear of leakage.

The presence of urge incontinence (and the worry of impending incontinence) should suggest the diagnosis of detrusor overactivity rather than sensory urgency-frequency syndrome.

- Little research exists concerning the incidence and epidemiology of this condition, although many believe its etiology to be psychological in origin and thus a learned behavior (e.g., improper toilet training).

- As the syndrome is classically a urodynamic diagnosis, evaluation is best made via a cystometric study followed by cystoscopy to rule out any intravesical pathology.

- Treatment modalities center on bladder retraining, psychotherapy, biofeedback, and sacral nerve electrical stimulation.

BIBLIOGRAPHY

Chancellor MB, Yoshimura N. Treatment of interstitial cystitis. *Urology.* 2004;63(Suppl 3a):85–92.

Dell JR, Parsons CL. Multimodal therapy for interstitial cystitis. *J Reprod Med.* 2004;49:243–252.

Gittes RF. Female prostatitis. *Urol Clin North Am.* 2002;29: 613–616.

Hanno PM. Interstitial cystitis and related disorders. In: Walsh PC, Retik AB, Vaughan ED, et al., eds. *Campbell's Urology.* Philadelphia, PA: WB Saunders; 2002:631–670.

Karram MM. Frequency, urgency, and painful bladder syndromes. In: Walters MD, Karram MM, eds. *Clinical Urogynecology.* St. Louis, MO: Mosby; 1993:285–298.

Liss PE, Aspevall O, Karlsson D, et al. Terms used to describe urinary tract infections—the importance of conceptual clarification. *APMIS.* 2003;111:291–299.

Lukban JC, Whitmore KE, Sant GR. Current management of interstitial cystitis. *Urol Clin North Am.* 2002;29:649–660.

Mattox TF. Interstitial cystitis in adolescents and children: a review. *J Pediatr Adolesc Gynecol.* 2004;17:7–11.

Metts JF. Interstitial cystitis: urgency and frequency syndrome. *Am Fam Physician.* 2001;64(7):1199–1206.

Nickel JC. Interstitial cystitis: a chronic pelvic pain syndrome. *Med Clin North Am* 2004;88:467–481.

Parsons CL, Tatsis V. Prevalence of interstitial cystitis in young women. *Urology.* 2004;64(5):866–870.

Scotti RJ, Ostergard DR. Urethral syndrome. In: Ostergard DR, Bent AE, eds. *Urogynecology and Urodynamics: Theory and Practice.* Baltimore, MD: Williams & Wilkins; 1996:339–359.

Theoharides TC, Sant GR. Immunomodulators for the treatment of interstitial cystitis. *Urology.* 2005;65:633–638.

Wall LL, Norton PA, DeLancey JOL. Sensory disorders of the bladder and urethra: frequency/urgency/dysuria/bladder pain. In: Wall LL, Norton PA, Delaresy JOL. *Practical Urogynecology.* Baltimore, MD: Williams & Wilkins; 1993:255–273.

Wesselmann U, Burnett AL, Heinberg LJ. The urogenital and rectal pain syndromes. *Pain.* 1997;73:269–294.

QUESTIONS

1. A 43-year-old nulligravid woman is referred to the office from the emergency department after presenting with a 3-month history of lower pelvic pain and persistent urinary frequency and urgency with frequent nocturia. The patient notes that her diffuse pelvic pain is usually relieved with voiding but is often triggered by sexual intercourse. She reports a medical history significant for SLE, recent onset of generalized anxiety disorder, and numerous food allergies. A review of a urine culture taken in the emergency department 1 week ago shows no abnormal findings. This patient's expanded medical and social history would most likely contain which of the following:
   (A) a history of sexual abuse as a child
   (B) recent trauma to the pelvic area secondary to a motor vehicle accident
   (C) a sister with a recent onset of similar symptoms
   (D) worsening of symptoms immediately after the end of her menses
   (E) improvement of symptoms after the consumption of orange juice

2. A 61-year-old woman, gravida 3, para 3, is referred from her general gynecologist with a presumptive diagnosis of IC. This diagnosis was based on her constellation of symptoms, her urinary history per a voiding diary, and normal urinalysis and culture. The patient is being referred because her symptoms have persisted despite pharmacological treatment with alpha-adrenergic antagonists and oral steroids. A cystoscopic evaluation under anesthesia reveals submucosal ulcerations and the pathology report from an intravesical biopsy indicates extensive mast cell infiltration. The most appropriate mode of treatment at this time is which of the following:
   (A) increase the dosage of the alpha-adrenergic antagonists and steroids
   (B) complete cystectomy with urinary diversion
   (C) reassurance and referral to a psychologist for behavioral and psychotherapy
   (D) hydrodistention and oral treatment with PPS
   (E) broad-spectrum antibiotic coverage

3. A 24-year-old female presents to the emergency department with a recent onset of severe dysuria, frequency, urgency, and episodes of urge incontinence. She also notes recent dyspareunia, yet denies any episodes of nocturia. A urinalysis per a catheter specimen shows no abnormalities. The nurse mentions in passing, however, that the patient had just voided prior to the placement of

the catheter, and that the postvoid residual seemed to be abnormally high. On physical examination, the patient has significant suprapubic tenderness. Given the patient's clinical presentation, which of the following circumstances would suggest that this patient has the urethral syndrome rather than IC:

(A) onset of severe urinary frequency and urgency

(B) denial of any episodes of nocturia

(C) a normal urinalysis

(D) suprapubic tenderness on physical examination

(E) recent dyspareunia

4. An 18-year-old woman with urethral syndrome is seen in clinic for her regularly scheduled appointment. She was first diagnosed with the condition several months ago when she unexpectedly started having suprapubic pain, dyspareunia, persistent urinary frequency problems, and intermittent incontinence. Numerous treatment strategies have been implemented without success, including urethral massage, estrogen creams, tricyclic antidepressants, and electrical stimulation. She has been told by a family friend that her condition is serious and that she will likely require extensive surgery. Which of the following responses concerning her prognosis is most appropriate in this situation:

(A) Her friend is correct and the need for reconstructive surgery is almost certain.

(B) Most patients with urethral syndrome require lifelong medication-based therapy.

(C) There is a 1 in 25 risk that she could develop bladder cancer in the near future.

(D) There is a high probability that her children will have a similar problem.

(E) The majority of patients with urethral syndrome have a spontaneous remission.

5. A 55-year-old nulligravid woman is attending her yearly gynecological office visit when she mentions that lately she needs to void much more often during the day than in past years. She notes that she constantly feels the need to urinate, although she denies any symptoms of dysuria, dyspareunia, incontinence, or suprapubic pain. On further questioning, the patient states that although she persistently feels the need to urinate, she does not fear incontinence. The patient's physical examination is unremarkable and a urinalysis in the office shows no evidence of a UTI. Assuming sensory urgency-frequency syndrome as one of the differential diagnoses, which of the following is the best confirmatory study or test:

(A) a cystometric urodynamic study followed by cystoscopy

(B) successful treatment with anticholinergics and alpha-adrenergic antagonists

(C) a urine electrolyte panel

(D) postvoid urinary residual volumes

(E) intravesicular instillation of potassium chloride

ANSWERS

1. *(C).* Many epidemiological studies have shown that patients with IC often have a first-degree relative with similar symptoms. Concerning choice A, there is no evidence that sexual abuse as a child is an etiological agent for IC. Further, recent trauma to the pelvic area, choice B, would likely suggest a diagnosis of urethral syndrome rather than IC. Choice D is incorrect because IC is usually worse immediately before menses rather than immediately after. This finding has led some authors to suggest that hormonal fluctuations may be one of the etiological agents. The opposite of choice E is correct, that is, the consumption of citrus fruits and drinks, such as orange juice, has a tendency to exacerbate rather than improve symptoms of IC.

2. *(D).* Treatment of IC requires a multimodal approach that is individualized for each patient. This patient has evidence of a disrupted GAG layer and mast cell infiltration. Hydrodistention has been shown to help with mast cell infiltration by causing extensive degranulation. Similarly, oral PPS is an FDA-approved medication which will promote the growth of the intravesical GAG layer. Choice A is incorrect because alpha-adrenergic antagonists and steroids have shown to provide little relief for patients with IC and would be more suitable for a patient with the urethral syndrome. Complete cystectomy and urinary diversion, choice B, is highly controversial and is considered a last resort if all treatment modalities fail. Choice C, reassurance and psychological treatment, while perhaps helpful, is not the most appropriate step in treating this patient's symptoms and would be most helpful in treating sensory urgency-frequency syndrome. Choice E, antibiotic treatment, is also not appropriate, as this patient had a negative urine culture.

3. *(B).* The patient presents with many symptoms that could lead to a diagnosis of either IC or the urethral syndrome. Severe urinary frequency and urgency, choice A, a normal urinalysis, choice C, suprapubic

tenderness, choice D, and recent dyspareunia, choice E, are all symptoms that can be present in both IC and the urethral syndrome. Nocturia, however, is often present in patients with IC but is classically absent in patients with the urethral syndrome, choice B. The fact that this patient has both incontinence of urine and a high postvoid residual is also suggestive of the urethral syndrome rather than IC.

4. *(E)*. Unlike IC, which can often be chronic in nature, urethral syndrome has been shown to have a very high rate of spontaneous remission. The opposite of choice A is correct, that is, invasive treatments are not recommended for urethral syndrome. Although treating the symptoms of urethral syndrome is often based on trial and error, these patients do not usually require lifelong medications (choice B). Further, there are no data that suggest such patients have a higher incidence of bladder cancer (choice C). Similarly, there is not any evidence that the condition has a heritable component (choice D); this is in contrast to IC.

5. *(A)*. Due to the fact that the syndrome is an urodynamic diagnosis, evaluation is best made via a cystometric study. Anticholinergics and alpha-adrenergic antagonists are used to treat the urethral syndrome, not sensory urgency-frequency syndrome (choice B). Choice C is incorrect because abnormal urine electrolyte results are not coincident with this syndrome and should suggest alternative differential diagnoses. Similarly, abnormal postvoid residual volumes would instead suggest the urethral syndrome (choice D). Concerning choice E, intravesicular instillation of potassium chloride is a method of diagnosing IC.

27 BYPASS MECHANISMS: VESICOVAGINAL, URETHEROVAGINAL, AND URETEROVAGINAL FISTULAS

Bogdan A. Grigorescu

DEFINITION

• A fistula is an abnormal communication between two epithelial-lined organs. A urogenital fistula is an abnormal communication between the vagina and the urethra, bladder, uterus, or ureters.

INCIDENCE

• In the developing nations, the true incidence of urinary fistula is unknown. In 1989, the WHO estimated that there are >2 million women worldwide affected by obstetric fistulas (mainly vesicovaginal and rectovaginal fistulas or both) and >100,000 new cases are reported each year. However, these data are based on women seeking treatment → gross underestimate. Most women with fistulas live in remote rural areas and do not have access to curative services.

• In contrast to the developing nations, in the developed countries, most genitourinary fistulas develop following pelvic surgery.

• In a study on the incidence of urinary tract injuries, the total incidence of *ureteral injury* after 62,379 hysterectomies → 0.1% (1.39% after laparoscopic hysterectomy, 0.04% after total abdominal hysterectomy, 0.03% after supracervical abdominal, and 0.02% after vaginal hysterectomy surgery). The incidence of *bladder injury* → 0.13%. The incidence of vesicovaginal fistulas → 0.08% after all hysterectomies (0.22% after laparoscopic hysterectomy, 0.1% after total abdominal hysterectomy, 0.02% after vaginal hysterectomy, and 0% after supracervical hysterectomy). The rate of fistula development following radical hysterectomy or radiation for gynecological malignancies → between 1% and 4%, while the incidence of fistula formation after pelvic exenteration → around 10%.

ETIOLOGY

• In developing countries, over 90% of fistulas → from obstetrical causes—obstructed labor, ↓ access to obstetrical care. In obstructed labor, the ↑ compression of tissues of the genital tract between the fetal head and the bony pelvis lead to tissue necrosis, followed by sloughing, perforation, and fistula formation. Traditional surgical practices → large percentage of genitourinary fistulas among the Hausa, Fulani, and Kanuri tribes of northern Nigeria. Thus, gishiri (a traditional cut made with a razor blade or knife through the vaginal introitus) and circumcision (especially pharaonic incision, the removal of labia minora, most of labia majora, mons pubis, and often the clitoris) → formation of vesicovaginal and rectovaginal fistulas.

• In the developed countries, >70% of cases → from direct injury to the lower urinary tract during pelvic surgery, (e.g., hysterectomy).

• Obstructed labor is the most common cause of urethrovaginal fistula in the developing nations, whereas elective urethral and vaginal procedures associated with urethral injury (e.g., urethral diverticulum excision, plication of the urethra, and vaginal and retropubic needle suspension) are the most common causes of urethrovaginal fistulas in the United States.

- Other causes of urogenital fistulas include cancer affecting the lower genital tract, pelvic radiation, endometriosis, genital tract infection, foreign body (e.g., pessary) and rarely congenital urinary fistula (e.g., ectopic ureter and urethral duplication).

- Radiation therapy with ionizing radiation → in obliterative endarteritis and can lead to fistula formation months to years after treatment of the underlying malignancy. Malignancy by itself → genitourinary fistula formation. Cervical, vaginal, and rectal cancers are the most frequent malignancies associated with fistula formation. However, urothelial tumors are rarely associated with fistula formation, short of treatment with radiation therapy or surgery.

CLASSIFICATION

- There is no internationally accepted classification of urogenital fistulas. A classification based on anatomical site and the organs affected is described here:
- Simple—vesicovaginal, ureterovaginal, urethrovaginal
- Complex—urethrovesicovaginal, vesicouterine, and other genitourinary fistulas

CLINICAL PRESENTATION

- Patients with genitourinary fistulas present with urinary incontinence, use of a ↑ number of diapers and pads to prevent soiling, ↓ sensation of bladder fullness, and irregular voiding pattern. Patients with colovesical or colovaginal fistulas → pneumaturia and urinary infections. Rarely encountered, urethrocutaneous fistulas will manifest with leakage of urine onto the skin surface.

- In developing countries, the time of presentation is influenced greatly by the access to health care. Thus, a review of Nigerian patients showed that the average time for symptoms presentation was 5 years after the causative pregnancy.

- Most genitourinary fistulas will present between 5 and 14 days after the injury, however, in cases of direct surgical injury, leakage may occur from the first postoperative day, or soon after removal of the bladder catheter.

- In cases of extensive tissue loss, as in radiation or obstetric fistulas, the clinical findings lead to a clear diagnosis. However, in the case of postsurgical fistulas, the presenting symptoms may be atypical and the lesion small and difficult to detect, making the diagnosis

more difficult. In rare cases, patients with clinically detectable fistulas may deny urinary incontinence due to the levator muscle ability to occlude the vaginal walls below the level of the fistula.

- Small urethrovaginal fistulas distal to the sphincter mechanism will frequently be asymptomatic, however, proximal urethral fistulas cause symptoms of stress incontinence caused by impairment of bladder neck continence mechanism. Patients with urethrovaginal fistulas resulting from trauma (e.g., forceps delivery or automobile accidents) have loss of urine immediately or within the first 24 hours after injury.

- Ectopic ureter may drain into the vagina or urethra and must always be in the differential diagnosis in patients with a lifetime history of urinary incontinence.

- Patients with vesicocervical or vesicouterine fistulas subsequent to cesarean section may maintain continence at the uterine isthmus or have intermittent urine leakage, with cyclical hematuria during menses (menouria) and amenorrhea—Youssef syndrome.

DIAGNOSIS

- The purpose of investigation:
  ○ To prove that the leakage is urinary
  ○ To investigate that the leakage is urethral or extraurethral
  ○ To locate the site of leakage
- Vaginal examination
  ○ The vulva and perineum are wet, and accompanied by urine odor, and skin excoriation.

DIAGNOSTIC TESTING

- *Laboratory analysis*—postoperatively, the drainage of serum from a pelvic hematoma may simulate a vesicovaginal or ureterovaginal fistula. The fluid is collected and biochemical analysis of the urea content demonstrates a urine or serum etiology of the liquid. Urine cultures and sensitivity (UC&S) should be obtained and appropriate antibiotic regimen instituted. The phenazopyridine hydrochloride (Pyridium; Parke-Davis, Morris Plains, NJ) test can be used to diagnose the presence of urine in the vaginal discharge. The test consists of oral ingestion of phenazopyridine hydrochloride and insertion of a vaginal tampon. Staining of the tampon diagnoses the fluid as urine.

- *Dye tests*—vesicovaginal fistula is demonstrated by instilling a diluted solution of 250 mL of indigo carmine, methylene blue, or sterile infant's formula into the bladder through a transurethral Foley catheter. A vesicovaginal fistula is demonstrated by leakage of dyed liquid or milk into the vagina. If the test is inconclusive, or if the fistula is small, several cotton tampons are placed along the course of the vagina and the patient ambulates for 30 minutes. Staining of the tampon next to the vaginal wall indicates a fistula.

- *Moir's cotton ball or tampon test* is used to detect ureterovaginal fistula. After the negative dye test, the bladder is drained of the blue dye, and a tampon or multiple cotton balls are inserted in the vagina. About 2.5–5 mL of indigo carmine is injected intravenously. Then, the patient walks for 10–15 minutes and the tampon is removed from the vagina and examined for dye; + of dye on the tampon in contact with vaginal apex suggests a ureterovaginal fistula.
- *Water and air (flat-tire) test* is useful for diagnosis of small vesicovaginal fistulas. The patient is in the knee-chest position and the vagina is filled with sterile water or normal saline. The bladder is filled with air or carbon dioxide through a transurethral catheter. The presence of a vesicovaginal fistula is demonstrated by bubbles passing through the liquid in the vagina.
- *Endoscopic evaluation*: Cystourethroscopy shows the number, site, size, and exact location of fistulas. It is important to determine the proximity of fistulas in relation to the ureteral orifices, urethral sphincter, and the bladder neck, as well as assessment of the tissue edema, scarring, and induration, which can affect the optimal timing of the surgical repair. In cases of large fistulas, water cystoscopy may be difficult to perform. It is important to biopsy the edge of fistulas resulting from radiation treatment or recurrent malignancy to exclude malignant change. Moreover, in endemic areas where tissue biopsy may show evidence of schistosomiasis or tuberculosis, treatment must be started prior to surgical repair.
- *Sigmoidoscopy*: It is important to diagnose and treat inflammatory bowel disease (IBD) in any patient with complex or recurrent urinary fistulas.
- *Biopsy of the fistula site*: It is important in patients with a history of pelvic malignancy to assess the risk of local recurrence.

IMAGING

- Imaging techniques show the precise anatomical location of the fistula and the surrounding structures. The most useful imaging techniques involve intravenous (or excretion) urography and intravenous pyelography (IVP) or ureterography, cystography, misturating cysto-urethrography, computed tomography (CT), magnetic resonance imaging (MRI), barium enemas, and fistulography.

- Excretion urography, with a reported sensitivity of only 33%, is an essential investigation of ureteral fistulas, especially when they are a result of a malignant process, or of radiation therapy or surgery. The presence of a periureteric flare on intravenous urography is diagnostic of dye extravasation. Typically, ureteral fistulas are characterized by ureteral dilatation, and their association with a known vesicovaginal fistula may indicate a complex ureterovesicovaginal fistula.
- Retrograde pyelography has ↑ sensitivity at detecting the precise site of the ureterovaginal fistula and it may be performed simultaneously with retrograde or percutaneous ureteral stenting.
- Cystography is helpful in diagnosing complex fistulas, however, it is generally not a sensitive test for diagnosis of vesicovaginal fistulas. A combination of IVP and cystography is diagnostic for most vesicovaginal fistulas. Lateral film projections are performed to differentiate contrast within the vagina or uterus from the contrast-distended bladder.
- Voiding urethrography is essential for diagnosis of urethrovaginal fistulas and their differentiation from urethrovaginal reflux.
- Sonography may also be useful in the diagnosis of vesicovaginal fistulas. In one study, color Doppler ultrasound with a microbubble contrast agent detected fistulous tracts in 11 of 12 cases.
- Fistulography (sinography) is the most direct means of visualizing a fistula. Fistulography is a special x-ray imaging technique that involves the injection of dye → intervening fistulous tract. This technique is the imaging modality of choice in the diagnosis of urethrocutaneous fistulas. The nature of the fistulous tract may become apparent from the radiological appearance on fistulography (e.g., a loop of bowel will display haustrations).
- Hysterosalpingography may be used to diagnose complex genitourinary fistulas (e.g., vesicouterine fistulas).
- CT and MRI are used to assess complex fistulas in patients with urogenital fistulas associated with gynecological cancers. CT scan shows a postoperative urinoma caused by ureteral laceration during surgery and urine extravasation into the retroperitoneal and peritoneal space (ureteroperitoneal fistula).

MANAGEMENT

- The best treatment of genitourinary fistulas is their prevention.
- In the developing world, ↑ education of girls, women, and community leaders and improved economic opportunities delay childbearing and ↑ awareness of obstetric fistulas. Fistula prevention programs in sub-Saharan Africa can provide access to emergency

obstetric care, including safe cesarean sections for women with obstructed labor. It has been shown that at least 5% of deliveries must be done by cesarean section to reduce maternal morbidity and mortality. In the majority of sub-Saharan Africa, the cesarean section rates were <5% (<2% in half of them).

- Several operative and preoperative techniques can be applied, which will help prevent lower urinary tract injuries:
  ○ Proper operative field setup including patient positioning in stirrups, prepping, and sterile draping to allow for double access (e.g., laparoscopic-assisted vaginal hysterectomy, or LAVH drapes), thus allowing ready access to both the abdominal and vaginal areas
  ○ Continuous bladder drainage by a two- or three-way (14 or 16 French) transurethral balloon catheter, which allows for intraoperative bladder filling with sterile water, normal saline, or a dye (e.g., indigo carmine). The presence of dye in the operative field will help the surgeon to find the extend and location of urinary tract injury
  ○ Provide ample exposure, lighting, suctioning of the operating area, and assure adequate hemostasis
  ○ Skeletonization of large tissue pedicles before clamping, cutting, and suturing
  ○ Retraction of the bladder out of the operative field (e.g., using a Harrington or Deaver retractor) and avoid excessive use of electrocautery in the vicinity of the bladder and ureter
  ○ Identification of the ureteral course in the pelvis and gentle retraction of ureters during radical hysterectomy (e.g., using a Penrose drain around the ureteral lumen)
  ○ Development of extraperitoneal spaces and execution of sharp dissection along anatomic planes
  ○ If indicated, intraoperative testing for urinary tract injuries may be accomplished with cystoscopy or cystotomy. Cystoscopy is performed with sterile water, normal saline, or hypertonic glucose (i.e., 10–50%), and it is important to examine the bladder wall for injuries and foreign bodies (e.g., sutures and stitches). The administration of 5 mL of indigo carmine or methylene blue intravenously will result in bilateral excretion of blue-dyed urine from bilateral ureteral orifices into the bladder, if both ureters are patent and are functioning normally.

- Routine preoperative IVP and preoperative placement of ureteral catheters have not been shown to ↓ the incidence of surgical injury to the bladder and ureters. Moreover, ureteral catheters may cause mucosal injury and may ↑ ureteral diffness which → ureteral devascularization or laceration. If scarring or obesity makes intraoperative ureteral identification impossible, ureteral catheters may be placed by transurethral cystoscopy or by a cystotomy in the dome of the bladder.

- If bladder is injured with monopolar cystotomy, double-layered bladder repair with an absorbable suture is preferred to single-layer repair for the prevention of vesicovaginal fistulas.
- If the ureter is injured during the surgery, ureteral injuries heal better and with fewer complications if they are recognized and repaired during the initial operation.
- Successful correction of urogenital fistulas can be affected by several factors:
  ○ Timing of repair (immediate vs. 8–12 weeks waiting period)
  ○ Type of management (nonsurgical vs. surgical treatment),
  ○ Route of repair (vaginal vs. abdominal approach)
  ○ Technique of repair (layered repair vs. Latzko's procedure)
- Other important issues that lead to successful fistula closure are the experience of the surgical team, the condition of tissues surrounding the fistula, the general clinical condition of the patient, the cause of the fistula (obstetric vs. surgery vs. radiation therapy for cancer), the type of fistulas (simple vs. complex), the type of suture used, the use of antibiotics, and proper postoperative management.
- Multispecialty approaches are important to ensure the best line of treatment and involve gynecologists, urologists, and diagnostic and interventional radiologists.
- It is important that the patients with urogenital fistulas be counseled by surgeons, nursing staff, and counselors experienced with this condition.
- Support groups can play an important role in maintaining patient morale, particularly when the clinical circumstances require a delay in definitive treatment.

TIMING OF REPAIR

- The timing of repair is the most contentious issue of fistula management. Traditionally, clinicians advocate a delay in surgical management of >8–12 weeks from the onset of fistula to allow for ↑ inflammation, tissue sloughing, and edema. Proper patient selection is very important in determining the timing of definitive treatment. The timing of restorative surgery is based on the type of causative procedure (obstetric vs. surgery) and the disease for which the original operation was performed (pelvic inflammatory disease [PID], gynecological cancer, the administration of radiation therapy). In radiation fistulas, there is ↑ tissue sloughing and it is necessary to wait *at least* 12 weeks before attempting surgical repair. Recent data show that immediate management of obstetric fistulas proves ↑ effective with regard to surgical repair and continence. In a prospective study, 1716 patients with fistula duration of 3–75 days after vaginal delivery were treated immediately by catheter and/or early surgical repair. The total closure rate → 98.5% and 95.2% of patients were successfully treated at first attempt. Moreover, 93.2% of patients achieved urinary continence. Surgical repair is best avoided during menstruation to avoid the ↑ tissue vascularity.

NONSURGICAL MANAGEMENT

- Bypassing the affected fistulous urinary tract with urinary catheterization or ureteral stenting may help heal the defect. In a prospective study of 1716 Nigerian patients with fresh obstetric fistulas, 15.4% were healed by catheterization only.
- Vesicovaginal fistulas up to 3 mm in diameter can be successfully treated by electrosurgical coagulation of the fistulous tract and prolonged bladder catheterization.
- In a study of primary treatment of ureterovaginal fistulas only with percutaneous nephrostomy, 55% of patients had persistent fistulas and 18% had ureteral strictures.
- Traditionally, ureterovaginal fistulas were treated by an open surgery, primary ureteroneocystotomy (see further), because of the ureteral stenosis and stricture formation in a large percent of injured ureters. Endourological techniques are emerging as the primary choice for treatment of ureterovaginal fistulas. Improvements in ureteral stents (e.g., double-J ureteral stents), ureteroscopes, guide wires, and endourological techniques have ↑ the successful treatment of ureterovaginal fistulas by ureteral stents. In one study → 82% of ureterovaginal fistulas less than 1 month old and 33% of older fistulas were treated successfully with ureteral stenting and the antegrade stent insertion was the treatment of choice. Another study → healing of all ureterovaginal fistulas in whom a self-retaining internal stent was placed in a retrograde or anterograde manner for a minimum of 4–8 weeks (mean 5.5 weeks), with only one case complicated by ureteral stricture (14%), which was also repaired endoscopically.
  - Route of repair: Most gynecological surgeons favor vaginal approach whereas some urological surgeons advocate the abdominal surgical repair. Indications for abdominal repair are
    - Indurated vaginal epithelium 2 cm in circumference surrounding the fistula
    - A vaginal vault fistula with inadequate vaginal exposure (high fistula, long, narrow vagina)
    - The presence of ureterovaginal fistulas
    - Complex urogenital fistulas involving the uterus or the bowel

- Pelvic malignancy
- Prior pelvic radiation therapy
  - The size, number, and history of previous operative repair do not rule out a vaginal approach. In a study with 68 patients over a span of 25 years, vesicovaginal and urethrovaginal fistulas were repaired transvaginally with 70% success at first attempt and 92% success after two attempts. However, only 58% of fistulas were closed successfully after transabdominal or combined approaches. Moreover, the transvaginal approach → in ↑ hemostasis, required ↓ operative time and ↓ hospitalization than the transabdominal approach.
  - Prophylactic antibiotics:
    - While some clinicians use antibiotics only in the treatment of specific urinary tract infections (UTIs), most surgeons recommend prophylactic broad-spectrum antibiotics in all patients. In a blind, randomized controlled study of antibiotic prophylaxis (ampicillin 500 mg intraoperatively) during vesicovaginal fistula repair, antibiotic prophylaxis did not ↓ the rate of failed repair (OR 2.1, 95% CI, 0.75–6.1), or the rate of objective incontinence. However, women in the antibiotic prophylaxis group received ↓ postoperative antibiotics and had a ↓ rate of UTI on postoperative day 10.
  - Palliation and skin care:
    - It is important to optimize the quality of vaginal tissue surrounding the fistula and to make the patient as comfortable as possible during the waiting period from diagnosis to repair. Thus, patients should be provided with an adequate amount of incontinence pads to allow them to function socially. Ammoniacal dermatitis is treated with zinc oxide topical ointment and sitz baths. Systemic or local estrogen is used in postmenopausal or oophorectomized patients to improve urogenital tissue integrity.
  - Anesthesia and patient positioning:
    - Small fistulas may be repaired under local anesthesia with or without conscious sedation. However, most fistulas require general anesthesia, and epidural and spinal anesthesia have also been used with success.
    - Depending on the proximity of the fistula on the vagina wall, the patient may be positioned accordingly. For proximal urethral or bladder neck fistulas, Lawson's position—the patient is prone on the operative table, with knees separated and ankles raised in stirrups and the table in reversed Trendelenburg's position. In cases of high vaginal fistulas, a lithotomy position is used with the operative table in Trendelenburg's position.

○ Instruments and suture materials:

- Useful instruments are the Chaser Moiré 30° angled-on-flat and 90° curved-on-flat scissors, Church or Kelly fistula scissors, Sims skin hooks to help keep the tissues under tension during dissection, Allis forceps, Sims or Breisky retractors, fine-tipped suction tips, and long-handled scalpels with no. 11 and 15 blades. The curved needle holder may be useful in areas that are difficult to reach and with limited exposure.

- Most surgeons prefer absorbable sutures. A 2-0 and 3-0 polyglactin (Vicryl) suture on CT-2 needle is preferred for the bladder and vagina repair. An alternative is the use of fine monofilament nylon for vaginal closure and delayed removal after 3–4 weeks. A 4-0 polydioxanone (PDS) suture is preferred for ureteral repairs.

MANAGEMENT OF VESICOVAGINAL FISTULAS

• *Latzko's procedure* is indicated for vesicovaginal fistulas located at the vaginal apex. These vesicovaginal fistulas are usually small and result from a vaginal or abdominal hysterectomy. Latzko's procedure is an apical colpocleisis, it avoids surgery on the fistula itself or the bladder and it can be done shortly after the diagnosis of vesicovovaginal fistula. The following steps are involved in the Latzko's procedure:

1. Patient placed in lithotomy position
2. Placement of four stay sutures around vaginal apex at 12, 3, 6, 9 o'clock more than 2 cm from the margins of the fistula
3. Tension is applied to the four stay sutures and a circle is drawn with a radius of approximately 2 cm from the edge of the fistula
4. Hydrodistention with normal saline or a diluted solution of a vasoconstrictive agent helps dissect the vaginal epithelium from around the underlying fibromuscular wall of vagina
5. Dissection of vaginal squamous epithelium from within the circumference of the circle drawn in step 3.
6. The fibromuscular wall of the vagina is closed over the fistulous tract with one layer of interrupted absorbable suture (3-0 or 4-0 chromic) followed by two layers of interrupted delayed-absorbable 3-0 or 4-0 polyglactin (Vicryl) suture.
7. Testing the bladder water tightness with the injection of 300 cc of sterile milk or indigo carmine dyed water into the bladder and repairing any site of leakage with interrupted delayed-absorbable sutures.

8. Approximation of vaginal epithelium using delayed-absorbable sutures (e.g., 2-0 polyglactin suture).

• *Layered vaginal repair:* In the presence of distal and larger vesicovaginal, urethrovaginal, or urethrovesicovaginal fistulas along the anterior vaginal wall, the Latzko's procedure may result in ↑ loss of vaginal length and a layered vaginal repair is indicated. To ↓ tissue loss and bleeding, the fistulous opening into the bladder and its fibrous ring is left intact and all suture lines must be tension free. The following steps are involved in the layered vaginal repair:

1. Patient placed in lithotomy position
2. Making a vertical incision encircling the fistulous opening lateral to the scar tissue
3. Wide mobilization of the vaginal mucosa from the bladder wall
4. Placement of a first layer of absorbable (e.g., 3-0 or 4-0 chromic) sutures in the submucosa of the bladder, which closes the fistula by inverting the bladder mucosa into the lumen of the bladder.
5. Closure of the opening into the bladder
6. Layered closure of the bladder muscularis and repair of fibromuscular wall of the vagina using interrupted delayed-absorbable (e.g., 3-0 polyglactin) sutures.
7. Testing the bladder water tightness with the injection of 300 cc of sterile milk or indigo carmine dyed water into the bladder and repairing any site of leakage with interrupted delayed-absorbable sutures.
8. Approximation of vaginal epithelium using delayed-absorbable sutures (e.g., 2-0 polyglactin suture).

• *Abdominal repair:* The abdominal approach is indicated for high, fixed, poorly accessible fistulas in the vaginal vault, ureterovaginal fistulas, complex urogenital fistulas involving the uterus or the bowel, pelvic malignancy, or prior pelvic radiation therapy. The following technique is used for the abdominal repair of vesicovaginal fistulas:

1. Making a lower abdominal midline incision
2. Creation of a sagittal cystotomy to provide access to the site of the fistula
3. Placement of ureteral stents through the cystotomy
4. Sharp dissection of the base of the bladder from the anterior vaginal wall
5. Excision of the fistulous tract in the bladder and vagina
6. Approximation of vaginal mucosa with two layers of running 3-0 delayed-absorbable suture (e.g., 3-0 polyglactin or polyglycolic acid) and removal of ureteral stents. The ureteral stents are left in place for 1 week to ↓ edema in cases where the ureters are close to the edge of incision.
7. Closure of cystotomy in two to three layers: one layer of absorbable 3-0 delayed-absorbable suture

(e.g., 3-0 polyglactin) to approximate the submucosa and one to two layers of same suture to imbricate the adjacent muscularis layer

8. Suturing an omental pedicle or peritoneum to the anterior vaginal wall will separate the vaginal and bladder repairs. An omental pedicle may be useful in larger, complex fistula procedures or for radiation-induced fistulas where additional blood supply is brought via the omental pedicle.

MANAGEMENT OF URETHROVAGINAL FISTULAS

- Simple urethrovaginal fistulas situated proximal to the bladder neck may not produce urinary incontinence and may not require surgical repair. However, if symptomatic, fistulas situated close to the bladder neck may be technically more challenging to cure. Surgical repair of such fistulas → in stress urinary incontinence caused by tissue fibrosis, immobility, and poor contractility of the urethral musculature. Generally surgical repair of urethrovaginal fistulas is deferred until 8–12 weeks after the initial surgery, which caused the injury. The following surgical technique is used for repair of urethrovaginal fistulas:
  ○ Patient placed in lithotomy position
  ○ Making a linear midline incision which will encircle the urethrovaginal fistula, thus separating the anterior vaginal wall from pubocervical fascia
  ○ Mobilization of anterior vaginal wall laterally off the pubocervical fascia in a manner similar to a modified Kelly anterior colporrhaphy
  ○ Excision of the fistula tract and associated scar tissue, thus preparing the edges of the urethra for reapproximation
  ○ Approximation of the edges of the mucosa and submucosa of the urethra in an extramucosal fashion, tension free with 3-0 of 4-0 delayed-absorbable suture (e.g., 3-0 polyglactin). The placement of a small-caliber urethral catheter (e.g., 12–14 French) will aid in precise placement of sutures close to the fistulous tract.
  ○ Placement of a second inverting line of sutures past the proximal and distal ends of the original suture line, thus plicating snugly and tension free the bladder neck pubocervical septum and inverting the initial suture layer
  ○ Approximation of the vaginal mucosa in a tension-free manner with delayed-absorbable sutures (e.g., 2-0 polyglactin suture).
- In patients who underwent a successful surgical repair of urethrovaginal fistula, but who have symptoms of stress urinary incontinence, it may be indicated to perform a retropubic urethrovesical suspension at a later time.

INTERPOSITION GRAFTS

- Interposition grafts have the purpose of supporting fistula repair by filling the dead space and bringing in additional blood supply to devitalized tissues, important especially for the repair of fistulas resulting from radiation therapy:
- Martius graft—consists of labial fat and bulbocavernous muscle passed subcutaneously and has the role of maintaining competence of the urethral and bladder neck fistula repair by ↓ scarring
- Gracilis muscle is passed subcutaneously or via the obturator foramen
- Omental pedicle grafts are used mostly for repair of postradiation fistulas. They are dissected from the grater curvature of the stomach and are rotated and brought into the pelvis along with the gastroepiploic artery
- Peritoneal flap graft provides an extra layer for transperitoneal repair procedures and it consists of a flap of peritoneum usually from the paravesical area.

MANAGEMENT OF URETEROVAGINAL FISTULAS

- Commonly, ureterovaginal fistulas are caused by ureteral damage during pelvic surgery. The routine preoperative placement of ureteral catheters and routine preoperative IVP have not been shown to prevent ureteral injuries.
- Most often, ureterovaginal fistulas involve the distal ureter and are located within 4–5 cm of the ureterovesical junction.
- Endourological techniques are emerging as the primary choice for treatment of ureterovaginal fistulas. The following illustrates the technique of ureteral stent placement:
  ○ First cystoscopy is done to assess ureteral openings into the bladder and IVP is performed to rule out ureteral obstruction. Cystoscopic-assisted retrograde ureteral stenting is attempted; if ureteral obstruction is present, ipsilateral percutaneous nephrostomy is placed to avoid kidney failure. Consequently, antegrade ureteral catheterization can be achieved via the percutaneous nephrostomy and the ureteral catheter is advanced and a ureteral stent is placed to overlap the ureteral fistula. If the ureteral stent corrects the leakage of urine, it is left in place for 1 month to allow time for healing of ureterovaginal fistula. After 1 month, the ureteral catheter is removed and IVP is performed. If the IVP is normal, it is repeated in 3 months to ensure absence of ureteral extravasation and to rule out ureteral stenosis. If ureteral leakage still occurs, then surgery is indicated.

- The most appropriate treatment for distal ureterovaginal fistulas that fails to heal after ureteral stenting is ureteroneocystostomy, using an abdominal approach. Ureterovaginal fistulas located in the upper ureter are most commonly treated by ureteroureterostomy.
- Ectopic ureter may drain into the vagina or urethra and is treated by ureteral reimplantation into the bladder (ureteroneocystostomy) or into the ipsilateral ureter.
- Surgical repair is delayed for 3 months after surgery, except in the case where the injury is recognized within the first 48 hours postoperatively. UTIs must be treated prior to surgery and most surgeons recommend prophylactic treatment with antibiotics.
- The following surgical technique is used for ureteroneocystotomy:
  1. Mobilization of the ureter from its peritoneal covering and the affected ureter is transected obliquely at a point where the ureter is intact and has a good blood supply.
  2. The dome of the bladder is incised vertically in the midline close to the trigone, and the fundus of the bladder is displaced toward the proximal portion of the ureter that will be implanted into the bladder.
  3. Ligation or resection of the distal portion of the transected ureter close to the bladder.
  4. Attachment of a fine suture to the proximal end of the transected ureter.
  5. Creation of an opening in the mucosa of the bladder with a scalpel, in the proximity of the original ureteral opening, passing of a tonsil clamp or hemostat through this opening. To prevent ureteral reflux, the tonsil clamp is then tunneled between the bladder mucosa and muscularis for 1 cm laterally toward the pelvic wall and an opening is made into the bladder from the outside over the tips of the clamp. The opening in the bladder is stretched with a hemostat clamp to prevent stenosis.
  6. The suture attached to the proximal end of the ureter in step 5 is pulled through the cystotomy and through the tunnel between the bladder mucosa and muscularis created earlier, thus tunneling the distal ureter within the bladder wall in order to prevent ureteral reflux.
  7. The ureteral opening is sutured to the bladder mucosa with interrupted absorbable (e.g., 3-0 or 4-0 chromic) sutures, incorporating the full thickness of the ureteral wall. It is crucial to the success of the operation that the anastomosis between the end of the ureter and the bladder is tension free. The bladder can be mobilized by freeing it from the retropubic space. Moreover, the tension-free anastomosis of the ureteroneocystotomy can be maintained by suturing the bladder fundus to the psoas muscle (e.g., psoas hitch) with permanent sutures.
  8. The adventitial sheath of the ureter is attached to the bladder adventitia with delayed-absorbable (e.g., 3-0 or 4-0 polyglactin or polyglycolic acid) sutures in order to further take the tension off the anastomosis line
  9. The incision in the dome of the bladder is closed with one layer of running delayed-absorbable (e.g., 3-0 or 4-0 polyglactin or polyglycolic acid) suture. A second layer of delayed-absorbable (e.g., 3-0 or 4-0 polyglactin or polyglycolic acid) suture is used to close the bladder muscularis and the serosa.
  10. A suction drain is placed in the proximity of the ureteroneocystotomy to protect the anastomosis from serum or urine.
  11. The anastomosis site may also be protected by covering it by pelvic peritoneum.
  12. Placement of transurethral and suprapubic (e.g., Foley or Malecot) catheters for at least 24 hours ensures the flow of urine and reduces the possibility of a blood clot obstructing a single catheter.
- Ureteroneurostomy is the procedure of choice for ureterovaginal fistulas which involve the proximal two-thirds of the ureter. Ureteroenterostomy is an end-to-end anastomosis of the proximal and distal portions of the ureter and it will be successful if the ureteral blood supply is adequate and if the resection of the affected segment of the ureter does not shorten the ureter.
  - The fistulous portion of the ureter is removed and the proximal and distal ends are freshened to ensure good blood supply. The ureteral ends are first spatulated to prevent ureteral stricture formation. Anastomosis is performed over a stenting ureteral catheter using 4–5 through-and-through fine-interrupted absorbable or delayed-absorbable suture material with the stitches set 2 mm back from the edge of the proximal and distal ureter.
  - The anastomosis site is then extraperitonealized and drained with a suction drain to prevent any urine or serum accumulation that may impede healing of the repair.
- Rarely, other options for proximal ureterovaginal fistulas exist and include transureteroureterostomy (end-to-site anastomosis), temporary cutaneous ureterostomy (proximal ureter is brought out and sutured to the skin edge of the flank when extensive blood loss occurs and the clinical condition of the patient mandates speedy termination of the surgery), and ileal transplant (replacing the fistulous segment of the ureter with a transplanted defunctionalized segment of the ileum).

COMPLEX GENITOURINARY FISTULAS

- Involve a number of abnormal communications between the ureters, bladder, urethra, uterus, vagina, colon, and skin. These complex fistulas are managed by vaginal or abdominal surgery keeping into account the general principles of fistula repair mentioned earlier.

POSTOPERATIVE COMPLICATIONS (ARE GROUPED INTO EARLY OR LATE)

- Early complications are bleeding, bladder spasms, wound dehiscence, and wound infection.
- Late complications are stress urinary incontinence (occurs in at least 10% of patients with urogenital fistulas), vaginal stenosis, ureteral stricture and stenosis, and small capacity bladder, dyspareunia.

POSTOPERATIVE MANAGEMENT

- Fluid balance: Strict fluid input/output (I/Os) are measured. Maintain a daily fluid intake of at least 3 L and a urine output of 100 mL/h to prevent formation of blood clots around the site of fistula repair.
- Bladder catheterization: Continuous bladder drainage is critical to the healing process of fistula repair. This can be accomplished by using both a suprapubic and a transurethral catheter of large enough caliber to accommodate the passage of blood and small clots. After ureteroneocystostomies and ureterostomies, both ureteral and bladder catheters should be used to prevent stricture at the site of anastomosis and to protect the cystotomy site.
- Antibiotic use: Perioperative prophylactic antibiotics for genitourinary fistula repair are advised by most surgeons. Postoperatively, antibiotic cover is recommended for all intestinovaginal fistulas and if antibiotics are not used after genitourinary fistula repair, it is advised that catheter urine specimens are collected for UC&S tests every 48 hours and UTI must be treated with appropriate antibiotics.
- Thromboprophylaxis: ↓ patient activity is advised in the postoperative period to ensure adequate catheter drainage. It is recommended that patient be treated with thromboembolism prophylaxis (e.g., low molecular heparin products).
- Bladder training: The bladder capacity is functionally decreased and patients will commonly complain of urinary urgency. To prevent bladder distension, patients should be encouraged to ↓ fluid intake and to perform timed voids every hour while awake and 2× during the nighttime. Painful bladder spasms may be treated with anticholinergic therapy.

- Use of vaginal tampons, pessaries, and intercourse should be avoided for 8–12 weeks after genitourinary fistula repair.

PROGNOSIS AND CONCLUSIONS

- Cure of genitourinary fistula is defined as successful closure after the first attempted intervention or surgery and varies from 60% to 100%, with a mean success rate of 91%.
- In patients exposed to radiation therapy, the success rate ranges from 40% to 100% and many patients are treated by urinary diversion.
- The transvaginal approach to vesicovaginal fistula repair results in more than 90% success rate, is ↓ invasive and is ↑ amenable to an early repair than the abdominal approach.
- The success percent of genitourinary fistula repair ↓ progressively with subsequent unsuccessful procedures. In a series of 2484 mostly obstetric fistulas, the success rate ↓ from 81.2% after the first procedure to 65% after two or more procedures.
- Endourological techniques are emerging as the primary choice for treatment of ureterovaginal fistulas and only refractory fistulas that fail ureteral stenting or fistulas resulting from radiation therapy or malignancy are amenable to abdominal repair.

BIBLIOGRAPHY

Angioli R, Penalver M, Muzii L, et al. Guidelines of how to manage vesicovaginal fistula. *Crit Rev Oncol Hematol.* 2003;48(3):295–304.

Avritscher R, et al. Fistulas of the lower urinary tract: percutaneous approaches for the management of a difficult clinical entity. *Radiographics.* 2004;24:S217–S236.

Bent AE, Ostergard DR, Cundiff GW, et al. *Ostergard's Urogynecology and Pelvic Floor Dysfunction.* 5th ed. Lippincott Williams & Wilkins; 2003:433.

Blaivas JG, Heritz DM, Romanzi LJ. Early versus late repair of vesicovaginal fistulas: vaginal and abdominal approaches. *J Urol.* 1995;153(4):1110–1112; discussion 1112–1113.

Cardozo L, Staskin D. *Textbook of Female Urology and Urogynecology.* Oxford: ISIS Medical Media; London, UK: 2001:286–297, 692–719.

Copeland LJ, Hatch KD, Fowler JM. In: Copeland LJ, ed. *Textbook of Gynecology.* Philadelphia, PA: W.B. Saunders; 2000:1093–1103.

Cunningham FG, Gant NF, Leveno KJ, et al. *Williams Obstetrics.* 21st ed. New York: McGraw-Hill; 2001:443.

DeBaere T, Roche A, Lagrange C. Combined percutaneous anterograde and cystoscopic retrograde approach in the treatment of distal ureteral fistulae. *Cardiovasc Intervent Radiol.* 1995;18:349–352.

Donnay F, Well L. Obstetric fistula: the international response. *Lancet.* 2004;363:71–72.

Elkins TE, Fitzpatrick CK. In: Walters MD, Karram MM, eds. *Clinical Urogynecology.* St. Louis, MO: Mosby; 1993: 330–353.

Goodwin WE, Scardino PT. Vesicovaginal and ureterovaginal fistulas: a summary of 25 years of experience. *Trans Am Assoc Genitourin Surg.* 1979;71:123–129.

Haarki-Siren P, Sjoberg J, Tiitinen A. Urinary tract injuries after hysterectomy. *Obstet Gynecol.* 1998;92:113–118.

Hadley HR. Vesicovaginal fistula. *Curr Urol Rep.* 2002;3(5): 401–407.

Hilton P, Ward A. Epidemiological and surgical aspects of urogenital fistulae: a review of 25 years experience in Nigeria. *Int Urogynecol J Pelvic Floor Dysfunct.* 1998;9(4):189–194.

Hurt GW. Urogynecologic surgery. *The Master's Techniques in Gyncologic Surgery.* 2nd ed. Lippincott Williams & Wilkins; 2000:141–148.

Lee RA. Urinary fistula. In: Webb MJ, ed. *Mayo Clinic Manual of Pelvic Surgery.* 2nd ed.Philadelphia, PA: Lippincott Williams & Wilkins; 2000:117–123.

Murray C, Lopez, A. *Health Dimensions of Sex and Reproduction.* Geneva: WHO; 1998.

PROLOG. *Gynecology and Surgery.* 5th ed. Washington DC: The American College of Obstetricians and Gynecologists; 2004:128.

Schmeller NT, Gottinger H, Schuller J, et al. Percutaneous nephrostomy as primary therapy of ureterovaginal fistula. *Urologe A.* 1983;22(2):108–112.

Selzman AA, Spirnak JP, Kursh ED. The changing management of ureterovaginal fistulas. *J Urol.* 1995;153(3, pt 1):626–628.

Sokol AI, Paraiso MF, Cogan SL. Prevention of vesicovaginal fistulas after laparoscopic hysterectomy with electrosurgical cystotomy in female mongrel dogs. *Am J Obstet Gynecol.* 2004;190(3):628–633.

Stovsky MD, Ignatoff JM, Blum MD, et al. Use of electrocoagulation in the treatment of vesicovaginal fistulas. *J Urol.* 1994;152(5, pt 1):1443–1444.

Tomlinson AJ, Thornton JG. A randomised controlled trial of antibiotic prophylaxis for vesico-vaginal fistula repair. *Br J Obstet Gynaecol.* 1998;105(4):397–399.

Volkmer BG, Kuefer R, Nesslauer T, et al. Colour Doppler ultrasound in vesicovaginal fistulas. *Ultrasound Med Biol.* 2000;26:771–775.

Waaldijk K. The immediate management of fresh obstetric fistulas. *Am J Obstet Gynecol.* 2004;191(3):795–799.

WHO. The prevention and treatment of obstetric fistulae: report of a technical working group, WHO/FHE/89.5: Geneva: Division of Family Health, WHO; 1989.

Yu NC, Raman SS, Patel M, et al. Fistulas of the genitourinary tract: a radiological review. *Radiographics.* 2004;24: 1331–1352.

QUESTIONS

1. A 52-year-old $G_3P_2A_1$ comes back to the office for postoperative check. The patient complains of constant leakage of urine and dysuria. She is 2 weeks' status post exploratory laparotomy and total abdominal hysterectomy with bilateral salpingo-oopherectomy (TAH/BSO) for stage Ia Grade 1 endometrial carcinoma confirmed by final pathology. These symptoms have started 3 days before the visit and she wears a heavy pad at all times. Abdominal examination shows a well-healed abdominal incision, no significant abdominal tenderness, and normal bowel sounds. Pelvic examination shows well-supported vaginal walls and a small amount of fluid at the vaginal cuff. Urine dipstick is positive for bacteria, nitrates, and leukocytes. The most appropriate next test for the diagnosis of this patient is

   (A) Intravenous pyelogram (IVP)
   (B) Bladder methylene blue dye test
   (C) Urine culture and sensitivity
   (D) Filling cystometry
   (E) CT scan of abdomen and pelvis

2. A 32-year-old G_3P_3 underwent TAH/BSO 6 months ago for severe endometriosis unresponsive to medical treatment. Patient's postoperative course was complicated by a right distal ureterovaginal fistula. She underwent unsuccessful ureteral stenting 4 months ago, however, she continues to leak urine per vagina continuously and she wears a heavy pad at all times. Urine dipstick shows no leukocyte, nitrates, or bacteria and urine culture shows no growth. Patient is physically active, otherwise healthy, and desires complete resolution of symptoms. What is the most appropriate surgical treatment for her distal ureterovaginal fistula?

   (A) Ureteroureterostomy
   (B) Ureteroneocystostomy
   (C) Latzko's procedure
   (D) Right percutaneous nephrostomy
   (E) Expectant management

3. A 24-year-old G_1P_1 status postcesarean section 1 week ago for failure to progress in labor presents with small but constant leakage of urine. Patient was in labor for 8 hours, had epidural analgesia, progressed to a dilatation of 10 cm and after 3 hours of pushing with no fetal descent was counseled and offered cesarean section. Her bladder was catheterized just prior to surgery and Foley catheter was discontinued postoperative day 1 and was discharged postoperative day 3 with no urinary complaints. Patient has no dysuria and normal bowel movements. A vesicovaginal fistula is demonstrated by injecting methylene blue dye into the bladder. IVP shows no periureteric flare. Cystourethroscopy reveals a 2 mm size vesicovaginal fistula in the base

of the bladder. The best management for this patient's vesicovaginal fistula is

(A) Latzko's procedure

(B) Latzko's procedure with a Martius graft

(C) Layered vaginal repair

(D) Continuous bladder drainage with a Foley catheter for 10 days

(E) Abdominal repair of vesicovaginal fistula

4. A 39-year-old G2P2 with a prior history of colectomy for ulcerative colitis underwent a TAH/BSO for a right-sided complex adnexal mass. The procedure was complicated by multiple adhesions around the right pelvic sidewall. Postoperative course was complicated by right-sided abdominal pain, creatinine concentration of 1.9 mg/dL, blood urea nitrogen (BUN) concentration of 32 mg/dL. Complete blood count (CBC) was stable at 10.2. Preoperative creatinine concentration was 0.9 mg/dL and BUN concentration was 10 mg/dL. The most likely findings noted on a CT scan of abdomen and pelvis would be

(A) Ureterovaginal fistula

(B) Vesicovaginal fistula

(C) Ureterocutaneous fistula

(D) Right-sided hydronephrosis

(E) Ureteroperitoneal fistula (urinoma)

5. A 45-year-old G4P4 comes to the office complaining of continuous urinary leakage. She is status postradiation therapy for stage IIb cervical cancer that she completed 4 months ago. She has no dysuria and urinalysis snows no leukocytes, nitrates, or bacteria. IVP shows no periureteric flare and no extravasation of contrast. Pelvic examination shows an obliterated, erythematous vaginal cuff with a moderate amount of fluid, and well-supported vaginal walls. A vesicovaginal fistula is demonstrated by injection of methylene blue dye into the bladder and cystourethroscopy reveals a 3-cm size vesicovaginal fistula in the trigone of the bladder. Patient underwent bilateral nephrostomy placement. The best surgical management of this patient's vesicovaginal fistula is

(A) Immediate layered vaginal repair

(B) Layered vaginal repair in 12 months

(C) Abdominal repair with an omental pedicle graft in 12 months

(D) Immediate abdominal repair with an omental pedicle graft

(E) Latzko's repair of vesicovaginal fistula

6. A 58-year-old G1P0A1 underwent TAH/BSO and pelvic retroperitoneal lymph node dissection for stage 2b ovarian cancer and she is POD #4. Patient

is complaining of greater-than-expected right-sided abdominal pain. CT scan of the abdomen and pelvis which shows right-sided hydronephrosis and hydroureter. Serum creatinine concentration is 2.9 mg/dL and preoperative serum creatinine concentration was 0.9 mg/dL. The best next treatment option for this patient is

(A) Cystoscopic-assisted retrograde ureteral stenting

(B) Immediate laparotomy and reexploration

(C) Inpatient close observation and repeat CT scan in 2 days

(D) Percutaneous nephrostomy

(E) Percutaneous nephrostomy and ureteral stenting

ANSWERS

1. *(B)*. A vesicovaginal fistula is demonstrated by instilling a diluted solution of 250 mL of indigo carmine, methylene blue into the bladder through a transurethral Foley catheter. A vesicovaginal fistula is demonstrated by leakage of dyed liquid into the vaginal tampon. If the tampon is dyed, this demonstrates a vesicovaginal fistula. If not dyed, an IVP may be performed to rule out ureterovaginal fistula. Or, alternatively, after the negative dye test, the bladder is drained of the blue dye, and a tampon is inserted in the vagina. About 2.5–5 mL of indigo carmine is injected intravenously. Then, the patient walks for 10–15 minutes and the tampon is removed from the vagina and is examined for dye. + of dye only on the tampon suggests a ureterovaginal fistula. Filling cystometry is not useful for this patient and UC&S will rule out UTI, but it will not help resolve in identifying this patient's fistula.

2. *(B)*. The most appropriate treatment for distal ureterovaginal fistulas that fails to heal after ureteral stenting is ureteroneocystostomy using an abdominal approach. Ureterovaginal fistulas located in the upper ureter are most commonly treated by ureterouretersostomy. Treatment of ureterovaginal fistulas only with percutaneous nephrostomy may result in persistent fistulas and ureteral strictures. Latzko's procedure is used for treatment of vesicovaginal fistulas.

3. *(D)*. Bypassing the affected fistulous urinary tract with urinary catheterization or ureteral stenting may help heal the defect. Between 15% and 50% of small vesicovaginal fistulas heal by conservative management with Foley catheter drainage. Vesicovaginal fistulas up to 3 mm in diameter have been successfully treated by electrosurgical coagulation

of the fistulous tract and prolonged bladder catheterization. Surgical correction is indicated only if conservative management fails.

4. *(E)*. This patient has symptoms of urinoma caused by ureteral injury during surgery with subsequent extravasation into the peritoneal/retroperitoneal space. CT and MRI are used to assess complex fistulas in patients with urogenital fistulas associated with gynecological cancers. CT scan shows a postoperative urinoma caused by uterine laceration during surgery and urine extravasation into the retroperitoneal and peritoneal space (ureteroperitoneal fistula).

5. *(C)*. This patient underwent radiation therapy for cervical cancer and it is indicated to perform an abdominal repair. Omental pedicle grafts are used mostly for repair of postradiation fistulas. They are dissected from the grater curvature of the stomach and are rotated and brought into the pelvis along with the gastroepiploic artery to provide an additional blood supply to the tissues undergoing surgical repair. In radiation fistulas there is ↑ tissue sloughing and it is necessary to wait at least 12 months before attempting surgical repair. Biopsy of the fistula edge is necessary to rule out cancer recurrence. During the waiting period, patient can have bilateral nephrostomies placed to increase decreased symptoms of constant urinary leakage and ↑ quality of life. An immediate layered vaginal repair is contraindicated in this case.

6. *(A)*. This patient likely suffered a ureteral intraoperative injury, which needs to be managed immediately to avoid kidney failure. First cystoscopy is done to assess ureteral openings into the bladder. Cystoscopic-assisted retrograde ureteral stenting (e.g., double-J ureteral stents) is attempted and if ureteral obstruction is present, and a stent cannot be introduced past the ureteral lesion, ipsilateral percutaneous nephrostomy is placed to avoid kidney failure. Consequently, anterograde ureteral catheterization can be tried via the percutaneous nephrostomy and the ureteral catheter is advanced. A ureteral stent is then placed to overlap the ureteral fistula. If the ureteral stent corrects the leakage of urine, it is left in place for 1 month to allow time for healing of ureterovaginal fistula. After 1 month, the ureteral catheter is removed and IVP is performed. If the IVP is normal, it is repeated in 3 months to ensure absence of ureteral extravasation and to rule out ureteral stenosis. If ureteral leakage still occurs, then surgery is indicated. Inpatient close observation and repeat CT scan in 2 days may further worsen hydronephrosis and is contraindicated in this patient.

28 URETHRAL DIVERTICULA
John J. Kim and Sam Siddighi

INTRODUCTION

- An epithelium-lined pouch results either of a distention of a segment of urethra or protrudes off the urethra.
- Generally located posteriorly anywhere along the urethra.
- Essentially, it is a fluid-filled pouch with direct communication with urethra.
- Most are false diverticula (lack of muscular layer).
- Paraurethral glands arise embryologically from urethra.
- Some diverticula have more than one orifice.

ETIOLOGY

- Infectious (gonococcus, *Escherichia coli*, *Chlamydia*, *Trichomonas*, recurrent vaginitis): thought to be #1 cause
  ○ Pathogenesis: infection of periurethral gland → obstruction → retention of secretions → dilation → ruptures into urethral lumen
- Congenital (remnant of Gartner's of müllerian duct cysts)
  ○ Diverticula can be found proximally in the urethra and may be lined with colonic epithelium; this suggests possibility of congenital etiology
- Trauma (e.g., birth trauma, urethral dilation, stress urinary incontinence [SUI] surgery, and other iatrogenic causes)

DIFFERENTIAL DIAGNOSIS

- For detailed review, see Chap. 39, Vulvovaginal and Urethral Disorders.
- Vaginal wall inclusion cyst
- Dilated Skene's glands
- Gartner's duct remnants
- Endometriosis
- Leiomyoma
- Bladder diverticulum
- Urethrocele
- Suburethral abscess

INCIDENCE

- Davis and Telinde reported an 8% rate in the 1950s.
- Anderson in Denmark reported a 3% rate in the 1960s.
- University of Copenhagen reported 15 women in 9-year period in the 1990s.
- Progressive decline maybe due to earlier diagnosis and treatment of infections.

- Currently quoted from 0.6 to 8%.
- Occurs most frequently in women in fifth decades of life.
- Most urethral diverticula are found in the distal two-third of the urethra.
- ≈50% of the time there are multiple diverticula and not just one.
- Diverticula are seen more in the peripartum period than the nonpregnant state.

SYMPTOMS AND SIGNS

- Urinary incontinence (especially SUI): the most common complaint
- Asymptomatic recurrent urinary tract infections (UTIs): the second most common complaint
- Dysuria
- Urgency
- Vaginal mass
- Dyspareunia
- Postmicturition leakage
- Hematuria
- Frequency
- Pain
- Palpable, tender suburethral mass
- Classically, the three Ds (**D**ysuria, **D**ribbling, and **D**yspareunia)

DIAGNOSIS

HISTORY

- Recurrent UTIs, incontinence, and chronic dysuria are the most common presenting symptoms. Also urethral pain, dyspareunia, and postvoid dribble not responsive to medical therapies should be suggestive.

PHYSICAL EXAMINATION

- Most commonly described sign of a urethral diverticulum is anterior vaginal mass and the ability to milk it of pus or urine.
  - Davis and Telinde used this method and diagnosed urethral diverticula correctly in 63% of their cases.

TESTS

- Urinalysis
  - Hematuria, pyuria, and evidence of UTIs
- Urethrocystoscopy (using 0 degree urethra/70 degree bladder)
  - Thought to be inadequate for diagnosis. The opening to the diverticula may be too small to be seen endoscopically; 30–40% false negative rate. Additionally, it may not reveal number of diverticula if multiple diverticula are present.

- Occlusion of bladder neck by pushing up through vagina may increase ability to diagnose because it creates more pressure in the urethra → leading to dilation of diverticula.
  - Pediatric cystoscope is preferred. Injecting dye into suspected diverticula while observing with cystoscope can yield better visualization/localization.
- Positive pressure urethrography (PPUG)
  - Trattner double-balloon catheter is used.
    - Catheter with two balloons. One at the bladder neck and other at the external urethral meatus. Contrast is infused between balloons under pressure. Dye may leak.
    - Is uncomfortable for patients.
    - PPUG is indicated when other tests are negative and there is still a high suspicion.
  - Usually combined with voiding cystourethrogram (VCUG) to increase sensitivity.
- Ultrasonography
  - Transvaginal, perineal, and endoluminal
    - Operator dependant. More useful after diagnosis of diverticula is confirmed.
- VCUG: using anteroposterior (AP) and oblique views; has high sensitivity for diagnosis
- MRI
  - MRI has high sensitivity for detection of urethral diverticula.
- Urodynamics
  - Urodynamic testing is required if a patient who is suspected of having urethral diverticula also has urinary incontinence.
  - Relationship of diverticulum to maximum urethral closure pressure (MUCP) is helpful in choosing corrective surgical procedure.

TREATMENT

1. Surgical
   - Complete or partial diverticulectomy: A classic approach is to identify the location of the diverticulum by radiographic or endoscopic techniques. (There may be multiple diverticula.) Prophylactic antibiotics are given. The Trattner double-balloon catheter is placed into the urethra and inflated. Dye is then injected and kept in place until the sac is entered. An incision is made in the anterior vaginal wall in either a vertical incision or in an upside down "U" shape. The diverticulum is then dissected free of the pubocervical fascia. A longitudinal incision is made over the diverticular sac. The fascial tissue over and around the diverticulum is carefully dissected and mobilized. Once the neck of the diverticulum is identified, wide excision of diverticulum is performed. If the entire sac cannot be identified, then a longitudinal incision is performed. Urethrocele should be performed and the diverticulum

explored to note the presence of other diverticular openings. Then the sac is excised at the neck leaving behind part of the diverticulum. The defect in the urethra is closed (in multiple layers) using 4-0 chromic or polyglycol over the Foley catheter. *Try to minimize stress on the suture line and attempt to maintain excellent hemostasis.* Next, the incision is closed with 3-0 polyglycol. This "vest-over-pants" closure of the periurethral fascia is to avoid overlapping sutures and reduce the incidence of urethrovaginal fistulas. The vagina is generally packed for 1 day. Foley catheter or suprapubic catheter is left in place for 1 week.

- Most diverticula are located on the ventral side of the urethra (i.e., suburethral). Some are located laterally or dorsally. Dorsally located diverticula are amputated at the neck and allow the tissues of the urethra to retract with placement of a Foley catheter for 6–7days.
- A Martius graft maybe beneficial to prevent wound breakdown and fistula.
- Most authors agree that complete or partial excision is recommended. Some though believe that a marsupialization procedure (the Spence procedure) can also be curative.
  - Spence (aka marsupialization): Can be used for diverticula when the sac is located distally (distal to midurethral MUCP). One blade of the scissor is placed in the urethra and the other in the vagina. This is used to divide the floor of the diverticulum and the vaginal epithelium. Running locked suture around the cut edge is placed. This coapts the lining of the sac with the adjacent vaginal epithelium. The bladder neck and urethra proximal to the diverticular orifice are left untouched. No catheter is necessary. Complications are urine spraying and dyspareunia.
  - Suburethral sling procedure—may be performed in addition to diverticular repair in a patient who has urethral diverticulum + SUI on urodynamic testing.
2. Postoperative management: Consists of leaving a Foley catheter in place (some also recommend a concurrent suprapubic catheter) for 1–2 weeks. Then obtaining a VCUG. If there is a small amount of extravasation, leave the catheter in place (or pull the Foley and leave the suprapubic) then repeat VCUG in 1 week. Then perform a voiding trial. Antibiotics should be given intraoperative and while the catheters are in place.
3. Complications include recurrence of urethral diverticulum recurrence of urethral diverticulum (#1 complication), recurrent UTI, postoperative SUI, urethral stricture, and urethrovaginal fistula formation. If fistula formation occurs, many authors believe that reoperation should not occur for a minimum of 3 months. Success rates for any of the techniques discussed earlier are >90%.

4. Nonsurgical management: If symptoms are not significant, a small diverticula can be followed by conservative methods including observation, postmicturition compression, or injection therapy.

BIBLIOGRAPHY

Bent AE. Disorders affecting the urethra. In: Bent AE, Ostergard DR, Cundiff GW, et al., eds. *Ostergard's Urogynecology and Pelvic Floor Dysfunction*. Philadelphia, PA: Lippincott William & Wilkins; 2003:251–260.

Urethral diverticulum. In: Walsch PC, Wein JA, Kavonssi LR, et al. *Cambell's Urology*. 8th ed. Elsevier Sciences; 2002:1207–1214.

Urogynecology. In: Stenchever MA, Droegemueller W, Herbst AL, eds. *Comprehensive Gynecology*. 4th ed. 607–639.

Cundiff GW. Urethral diverticula. In: Cundiff GW, Bent AE, eds. *Endoscopic Diagnosis of the Female Lower Urinary Tract*. London: WB Saunders; 1999:43–51.

Ganabathi K, Leach GE, Simmern PE, et al. Experience with the management of urethral diverticulum in 63 women. *J Urol*. 1994;152:1445–1452.

Ginsburg DS, Genadry R. Suburethral diverticulum in the female. *Obstet Gynecol Surv*. 1984;39:1–7.

Kim B, Hricak H, Tanagho EA. Diagnosis of urethral diverticula in women: value of MR imaging. *Am J Roentgenol*. 1993;161:809–815.

Niemiec TR, Mercer LJ, Stephens JK, et al. Unusual urethral diverticulum lined by colonic epithelium with Paneth cell metaplasia. *Am J Obstet Gynecol*. 1989;160:186–188.

Summitt RL Jr, Stovall TG. Urethral diverticula: evaluation by urethral pressure profilometry, cystourethroscopy, and the voiding cystourethrogram. *Obstet Gynecol*. 1992;80:695–699.

Rock JA, Horowitz IR, Domergnez CE. Surgical conditions at vagina and urethra. In: Rock JP, Jones HW III. *Te Linde's Operative Gynecology*. 9th ed. Philadelphia, PA: Lippincott Williams & Wilkins; 893–924.

Urologic Clinics of North America: Contemporary Evaluation and Management of Female Urethral Diverticulum. Philadelphia, PA: WB Saunders; 2002;29(3).

QUESTIONS

QUESTIONS 1–4

Match the statement below with the word that best corresponds to it above. The answers may be used once, more than once, or not at all.

(A) Spence

(B) Diverticulectomy

(C) Urethroscopy

(D) MRI

(E) VCUG

(F) Complex cystometry

(G) PPUG

(H) Iatrogenic

(I) Infectious

(J) Congenital

1. Accumulation of secretions followed by rupture of cystic dilatation

2. Believed to be the most common etiology for urethral diverticula

3. Procedure of choice in patient with a history of bicornuate uterus and suspicion of a urethral diverticula

4. This procedure is diagnostic for urethral diverticulum but is associated with patient discomfort

5. A 53-year-old woman complains of involuntary loss of urine during straining efforts (coughing, laughing, getting up from a chair). Her past medical and surgical history is unremarkable. On pelvic examination, a cystic mass is found on the distal-lateral vaginal wall. There is no induration or tenderness on palpation of the mass. Milking of the urethra does not express any fluid. The most likely diagnosis is _____.

(A) SUI

(B) urethral diverticulum

(C) Skene's duct cyst

(D) urethral prolapse

(E) urethral caruncle

ANSWERS

ANSWERS 1–4

1. *(I)*, 2. *(I)*, 3. *(D)*, 4. *(G)*. The #1 cause of urethral diverticula is infectious (gonococcus, *E. coli*, *Chlamydia*, *Trichomonas*, recurrent vaginitis). Infection of periurethral gland leads to obstruction → dilation → and eventual rupture into urethral lumen. Since bicornuate uteri are associated with anomalies of the urinary tract and spine. Since there is suspicion that a urethral diverticulum may coexist with an intra-abdominal congenital anomaly, MRI is the study of choice. PPUG is sensitive for the detection of urethral diverticula but can cause pain when contrast is injected under high pressure.

5. *(A)*. This patient has symptoms of SUI and also happens to have an incidental asymptomatic vaginal inclusion cyst on pelvic examination. Epidermal inclusions cysts are located laterally on the distal vaginal wall. The physical examination is against a urethral diverticulum because of the location of the mass and absence of expressed fluid. A urethral prolapse appears as a beefy protruding mass (color: pink/red, violet, black) in the area of the external urethral orifice. A urethral caruncle is a small red mass arising from the posterior lip of external urethral meatus. Skene's duct cyst is a mass arising in the anterior lateral introitus. Often VCUG or urethroscopy must be done to differentiate Skene's duct cyst from a urethral diverticulum.

29 CHANGES IN THE URINARY TRACT DURING PREGNANCY AND PUERPERIUM

Yvonne G. Gollin

ANATOMIC CHANGES

UPPER URINARY TRACT

- The anatomic changes in the urinary tract during pregnancy are most significant in the collecting system, with a greater magnitude of change noted on the right side.
- The kidney is larger during pregnancy and increases in length from 1 to 1.5 cm and in weight from 259 to 307 g, with the right kidney enlarging more than the left. In general, this is accounted for by changes in vascular and interstitial volume.
- The renal pelvis also enlarges disproportionately, with the right renal pelvis measuring 15 mm (range 5–25) versus 5 mm (range 3–8) on the left.
- The right ureter is more dilated than the left purportedly secondary to dextrorotation of the uterus and a cushioning effect of the sigmoid colon on the left ureter. More than 90% of patients have some hydroureter toward the end of their pregnancy.
- Ureteral dilation is not seen below the pelvic brim suggesting a mechanical effect of the enlarging uterus. However, since ureteral dilation occurs by 8 weeks and is maximum in the middle of the second trimester, mechanical factors cannot completely explain the findings and suggest a hormonal contribution to the dilation.
- Dilation of the ureters below the pelvic brim, whether due to mechanical or hormonal factors, may be limited by their encasement in a connective tissue sheath (Waldeyer's sheath), which hypertrophies in pregnancy.
- The *iliac sign* refers to the radiographic filing defect noted where the iliac artery and ureter cross.

- At term, the ureters can hold 200 mL more than in the nonpregnant state.
- For most women, ureteral dilation resolves by the third month postpartum with persistent dilation in only 11%.

LOWER URINARY TRACT

- The functional length of the urethra increases in pregnancy from approximately 30 cm to a maximum of 35 cm in the third trimester and decreases to 28 cm in the postpartum period. Lengthening of the urethra during pregnancy most likely occurs as the bladder is displaced upward and forward.
- Since urethral closure pressure increases during pregnancy, theoretically improving continence, another mechanism must be operative to explain the increased incidence of stress incontinence in pregnancy.
- Bladder neck support and descent with Valsalva maneuver are adversely affected by pregnancy and, especially, vaginal delivery but there is no correlation with incontinence.
- Bladder capacity increases from 410 to 460 mL by midgestation, but declines to 272 mL in the late third trimester due to lower uterine segment relaxation and engagement of the fetal head in the pelvis. Bladder pressure also increases from 9 cm H_2O early in pregnancy to 20 cm H_2O later. In the postpartum period, capacity increases and pressure decreases as would be expected.

PHYSIOLOGIC CHANGES

- Kidney function in pregnancy can generally be characterized to be augmented. Despite the dramatic increases in glomerular filtration rate (GFR) and renal blood flow (RBF) and increased filtration of sodium, glucose, amino acids, and water-soluble vitamins, pregnant individuals retain the ability to excrete a water load and concentrate their urine when compared with nonpregnant women.

LABORATORY PARAMETERS

- A different scale of values should be used for blood urea nitrogen (BUN) and creatinine measurements in pregnancy as a consequence of the dramatic increase in filtered solute: BUN decreases from 13 to 9 mg/dL and creatinine from 0.7 to 0.5 mg/dL. Therefore, BUN/ creatinine concentrations above 13/0.8 suggest renal insufficiency.
- GFR increases 30–50% by the end of the first trimester with no late pregnancy fall. Because GFR increases 50% and RBF increases 80%, there is a decrease in the filtration fraction until the late third trimester. After that, the RBF decreases while the GFR does not, which normalizes the filtration fraction to 0.21.
- The GFR is estimated clinically by measuring creatinine clearance. Creatinine is secreted by the tubules, which leads to an overestimation of the GFR. Normal pregnancy values are 89–222 mL/min compared with 46–136 mL/min in nonpregnant women.
- Consistent with the increased solute filtered, urinary protein excretion is augmented in pregnancy with the threshold being 300 mg/dL in a 24-hour period.
- Routine urinalysis in pregnancy will reveal an increase in glycosuria thought to be a factor in the increased susceptibility during pregnancy to urinary tract infections. Physiologic aminoaciduria also occurs in pregnancy.

SALT HANDLING

- The augmented GFR has a significant impact on renal salt handling with an additional 10,000 mEq of sodium filtered and reabsorbed by the renal tubules every day. Despite this apparent natriuresis, there is a net gain in sodium accumulation throughout pregnancy of 950 mEq, which is most rapid in the third trimester.
- Favoring salt retention are increased levels of aldosterone, renin, angiotensin, estrogen, cortisol, and placental lactogen and physical factors such as the supine and upright positions. Progesterone normally causes natriuresis but in pregnancy is a major source of desoxycorticosterone production, which results in salt retention.

OSMOLARITY

- The decrease in plasma osmolarity of 10 mOsm/kg, which occurs in pregnancy, would provoke a dramatic diuresis in a nonpregnant woman. However, this does not occur in pregnancy because thirst and ADH release thresholds are each reset at a lower levels, allowing expected dilution and concentration of urine. ADH levels do not change but production increases as compensation for the degradation occurring due to placental vasopressinase.

FLUID BALANCE

- The pregnant woman experiences an increase in urine output concomitant with an apparently paradoxical increase in net fluid accumulation.
- The net increase in fluid accumulation in pregnancy is approximately 7 L of water which occurs despite the increase in GFR and is distributed between the extracellular space (20%) and pregnancy-related tissues (80%).
- The increased GFR has lead to an increase in urine output, which reaches a maximum in the second trimester of 2020 mL compared with 1475 in the postpartum period.
- Increased urine output leads to the complaint of frequency, which, defined as voiding more than seven times during the day and more than once at night, occurs as early as the first trimester and worsens with each trimester.
- Since bladder capacity increases in pregnancy, the increase in frequency is not thought to be due to a limited capacity until the third trimester when anatomic constraints from the fetal head cause a decrease in voided volumes.
- Nocturia occurs as a result of the mobilization of accumulated fluid during the daytime when it is manifest as dependent edema.

URINARY TRACT INFECTION

- Urinary tract infections are the most common bacterial infection which occur in pregnancy.
- The increased propensity to infection of the urinary tract in women compared to men has been primarily related to anatomic and physiologic differences with behavioral factors playing an important secondary role. The urethra in women is only 4 cm long and is in close proximity to the vagina and rectum. Sexual intercourse creates a pumping action, facilitating entry of microorganisms into the sterile environment of the bladder.
- Pregnancy further predisposes to urinary tract infection because of physiologic and anatomic changes including increased stasis, changes in pH, a decreased concentrating ability, and normalizing osmolarity. The decreased threshold for excretion of glucose and amino acids which occurs in pregnancy results in an excellent media for growth of organisms.

ASYMPTOMATIC BACTERURIA

- The incidence of asymptomatic bacteruria is approximately 2–10% with an additional 1–2% of women testing positive later in pregnancy.
- Asymptomatic bacteriuria is not more prevalent in pregnancy than in the nonpregnant woman. However, progression to pyelonephritis is increased largely due to the progesterone-induced smooth muscle relaxation of the ureter which facilitates bacterial access to the kidney.
- Many conditions increase the risk for both asymptomatic and symptomatic urinary tract infection and include childhood urinary tract infections with renal scarring, diabetes, a history of urinary tract infections, sickle cell trait and disease, anatomic abnormalities, and lower socioeconomic status.
- The most important complication of asymptomatic bacteruria is the progression to pyelonephritis which occurs in 28% (range 16–65%) compared with 1.4% in pregnant patients without asymptomatic bacteruria. Since treatment can reduce the progression to pyelonephritis by 80%, screening for asymptomatic bacteriuria at the first prenatal visit is the standard of care.
- Diagnosis of asymptomatic bacteruria requires the presence of $\geq 10^5$ CFU/mL on one midstream clean catch urine specimen. This provides a sensitivity of only 51% compared with the criteria of 10^2 CFU/mL with a sensitivity of 91%. (Newton). If a catheterized specimen is obtained, a colony count of 10^2 CFU/mL indicates infection.
- Common organisms found in cases of asymptomatic bacteruria include *Escherichia coli* (60–90%), *Klebsiella Pneumoniae, Enterobacter* (5–15%), and *Proteus* species (1–10%). The presence of group B streptococcus in the bladder suggests heavy vaginal colonization which has been associated with increased perinatal morbidity and mortality and necessitates intrapartum prophylaxis.
- Three-day treatment regimens have comparable efficacy to longer courses except for nitrofurantoin. When empiric therapy is given, resistance of *E. coli* to Ampicillin and Bactrim should be taken into account.
  ○ Cephalexin 500 mg PO bid to qid × 3 days
  ○ Amoxicillin 500 mg PO bid or 250 mg tid × 3 days (check resistance patterns)
  ○ Nitrofurantoin 100 mg PO bid × 7 days (avoid in glucose-6-phosphate dehydrogenase [G6PD] deficiency)
  ○ Bactrim DS 1 PO bid × 3 days (avoid near delivery)
- Treatment sterilizes the urine in 60–90% of cases. A test of cure is offered 2 weeks after the end of antibiotics to detect complicated cases which occur with asymptomatic renal infection, nephrolithiasis, and anatomic abnormalities of the urinary tract. Stones should be suspected if the urine pH is >6, suggesting *Proteus* infection, and in the presence of hematuria.
- Treatment of asymptomatic bacteruria reduces the risk of pyelonephritis, preterm delivery, and low birth weight.
- If recurrent bacteriuria is detected, underlying structural disease or renal infection should be suspected and has been found in 40% and 50% of patients, respectively.
- Preventive measures followed prior to pregnancy should be strictly adhered to during pregnancy and include avoidance of the female superior position, wiping front to back, voiding 5 minutes after sexual activity, and avoiding douching or bubble baths.

CYSTITIS

- Cystitis occurs in approximately 4% of the pregnant population and is defined as urgency, frequency, and dysuria without systemic symptoms of nausea, vomiting, fever, or flank pain.
- In contrast to asymptomatic bacteriuria, cystitis is not associated with an increased risk of preterm delivery, low birth weight, or pyelonephritis.
- Of the classic symptoms of acute cystitis, frequency and urgency are common in normal pregnancy and may not indicate pathology. Frequent voiding of normal amounts is less concerning than the complaint of frequency associated with minimal volumes. Dysuria is one of the most important symptoms, with a high positive predictive value but low sensitivity.
- A pregnant patient presenting with symptoms suggestive of acute cystitis should undergo a pelvic examination to exclude other causes of dysuria such as vaginitis or labial infections. More importantly, examination of the cervix is indicated as many patients with preterm labor and expansion of the lower uterine segment will present with urgency, frequency, and suprapubic discomfort.
- The risk factors for acute cystitis are similar to those for asymptomatic bacteruria in the antepartum period. However, events during labor, delivery, and the puerperium markedly increase the risk for acute cystitis. Numerous digital examinations and catheterization during labor and the back and forth action of the fetal head against the urethra during pushing increase the deposition of periurethral flora into the bladder. In the postpartum period, urinary retention from perineal trauma or secondary to anesthesia further increases the risk.
- The infectious agents associated with acute cystitis are similar to those causing asymptomatic bacteruria. Identification of the organism is important since

10–15% of acute cystitis in pregnancy is due to group B streptococcus.
- Treatment and follow-up are similar to that of asymptomatic bacteruria, with a test of cure offered within 2 weeks of the end of therapy. Relapse occurs in 20–30%, which requires retreatment and suppressive therapy (Nitrofuration 100 mg PO qhs). Alternatively, if the patient is not treated for suppression then biweekly evaluation for leukocyte esterase and nitrites is recommended.

PYELONEPHRITIS

- Pyelonephritis is the most common medical complication of pregnancy and occurs in 1–2% of patients. While asymptomatic bacteriuria is not more common in pregnancy, the increased stasis and dilation of the collecting system place the gravid patient at increased risk for pyelonephritis. Three-fourth of cases of pyelonephritis occur in women with antecedent asymptomatic bacteriuria.
- The majority of cases present antepartum with most of those occurring in the second and third trimesters. However, labor and delivery poses a unique risk as noted above for infection in the postpartum period which accounts for 10–25% of all cases of pyelonephritis.
- Symptoms such as nausea, vomiting, fever, chills, and flank pain and signs such as costovertebral angle tenderness differentiate cystitis from pyelonephritis. The most common symptoms are back pain and chills (82%) while less than half (40%) present with classic cystitis symptoms of dysuria, frequency, or urgency. Right costovertebral angle tenderness is more common than left (54% vs. 16%). The diagnosis is confirmed if $\geq 10^2$ colony-forming units (CFU)/mL are found in a catheterized specimen.
- Other laboratory parameters which are abnormal include an elevated creatinine in 20% of patients and alterations in creatinine clearance in up to half of the patients.
- Organisms responsible for pyelonephritis are similar to those causing asymptomatic bacteriuria and cystitis with the exception that gram-positive isolates do not generally cause upper infection.
- All pregnant patients with pyelonephritis should be admitted to the hospital and treated with intravenous antibiotics (Ampicillin or Cephalosporin). However, outpatient treatment of pyelonephritis in pregnant patients with lower risk of morbidity (e.g., low white blood cells [WBCs], afebrile, and good follow-up) has been shown to be successful. For inpatient management, addition of gentamicin is recommended for the 5–10% of patients who do not become afebrile within

48 hours with careful dosing adjustments if the creatinine is >1 mg/dL. Antibiotics are continued until the patient is afebrile for 24 hours. A total of 10–14 days of antibiotics are recommended and a test of cure offered 2 weeks after completion of therapy. Twenty to thirty percent of patients with pyelonephritis will have recurrence and suppressive antibiotics and increased surveillance are both acceptable regimens for follow-up.
- Uterine contractions in the setting of pyelonephritis occur in 86% of patients at the initiation of therapy. However, preterm contractions are not always associated with preterm labor. Differentiation is important because hydration and tocolysis in the setting of endotoxemia predisposes the pregnant patient to pulmonary edema and adult respiratory distress. If tocolysis is administered, judicious fluid management and magnesium administration is recommended because of the potential underlying renal dysfunction.
- Other complications of pyelonephritis include bacteremia in 15% of patients and ARDS or septic shock.

NEPHROLITHIASIS

- The incidence of nephrolithiasis is approximately 1/1500 pregnancies to 1/2500, which does not reflect an increase over the general population. It is more commonly seen in multiparas and in the second trimester.
- The increased calcium and uric acid excretion encountered in pregnancy theoretically increase the risk of stones, but this is countered by an increased urine output.
- Nephrolithiasis should be suspected when a patient presents with nausea, vomiting, and flank pain and both sides are equally affected. Alternatively, intermittent abdominal pain, hematuria, and frequent urinary tract infections can indicate nephrolithiasis. Microscopic hematuria is more common (60–90%) than gross hematuria.
- Ultrasound is commonly used in the diagnosis of nephrolithiasis, but the sensitivity is estimated at only 60%. Therefore, many experts advocate use of a limited intravenous pyelogram (IVP) with avoidance of fluoroscopy if fever and symptoms persist or obstruction is suspected. The fetal exposure has been estimated at 40 mrad to 1 rad.
- Most cases (66–85%) of nephrolithiasis respond to conservative management with analgesia and hydration. Stent placement or percutaneous nephrostomy are reserved for those cases failing conservative management. Recently, ureteroscopy and holmium:YAG laser lithotripsy have been suggested as safe since the energy is confined within 0.5 mm of the laser tip.

URINARY RETENTION

- The earliest urinary symptom of the postpartum patient is urinary retention, occurring in approximately 4% of women. Any anesthetic which results in decreased bladder sensation increase the risk of retention. Intermittent or continuous self-catheterization is the treatment of choice and is effective in almost all cases.

URINARY INCONTINENCE DURING PREGNANCY

- Urinary incontinence is an important woman's health issue with annual treatment costs of approximately $12.4 billion. Important risk factors for *long-term* incontinence are age and mode of delivery, with a decreased incidence in women delivering by cesarean section. Incontinence *during* pregnancy is affected by age, history of incontinence, and mode of delivery.
- The effects of pregnancy per se irrespective of the mode of delivery are ideally studied in primiparous women with no antecedent incontinence history. New-onset incontinence occurs in approximately one-third of primiparous women and is usually mild in nature. Resolution occurs in the majority of patients with new-onset incontinence with less than one-third having persistent symptoms in the immediate postpartum period. Onset of incontinence during pregnancy confers an increased risk of incontinence at 5 years when compared to women who remain continent throughout pregnancy.
- The incidence of incontinence during pregnancy is increased in multiparas compared with primiparas, most likely associated with the previous mode of delivery in multiparas. The incidence of incontinence in parous women delivered only by cesarean section is not known but would be the best estimate of the effect of pregnancy alone on the continence mechanism.
- Patients with incontinence prior to the first pregnancy can expect worsening of symptoms. The rate of incontinence prior to pregnancy in primiparous women in one study was 4% and three-fourth of these women continued to have symptoms throughout their pregnancy. The background rate of incontinence depends on maternal age and ranges from 10% to 20% in women between the ages of 20 and 40.
- Urge incontinence is also more common during pregnancy, with an estimate of 43% in the third trimester in one study compared with a prepregnancy incidence of 5%. Urinary leakage from urge incontinence should be considered in the differential diagnosis when a pregnant woman presents with the complaint of ruptured membranes, especially when it occurs nocturnally.

URINARY INCONTINENCE POSTPARTUM

- The mode of delivery has a significant impact on the development of incontinence in the postpartum period with less of a contribution from the same factors which affect incontinence during pregnancy, namely age and a history of antecedent incontinence. Vaginal delivery increases the risk of stress urinary incontinence 2.8 times compared with a cesarean section without labor. Among women undergoing a vaginal delivery, additional risk factors include macrosomia, operative delivery, and protracted second stage of labor.
- As noted above, the incidence of incontinence in the *immediate* postpartum period is best studied in primiparous patients. In one such study in which most patients were delivered vaginally, patients were classified into three categories: those with incontinence prior to pregnancy (4%), those with new-onset incontinence during pregnancy (29%), and those with new-onset incontinence only postpartum (7%). The incidence of incontinence after delivery actually *decreased* by two-thirds in patients in the first two categories suggesting that pregnancy significantly stresses the continence mechanism.
- Incontinence symptoms during pregnancy or the immediate postpartum period and at 3 months predict the development of symptoms at 5 years, even with intervening resolution of symptoms. However, even patients continent throughout their first pregnancy had a 19% risk of incontinence at 5 years.

BIBLIOGRAPHY

Donat S, Cozzi P, Herr H. Surgery of penile and urethral carcinoma. In: Walsh PC, Retik AB, Vaughan ED, et al., eds. *Campbell's Urology*. 8th ed. Philadelphia, PA: W.B. Saunders; 2002:2983–2991.

Brubaker L. Pelvic Organ Prolapse in Pregnant and Postpartum Women. In: Weber A., Brubaker L, Schaffer J. *Office Urogynecology*. New York: McGraw-Hill; 2004:425–433.

Farrell S, Allen V, Baskett T. Parturition and urinary incontinence in primiparas. *Obstet Gynecol*. 2001:97:350–356.

Fried A, Woodring JH, Thompson TJ. Hydronephrosis of pregnancy. *J Ultrasound Med*. 1983;2:225.

Goldberg RP, Lobel RW, Sand PK. The urinary tract in pregnancy. In: Bent AE, et al., eds. *Ostergard's Urogynecology and Pelvic Floor Dysfunction*. 5th ed. Philadelphia, PA: Lippincott Williams & Wilkins; 2003:225–242.

Graham JM, Oshiro BT, Blanco JD, et al. Uterine contractions after antibiotic therapy for pyelonephritis in pregnancy. *Am J Obstet Gynecol*. 1993;168:577–580.

Hunskaar S, Burgio K, Diokno A, et al. Epidemiology and natural history of urinary incontinence in women. *Urology*. 2003; 62(Suppl. 4A):16–23.

Katz AI, Davison JM, Hayslett JP. Effect of pregnancy on the natural history of kidney disease. *Contrib Nephrol.* 1981;25:53–60.

Davison JM, Katz AJ. Lindheimer MD. Kidney disease and pregnancy: obstetric outcome and long-term renal prognosis. *Clin Perinatol.* 1985;12(3):497–519.

Newton ER. The urinary tract in pregnancy. In: Karram MM, Walters MD, eds. *Urogynecology and Reconstructive Pelvic Surgery.* 2nd ed. St. Louis, MO: Mosby; 1999:399–417.

Schulman A, Herlinger H. Urinary tract dilatation in pregnancy. *Br J Radiol.* 1975;48(572):638–645.

Smaill F. Antibiotics for asymptomatic bacteriuria in pregnancy (Cochrane Review). In: *The Cochrane Database of Systematic Reviews 2001.* Issue 2.Art.No.:CD000490. Oxford: Update Software.

Viktrup L, Lose G. The risk of stress incontinence 5 years after first delivery. *Am J Obstet Gynecol.* 2001;185:82–87.

Wilson L, Brown JS, Shin GP, et al. Annual direct cost of urinary incontinence. *Obstet Gynecol.* 2001;98:398–406.

QUESTIONS

1. All of the following renal parameters are normal in pregnancy except:
   (A) Creatinine of 1.0 mg/dL
   (B) Twenty-four-hour urinary protein <300 mg
   (C) BUN 5 mg/dL
   (D) Osmolarity 280 mOsm/kg

2. Which of the following statements is true?
   (A) The incidence of asymptomatic bacteriuria and pyelonephritis are increased in pregnancy.
   (B) The incidence of asymptomatic bacteriuria and pyelonephritis are both decreased in pregnancy.
   (C) The incidence of asymptomatic bacteriuria is decreased and pyelonephritis is increased in pregnancy.
   (D) The incidence of asymptomatic bacteriuria is unchanged but the incidence of pyelonephritis is increased in pregnancy.

3. Which of the following organisms is associated with the most perinatal morbidity and mortality if found in a patient with asymptomatic bacteriuria?
   (A) *E. coli*
   (B) *Enterococcus*
   (C) *Staphylococcus*
   (D) Group B streptococcus
   (E) *Chlamydia*

4. Labor and delivery pose a unique risk for introducing infection because of all of the following except:
   (A) Frequent digital examinations
   (B) Use of the Foley catheter
   (C) Increase in periurethral tears
   (D) Anesthesia-related urinary retention and stasis

5. Vaginal delivery increases the risk of incontinence compared with elective cesarean section:
   (A) Tenfold
   (B) Threefold
   (C) Twenty-fold
   (D) Does not increase the risk

ANSWERS

1. *(A).* A different scale of values should be used for BUN and creatinine measurements in pregnancy as a consequence of the dramatic increase in filtered solute: BUN decreases from 13 to 9 mg/dL and creatinine from 0.7 to 0.5 mg/dL. Therefore, BUN/ creatinine concentrations above 13/0.8 suggest renal insufficiency.

2. *(D).* Asymptomatic bacteriuria is not more common in pregnancy than in the nonpregnant woman. However, progression to pyelonephritis is increased largely due to the progesterone-induced smooth muscle relaxation of the ureter which facilitates bacterial access to the kidney.

3. *(D).* Common organisms found in cases of asymptomatic bacteruria include *E. coli* (60–90), *K. pneumoniae, Enterobacter* (5–15%), and *Proteus* species (1–10%). The presence of group B streptococcus in the bladder suggests heavy vaginal colonization which has been associated with increased perinatal morbidity and mortality and necessitates intrapartum prophylaxis.

4. *(C).* Events during labor, delivery, and the puerperium markedly increase the risk for acute cystitis. Numerous digital examinations and catheterization during labor and the back and forth action of the fetal head against the urethra during pushing increase the deposition of periurethral flora into the bladder. In the postpartum period, urinary retention from perineal trauma or secondary to anesthesia further increases the risk.

5. *(B).* The mode of delivery has a significant impact on the development of incontinence in the postpartum period with less of a contribution from the same factors which affect incontinence during pregnancy, namely age and a history of antecedent incontinence. Vaginal delivery increases the risk of stress urinary incontinence 2.8 times compared with a cesarean section without labor. Among women undergoing a vaginal delivery, additional risk factors include macrosomia, operative delivery, and protracted second stage of labor.

30 "SELECTIVE" CESAREAN SECTION FOR PREVENTION OF PELVIC FLOOR DISORDERS, PROS AND CONS

Sam Siddighi and Barry S. Block

INTRODUCTION

- Cesarean section (aka abdominal delivery)—combination of laparotomy and hysterotomy. Delivery of the fetus after making an abdominal incision and then a uterine incision.
- The origin of the term "cesarean" is unknown. There are three hypotheses: (1) Lex cesarean = Roman law in eighth century B.C. decreeing that this operation be performed on women dying during childbirth; (2) partus caesareus = from the Latin verb caedere which means to cut; (3) Julius Cesar may have been born by cesarean section thus named after him (although unlikely).
- Review of current indications for cesarean section
  - Dystocia: cephalopelvic disproportion, failure to descend, arrest of descent or dilation, failure to progress in labor due to fetal malposition or posture, failed trial of forceps or vacuum
  - Contraindications to labor: placenta previa, vasa previa, malpresentation of fetus, active genital herpes, previous classic uterine scar, previous myomectomy with entrance into uterine cavity, previous uterine reconstruction, possibly certain treatable fetal malformations (spina bifida, meningomyelocele, and hydrocephalus), previous cesarean and patient refuses trial of labor (repeat), no previous deliveries and patient requests a cesarean section (elective), human immunodeficiency virus (HIV) + with high viral load (>1000 copies/mL)
  - Failed induction for maternal or fetal indications: isoimmunization, diabetes mellitus, nonreassuring antenatal testing (e.g., nonstress test [NST], biophysical profile [BPP], contraction stress test [CST], and Doppler), intrauterine growth restriction, preeclampsia, eclampsia, hemolysis, elevated liver, low platelet [HELLP] syndrome
  - Emergent conditions: placental abruption with heavy hemorrhage and instability, umbilical cord prolapse, nonreassuring fetal heart rate tracing, uterine rupture, impending maternal death (cardiopulmonary resuscitation [CPR] for > 4 min)
- Elective cesarean (aka *maternal-choice*, cesarean delivery *on-demand*, and *designer*, preplanned cesarean)—an elective cesarean delivery is one that is performed before the onset of labor (scheduled) due to patient request for such a delivery rather than an indication. Therefore, elective cesareans may be performed for nonmedical reasons.
- Selective cesarean (aka *prophylactic* cesarean)—a cesarean section before the onset of labor (scheduled) for a selected population of patients at high risk for some morbidity. First recorded prophylactic cesarean delivery at term was in 1985. The American College of Obstetricians and Gynecologists (ACOG) Practice Bulletin Number 22, November 2000 states that, "Although the diagnosis of fetal macrosomia is imprecise, prophylactic cesarean delivery may be considered for suspected fetal macrosomia with estimated fetal weights greater than 5000 g in women without diabetes." This is an example of a "selective" cesarean delivery, although it is considered by many as an indication. Even though, more than 400 cesarean deliveries would need to be performed to prevent one case of permanent brachial plexus injury, ACOG supports performing a cesarean section for the high-risk population.
- Therefore, performing a primary cesarean section for a population of patients at high risk of labor-related pelvic floor disorders such as fecal incontinence, urinary incontinence, and pelvic organ prolapse is also an example of selective cesarean delivery.

ARGUMENTS AGAINST ELECTIVE CESAREAN SECTION

- Maternal mortality is higher (two to four times) for a cesarean delivery than for a vaginal delivery. However, this statement does not take into account the type of cesarean (elective, selective, and indicated).
- Elective cesarean is not like other elective surgery (e.g., plastic surgery) because the mother is not only assuming the risk for herself but also for the fetus.
- Iatrogenic respiratory distress syndrome (RDS) in the neonate may increase since obstetricians may perform a delivery either before 39 weeks or with uncertain gestational age and the fetal lungs may be immature. Additionally, attempting to prevent RDS by performing amniocentesis for fetal lung maturity is itself problematic since amniocentesis is associated with fetal morbidity and mortality.
- Cesarean section is not a risk-free surgery and morbidity to mother and baby increases with a repeat cesarean section. Although the average number of children per woman in the United States is 2.013 (in 2002), many women become pregnant more than two

times throughout their lives. Repeat cesarean sections have increased maternal morbidity.

- ○ Risks of initial cesarean section: Risks include but are not limited to infection (wound, uterine, and urinary tract), febrile morbidity, thromboembolic phenomenon (which may lead to death), injury to structures (bladder, bowel, ureter, major blood vessels, and nerves), injury to the fetus (laceration), risks associated with general anesthesia (aspiration, intubation errors, inadequate ventilation, and respiratory failure), spinal anesthesia (local anesthetic toxicity, maternal hypotension which can cause transient fetal respiratory acidosis, and inadvertent high spinal or epidural), uterocervical lacerations leading to profuse bleeding, hemorrhage requiring a blood transfusion, hysterectomy, delayed bonding with and delayed breastfeeding infant, and possible reaction to medications.
- ○ Risk in future pregnancies: Increase in incidence of all of the following: uterine rupture (<1% with one low transverse uterine incision); risk of placenta previa (if 1 previous cesarean section: relative risk (RR) = 4.5 and if ≥ 4 previous cesarean sections: RR = 44.9), risk of placenta accreta (if previa + 1 previous cesarean section: 24% and if previa + 2 previous cesarean sections: 47%), risk of placental abruption (30%), and even risk of ectopic pregnancy. Few of the preceding are associated with preterm labor and low birth weight, requirement of blood transfusion, posthemorrhagic anemia, disseminated intravascular coagulation (DIC), need for an emergency hysterectomy (accreta/increta/percreta are #1 indication for cesarean hysterectomy), fetal morbidity, and even death are possible.
- ○ Risk of repeat cesarean section: Abdominal and pelvic adhesive diseases (which increase morbidity during future surgery and may lead to infertility) and need for a hysterectomy increases with history of more than two cesarean sections. Maternal mortality also increases with higher-order repeat cesarean deliveries because of the aforementioned complications.
- • Cesarean deliveries are associated with longer hospital stays, longer recovery periods, more rehospitalizations, and longer disability.
- • Some experts claim that data that support performing cesarean sections for prevention of pelvic dysfunction later in life is weak because of the following:
  - ○ Loss to follow-up: One of the difficulties with a prospective study is that patients will be lost to follow-up. This causes an overestimation of a disease process. Patients who are lost to follow-up are more likely to lack urinary and fecal incontinence and thus less likely to return to report normal findings. Conversely, those that do return for follow-up

are more likely to have problems and therefore since more of these patients are accounted for in the data, we tend to overestimate the prevalence of fecal and urinary incontinence.

- ○ Lack of long-term outcome data: Data from which conclusions are being made of "long-term" effects of vaginal delivery on the pelvic floor are actually short-term follow-up (i.e., only 2 months, 10 months, or 1 year). There is evidence that the prevalence of incontinence decreases as the interval from vaginal delivery to time of analysis of the outcome (e.g., incontinence) increases. Also, nerve latencies normalize in the majority of women several months after vaginal delivery. In other words, cesarean delivery may only have an immediate protective effect which is gone before 1 year postpartum. Additionally, one large, population-based study did not find an association between cesarean delivery and significant reduction in pelvic floor disorders over long term compared with spontaneous vaginal delivery. Based on a retrospective study by Iosif et al., <4–5% of patients who had 1 or 2 cesarean deliveries up to 6 years earlier, developed stress incontinence. Furthermore, some epidemiological data looking at parity (which is a long-term measure) have either failed to identify it as an independent risk factor for incontinence or have shown it to be a weak risk factor.
- ○ Lack of clinical significance: Example 1: increased pudendal nerve latency is statistically significant (0.1 ms difference) but not clinically relevant, Example 2: anal sphincter disruption measured by transanal ultrasonography usually does not translate into clinically relevant fecal incontinence.
- ○ One long-term retrospective study contradicts common belief that cesarean section is protective against flatal and fecal incontinence in that the episiotomy, sphincter rupture, and cesarean section group all had similar prevalence of incontinence.
- ○ Women who deliver by cesarean section may also develop moderate to severe incontinence and pelvic support problems later in life.
- ○ The protective effect of nulliparity on urinary incontinence, if any, disappears by age 50–60 because older women have the same rate of incontinence regardless of their delivery type.
- • "Don't jump on the bandwagon": As seen in the past, medical fashions come and go. An intervention that seems "common sense" or popular may fail to deliver promised results (home uterine monitoring) or may even cause harm (e.g., diethylstilbestrol [DES]-related health risk).
- • Surveys reveal that high percentage of obstetricians (62–81%) in the United Kingdom, Israel, Canada, Ireland, and New Zealand would honor patients'

requests for an elective cesarean delivery. Additionally, 7–30% of obstetricians preferred cesarean for themselves or their partners. Perineal injury was the #1 cited reason for cesarean delivery among obstetricians.

• A recent survey revealed that the majority of urogynecologists and perinatologists (American Urogynecologic Society [AUGS] + Society for Maternal–Fetal Medicine [SMFM] = 65.4%) would perform an elective cesarean section. Significantly greater percentage of urogynecologists (AUGS = 80.4%) would perform an elective cesarean section as compared to perinatologists (SMFM = 55.4%).

• Backlash against/reaction to increasing number of indications for cesarean section such as (1) persistent breech presentation of singleton at term, (2) only one low transverse uterine scar and avoiding prostaglandins for induction of labor, (3) decline of vaginal birth after cesarean section (VBAC; 23% decrease).

• Beneficence-based clinical judgments: Since vaginal delivery is a safer method of delivery (i.e., lower maternal mortality), respecting his or her own professional integrity and conscience (respecting his or her own autonomy), the physician should inform the patient that he or she is unable to honor her request and refer or transfer her to a provider who can. Respecting the patient's autonomy assumes that the layperson is capable of choosing among medical alternatives and transforms the physician into a mere technician.

• Justice-based clinical judgment: A small decrease in the rate of urinary incontinence (from 33 to 29% in one study) would increase the cesarean rate by threefold. Thus, cesarean delivery would benefit only a few but put the majority of pregnant women at risk.

• Patients with financial capability, influence, popularity are choosing elective cesarean sections for non-medical reasons (*in vitro* fertilization [IVF] patients and celebrities who are *Too posh to push*). This name was derived from Victoria Beckham (Posh Spice). Other celebrities rumored to have delivered by early cesarean to avoid last 2 weeks of abdominal stretching include Elizabeth Hurley, Claudia Schiffer, Elle Macpherson, Madonna, Catherine Zeta Jones, and Celine Dion.

• Physicians receive better reimbursement for a cesarean delivery versus a vaginal delivery. In Brazil, the cesarean section rate in the private sector, among more educated, and among those who have had more prenatal visits is very high, approaching 70–90%. Other countries such as Chili, Columbia, Mexico, and China also have high rates of cesarean delivery.

• In the United States, cesarean rates are the highest in the Northeast and among the more educated.

• Physician convenience: Private physicians are more likely to do a cesarean to expedite delivery in order to get back to their busy schedule or to avoid spending their social time doing work in the hospital.

• Physicians who believe they are avoiding litigation or saving time and effort fighting complaints by respecting the mother's autonomy.

• Patients may have many reasons to want a cesarean section at a particular time. Examples of auspicious deliveries are: Holiday baby, Chinese New Year, before January 1 for tax purposes, busy careers, fear of labor, fear of pain, fear of loss of control over childbirth, not wanting to deliver at 3 A.M., and belief of better preservation of sexual function.

• The World Health Organization (WHO) strives to keep cesarean section rate 10–15% in developed countries rather the reported 26.1% in the Unites States in 2002 or even higher rates in other countries.

ARGUMENTS FOR "SELECTIVE" CESAREAN SECTION

• Many interventions which were unpopular at their inception are now standard of practice (emergency contraception).

• Cesarean section are among the most common surgical procedures performed in the United States and the risks to both the mother and baby have decreased over time as improved surgical, anesthetic, blood banking, and treatment of infectious diseases are available.

• Data showing higher rates of maternal mortality associated with cesarean section may not apply to elective cesarean sections performed today because (1) standard of care has improved over time, risk associated with surgery have diminished, and relative risk of death has decreased dramatically, (2) it is difficult to select cesarean sections performed for elective versus emergent reasons (medical or obstetric complications) from the studies. Additionally, many deaths attributed to cesarean delivery may have been avoided if complicated labors did not precede the cesarean section, (3) one recent study showed a lower maternal mortality from a scheduled cesarean delivery versus a vaginal delivery.

• Autonomy-based clinical judgment: In current thinking, there is a prominent role for respect of a pregnant woman's autonomy. If a patient has serious concerns about pelvic floor dysfunction (PFD) and her beliefs are well supported, then cesarean should be performed either by her physician or a referral should be made in order to avoid paternalistic behavior.

• A scheduled cesarean section (elective, selective, or indicated) avoids an emergency cesarean section which is associated with a manyfold increase in maternal morbidity and mortality. Avoidance of emergency cesarean also enhances satisfaction in the process of childbirth.

- Since rates of stillbirths, aspiration of meconium, cord accidents, and abruptions increase after 39 weeks of gestation, a scheduled cesarean section can potentially decrease fetal morbidity and mortality.
- Avoidance of vaginal delivery can decrease mother to child transmission of infectious diseases (e.g., HIV, hepatitis B virus [HBV], hepatitis C virus [HCV], and human papillomavirus [HPV]), especially since many women with these infections can be asymptomatic yet shedding viruses.
- Scheduled cesarean section can reduce intrapartum intracranial injury which is the highest with failed instrument vaginal delivery (especially vacuum + forceps) > trial of labor leading to cesarean section > and lowest for scheduled cesarean section (no trial of labor).
- According to some, one-quarter of cerebral palsy arises during intrapartum period (e.g., intrapartum fever), avoidance of labor entirely may decrease risk of cerebral palsy since labor is prerequisite in those cases.
- Avoidance of vaginal delivery can decrease birth injuries (e.g., clavicle and humeral fractures and brachial plexus injuries).
- Although cesarean delivery may delay breastfeeding for a few hours, it has no adverse effect on eventual breastfeeding and mother–infant bonding.
- A scheduled cesarean delivery allows easier allocation of staff (to ensure an adequate number of properly trained staff is available) and is likely to avoid the problem of fatigue in providers. Both of these factors can contribute to increased morbidity.
- The costs of vaginal delivery with Pitocin (oxytocin) is comparable to that of a cesarean. In the Northeast, normal vaginal delivery costs $6800 while elective repeat cesarean costs $7700. A failed trial of labor costs $2000 more than an elective cesarean.
- The costs of future reconstructive pelvic surgery and treatment of pelvic floor dysfunction are enormous given that the lifetime risk for prolapse and anti-incontinence in the population is 11.1% and ≈30% of these will need repeat surgeries (which have a higher morbidity and thus more costly).
- Today women live longer and have fewer children; therefore, quality-of-life issues (e.g., protection against pelvic floor dysfunction) are more important. According to the recent National Vital Statistics Report, women in the United States had 2.044 children in 2003 (highest = Hispanic > White > Black > Asian/Pacific Islander > American Indian). Life expectancy for women in the United States in 2001 was 79.8 years. "Elective cesarean delivery in healthy women who plan to have small families is now safe enough to warrant individual consideration of such patient requests." One primary and one repeat cesarean section may be cheaper and have lower morbidity if it reduces the probability of future costly pelvic reconstructive surgery and its associated morbidity.
- There is sufficient evidence that vaginal delivery and increased parity may lead to damage to pelvic floor structures. This damage to the nerve, muscle, and connective tissue may become more apparent as the population ages.
  - Vaginal delivery can cause damage to pelvic nerves (i.e., compression from the fetal head during descent and stretching of nerves like the pudendal). (1) Studies have shown increased pudendal nerve terminal motor latency (PNTML) and decreased anal pressures after spontaneous vaginal delivery (60% of which recovered by 2 months; however, a third of those returning for follow-up 5 years after delivery still had evidence of nerve damage). Pregnancy itself caused no changes in PNTML. Latencies were worse for forceps delivery, higher parity, and patients with longer second stage of labor. PNTML also correlate with increasing parity. (2) There is probably more injury than we are aware because a prolonged latency only reflects injury to the largest, heavily myelinated nerves. Latencies may be normal if only smaller nerve fibers are injured, thus subtle injuries are not detectable by nerve terminal motor latency testing. Needle electromyography (EMG) is more sensitive. There is loss of pelvic floor strength and EMG abnormalities in 80% of vaginal delivery group 2 months after delivery but in none of the patients in the cesarean section group. (3) Single-fiber EMG can quantify ratio of nerve to muscle fiber (N/F = fiber density). An increase in fiber density is evidence of nerve injury and successful reinnervation. There was an increase in fiber density after vaginal delivery in 80% of women (especially in multiparous and those with stress urinary incontinence [SUI] and prolapse). No signs of reinnervation were found after elective cesarean section.
  - Vaginal delivery can contribute to future pelvic muscle and fascial weakness (i.e., distention during delivery can cause trauma to levator ani muscles and endopelvic fascia). (1) Delayed pudendal nerve conduction leads to decreased levator ani tone and lower reflex contraction speed, strength, and duration. Therefore, when there is recurrent increase in intra-abdominal pressure (chronic obstructive pulmonary disease [COPD] or chronic constipation), reflex contraction which closes the genital hiatus and lifts the pelvic organs in a cephalad-posterior direction does not occur as previously and this places stress on the connective tissue support. Over time, the connective tissue may weaken, stretch, and/or break. (2) Vaginal delivery, particularly forceps-assisted delivery, is associated with greater pelvic organ mobility and

descent than cesarean delivery. (3) There is a higher proportion of Type 3 collagen versus Type 1 collagen in women with pelvic prolapse and incontinence. Perhaps injury to pelvic floor connective tissue after vaginal delivery is repaired with a weaker Type 3 collagen rather than original Type 1 collagen. More data are needed on this matter. (4) Pelvic floor muscle strength also decreases after vaginal delivery (assessed by vaginal cones and squeeze pressure measurements). (5) Levator ani defects are observed in 20% of primiparous on MRI versus in none of nulliparous women studied. (6) Two recent large studies have found a relationship among parity, age, and an increased risk of pelvic organ prolapse and subsequent surgery for it.

○ Vaginal delivery can lead to flatal and fecal incontinence (strong association). (1) Studies using anal ultrasonography have found that more than a third of primiparous women who returned for follow-up had evidence of anal sphincter tears which persisted in most of them 6 months after delivery. None of the cesarean delivery patients had anal sphincter tears. Occult sphincter defects occur in 33% of primiparous versus only 4% of multiparous. The first vaginal delivery has the greatest risk for damaging the anal sphincter. Damage is worse for those who had forceps delivery (8/10 of forceps deliveries had evidence of sphincter tears) and those who received midline episiotomy. Although controversial, some studies have shown duration of second stage, large birth weight, and occipito-posterior positions, and labor induction as also being associated with greater damage to the anal sphincter. Additionally, symptoms of fecal incontinence were seen in 5% of primiparous and 4% of multiparous after vaginal delivery but in none of the cesarean delivery patients. Data regarding decreased pudendal motor latencies and anal squeeze pressures were also substantiated in this study. In another study that followed 259 women delivered at one hospital, none of the 31 delivered by cesarean section reported fecal incontinence compared to 13% of primiparous that delivered vaginally. Anal sphincter tears were found 3 months postpartum in 38% of vaginal deliveries versus 3% of cesarean deliveries. (2) In another study, 62% of those with sphincter tears complained of fecal incontinence 8 years after vaginal delivery versus only 25% who delivered vaginally but who did not have evidence of sphincter disruption. (3) Resting anal sphincter pressures decrease after vaginal delivery up to 6 months. Squeeze anal sphincter pressures also reduced but not as much as resting pressures. (4) Anal canal sensation was reduced after vaginal birth up to 6 months but not after cesarean section. (5) After vaginal delivery, <6% develop new fecal incontinence but this rose to <50% in vaginal deliveries complicated by anal sphincter rupture. Vaginal deliveries subsequent to delivery with sphincter rupture and fecal incontinence result in recurrent fecal incontinence in 39% and permanent fecal incontinence in 4%. (6) Forty-two percent of women with occult external anal sphincter damage after first vaginal delivery developed fecal incontinence after second vaginal delivery.

○ Vaginal delivery can contribute to SUI. (1) One study found that 53% of primiparous and 85% of multiparous patients had urodynamic stress incontinence during pregnancy but this decreased to 47% after vaginal delivery. However, of the women who had urodynamic stress incontinence during pregnancy and who underwent cesarean section, none had stress incontinence following this mode of delivery. Other investigators have obtained results leading to the same conclusions. (2) Another researcher found that in women without symptoms during pregnancy, 13% of the patients who underwent vaginal delivery developed SUI versus none of the patients delivered by cesarean section. This number decreased to 3% at 1-year follow-up. However, at 5-year follow-up of the majority of the original study participants, 30% had moderate to severe stress incontinence. Additionally, 19% of the women without any symptoms after delivery had stress incontinence 5 years later and of those with symptoms 3 months after vaginal delivery, 92% were incontinent at 5 years. (3) Investigators have found decrease in urethral closure pressure, functional urethral length, pressure transmission ratio (PTR), bladder neck support (increase in bladder neck mobility), and position of the perineum after vaginal delivery but none of these changes were noted after cesarean section. (4) Several population-based trials, the largest of which included more than 10,000 women in Sweden, have shown a consistent relationship between increased parity from vaginal birth and genuine stress incontinence. One study found that there was an almost linear increase in the odds ratio (OR) for genuine stress incontinence as the number of vaginal deliveries increased (OR = 2.2 after 1 vaginal delivery; OR = 3.9 after 2 vaginal deliveries; OR = 4.5 after 3 vaginal deliveries). A recent, large study found that compared to patients delivered by cesarean section, those delivered by vaginal delivery have two times higher incidence of SUI.

○ Women with greater parity (P_2 or P_3) have left-right asymmetry of pelvic floor contractions on MRI.

○ In developing countries, prolonged labor and vaginal birth are associated with an epidemic of vesicovaginal fistulas.

CONCLUSIONS

- Childbirth increases the risk of pelvic floor disorders in young and middle-aged women.
- Most parous women do not undergo surgery for pelvic floor disorders.
- SUI occurs in many women after pregnancy and delivery.
- Vaginal delivery roughly doubles the chance of future SUI.
- Cesarean delivery slightly increases the chance for future urge incontinence.
- Women with transient postpartum incontinence are at greatest risk for future (i.e., >5 years after delivery) persistent SUI.
- Latent injuries to the pelvic floor become more apparent as the population ages.
- The first vaginal delivery causes the greatest damage to the anal sphincter and subsequent vaginal deliveries contribute to cumulative pudendal nerve damage.
- Surgery to correct anatomical disruption in the pelvic floor may fully restore anatomy, but it does not fully restore function (i.e., function of nerves, muscles, and surrounding organs).
- With current technology, elective scheduled cesarean section is safe and thus should be considered if certain criteria are met (see Section, A Reasonable Approach).

A REASONABLE APPROACH

- The topic of elective cesarean delivery is controversial.
- ACOG Technical Bulletin Number 289 stated that, "Elective cesarean delivery in healthy women who plan small families is believed safe enough to warrant individual consideration when requested by the patient."
- This technical bulletin was later withdrawn because of outside pressure. However, on February 14, 2004 in response to an article written on February 8, 2004 in the Washington Post, which denounced ACOG's position on elective cesarean, ACOG responded in essentially the same manner as the Technical Bulletin Number 289.
- A request for a selective cesarean section for prevention of disorders of pelvic dysfunction deserves careful individual consideration.
- It is best to begin conversation with patients regarding delivery options early on in their pregnancy. Patients need not be offered an elective cesarean as part of prenatal counseling or antepartum management. Similarly, requests for an elective cesarean need not be considered decisive in performance of a cesarean section.
- The physician should be up-to-date on literature and issues concerning elective cesarean section so that he or she can educate the patient to make an informed decision. The patient should be free to ask questions and voice any concerns.
- There may be things the patient can do to reduce her risk of pelvic floor damage. She can be encouraged to do the following:
  - Perform regular pelvic floor exercises because it helps regain pelvic floor function after vaginal delivery.
  - Lose weight because obesity is associated with greater pelvic floor morbidity.
  - Exercise (more than three times per week, jogging, or cycling) as this is associated with less high-degree anal sphincter tears.
  - Stop smoking as it interferes with tissue healing.
  - Treat COPD and other causes of chronic coughing.
  - Minimize activities that chronically and repetitively increase intra-abdominal pressure (e.g., job requiring regular heavy lifting).
  - If vaginal delivery is attempted, avoid midline episiotomy and forceps delivery (if protection of the pelvic floor is a major concern). Note that while maternal morbidity is higher with forceps delivery (pelvic floor damage, more third and fourth degree lacerations), neonatal morbidity (cephalohematoma, retinal hemorrhage, and suckling difficulty) is slightly increased with vacuum extraction. Neonatal morbidity in the form of facial injury (corneal and ocular) is more common with forceps deliveries.
  - Although controversial, there is some evidence for the following:
    - Flexion and counterpressure to baby's head, perineal massage, warm compresses, and upright or lateral birth positions may reduce episiotomies and sphincter lacerations.
    - Avoidance of epidural anesthesia may reduce vacuum/forceps deliveries for prolonged second stage and thus reduce episiotomies also.
- Markers of collagen weakness are not predictive of future pelvic floor dysfunction (e.g., joint hypermobility, varicose veins, and hemorrhoids). However, women with collagen vascular disorders (e.g., Ehler-Danlos and Marfan's) do have a increased risk of pelvic organ prolapse).
- Scheduled, "selective" cesarean section may be reasonable for the following reasons: (1) a patient who desires pelvic floor protection (patient initiated request) and the request is well supported (i.e., for serious concerns regarding PFD), (2) a patient who has already some form of PFD (e.g., any fecal incontinence after anal sphincter laceration and primary repair), (3) a patient who has several risk factors for disorders of the pelvic floor (parity, obesity, smoking, COPD, chronic constipation, diabetes, occupation or

involved in activities that require long-term, repetitive lifting or straining; already has incontinence/prolapse or was treated for it in the past; recurrent hernias, connective tissue disorder such as defective type of collagen or elastin [Marfan's and Ehler-Danlos]; strong family history of connective tissue disorder), (4) a healthy woman who plans on having a small family (no more than two children in her lifetime), (5) only after appropriate counseling and allaying of fears or anxieties regarding vaginal birth, and (6) after informed consent of the patient making no guarantees of pelvic floor protection.

- Perhaps in the future, we may be able to perform a simple test such as a needle biopsy of tissue collagen or muscle during a prenatal visit or a test of the electrical integrity of the pelvic nerves, then numerically assess its strength and integrity, and then use this number in addition to knowledge of aforementioned risk factors (like cholesterol recommendations) to make recommendations regarding cesarean section.

BIBLIOGRAPHY

Abramowitz L, Sobhani I, Ganansia R, et al. Are anal sphincter defects the cause of anal incontinence after vaginal delivery? *Dis Colon Rectum.* 2000b;43(5):590–598.

Albers LL, Anderson D, Cragin L, et al. Factors related to perineal trauma in childbirth. *J Nurse Midewifery.* 1996;41:269–276.

Aylin P, Bottle A, Jarman B. Social class and elective caesareans in the English NHS. *Br J Hosp Med.* 2004;328:1399.

Chaliha C, Kalia V, Stanton SL, et al. Antenatal prediction of postpartum urinary and fecal incontinence. *Obstet Gynecol.* 1999;94:689–694.

Chaliha C, Sultan AH, Bland JM, et al. Anal function: effect of pregnancy and delivery. *Am J Obstet Gynecol.* 2001;185(2):427–432.

Chiarelli P, Brown W, McElduff P. Leading urine: prevalence and associated factors in Australian women. *Neurourol Urodyn.* 1999;18:567–571.

Dietz HP, Bennet MJ. The effect of childbirth on pelvic organ mobility. *Obstet Gynecol.* 2003;102:223–228.

Echt M, Berneaud W, Montgomery D. Effect of epidural analgesia on the primary cesarean section and forceps delivery rates. *J Reprod Med.* 2000;45:557–561.

Gardosi J, Sylvester S, Lynch C. Alternative positions in the second stage of labour: a randomized controlled trial. *Br J Obstet Gynaecol.* 1989;96:1290–1296.

Gonen R, Tamir A, Degani S. Obstetricians' opinions regarding patient choice in cesarean delivery. *Obstet Gynecol.* 2002;99:577–580.

Gupta JK, Nikodem VC. Woman's positions during second stage of labour. *Cochrane Database Sys Rev.* 2000;2:CD002006.

Hopkins K. Are Brazilian women really choosing to deliver by cesarean? *Soc Sci Med.* 2000;51(5):725–740.

Labreque M, Eaon E, Marcoux S, et al. Randomized controlled trial of prevention of perineal trauma by perineal massage during pregnancy. *Am J Obstet Gynecol.* 1999;180:593–600.

Land R, Parry A, Rane A, et al. Personal preferences of obstetricians towards childbirth. *Aust N Z J Obstet Gynaecol.* 2001;41:249–252.

Landon CR, Smith ARB, Crofts CE, et al. Biomechanical properties of connective tissue in women with stress incontinence of urine. *Neurourol Urodyn.* 1989;8:369–370.

Mant J, Painter R, Vessey M. Epidemiology of genital prolapse: observations from the Oxford Family Planning Association Study. *Br J Obstet Gynaecol.* 1997;104:579–585.

Minkoff H, Chervenak FA. Elective primary cesarean delivery. *N Engl J Med.* 2003;348:946–950.

Minkoff H, Powderly KR, Chervenak F, et al. Ethical dimensions of National Center for Health Statistics National Vital Statistics Reports. 2003;52(3). Available at: www.cdc.gov/nchs.

Minkoff H, Powderly KR, Chervenak F, et al. Ethical dimensions of elective primary cesarean delivery. *Obstet Gynecol.* 2004;103:387–392.

Norton P, Baker J, Shrap H, et al. Genitourinary prolapse: relationship with joint mobility. *Neurourol Urodyn.* 1990;9:321–322.

Nygaard IE, Cruikshank DP. Should all women be offered elective cesarean delivery? *Obstet Gynecol.* 2004;102(2):217–219.

Nygaard IE, Rao SSC, Dawson JD. Anal incontinence after anal sphincter disruption: a 30-year retrospective cohort study. *Obstet Gynecol.* 1997;89:896–901.

Pirhonen JP, Grenman SE, Haadem K, et al. Frequency of anal sphincter rupture at delivery in Sweden and Finland: results of difference in manual help to the baby's head. *Acta Obstet Gynecol Scand.* 1998;77:974–977.

Rortveit G, Daltveit AK, Hannestad YS, et al. for the Norwegian EPINCONT Study. *N Engl J Med.* 2003;348:900–907.

Samuelsson EC, Victor FTA, Tibblin G. Signs of genital prolapse in a Swedish population of women 20-59 years of age and possible related factors. *Am J Obstet Gynecol.* 1999;180:299–305.

Sand PK, Grobman W. Does elective cesarean delivery prevent future urogenital abnormalities? *Female Patient.* 2002;27(5):18–28.

Sonnenberg E. Are Some Women "Too Posh to Push?" The Debate Continues Over Rising Rate of Cesarean Deliveries. Patton Law Practice. Available at: www.patton.lexipal.com.

Viktrup L, Lose G. The risk of stress incontinence 5 years after first delivery. *Am J Obstet Gynecol.* 2001;185(1):82–87.

Walsh CJ, Mooney EF, Upton GJ, et al. Incidence of third-degree perineal tears in labour and outcome after primary repair. *Br J Surg.* 1996;83:218–221.

Williams MC, Knuppel RA, O'Brien WF, et al. A randomized comparison of assisted vaginal delivery by obstetric forceps and polyethylene vacuum cup. *Obstet Gynecol.* 1991;78:789–794.

Wood J, Amos L, Rieger N. Third-degree anal sphincter tears: risk factors and outcome *Aust N Z J Obstet Gynaecol.* 1998;38:414–417.

World Health Organization's Indicators to Monitor Maternal Health Goals. Available at: www.who.int/Accessed.

Wu JM, Hundley AF, Visco AG. Elective primary cesarean delivery: attitudes of urogynecology and maternal-fetal medicine specialists. *Obstet Gynecol.* 2005;102(2):301–306. Available at: www.popcouncil.org; www.vbac.com.

Xanos ET, Holtzman SL, Julian TM. Long-term study of anal sphincter disruption during childbirth. *J Pelvic Surg.* 2000; 6:140–144.

QUESTIONS

QUESTIONS 1–3

Match the statement below with one of the three words above. Each answer may be used once, more than once, or not at all.

(A) Indicated

(B) Elective

(C) Selective

1. A patient who is herpes simplex virus positive, lacks prodromal symptoms, lacks lesions, but is afraid of asymptomatic viral shedding in the vaginal canal. She wants to minimize any risk of neonatal infection.

2. A 34-year-old primigravid who has high sensitivity to pain.

3. A 35-year-old Chinese couple who want their baby born on a specific calendar date because it is auspicious.

4. Avoidance of _____ has the greatest protective effect on the anal sphincter.

(A) midline episiotomy

(B) forceps-assisted delivery

(C) vacuum-assisted delivery

(D) upright birth positions

(E) epidural

5. A 25-year-old gravida 3, para 2 at 30 weeks of gestation has been researching and inquiring about a cesarean section at every visit. She tells you that she does not plan to have any more children. She is healthy except for a history of asthma with three lifetime hospitalizations. Her surgical history is remarkable for one previous emergency cesarean delivery for fetal bradycardia and an appendectomy. Her family history is remarkable for osteoporosis diagnosed in her mother at age 50. She used to smoke one pack of cigarette every 2 days prior to pregnancy. She delivers furniture for a living. According to this chapter, the strongest factor in her history which makes her less than an ideal candidate for a selective cesarean delivery is _____.

(A) lung disease

(B) surgical history

(C) family history

(D) age

(E) occupation

ANSWERS

ANSWERS 1–3

1. *(C)*, 2. *(B)*, 3. *(B)*. In question 1, the patient desires cesarean delivery and has a valid medical risk factor. Questions 2 and 3 are examples of elective delivery.

4. *(A)*. Medial episiotomy has a high chance of extending into the external anal sphincter. Although forceps-assisted delivery has a negative effect on external anal sphincter, the OR for a third or fourth degree laceration is less than that of midline episiotomy.

5. *(B)*. According to the Section, "A Reasonable Approach," selective cesarean delivery is appropriate for someone who is planning on having no more than two children. This patient already has two children. Additionally, a history of a previous emergency cesarean section, although not a contraindication, places her at greater risk for morbidity with subsequent cesarean sections. All of the other factors (i.e., asthma, young age, and job involving heavy lifting) are in favor of selective cesarean delivery. Family history of osteoporosis has not been established as a risk factor for pelvic floor dysfunction.

31 EPISIOTOMY

Yvonne G. Gollin and Sam Siddighi

INTRODUCTION

- Episiotomy is an incision into the perineal body performed during the late second stage of labor in an effort to facilitate delivery. Historically it was performed to *decrease* the risk of injury to the perineum and to preserve the pelvic floor and perineal muscle by shortening the second stage of labor. It is now apparent, however, that this incision *facilitates* further perineal injury, especially to the anal sphincter.

- Approximately one-third of women in the United States (year 2000) who give birth vaginally received an episiotomy.
- Unfortunately, episiotomy use is influenced by experience in training, professional local norms, and individual practitioner preferences.

INDICATIONS

- An episiotomy can be used with disorders of descent, use of forceps or vacuum, predicted macrosomia, breech delivery, or suspected imminent tears. If fetal distress is noted, an episiotomy can be used to hasten delivery.
- The routine use of an episiotomy has been questioned with recent data indicating that the use of an episiotomy for selected cases is associated with a decreased risk of posterior perineal trauma. An extensive review of randomized controlled trials evaluating restrictive versus routine use of episiotomy noted a reduction in posterior perineal trauma, need for suturing, and healing complications at 7 days with the restrictive use. There were no differences noted with regard to stress urinary incontinence, fecal incontinence, pelvic organ prolapse, postpartum perineal pain, or severe vaginal trauma.
- An episiotomy does not change pudendal nerve motor latency, pelvic floor muscle strength, pelvic floor denervation, or urethral closure pressures.
- Women who had restrictive episiotomy or no episiotomy (with intact perineum) start postpartum sexual intercourse earlier than those receiving routine episiotomy.
- Therefore, restrictive episiotomy is superior to routine episiotomy.

TIMING

- Although an episiotomy is usually performed when the fetal head is crowning, the exact timing is operator dependent.
- Purported advantages of a late episiotomy include less blood loss and a decreased incidence of posterior extension secondary to *recession of the rectum* away from the incision with advancement of the fetal head.
- However, a late episiotomy is associated with an increased risk of perivesicular tears.

TYPES OF EPISIOTOMIES

- There are two types of episiotomies: medial and mediolateral.
- The latter is performed, theoretically, in an effort to avoid inadvertent extension into the anal sphincter.

- There is an increased rate of extension into the anal sphincter with midline episiotomy compared to no episiotomy.
- Although mediolateral episiotomies do not prevent sphincter ruptures, they may be protective against severe sphincter lacerations compared to medial episiotomies.
- There is an increase in perineal pain and blood loss with the mediolateral episiotomy and the repair is more difficult.
- Medial episiotomy has become more common in the United States, but there are no well-controlled studies to dictate which type results in a better outcome.

PROCEDURE

- A medial episiotomy is performed while the fetal head has distended the vulva 2–3 cm, using a scissor oriented vertically toward the anus.
- Alternatively, a scalpel can be used with the purported advantage of minimizing trauma compared with the crushing/cutting effect of the scissor.
- It is important for the operator to distend the introitus and thin the perineum prior to incising.
- One clean cut rather than successive *snips* is ideal in order to produce a straight incision. The ideal length of the incision should be approximately one-half of the perineal length.
- The incision should be extended into the vaginal mucosa for 2–3 cm in order to prevent a ragged tear into the vagina.
- A mediolateral episiotomy is oriented 45° from the midline and can be on the right or left side depending on the operator's dominant hand. Most are on the patient's right side.

REPAIR

- Before repair, ensure proper lighting, adequate anesthesia (regional or general), use operating room if necessary, and maintain aseptic conditions.
- During repair use plenty of irrigation.
- The ideal suture has not been established. Recommendations made below come from several randomized, controlled trials in Europe showing less pain, less need for analgesia immediately postpartum, and decreased rates of dehiscence with polyglycolic acid sutures. However, polyglycolic acid was associated with greater sensation of "tightness" in comparison to chromic.
- The tissues, which require repair, include vaginal epithelium, perineal skin, transverse perineal muscles, and part of the bulbocavernosus muscles.

- If an episiotomy extends beyond the initial incision, it can be classified as follows: a first-degree tear involves only the superficial skin, a second degree extends through vaginal mucosa, a third degree involves the anal sphincter, and a fourth degree extends through the anal mucosa.
- A rectal examination is performed first to evaluate the area between midvagina and rectum which can have "buttonhole" defects secondary to protrusion of bony parts of the fetus, i.e., elbow, chin, and so forth.
- Traditionally, repair of a fourth-degree tear involved approximation of the anal mucosa with a running suture of 00 chromic inverting the mucosa into the bowel lumen. Now experts recommend using interrupted 3-0 or 4-0 delayed absorbable suture such as polyglycolic acid. Additionally, there is no evidence that placing sutures through the full thickness of rectal mucosa causes rectovaginal fistulas.
- The internal anal sphincter (IAS) is the white structure (after irrigation) between rectal mucosa and external anal sphincter (EAS). IAS provides 75–80% of anal tone. It can be retracted laterally and must be identified. A continuous imbricating layer using 3-0 or 4-0 polyglycolic acid should be used to approximate the IAS.
- In a third-degree repair, the retracted EAS muscles should be grasped with Allis clamps and *approximated* (either end-end or overlap technique) with several figure-eight sutures of 2-0 PDS or Maxon. Be sure to incorporate the concentric surrounding fascial elements of the muscle. There is no difference in outcome (fecal soiling, squeeze pressure, EAS defect on ultrasound) between end-to-end approximation of EAS versus overlap EAS immediately after obstetric disruption (i.e., primary repair). Most physicians prefer end-to-end approximation for primary repair as mobilization of EAS and suture pull-through muscle are concerns immediately after vaginal delivery. However, for secondary repair (i.e., months to years after vaginal delivery), overlapping technique is preferred by colorectal surgeons and experts in the field of Female Pelvic Medicine and Reconstructive Surgery (FPMRS).
- Broad-spectrum antibiotics (1–7 days) and stool softeners are common practices after repair of third- and fourth-degree lacerations.
- The initial suture (e.g., 2-0 polyglycolic acid) in a second-degree repair is placed above the vaginal apex to incorporate any retracted bleeders and to anchor the suture. A continuous, locking suture of vaginal epithelium and subepithelium is carried out to the level of the introitus and the suture held for later use. Successive interrupted sutures can be used to reapproximate the deeper transverse perineal muscles and the more superficial bulbocavernosus muscles. These latter sutures

restore perineal anatomy, especially allowing alignment at the introitus. Additionally, be sure to reattach the distal rectovaginal septum to the perineal body. The previously held vaginal suture can now be used as a superficial layer on the perineal skin going toward the anus. The direction is reversed at the apex on the skin and brought up to the introitus as a subcuticular running mattress suture.
- Continuous subcuticular closure of the perineal skin is better than interrupted transcutaneous closure.

COMPLICATIONS

- Blood loss from an episiotomy is estimated to be 253 mL with a range of 50–300 mL. As noted above, the earlier the episiotomy the greater the blood loss.
- There is increased risk of extension into the anal sphincter and increased perineal pain and dyspareunia with an episiotomy, although the rate of anterior and vaginal lacerations is lower.
- Additional complications related to third- and fourth-degree lacerations include infection, dehiscence, and rectovaginal fistula (see Chapter 21, Contraception).
  ○ Dehiscence or wound breakdown usually occurs within the first week of repair.
  ○ Symptoms and signs include pain/tenderness, purulent discharge, passage of flatus or stool from vagina.
  ○ Although traditionally, repair of dehiscence was delayed for several months, early repair can be successful after antibiotic treatment and aggressive wound debridement. In other words, resolution of infection and appearance of granulation tissue is important to success.
  ○ Additionally, bowel preparation, antibiotics, low-residue/high fiber diet, and stool softeners should be used.

REFERENCES

Baessler K, Bernhard S. Childbirth-induced trauma to the urethral continence mechanism: review and recommendations. *Urology.* 2003;62(4)Supplement 1:39–44.

Carroli G, Belizan J. Episiotomy for vaginal birth. *The Cochrane Database of Systematic Reviews 1999.* Issue 3. Art.No.: CD000081.DOI: 10.1002/14651858.CD000081.

Klein MC, Gautheir RJ, Robbins JM, et al. Relationship of episiotomy to perineal trauma and morbidity, sexual dysfunction, and pelvic floor relaxation. *Am J Obstet Gynecol.* 1994;171: 591–598.

O'Brien WF, Cefalo RC. Labor and delivery: In: Gabbe SG, Niebyl JR, Simpson JL, eds. *Obstetrics: Normal and Problem*

Pregnancies. 3rd ed. New York: Churchill Livingstone; 1996:374–375.

Plauche WC. Episiotomy and repair. In: Plauche WC, Morrision JC, O'Sullivan MJ, eds. *Surgical Obstetrics*. Philadelphia, PA: W.B. Saunders; 1998:365–371.

Rogers RG, Kammerer-Doak DN. Obstetric anal sphincter lacerations: an evidence-based review. *Female Patient*. 2002;27(5): 31–36.

QUESTIONS

1. All of the following are indications for episiotomy except:
   (A) Fetal distress
   (B) Anticipated forceps
   (C) Breech delivery
   (D) Routine use

2. Routine use of episiotomy is associated with all of the following except:
   (A) Decreased incidence of anterior and vaginal tears
   (B) Increased incidence of posterior perineal trauma
   (C) Increased need to suture
   (D) More healing complications

3. _____ is an essential step for the reestablishment of DeLancey Level III support. Some practitioners do not perform this step during repair of a second-degree repair.
   (A) Suturing of the vaginal mucosa in an interlocking manner

(B) Reconstruction of the perineal body
(C) Attachment of the rectovaginal fascia to the perineal body
(D) End-to-end apposition of the EAS
(E) Approximation of the rectal mucosa

ANSWERS

1. *(D)*. The routine use of an episiotomy has been questioned with recent data indicating that the use of an episiotomy for selected cases is associated with a decreased risk of posterior perineal trauma. An extensive review of randomized controlled trials evaluating restrictive versus routine use of episiotomy noted a reduction in posterior perineal trauma, need for suturing, and healing complications at 7 days with the restrictive use. There were no differences noted with regard to stress urinary incontinence, fecal incontinence, pelvic organ prolapse, postpartum perineal pain, or severe vaginal trauma.

2. *(A)*. The only benefit of routine episiotomy over restrictive episiotomy is the possibility of less anterior perineal trauma and vaginal tears.

3. *(C)*. Answers A and B are routine parts of a second-degree repair and are not steps which are forgotten. Answer D is only applicable to a third- and fourth-degree repair. Answer E is only applicable to a fourth-degree repair. Reattachment of the rectovaginal fascia to the perineal body is an important step which is sometimes deleted in the repair of a second-degree repair.

32 EFFECTS OF CANCER AND ITS TREATMENT ON THE LOWER URINARY TRACT, RECTUM, AND PELVIC FLOOR

Jeffrey S. Hardesty

EFFECTS OF CANCER ON THE PELVIC ORGAN SYSTEMS

- ○ Since there are four major organ systems (urinary, reproductive, digestive, and musculoskeletal) that share a restricted common space (pelvis) and have a common neurovascular supply it is no surprise that a cancer that involves any of these four systems will have some direct or indirect effect on the other three.
- ○ Physicians who specialize in female pelvic medicine need to be fully informed of the relationship of cancer and its treatment side effects on the pelvic organs.
- ○ Even though the malignancy itself may be cared for by oncologists, the complications of cancer therapy are often referred to urogynecologists for treatment.
- Surgical resection of pelvic tumors
  - ○ May result in intraoperative damage to the surrounding organs that require immediate repair, devascularization injuries that will need repair after the damage manifests itself, or by neuropathic injuries that later result in a dysfunction of the nearby organ systems that share common nerve pathways.
- Radiation therapy (RT)
  - ○ No matter how focused, RT will inevitably have some dose-dependent effect on all pelvic organ systems due to their close proximity.
  - ○ The most serious effects often appear many weeks, months, or even years after the RT has been completed.

- Chemotherapy
  - ○ May cause hemorrhagic cystitis, renal failure, promotion of bladder tumors, diarrhea, and constipation.
  - ○ May have indirect effect on pelvic floor by decreasing fertility.

SIDE EFFECTS OF CANCER TREATMENT BY RADICAL PELVIC SURGERY

- Complications from radical pelvic surgery (RPS), such as radical hysterectomy (RH), radical vulvectomy (RV), or abdominoperineal resection of rectum (APR), include intraoperative injuries, postoperative fistula formation, bladder dysfunction, urethral incompetence, and development of pelvic floor relaxation.
  - ○ Intraoperative injuries to ureters or bladder occur in 1–3% of patients undergoing RH.
    - Small crush injuries to ureter or ureteral lacerations require ureteral stent placement and absorbable suture repair.
    - Large injuries to ureter or complete transactions above the pelvic brim require stenting, excision of damaged portions of ureter, reimplantation via Boari flap or Demel technique, or primary anastomosis (ureteroureteral anastomosis).
    - Major ureteral injuries below the pelvic brim are best managed by ureteral reimplantation (ureteroneocystostomy) with bladder mobilization, and psoas hitch if needed.
    - Bladder injuries require two-layer absorbable suture closures preceded by evaluation for intactness of trigonal structures.
    - Bladder drainage with catheter for 5–14 days (or longer if bladder has been previously irradiated) is done after repair.
    - Postoperative urinary fistula formation occurs in 1–2% of patients undergoing RH.
    - Vesicovaginal fistula (VVF) becomes clinically evident within 10 days of the surgery in over two-thirds of cases while ureterovaginal fistula (UVF)

may take longer for the symptoms of constant urinary leakage to occur.

- VVF can be demonstrated by intravesical instillation of dye (methylene blue, indigo carmine, or sterile milk) with simultaneous vaginal speculum examination observation.
- If VVF test is negative then UVF can be demonstrated by vaginal tampon staining following oral Pyridium or IV indigo carmine.
- Cystoscopy and evaluation of upper tracts by intravenous pyelogram (IVP) or computed tomography (CT) should be done to confirm office findings, check for ureteral obstruction, and look for multiple fistulas.
- Bladder drainage and antibiotic coverage for 1 month allows for about 10% of postoperative VVF to close spontaneously.
- UVF should be treated by retrograde stenting if possible as this will often allow for spontaneous healing of the fistula.
- If retrograde stent cannot be passed then percutaneous nephrostomy with antegrade stenting is done.
- If antegrade stent cannot be passed then nephrostomy drainage tube should be placed.
- Surgical repair of VVF or UVF (see Chap. 27, Bypass Mechanisms: Vesicovaginal, Uretherovaginal, and Uretrovaginal Fistulas) should not be attempted until inflammation and infection from the original procedure has been resolved to optimize success rates.

○ Bladder dysfunction following RPS is a common and very troubling complication that can affect the patient's long-term quality of life (QOL).

- Almost all patients will have minor degrees of motor or sensory dysfunction post-RPS but 2–3% will have persistent dysfunction that requires chronic self-intermittent catheterization (SIC).
- Damage to autonomic or somatic nerve supply to the bladder during the required pelvic dissection or stretching and pressure damage to the detrusor muscle and its neurovascular supply with resultant hematoma and scar formation from prolonged retractor usage may cause loss of bladder function.
- Initial post-RPS (1 week to 6 months) bladder dysfunction is usually manifested by reduced bladder capacity, diminished bladder sensation, detrusor hypoactivity, overflow incontinence, and elevated postvoid residual volumes.
- Treatment is usually by teaching SIC once the patient is mobile.
- Bladder dysfunction that persists >6 months is characterized urodynamically by either persistent

acontractile bladder with increased bladder capacity or detrusor instability with reduced bladder compliance and capacity.

- Antimuscarinic medications and neuromodulation by pelvic electrostimulation therapy may give some help, but if normal bladder function does not return within 15 months of surgery then permanent dysfunction is expected.
- A delayed onset of bladder dysfunction may be the first sign of cancer recurrence and requires investigation with cystoscopy and imaging studies.

○ Urethral incompetence with resultant stress urinary incontinence is also seen at higher rates in patients post-RPS.

- A decrease in urethral functional length and urethral closure pressure has been documented to occur in 40% of patients undergoing RH and up to 90% in patients who underwent RV accompanied by distal urethral resection.
- Urine stream misdirection resulting in a bothersome spraying of urine occurs in up to 65% of patients who had RV.

○ Pelvic floor relaxation is more often reported in association with RV than with other types of RPS.

- Development of cystocele, rectocele, or uterine prolapse in patients who have undergone RV has been reported to occur in 17–26% of patients according to two large case series.
- Extensive scarring with loss of elasticity and problems with dyspareunia are more often reported with RV than with other types of RPS.

SIDE EFFECTS OF RADIATION THERAPY ON THE LOWER URINARY TRACT, RECTUM, AND PELVIC FLOOR

- Early onset radiation side effects are due to acute cellular damage. Since these are usually mild or transient they should not be classified as complications, but rather as anticipated treatment-related conditions.
- Late onset radiation side effects are due to gradual occlusion of capillaries by endarteritis with resultant tissue hypoxia and fibrosis that occurs as a reparative process involving nerves, vessels, and connective tissue.
- Cervical cancer is the most common indication for pelvic RT.
- Side effects of pelvic RT include radiation cystitis, recurrent hematuria, detrusor instability, decreased bladder

compliance and capacity, urethral incompetence, vaginal stenosis, radiation proctitis, bowel stricture or obstruction, hematochezia, and formation of VVF/UVF/RVF.

- Degree of radiation damage is dependent on total dose delivered and mode of delivery.
  - Total dose of up to 6500–7000 rads is unlikely to cause permanent or severe injury to lower urinary tract (LUT) or pelvic floor.
  - Dosages above 7500 rads are associated with a >20% likelihood of severe LUT injury requiring surgical intervention such as bladder augmentation or urinary diversion.
  - External beam irradiation is more likely to cause LUT damage than is intracavitary brachytherapy with afterloaded tandem and ovoids as more precise placement can be confirmed before installing the isotopes and shields.
  - Pelvic radiation side effects may be further reduced by the use of beams of differing radiation intensity to configure high-dose regions to target tissues in a technique known as intensity-modulated RT.
- Effects of RT on the LUT
  - Side effects of RT on the LUT may be divided into early and late reactions.
    - Early reactions occur in over two-thirds of patients treated with RT.
    - Early reactions are irritative symptoms that present as dysuria, frequency, and a predilection for urinary tract infection (UTI).
    - Early reactions usually respond to symptomatic treatment with bladder antispasmodics and antibiotics as indicated.
    - Late reactions present 6–24 months after RT in up to one-fifth of patients.
    - Late reactions include frequency, urge incontinence, hematuria, and nocturia (collectively called radiation cystitis) as well as development of VVF (in up to 5%) or UVF.
    - Late reactions may also cause urethral incompetence and development of intrinsic sphincteric deficiency with a fibrotic "drain pipe" urethra.
    - Late reactions also may cause a marked decrease in bladder compliance and capacity due to fibrosis with resultant bladder contracture.
    - Diagnostic workup for late reactions must include urinalysis/culture and sensitivity (UA/C&S), urine cytology, blood urea nitrogen (BUN), creatinine (Cr), imaging of upper tracts, and cystoscopy with superficial cold cup biopsy of any suspicious lesions.
    - In patients with late urologic complication post-RT, it must be remembered that recurrence or persistence of the pelvic neoplasm is several times more likely to be the cause of the symptoms.
  - Management of late RT side effects on the LUT range from conservative to radical depending on the severity of the symptoms and if fistula formulation or tumor recurrence has occurred.
    - Bladder irritative symptoms are treated with antimuscarinic medications, bladder retraining, and intravesical dimethyl sulfoxide (DMSO) instillations but cure rates are poor.
    - Augmentation cystoplasty or urinary diversion may be necessary for a severely contracted, fibrotic bladder.
    - Surgical repair of UVF/VVF post-RT usually requires interposition of a graft (Martius bulbocavernosus, omental, myocutaneous gracilis, or gluteal skin flap) to bring in fresh blood supply to the radiated area.
- Side effects of RT on the rectum and colon
  - The intestinal epithelial cells are relatively more sensitive to the effects of RT than other pelvic organs due to their rapid cell cycle time and abundance of mitotic activity.
  - Early reactions include greater frequency of stool, increased mucus production, diarrhea, rectal bleeding, and abdominal cramps.
  - Late reactions occurring 6–24 months post-RT include proctitis, sigmoiditis, ulceration, stenosis, obstruction, and fistula formation.
  - Other symptoms include hematochezia, chronic diarrhea, tenesmus, rectal urgency, and fecal incontinence.
  - Low residue diet, stool softeners, and fiber laxatives are helpful in managing milder symptoms.
  - Corticosteroid enema preparations (Cortifoam or Proctofoam) have also been used for ulcers and rectal bleeding.
  - Endoscopic application of neodymium:yttrium aluminum garnet (Nd:YAG) laser may help to control rectal bleeding.
  - If symptoms are severe, debilitating, and persistent surgical intervention should be cautiously considered, as complications from operating on irradiated bowel are high.
  - The rectum is the most common site for fistula formation to occur in the lower gastrointestinal (GI) tract and presents most often in patients who have received brachytherapy for cervical cancer.
- Side effects of RT on the pelvic floor
  - Dyspareunia, vaginal stenosis, and shortening of vaginal length post-RT can result in serious sexual dysfunction.
    - Local estrogen therapy and use of vaginal dilators may enhance sexual function significantly and improve QOL.

○ Pelvic floor relaxation is not associated with RT as the fibrosis that occurs may act to shore up potentially weakened supportive tissues.

EFFECT OF CHEMOTHERAPY ON THE LOWER URINARY TRACT, RECTUM, AND PELVIC FLOOR

- Urologic side effects of chemotherapy include renal failure, hemorrhagic cystitis, and promotion of bladder tumors.
  ○ Cisplatin is the chemotherapeutic agent most commonly associated with nephrotoxicity.
    ▪ Damage to renal tubules is the underlying mechanism for potentially irreversible renal failure.
    ▪ Electrolyte containing hydration during administration of cisplatin blunts the renal damage.
    ▪ Magnesium and calcium levels as well as renal function tests need to be monitored.
  ○ Mitomycin is also associated with nephrotoxicity and kidney failure.
  ○ Cyclophosphamide (CTX) may cause hemorrhagic cystitis.
    ▪ Direct irritation of the bladder urothelium from acrolein (a metabolite of CTX) is responsible.
    ▪ Administration of acetylcysteine sulfonate (Mesna) can prevent urothelial irritation by conjugating with acrolein without decreasing CTX efficacy.
    ▪ CTX is also associated with a four-time increase in later development of bladder neoplasms so unexplained hematuria in these patients requires investigation.
  ○ Ifosfamide is an alkylating agent similar to CTX that also releases the urothelial irritant acrolein as a metabolite.
    ▪ Mesna is indicated whenever this agent is used.
    ▪ Nephrotoxicity and renal failure may also occur with ifosfamide.
- Rectal side effects of chemotherapy
  ○ Diarrhea is associated with many chemotherapy drugs and occurs in up to 75% of patients receiving antineoplastic therapy.
    ▪ Irinotecan causes a secretory diarrhea that can be managed with antimotility agents, hydration, and administration of octreotide.
    ▪ Diffuse mucosal injury causing diarrhea is linked with cytarabine, dactinomycin, doxorubicin, 5-flurouracil, methotrexate, raltitrexed, and topotecan.
    ▪ Patients receiving chemotherapy are at increase risk for infections, so persistent diarrhea requires testing for *Clostridium difficile*.
- Constipation is seen in cancer patients receiving opioid analgesics or chemotherapy with vinca alkaloids.

○ Prophylactic bowel program with high fiber diet, stool softeners, and prn osmotic laxatives is necessary for these patients.
○ Protecting the integrity of the rectal mucosa in patients who are leukopenic or thrombocytopenic contraindicates the use of enemas for these patients.
- Pelvic floor side effects of chemotherapy
  ○ Direct effects on subsequent prolapse development is uncertain.
  ○ Deleterious actions on ovarian function and subsequent subfertility may have indirect benefits on pelvic floor function.

BIBLIOGRAPHY

Andrews CW, Goldman H. Chemical and physical disorders. In: Ming SC, Goldman H, eds. *Pathology of the Gastrointestinal Tract*. 2nd ed. Philadelphia, PA: Williams and Wilkins; 1998:195–223.

Ansink AC, van Tinteren H, Aartsen EJ, et al. Outcome, complications and follow-up in surgically treated squamous cell carcinoma of the vulva, 1995-1982. *Eur J Obstet Gynecol Reprod Biol*. 1991;42(2):137–143.

Calame RJ. Pelvic relaxation as a complication of the radical vulvectomy. *Obstet Gynecol*. 1980;55(6):716–719.

Disaia PJ, Creasman WT, eds. Colorectal and bladder cancer. In: Disia PJ, Creasman WT eds. *Clinical Gynecologic Oncology*. 5th ed. St. Louis, MO: Mosby; 1997:429–443.

Fischer DS, Knobf MT, Durivage HJ, et al. *The Cancer Chemotherapy Handbook*. 6th ed. St. Louis, MO: Mosby; 2003.

Koonings PP. The effects of gynecologic cancer and its treatment on the lower urinary tract. In: Walters MD, Karram MM, eds. *Urogynecology and Reconstructive Pelvic Surgery*. 2nd ed. St. Louis, MO: Mosby; 1999:387–398.

Mendex LF, Penalver M. Pelvic reconstruction after gynecologic cancer surgery. In: Rock JA, Jones HW III, eds. *Te Linde's Operative Gynecology*. 9th ed. Philadelphia, PA: Lippincott William and Wilkins; 2003:1537–1559.

Mutch DG, Grigshy PW, Markman M, et al. Management of late effects of gynecologic cancer treatment. In: Hoskins WJ, Young RC, Markman M, et al., eds. *Principles and Practice of Gynecologic Oncology*. 4th ed. Philadelphia, PA: Lippincott William and Wilkins; 2005:1193–1214.

Savides TJ, Jensen DM. Acute lower gastrointestinal bleeding. In: Friedman SL, ed. *Current Diagnosis and Treatment in Gastroenterology*. 2nd ed. New York: Lange Medical Books; 2003:70–82.

Welton ML. Anorectal diseases. In: Friedman SL, McQuaid KR, Grendall JH, eds. *Current Diagnosis and Treatment in Gastroenterology*. 2nd ed. New York: Lange Medical Books; 2003:452–479.

Zimmerm PE. Bladder dysfunction after radiation and radical pelvic surgery. In: Raz S, ed. *Female Urology*. 2nd ed. Philadelphia, PA: WB Saunders; 1996:214–218.

QUESTIONS

1. You are asked to evaluate a patient with stage 1_B squamous carcinoma of cervix who underwent RH 3 weeks ago. Her pathology reports showed metastatic disease involving the pericervical nodes so adjuvant RT is being considered. The patient is now doing SIC and has concerns about bladder function. You should advise her that
   - (A) Since she already has a bladder voiding dysfunction adjuvant RT poses no further risk to her urinary tract.
   - (B) The need for doing SIC may unpredictably decrease or stay the same whether or not she receives adjuvant radiation.
   - (C) Her life expectancy may be longer if she receives adjuvant radiation, but her QOL could be adversely affected.
   - (D) B and C
   - (E) All of the above

2. You are called to do an intraoperative consult by your gyn/onc colleague when he discovered that the senior resident assisting him had crushed the left ureter with a Heaney clamp at a point 3 cm from the ureterovesical junction. You should:
   - (A) Resect the crushed segment of ureter and perform an ureteroureteral anastomosis.
   - (B) Open up the intact bladder so that an infant feeding tube can be inserted into the left ureter.
   - (C) Create a Boari flap so that the intact portion of the ureter can be easily reimplanted after the damaged portion is excised.
   - (D) Evaluate the extent of the injury and pass a double J stent up the left ureter while performing cystoscopy.

3. A 37-year-old $G_6P_2A_4$ has completed a course of pelvic RT 6 months ago for stage 2_A squamous carcinoma of cervix. Her initial problems with bladder irritation resolved 1 month after completion of RT. However, she reports a continuous leakage of fluid with a uriniferous odor coming from her vagina over the last 10 days. You should:
   - (A) Immediately schedule her for repair of a VVF as it has now been 6 months since original surgery and therefore there is no need to wait for postsurgical inflammatory changes to resolve.
   - (B) Inject indigo carmine IV or have her swallow two tablets of Pyridium while wearing a vaginal tampon so that VVF can be distinguished from ureterovaginal fistula.
   - (C) Perform a vaginal speculum examination.
   - (D) Do cystoscopy and take deep biopsies from a visible ulcer found on posterior bladder wall just beyond the trigone.

ANSWERS

1. *(D)*. Choice A is incorrect. Adjuvant RT post-RH poses significantly increased risks for late onset complications involving the urinary tract such as fistulas and bladder contraction. Choice B is incorrect. At 3 weeks postoperation, it is impossible to predict how long her bladder voiding dysfunction will last or if it will ever resolve. Choice C is incorrect. Longevity versus QOL as well as potential risks and benefits of any prescribed treatment program need to be thoroughly discussed with all cancer patients.

2. *(D)*. Choice A is incorrect. Ureteral injuries close to the bladder are best treated by ureteral reimplantation (ureteroneocystostomy). Choice B is incorrect. A stent that is designed for long-term use needs to be used in this case as any crush injury requires more than a momentary check for ureteral patency. Choice C is incorrect. A Boari flap is a way to elongate the bladder so that ureteral injuries that occur above the pelvic brim can be reimplanted into the bladder. Choice D is correct. If the crush injury is not severe and the damaged section of ureter maintains a good blood supply the indwelling stent may be all that is needed.

3. *(C)*. Choice A is incorrect. Proper diagnosis of the cause of the continuous leakage and identification of the presence of a fistula versus urethral incompetence needs to be done prior to scheduling surgery. Since this is a relatively late onset urologic complication the possibility of tumor recurrence needs to be evaluated also. Choice B is incorrect. The correct sequence to distinguish between a VVF and UVF would be to first perform a vaginal speculum examination while instilling a dye into the bladder via the urethra to look for VVF then do the vaginal tampon testing with oral or IV dye administration if the test for VVF was negative. A vaginal speculum examination is needed to visualize the fungating mass extending from the cervix along the anterior vaginal wall and invading into the bladder that was causing the urine leakage in this patient. Choice D is incorrect. Cystoscopy is needed but taking deep biopsies from a posterior bladder ulcer may create a VVF if one was not already present.

33 PREVENTION, RECOGNITION, AND MANAGEMENT OF INJURIES TO THE LOWER URINARY TRACT DURING GYNECOLOGIC SURGERY

Kevin C. Balli

INTRODUCTION AND PERTINENT ANATOMY

- The reproductive and urologic systems develop in intimate proximity, and thus, must be considered jointly during any gynecologic surgery.
- Failure of constant vigilance regarding the urologic system is responsible for the majority of urinary tract injuries during gynecologic surgery.
- Knowledge of the relevant anatomy of the lower urinary tract is needed to prevent complications.
- Ureteral anatomy
  ○ Four-layer wall: transitional epithelium, mucosa, muscular layer, adventitial sheath
  ○ Blood supply: small branches from multiple large pelvic vessels supply a rich network to the adventitial sheath
  ○ Can be divided by the pelvic brim into abdominal and pelvic segments, each 12–15 cm in length
- Course of the ureter
  ○ The ureter exits the renal pelvis and courses retroperitoneally over the psoas muscle
  ○ Runs posterior to the infundibulopelvic vessels down to the level of the pelvic brim
  ○ Crosses into the pelvis over the bifurcation of the common iliac vessels
  ○ Courses retroperitoneally over the lateral pelvic sidewall, immediately ventral to the hypogastric artery down to the level of the uterine artery
  ○ Crosses under the uterine artery (water under the bridge) approximately 1.5 cm lateral to the internal cervical os
  ○ Descends through the cardinal ligament in the tunnel of Wertheim
  ○ Turns medially over the vaginal fornix to enter the base of the bladder
- Bladder anatomy
  ○ The bladder is divided into the base and the dome.
  ○ The base sits on the upper vagina and consists of the trigone and the detrusor loop.
  ○ The triangular trigone traces the area bounded by the entrance of the ureters and the exiting urethra.
  ○ The bladder dome is distensible with filling and its serosa is continuous with the vesicouterine peritoneum and the anterior abdominal wall peritoneum.
  ○ It receives its blood supply from the superior and inferior vesicle arteries.

INCIDENCE OF LOWER URINARY TRACT INJURY

- Overall, urinary tract injury is reported in 1–2% of all major gynecologic surgery.
- Traditionally, nearly 75% of urologic injury is thought to occur during gynecologic surgery; this is decreasing with the rise of injuries during more complex endoscopic urologic procedures.
- Ureteral injury:
  ○ The true incidence of ureteral injury is likely underestimated due to underreporting and silent renal death. Incidence varies with procedure, but is approximately 0.4% of major gynecologic surgeries.
  ○ Although rare, most studies show a significantly higher rate of injury in abdominal surgery compared to vaginal surgery.
- Bladder injury:
  ○ Reported incidence varies from 0.5% to 1.6%.
  ○ Injury is 3–5 × more likely during vaginal surgery as compared to abdominal surgery in most series.
  ○ The majority of bladder injuries occur during dissection of the bladder off the uterus, with a minority occurring during other procedures (i.e., anterior colporrhaphy and retropubic urethropexy), or retractor injuries.

RISK FACTORS

- Risks for lower urinary tract injury include previous surgeries (notably cesarean sections and myomectomy), nondescent vaginal hysterectomy, broad ligament or cervical myomas, intraoperative hemorrhage, cesarean hysterectomy, endometriosis, pelvic inflammatory disease, malignancy (especially ovarian cancer debulking), and prior pelvic radiation.

ABDOMINAL SURGERY

- Ureteral injury prevention
  ○ Develop *ureteral consciousness. Always* consider the position of the ureter during each step of gynecologic surgery.
  ○ Maintain knowledge of the most common sites of injury:

- Pelvic brim near ovarian vessels
- Uterine artery at the internal cervical os
- Pelvic sidewall near the uterosacral ligaments
- Tunnel of Wertheim
- Intramural portion of ureter
  - When dissecting the ureter away from other pelvic tissues, always dissect outside its adventitial sheath, thus preserving the blood supply. Devascularization leads to ischemic necrosis.
  - When using instruments that deliver energy to the tissues, pelvic surgeons must know the precise extent of lateral energy spread. Thermal injury during advanced laparoscopic surgery largely accounts for the recent rise in ureteral injury rates.
  - Placement of ureteral stents has not been shown to decrease ureteral injury. Likewise, routine preoperative imaging studies have not been shown to reduce operative urinary tract injury.
- Intraoperative diagnosis of ureteral injury
  - Most series report that between 50% and 90% of ureteral injuries are recognized and repaired at the time of the initial procedure. Immediate recognition and repair greatly decrease the long-term morbidity associated with these injuries.
  - Pelvic surgeons should consider universal stirrups and an indwelling three-way Foley catheter during anticipated difficult abdominal cases. This allows for rapid filling and emptying of the bladder, and prompt cystoscopy if needed.
  - Any suspicion of damage to the urinary tract *must* prompt intraoperative assessment.
  - Visualization of ureteral peristalsis does not exclude injury.
  - One ampule (5 mL) of indigo carmine dye is given intravenously. (No more than 2 ampules should be given during the procedure due to vasoactive properties.)
  - Dye spillage into the field indicates an open ureteral or bladder injury; its absence denotes no open injury but fails to exclude ligation, kinking, or crush injury.
  - Direct observation of dye passage from each ureteral orifice is necessary to ensure ureteral patency. This can be observed through cystoscopy or dome cystotomy.
- Ureteral stenting techniques
  - Stents may be placed from below using cystoscopy.
  - Alternatively, stents may be passed through a dome cystotomy or ureterotomy.
  - Generally double-J stents are utilized, with one end coiled in the renal pelvis, and one end in the bladder.
  - When used during injury repair, stents are usually removed at 4–6 weeks.
- Management of specific injuries
  - Ureteral kinking or ligation

- Kinking generally occurs when sutures are placed in close proximity to the ureter and tightened.
- This is most frequently encountered during cul-de-sac obliteration and apical suspension procedures.
- Diagnosis is made by cystoscopy and failure of ureteral dye passage.
- Suture removal and assessment of ureteral integrity is the first step in management. In the case of ligation and questionable ureteral integrity, a stent must be placed. Any devitalized ureteral segments must be resected and repaired as a transection.
  - Partial ureteral transection
    - Partial and complete transection is diagnosed by observation of dye passage into the surgical field from an open injury. Careful dissection of the ureter allows close inspection of the degree of transection.
    - Ureteral stents are placed through the partial ureterostomy.
    - Suture repair using full-thickness bites of 5-0 delayed absorbable suture is carried out. Avoid excess suture placement (more than three stitches are rarely needed), as this increases the chance of stricture.
    - Closed suction drainage is placed near the repair site and left in place until the ureteral stent is removed.
  - Complete ureteral transection above the pelvic brim
    - In general, injuries above the pelvic brim are not amenable to reimplantation due to their distance from the bladder.
    - The surgeon's choices for repair include (1) ureteroureterostomy, (2) transureteroureterostomy, (3) ureteroileal interposition, and (4) cutaneous ureterostomy. Whenever possible, most experts favor ureteroureterostomy.
    - Ureteroureterostomy is carried out over a ureteral stent placed by insertion into proximal and distal cut ends.
    - Both cut ends are trimmed and spatulated by making short longitudinal incisions along opposite sides. This allows greater circumference of luminal repair, thus decreasing the chance of stenosis. Care is taken not to interrupt the adventitial blood supply.
    - Four or five interrupted stitches of 5-0 delayed absorbable suture are placed around the repair site. Excess suture increases the chance of stenosis.
    - The surgeon must ensure the repair is tension free, either by mobilization of the bladder (described below), or renal mobilization. If tension-free repair is not possible, ileal interposition should be considered.

- Closed suction drainage should be used next to the repair site and continued until the stent is removed.
- Transureteroureterostomy doubles the number of urinary tract injuries and is best avoided according to expert opinion.
- Ileal interposition involves resecting a length of distal ileum and mobilizing it on its mesentery. An anastomosis is used to secure the remaining ilial segments. An end-to-side ileoureteral anastomosis is created at both ends by bringing the cut ends of ureter through the full thickness of antimesenteric bowel wall. The ileal ends are opened, and the ureteric ends are spatulated and sewn to the inside of the mucosal surface. The seromuscular layer of the ureter is sewn to the serosal surface of the ileum to reduce tension. The ileal ends are reclosed with interrupted 3-0 delayed absorbable suture and the segment is sutured to the psoas muscle. A closed suction drain is placed.
○ Complete ureteral transection below the pelvic brim
- Damage to the ureter below the pelvic brim, involving the last 4–6 cm, allows for potential bladder reimplantation.
- Tension-free principles must apply, and alternative methods should be used if this cannot be achieved with bladder mobilization, psoas hitch, or Boari flap construction.
- The bladder is mobilized with sharp dissection into the space of Retzius, transecting the attachments to the back of the symphysis.
- A dome cystotomy is created in the extraperitoneal portion of the bladder, and it is displaced laterally toward the ureteral injury.
- If a tension-free repair cannot be created, a psoas hitch or Boari flap is created.
  • Psoas hitch: The bladder is elevated toward the ipsilateral psoas muscle and secured with several interrupted sutures to the belly of the psoas muscle. Care must be taken to keep the sutures superficial and medial to avoid damage to the genitofemoral and femoral nerves which traverse the psoas muscle.
  • Boari flap: A U-shaped flap of bladder wall is created in the dome of the mobilized bladder and opened toward the injured ureter. This flap is then closed in a tubular fashion, creating an extension of the bladder.
- A 2-cm submucosal tunnel is sharply created near the trigone (or in the extended flap) as an antireflux measure.
- The cut proximal ureteral end is brought sharply through the bladder wall at the site of the submucosal tunnel. It is then passed through the tunnel, the end is spatulated open and then sutured to the mucosal surface. The seromuscular layer is secured to the bladder serosa with several interrupted sutures, a stent is passed, and the cystotomy is closed.
- Absence of tension is assured, and a closed suction drain is employed near the anastomosis site.
• Postoperative diagnosis and management
  ○ Although the best outcomes are seen with intraoperative detection and repair, some injuries must be managed when discovered postoperatively. A high index of suspicion must be maintained as prompt management improves outcomes.
  ○ Common symptoms of ligation are persistent postoperative flank pain, ileus, and fever.
  ○ A rise in serum creatinine of 0.8 mg/dL can be seen in the first several postoperative days after unilateral ureteral ligation.
  ○ Within days, imaging may detect a urinoma after complete ureteral transection, or rupture of a ureteral ligation. Alternatively, urine may leak from the vaginal cuff, forming a ureterovesical fistula.
  ○ Prompt intravenous (IV) pyelography combined with cystoscopy generally confirms the diagnosis.
  ○ Initial attempts are made to pass a ureteral stent cystoscopically, which if passed, should remain in place for 4–6 weeks. If a stent cannot be passed into the renal pelvis, a decision must be made to proceed with early repair, or delay repair until inflammation has subsided.
  ○ Most experts recommend early repair be carried out if injury is discovered in the immediate postoperative period. If not, percutaneous nephrostomy should be performed without delay to protect the ipsilateral kidney.
• Injury to the bladder
  ○ Prevention and diagnosis
    - Proper knowledge of bladder anatomy and careful sharp dissection of the bladder off the lower uterine segment and upper vagina are the cornerstones of injury prevention.
    - Previous radiation, distorting cervical myomas, or multiple previous cesarean sections can increase the risk of bladder injury. If injury is anticipated or suspected, 5 mL of indigo carmine dye should be given through the IV to facilitate an unequivocal diagnosis.
  ○ Management
    - Closure of bladder injuries is generally more straightforward than ureteral injuries.
    - A two- or three-layer closure using interrupted or running 3-0 delayed absorbable suture is sufficient for most injuries.
    - The first layer is placed through and through, closing the injury from beyond its furthest extent. The second (and possibly third) should imbricate the first layer, thus relieving tension.

- After repair, the bladder is filled with 300 cc saline to check for adequate closure.
- Repair of injuries to the base of the bladder must always include inspection for proximity to the ureteral orifices. Even when the ureter is not involved, one must take care not to cause a kink with the suture placement.
- Dome injury repairs should be extraperitonealized whenever possible. Bladder drainage should be used for 7–14 days, or until a cystogram shows no extravasation.

VAGINAL SURGERY

- Bladder injury
  - Prevention
    - Always use careful, sharp dissection of the bladder off the cervix—a gauze covered finger is too blunt, and may injure the bladder.
    - Maintain excellent hemostasis during bladder dissection.
    - In cases of difficult dissection, consider placing a uterine sound through the urethra to delineate the bladder reflection. Alternatively, the surgeon may access the posterior colpotomy, place a finger behind the uterine fundus, and palpate the anterior cul-de-sac to determine the extent of the bladder. Methylene blue dye, placed in the bladder through the urethra may help stain the tissues blue to better visualize the bladder wall.
    - When the vesicouterine peritoneum is encountered, do not push it away. Carefully pull it caudally and make a small, sharp incision. Only when the intraperitoneal contents can be seen through this incision should it be extended, and a retractor placed under the bladder.
  - Diagnosis
    - Diagnosis is facilitated as mentioned above by either back filling the bladder with dye, or injecting indigo carmine dye in the IV and clamping the Foley catheter. This technique should be routine, as difficult bladder dissections are often unanticipated.
  - Management
    - Once an injury is diagnosed, cystotomy should be used to redirect the plane of dissection. Once the surgery is complete, the injury is examined *cystoscopically* and proximity to the ureteral orifices is determined. Once ureteral integrity is assured, bladder repair is undertaken as described above, taking care not to kink the ureters during the repair process.
    - Bladder drainage is used for 7–14 days.

- Ureteral injury
  - Prevention
    - The bladder should be elevated out of harm's way and ligation of the uterosacral and transverse uterine ligaments should be performed using small pedicles.
    - Use precise suturing when closing the vaginal cuff, avoiding deeply placed, blind sutures.
    - Extreme care should be taken during high uterosacral ligament suspensions of the vaginal cuff. Most experts recommend routine cystoscopy after all apical suspension or cul-de-sac obliteration procedures.
  - Diagnosis
    - Injury to the distal (intramural) portion of the ureter generally is diagnosed with a concomitant bladder injury by cystoscopy.
    - Pelvic sidewall ureteral injury or kinking during apical suspension or cuff closure can only be diagnosed with cystoscopy. As mentioned, routine cystoscopy is often recommended following more complex vaginal surgery. Otherwise, the injury will be diagnosed postoperatively as noted above.
  - Management
    - When cystoscopy fails to demonstrate patent ureters after any vaginal surgery, some or all of the sutures must be removed and cystoscopy repeated. Generally, sutures placed during the vault suspension procedure or the cul-de-sac obliteration are removed, one at a time, and a check for ureteral flow is performed. Once flow is reestablished, the suspension is repeated in a more suitable location (often more superficial and distal), and cystoscopy is repeated.
    - Simple injuries to the trigone of the bladder, which involve the ureter, can often be repaired vaginally with primary bladder suturing and ureteral stenting.
    - More extensive injuries in the lower 3 cm of ureter can sometimes be identified and repaired vaginally. A ureteral catheter is passed as far as possible, and the site of injury identified. Depending on the distance and tension, a delegation or a ureteroneocystostomy can be performed near the trigone.
    - If proper repair and integrity cannot be assured from below, a transabdominal repair should be considered.

BIBLIOGRAPHY

Carley ME, et al. Incidence, risk factors and morbidity of unintended bladder or ureter injury during hysterectomy. *Int Urogynecol J Pelvic Floor Dysfunct.* 2002;13(1):18–21.

Gowri D, et al. Urological injuries during hysterectomies: a 6-year review. *J Obstet Gynaecol Res.* 2004;30(6):430–435.

Harkki-Siren P, et al. Urinary tract injuries after hysterectomy. *Obstet Gynecol.* 1998;92(1):113–118.

Hurt WG. Gynecologic injury to the ureters, bladder, and urethra. In: Karram MM, Walters MD, eds. *Urogynecology and Reconstructive Pelvic Surgery.* St. Louis, MO: C.V. Mosby; 1999:377–386.

Liapis A, et al. Ureteral injuries during gynecological surgery. *Int Urogynecol J.* 2001;12:391–394.

Maggio M, Karram MM. Ureteral surgery. In: Baggish MS, Karram MM, eds. *Atlas of Pelvic Anatomy and Gynecologic Surgery.* Philadelphia, PA: W.B. Saunders; 2001:254–262.

Makinen J, et al. Morbidity of 10,110 hysterectomies by type of approach. *Hum Reprod.* 2001;16(7):1473–1478.

Mathevet P, et al. Operative injuries during vaginal hysterectomy. *Eur J Obstet Gynecol Reprod Biol.* 2001;97:71–75.

Montz FJ, Bristow RE, Del Carmen MG. Operative injuries to the ureter: prevention, recognition, and management. In: Rock JA, Jones HW, eds. *Te Linde's Operative Gynecology.* 9th ed. Philadelphia, PA: Lippincott Williams & Wilkins; 2003:1081–1098.

Thompson JD. Operative injuries to the urinary tract. In: Nichols DH, ed. *Reoperative Gynecologic Surgery.* St. Louis, MO: Mosby Year Book; 1991:163–210.

QUESTIONS

QUESTIONS 1–3

A 47-year-old woman is undergoing abdominal hysterectomy for symptomatic leiomyomas. While the bladder is being dissected off of the uterus, a small rent is created in the bladder. As a urogynecologist, you are consulted over the phone.

1. The most important question to ask the surgeon is _____.

   (A) "How big is the laceration?"
   (B) "In what part of the bladder is the laceration?"
   (C) "How big is her uterus?"
   (D) "How much blood have you lost so far?"
   (E) "Have you transected the uterosacral ligaments yet?"

2. You arrive in the operating room and begin the repair. The type of suture and the number of layers used for closure is/are _____ and _____, respectively.
   (A) Permanent suture; two layers
   (B) Permanent suture; one layer
   (C) Delayed absorbable suture; three layers
   (D) Absorbable suture; one layer
   (E) Absorbable suture; three layers

3. Your gynecology colleague asks for your advice regarding what he should have done differently during hysterectomy. You tell him _____
   (A) Do not empty the bladder until dissection of the lower uterine segment from the bladder is finished.

   (B) Use your bovie to create a plane between the lower uterine segment and bladder, then gently push the bladder down with your finger.
   (C) Perform sharp dissection with scissors and do not deviate laterally on the lower uterine segment.
   (D) Create a plane between the lower uterine segment and bladder, then push the bladder down using a sponge stick.
   (E) Perform a supracervical hysterectomy whenever you can to minimize risk of bladder injury.

QUESTIONS 4–5

Choose the answer which is the most appropriate management for the injury described below. Each answer may be used once, more than once, or not at all.

   (A) Ureterorectostomy
   (B) Ureteroneocystostomy
   (C) Transureteroureterostomy
   (D) Cutaneous ureterostomy
   (E) Interposition of bowel segment

4. Transection of the ureter at the junction of the uterine artery and ureter

5. Large segment of the ureter is injured from bladder to pelvic brim

ANSWERS

1. *(B).* It is extremely important to establish the location of the bladder injury first. Bladder dome injuries are easy to repair. However, injuries in the bladder base, especially the trigone, deserve ureteral stenting after the repair to ensure that the repair did not compromise ureteral patency.

2. *(D).* The optimal technique is one- or two-layered closure with regular absorbable suture. There is no evidence that two layers are superior to one-layered closure. Permanent suture is not the best option because it may lead to recurrent cystitis and stone formation in the bladder.

3. *(C).* The best way to dissect the bladder off the lower uterine segment is with sharp dissection instead of blunt dissection (sponge stick or finger dissection) because it minimizes injury to the bladder. Some surgeons like to catheterize the bladder after performing an anterior colpotomy during a vaginal hysterectomy (*not* abdominal hysterectomy) so that they can be aware if cystotomy occurs. The risks and benefits of retaining or removing the cervix should be discussed with the patient. Supracervical hysterectomy should

not be performed injudiciously on everyone just to prevent bladder injury.

ANSWERS 4–5

4. *(B)*, 5. *(E)*. Major injuries (e.g., transaction) of the ureter within 5 cm of the bladder are best repaired by ureteroneocystostomy. Basically, the submucosal tunnel is created in the bladder. The ureter is passed through the tunnel and sutured to the bladder serosa and mucosa. The serosa of the bladder is sutured to the psoas muscle to stabilize the anastomosis. When a large segment of urether has been injured or removed, interposition of a bowel segment may be appropriate.

34 THE EFFECT OF ESTROGEN AND SERMS ON THE LOWER URINARY TRACT AND PELVIC FLOOR

Kendra Jones and Sam Siddighi

INTRODUCTION

- Menopause: Cessation of ovarian function, characterized by lack of menses for 1 year.
  - It is a normal process of aging that is genetically predetermined.
  - Menopause is the total loss of ovarian follicular function and is a clinical, retrospective diagnosis and not a laboratory one.
    - Women have a finite egg supply at birth ($\approx 10^6$) and this supply decreases throughout life:
      - At birth $\approx$ 1,000,000
      - Puberty $\approx$ 300,000
      - Age 21 $\approx$ 100,000
      - Age 38 $\approx$ 25,000
      - Menopause $\approx$ "0"
    - As age $\uparrow \rightarrow$ ovarian follicle number $\downarrow \rightarrow$ granulose cells (of follicles) inhibin $\downarrow \rightarrow$ less suppression of pituitary by inhibin $\rightarrow$ follicle-stimulating hormone (FSH) $\uparrow \rightarrow$ low estrogen levels (in postmenopause).
    - However, laboratory studies (e.g., FSH) are not useful in documenting menopausal transition because of hormonal fluctuations.
    - Menopausal transition (formerly, perimenopause) is the period (usually 2–6 years) before actual menopause and ends 12 months after the last menstrual period.
      - Median age of onset = 47.5 (data from World Health Organization [WHO] list median age = 51.3).
      - During this period, menstrual cycle changes (e.g., skipped periods) occur and patients may experience vasomotor instability (e.g., hot flushes and perspiration), mood changes, sleep disturbances, and changes in the genitourinary (GU) tract and pelvic floor.
- Menopause can result in weakening of connective tissue because of impairment in the synthesis and metabolism of collagen $\rightarrow$ may contribute to pelvic organ prolapse (POP).

ESTROGEN

- Estrogen (E) is a steroid hormone which binds estrogen receptors (ER) throughout the body.
  - Two types of ER have been isolated by molecular techniques (ER-alpha and ER-beta)
  - Receptors are located in the nucleus
  - Mechanism of action: E+ER in nucleus $\rightarrow$ E–ER conformational change $\rightarrow$ displacement of inactivating protein (Hsp 90) $\rightarrow$ binding to specific area on DNA $\rightarrow$ transcription of gene (mRNA) depending on shape formed after conformational change (tamoxifen forms different shape than estrogen) and on ER (alpha vs. beta)
  - Example: E $\rightarrow$ collagen mRNA $\rightarrow$ collagen synthesis
- Low estrogen can lead to genital atrophy.
  - Prolonged decreased estrogen $\rightarrow \downarrow$ blood vessels (genital paleness)
  - Thin epithelium (apoptosis), muscle density $\downarrow$, and decreased elasticity of connective tissue change (apoptosis)
  - $\downarrow$ lubrication (i.e., $\uparrow$ dryness and dyspareunia—is the most common sexual complaint in older women) and $\uparrow$ pH (atrophic and bacterial vaginitis and recurrent urinary tract infections [UTIs])
  - Loss of vibration and pressure sensation
  - $\uparrow$ symptoms of dysuria, frequency, urgency, nocturia, and incontinence
- Low estrogen can lead to negative clitoral changes.
  - Decrease in clitoral perfusion and engorgement during desire phase
  - Shrinkage in size of clitoris

○ Decrease in nerve fibers innervating cavernosal smooth muscle of clitoris
○ Decline sensation of touch, vibration, and cold of clitoris

POSITIVE EFFECTS OF ESTROGEN ON THE GU TRACT AND PELVIC FLOOR

• Intuitively it makes sense that estrogen has positive effects on the health and function of the GU tract and the pelvic floor.
• Embryologically, the genital and urinary tracts have a common origin, the urogenital sinus.
• ER location
  ○ A high density of ER is located in the pubococcygeus muscle, uterosacral ligament, urethra, bladder, trigone, and blood vessels in pelvis.
    ▪ Urethra has four estrogen-sensitive layers: Layers of the urethra starting from the lumen outward: epithelium (1) → loose connective tissue (2) (lamina propria) → submucosa (3) (vasculature) → thick longitudinal muscle (4) → thin circular muscle→ sphincter urethrae (if proximal urethra) or compressor urethrae/urethrovaginal sphincter (if distal urethra).
      • Epithelium: Estrogen improves maturation index (MI) of vaginal and urethral squamous epithelium (i.e., ↑ superficial cell/parabasal cell ratio). The distal end of the urethral epithelium is squamous while the proximal end is transitional. The location of the squamous–transitional junction depends on a person's age, hormonal status, and possibly sexual activity. In reproductive years the junction is closer to the bladder (and sometimes covering the trigone), while in menopause it is the opposite
      • Connective tissue (lamina propria, submucosa)
      • Striated urethral sphincter (sphincter urethrae, compressor urethrae/urethrovaginal sphincter) and smooth muscle (longitudinal and circular muscles)
      • Vasculature (submucosa)
    ▪ Uterosacral ligament → estrogen is responsible for the synthesis of strong collagen (collagen Type I). Women who develop POP and urinary incontinence (UI) heal with a higher percentage of weaker collagen (collagen Type 3).
    ▪ Blood vessels in pelvis → treatment of atrophic vaginitis leads to improved blood flow to GU tract (vaginal lubrication ↑, dyspareunia ↑).
  ○ Fibroblasts which secrete collagen are stimulated by estrogen → positive collagen synthesis and/or negative collagen degradation.

• During urodynamic studies, sensory threshold of the bladder is increased by estrogen.
• Early, uncontrolled, small study prior to widespread use of urodynamics (in 1941) found that IM estrogen improved symptoms of incontinence, nocturia, urgency, frequency, and dysuria.

ORAL COMBINED HORMONE THERAPY DOES NOT TREAT URINARY INCONTINENCE

• Recent high quality studies have not found improvement in objective outcome measures when comparing hormone therapy (HT) (estrogen + progesterone) to placebo for treatment of UI.
  ○ One level 1 study of hypoestrogenic female with urge urinary incontinence (UUI) or SUI: conjugated equine estrogen + medroxyprogesterone (cyclic) versus placebo → no subjective or objective differences were found (quality of life [QOL], perception of clinical improvement or incontinence episodes, volume of urine loss).
  ○ Meta-analysis of several controlled studies: Patients with SUI had significant subjective improvement (of incontinence, urgency, and frequency), but not objective improvement (volume of urine lost and maximal urethral closure pressure [MUCP]).
  ○ Large level 1 study: estrogen versus estrogen + progesterone versus placebo
    ▪ Estrogen versus placebo groups had similar improvement rate of UI.
    ▪ Estrogen + progesterone group had worse UI than placebo group (39% vs. 27%).
• One must be careful when making conclusions about the effects of estrogen on UI based on these studies because:
  ○ Route of estrogen: Local estrogen was not used in the large level 1 study.
  ○ The type and dose of estrogen used may be important.
  ○ Local estrogen alone (without progesterone) is beneficial.
  ○ There has been no study to address the use of estrogen to prevent UI (prophylaxis rather than treatment).

EFFECTS OF SERMS ON GU TRACT AND PELVIC FLOOR

• Selective estrogen receptor modulators (SERMs)
  ○ SERMs are synthetic compounds which have positive estrogenic effects (agonistic) in some tissues and no effects in other tissues (antagonistic).

- Tamoxifen
  ○ Tamoxifen has not been associated with POP.
  ○ Has estrogenic effects on the vagina (lower vaginal pH and MI).
  ○ Is associated with increased vaginal discharge.
- Raloxifene
  ○ Large level 3 study: raloxifene versus placebo → raloxifene group 50% less likely to undergo surgery for POP.
  ○ Raloxifene has not been associated with vaginal atrophy.
- Levomeloxifene
  ○ Large level 1 study: levomeloxifene versus placebo → study was stopped because levomeloxifene group had much higher incidence of UI and POP.
  ○ Patients on raloxifene and tamoxifen showed a ↑ cotton swab defection during resting and straining.

CONCLUSION

- By itself, estrogen does not treat UI in those who have it already; however, when combined with an alpha-adrenergic agonist or with pelvic floor exercises, estrogen has been shown to be effective for the treatment of SUI.
- Oral estrogen + progesterone should not be used to treat UI because this combination is a risk factor for UI.
- Local estrogen may be used to improve irritative symptoms (e.g., urgency and frequency) and to increase the quality of support tissue.
- A study of local estrogen without progesterone in hysterectomized women (therefore no risk of endometrial hyperplasia) for the prevention of UI is needed.

BIBLIOGRAPHY

Andersson K-E, Chapple CR, Wein AJ. Pharmacologic treatment of urinary incontinence. In: Bourcier AP, McGuire EJ, Abrams P, et al., eds. *Pelvic Floor Disorders*. Philadelphia, PA: Elsevier; 2004: 373–391.

Beisland HO, Fossberg E, Moer A, et al. Urethral sphincteric insufficiency in postmenopausal females: treatment with phenylpropanolamine and estriol separately and in combination. A urodynamic and clinical evaluation. *Urol Int.* 1984; 39:211–216.

Bergmann A, Karram MM, Bhatia NN. Changes in urethral cytology following estrogen administration. *Gynecol Obstet Invest.* 1990;29:211.

Brincat M, Moniz CF, Kabalan S, et al. Decline in skin collagen content and metacarpal index after the menopause and its prevention with sex hormone replacement. *Br J Obstet Gynaecol.* 1987;94:126–129.

Fantl JA, Cardozo LD, McClish DK, et al. Estrogen therapy in the management of urinary incontinence in postmenopausal women: a meta-analysis. First report of the Hormones and Urogenital Therapy Committee. *Obstet Gynecol.* 2000;36:83.

Ishiko O, Hirai K, Sumi T, et al. Hormone replacement therapy plus pelvic floor muscle exercise for postmenopausal stress incontinence: a randomized, controlled trial. *J Reprod Med.* 2001;46:213.

Klutke JJ, Bergman A. Nonsurgical treatment of stress urinary incontinence. In: Bent AE, Ostergard DR, et al., eds. *Ostergards's Urogynecology and Pelvic Floor Dysfunction.* Philadelphia, PA: Lippincott William & Wilkins; 2003: 447–455.

Norton PA. Pelvic floor disorders: the role of fascia and ligaments. *Clin Obstet Gynecol.* 1993;36(4):926–938.

Nygaard IE, Kreder KJ. Pharmacologic therapy of lower urinary tract dysfunction. In: Weber A, ed. *Clinical Obstetrics and Gynecology—Incontinence 2004*, Philadelphia, PA: Lippincott William & Wilkins; 2004:83–92.

Salmon UJ, Wlater RI, Geist SA. Th use of estrogens in the treatment of dysuria and incontinence in postmenopausal women. *Am J Obstet Gynecol.* 1941;42:845–851.

QUESTIONS

QUESTIONS 1–2

Match the statement below with the compound(s) above that best corresponds to the description. Each answer may be used once, more than once, or not at all.

(A) estradiol + medroxyprogesterone acetate
(B) estradiol
(C) tamoxifen
(D) raloxifene
(E) levomeloxifene

1. Use of this compound(s) is associated in increased POP and UI.
2. Oral therapy with this compound(s) is associated with higher UI.
3. Local estrogen therapy in postmenopausal women decreases the likelihood of lower UTI and has been shown to improve _____.

(A) urgency
(B) maximum urethral closure pressure
(C) functional urethral length
(D) volume of urine lost during incontinence
(E) overall well-being

ANSWERS

ANSWERS 1–2

1. *(E)*, 2. *(A)*. Large level 1 study demonstrated that levomeloxifene is worse than placebo. The study was stopped because levomeloxifene group had much higher incidence of both UI and POP. In one large level 1 study of estrogen versus estrogen progesterone versus placebo, it was shown that estrogen versus placebo groups had similar improvement rate of UI and that estrogen progesterone group had worse UI than placebo group (39% vs. 27%).
3. *(A)*. Local estrogen therapy improves subjective, irritative symptoms such as urgency and frequency but does not affect objective measures (volume of urine lost and MUCP). Oral estrogen improves overall sense of well-being.

35 EMBRYOLOGY PERTAINING TO FPMRS

Marianna Alperin and Sam Siddighi

INTRODUCTION

- The development of the female reproductive tract begins at 3 weeks of gestation and continues into the second trimester of pregnancy. The process is complex and involves cellular differentiation, fusion, canalization, and apoptosis.
- All malformations result from the failure of canalization, fusion, programmed cell death, or agenesis. In order to better remember and sort the disorders leading to the malformations, a pneumonic *café* can be used. It stands for disorders of *canalization, agenesis, fusion,* and *embryonic cell disorders.*

GONADS

- Development of the gonads results from migration of primordial germ cells to the genital ridge.
- Several genes, including steroidogenic factor 1 (SF1) and Wilms' tumor 1 (WT1), are critical for the development of the genital ridge into bipotential gonad.

- For the first 2 months of gestation, the two sexes develop in an identical fashion.
- Chromosomal sex determines the differentiation of the indifferent gonad into an ovary or a testis, beginning at week 6.
- The SRY gene, which is the sex-determining region, is located on the short arm of the Y chromosome. It is required for the development of the primitive gonad into a testis.
- SOX9 is the gene functioning downstream from SRY. It encodes transcription factor related to SRY and is also essential for testicular development.
- SF1 and WT1 play a role in the development of the testis as well.
- The genes involved in the development of the ovary are largely unknown to this date.
- The first sign of ovarian differentiation is the absence of Sertoli cells at 6–7 weeks of gestation.
- Ovarian cortex develops by 12 weeks and after 13 weeks the ovarian primordial follicles can be identified.
- The hormonal milieu will be determined by whether ovary or testis is formed. The type of hormone secreted and response of the end organ to that hormone determine phenotypic sex.
  - Leydig cells and Sertoli cells of the testes secrete testosterone and antimüllerian hormone, respectively.
  - These hormones induce differentiation of the primordial genitals into male phenotype, given normal androgen metabolism takes place and androgen receptors are present on the end organs.

URINARY SYSTEM

- The urinary system develops in three consecutive stages:
  - Pronephros—is transient and nonfunctioning structure that develops from the intermediate mesoderm in the cervical region and then regresses at about 4 weeks of gestation.
  - Mesonephros—develop from the paravertebral mesoderm of the upper thoracic to lumbar region, are also not functional. It replaces pronephros at gestational week 5.
  - Metanephros—renal metanephric development occurs from the interactions of the ureteric bud, which is a remnant of the mesonephros, and metanephric blastema. Organogenesis, induced by this interaction, causes formation of the nephrons, collecting tubules, calyces, the renal pelvis, and the ureter.
- The first functioning renal unit is developed when the connection between the nephrons and the collecting system is established.
- The metanephros forms the permanent kidney, which contains glomeruli and tubules.

- The kidney begins to function at 6–10 weeks of gestation and produces urine at approximately 11 weeks.
- The definitive kidney then migrates cephalad to its permanent position in the lumbar region.
- A separate structure termed the urogenital sinus gives rise to the bladder; therefore, bladder is present in fetuses with renal agenesis.

EXTERNAL GENITALIA

- The development of the external genitalia occurs between the 8th and 12th weeks of gestation.
- The genital tubercle, the genital swellings, and the genital folds give rise to the external genitalia and urethra of both sexes.
  - In females, the genital tubercle becomes the clitoris
  - The genital swellings become the labia majora
  - The genital folds become the labia minora
- The causes of ambiguous genitalia fall into one of the three main categories: virulized female infant, undervirulized male infant, and mixed sex chromosome pattern.
- The main etiologies responsible for the female virulization include congenital adrenal hyperplasia (CAH), exposure to maternal androgens, SRY translocation, SOX9 duplication, and true hermaphroditism.
- The top differential diagnoses of undervirulized karyotypically male infants include gonadal dysgenesis, androgen insensitivity syndrome, and 5-alpha reductase deficiency.

INTERNAL GENITAL TRACT

- The two sets of ducts, the wolffian and müllerian, which are present in early embryos of both sexes, give rise to the internal urogenital tracts.
- In males, the müllerian ducts' regression mediated by antimüllerian hormone is completed by the 8th gestational week. The wolffian ducts, under the influence of testosterone, develop into the epidi-dymides, vasa deferentia, seminal vesicles, and ejaculatory ducts.
- In females, the wolffian ducts persist only in vestigial form.

UTERUS AND FALLOPIAN TUBES

- The female genital tract is derived from the müllerian ducts, urogenital sinus, and vaginal plate.
- The müllerian ducts first appear at approximately 6 weeks of gestation. They elongate caudally, cross the metanephric ducts medially, and meet in the midline.

- Around 12 weeks, the caudal portion of the müllerian ducts fuses to form the uterovaginal canal, which inserts into the dorsal wall of the urogenital sinus, which is separated from the rectum by the urorectal septum by 7th week, at Müller's tubercle.
- The two müllerian ducts initially are lined up side by side and are composed of solid tissue.
- Subsequently, each duct undergoes internal canalization and two channels divided by a septum are produced.
- The septum is reabsorbed in a cephalad direction by 20 weeks.
- These fused portions of the müllerian ducts develop into uterus and vagina.
- The cranial portions, however, remain unfused and give rise to the fimbria and fallopian tubes.

VAGINA

- Vaginal plate is formed from the proliferation of the endodermal cells, which form sinovaginal bulbs at the site of contact of müllerian ducts with the urogenital sinus.
- Thus the upper-third of the vagina together with the cervix is formed from the müllerian system and the lower portion is derived from the urogenital sinus.
- By 20 weeks of gestation canalization occurs, producing the lumen of the lower vagina via degeneration of the central cells of this vaginal plate.
- The vaginal lumen is separated from the urogenital sinus by the membrane called hymen.
- The central epithelial cells of the hymen degenerate before birth and only a thin fold of mucous membrane persists around the vaginal introitus.

BIBLIOGRAPHY

Emans SJ, Laufer MR, Goldstein OP. *Pediatric and Adolescent Gynecology.* 5th ed, Philadelphia, PA: Lippincott, William and Wilkins; 2005; Chap. 10:334.

Gell JS. Mullerian anomalies. *Semin Reprod Med.* 2003;21(4): 375–388.

Glassberg KI. Normal and abnormal development of the kidney: a clinician's interpretation of current knowledge. *J Urol.* 2002; 167:2339.

Hamilton WJ, Boyd JD, Mossman HW. *Human Embryology.* Baltimore, MD: Williams & Wilkins; 1959:267–314.

Moore KL, Persaud TVN. *The Developing Human, Clinically Oriented Embryology.* 7th ed. Philadelphia, PA: Lippincott, William and Wilkins; W.B. Saunders; 2003:255–328, 77–99.

Voutilainen R. Differentiation of the fetal gonad. *Horm Res.* 1992;38(Suppl. 2):66–71.

Warkany J. *Congenital Malformations.* Chicago, IL: Year Book Medical Publishers, Inc; 1971;1067–1097.

Warne GL, Kanumakala S. Molecular endocrinology of sex differentiation. *Semin Reprod Med.* 2002;20(3):169–180.

QUESTIONS

Match each of the anatomic regions below with its derivative above. If more than one answer is correct, use the answer which is later in embryologic development. Each answer may be used once, more than once, or not at all.

(A) Urogenital sinus
(B) Müllerian
(C) Wolffian
(D) Gubernaculum
(E) Mesenchyme
(F) Cloaca
(G) Allantois
(H) Hindgut
(I) Labioscrotal swellings
(J) Neural crest
(K) Endoderm
(L) Ectoderm

1. Bartholin's gland
2. Rectovaginal fascia
3. Distal urethra
4. Obturator internus muscle
5. Uterosacral ligament
6. Proximal-most vagina
7. Distal anal canal
8. Round ligament
9. Ureter
10. Ischiocavernosus muscle
11. Pudendal nerve
12. Trigone of the bladder

ANSWERS

1. *(A),*
2. *(E),*
3. *(A),*
4. *(E),*
5. *(E),*
6. *(B),*
7. *(L),*
8. *(D),*
9. *(C),*
10. *(F),*
11. *(J),*
12. *(C).* See Table 35-1.

TABLE 35-1. Embryologic Precursors to Structures Relevant in Urogynecology

UROGYNECOLOGY AND EMBRYOLOGY	GIVES RISE TO
Indifferent gonad	Ovary
Gubernaculum	Ovarian ligament, round ligament
Mesonephric tubules	Epoophoron, paroöphoron
Mesonephric duct = wolffian	Gartner's duct, ureter, trigone of bladder, pelvis, kidney collecting tubules
Paramesonephric duct = müllerian	Hydatid of Morgagni, uterus
Urogenital sinus	Bladder, urethra, distal two-thirds vagina, urethral and paraurethral glands, Bartholin's gland (greater vestibular gland)
Urogenital sinus tubercle	Hymen
Phallus	Clitoris
Urogenital folds	Labia minora
Labioscrotal swellings	Labia majora
Cloaca and cloacal sphincter (distal-most part of cloaca)	Rectum, anus, and urogenital sinus; anterior cloacal sphincter → superficial transverse perineal muscle, bulbospongiosus, ischiocavernosus muscle Posterior cloacal sphincter → external anal sphincter
Fusion point of urorectal septum + cloacal membrane	Perineal body
Allantois	Continuous with and ventral to cloaca; forms as outpouching from yolk sac; in early embryonic life it serves as reservoir for urine and is place of blood cell formation; later embryonic life becomes urachus → median umbilical ligament; vessels inside allontois give rise to umbilical arteries
Hindgut	Continuous with and dorsal to cloaca; gives rise to half transverse colon, descending and sigmoid colon, rectum, and upper two-thirds anal canal
Pectinate line	Demarcation between endoderm and ectoderm; the upper two-thirds of anal canal is hindgut (endoderm) while the lower one-third of anal canal is proctodeum (ectoderm)
Neural crest cells	Spinal nerves (e.g., pudendal nerve)
Myotomes (mesoderm)	Pelvic floor muscles (levator ani, coccygeus, obturator internus)
Mesenchymal cells (ameboid cells from surface of primitive streak)	Most connective tissue (cardinal ligament, uterosacral ligament, rectovaginal fascia), mesoderm
Epiblast	Endoderm + ectoderm
Endoderm	Epithelial lining of respiratory, GI tract, and glands
Ectoderm	Epidermis, CNS, PNS, retina
Mesoderm	Smooth muscle coat, connective tissue, vessels, blood cells, bone marrow, striated muscle, excretory organs

ABBREVIATIONS: CNS, central nervous system; GI, gastrointestinal; PNS, peripheral nervous system.

36 CONGENITAL ANOMALIES OF THE FEMALE REPRODUCTIVE AND URINARY TRACT, AN ANATOMICAL APPROACH

Marianna Alperin

INTRODUCTION

Anomalies of the reproductive and urinary tracts can lead to the multitude of complications including poor obstetric outcomes, infertility, severe pain, wide array of infections, and social implications. This chapter will provide a concise review of the relevant embryology of the female reproductive and urinary tracts in order to facilitate understanding of the individual anomalies. It will provide an organ-based review of the significant abnormalities, their most common presentations, and treatment options.

The development of the female reproductive tract begins at 3 weeks of gestation and continues into the second trimester of pregnancy. The process is complex and involves cellular differentiation, fusion, canalization, and apoptosis. All malformations result from the failure of canalization, fusion, programmed cell death, or agenesis. In order to better remember and sort the disorders leading to the malformations a pneumonic *CAFE* can be used. It stands for disorders of *canalization, agenesis, fusion,* and *embryonic cell disorders*.

CONGENITAL ANOMALIES

- The etiology of the congenital anomalies of the müllerian ducts and urogenital sinus is not known at this time.
- Most patients, when such anomalies are isolated, will have a normal karyotype and the inheritance is likely polygenic and multifactorial. Viruses and teratogens have been implicated in some cases.
- The true incidence of these malformations is unknown because asymptomatic patients are not diagnosed most of the time.

ANOMALIES OF THE HYMEN

- Hymenal anomalies fall in the category of failed *canalization*.

- Incomplete degeneration of the central portion of the hymen can result in imperforate, microperforate, septate, and cribriform hymens.

IMPERFORATE HYMEN

- An imperforate hymen is one of the most common obstructive congenital anomalies in females. If noted at birth, it can present as a bulge in the introitus due to mucocolpos from vaginal secretions stimulated by maternal estrogen. After menarche girls usually present with a history of cyclic low abdominal, back or pelvic pain. Bulging hymen has a bluish hue secondary to hematocolpos.
- Microperforate, septate, and cribriform hymens can predispose to vaginal infections and postmenstrual spotting secondary to incomplete drainage. Women can also have difficulty with intercourse and tampon insertion.

TREATMENT

- Surgical repair is indicated for symptomatic patients. The best timing is after tissue had been primed by estrogen (after puberty).
- Repair consists of an excision of the hymenal tissue and evacuation of muco or hematocolpos. A normal size introitus is created and vaginal mucosa is sutured to the hymenal ring to prevent adhesion and recurrence of the obstruction.

CLOACAL ANOMALIES

- The cloaca is a primitive structure from which by the 6th week of gestation the rectum and urogenital sinus develop.
- Cloacal exstrophy refers to exstrophy of the urinary bladder and small or large intestine, anal atresia, and anomalous genitalia. It is a rare event, occurring in 1 in 200,000–400,000 live births.
- Several theories for the development of cloacal exstrophy have been proposed including the caudal-displacement theory, an abnormally large cloacal membrane creating a midline infra-abdominal defect, and the imbalance between cell proliferation and apoptotic cell death. The detailed description of the above theories is beyond the scope of this chapter.

TREATMENT

A series of complex reconstructive surgeries is necessary for the management of newborns with cloacal exstrophy.

BLADDER EXSTROPHY

- Bladder exstrophy is caused by a premature rupture of the cloacal membrane secondary to the failure of medial migration of abdominal mesenchyme. The local field defect results in failure of development of the lower abdominal wall, genital tubercles, and pubic rami; therefore, females with bladder exstrophy have epispadias and a bifid clitoris.
- Vesicoureteral reflux is commonly present due to the abnormal course of the distal ureter. The incidence is approximately in 1 in 40,000 live births with male to female ratio of 2.5:1.

TREATMENT

- Bladder exstrophy is treated surgically in stages. The three operations include bladder closure, epispadias repair, and bladder neck reconstruction.

  Most other congenital anomalies of the urinary tract are discovered during evaluation of the reproductive organs. Renal anomalies are found in 20–30% of women with müllerian defects. The basis for this association lies in embryology: development of paramesonephric structures requires prior appearance of mesonephric ducts. Renal anomalies include renal duplication, solitary kidney, hydronephrosis, anomalous position or shape of the kidney. Patients with ectopic ureter can present with constant wetness of the perineum. Once renal and reproductive tracts' anomalies have been discovered, the evaluation of central nervous system (CNS), skeletal, and cardiac systems should follow.

ANOMALIES OF THE VAGINA

TRANSVERSE VAGINAL SEPTUM

- A transverse vaginal septum results when there is failure of *canalization* of the urogenital sinus and müllerian ducts.
- The incidence is approximately 1 in 30,000 to 1 in 80,000 women.
- The septum has been noted at various levels in the vagina with the following distribution: 45% in the upper vagina, 35–40% in the middle, and 15–20% in the lower vagina.
- Primary amenorrhea is a common presentation, accompanied by cyclical pain, just as with imperforated hymen. However, bulge will likely not be present on the examination secondary to the thickness of the septum but a mass, which represents hematocolpos, can often be palpated on rectovaginal examination.

- Ultrasound or magnetic resonance imaging (MRI) is integral in defining the exact location and thickness of the septum.

TREATMENT

- A surgical excision of the septum followed by an end-to-end anastomosis of the upper and lower vaginal mucosa restores normal anatomy.
- Hematocolpos should not be evacuated prior to surgery because menstrual blood acts as a natural tissue expander, thus increasing the amount of upper vaginal tissue available for the reanastomosis.

LONGITUDINAL VAGINAL SEPTUM

- Longitudinal septa are the result of failure of *fusion* and are typically associated with uterine anomalies.
- The septum may be partial or complete.
- Patients may complain of dyspareunia or difficulty with tampon insertion.
- Cyclic pain and palpable mass on the bimanual examination can be noted if an obstructed hemivagina is present. Such cases are usually associated with ipsilateral renal agenesis.

TREATMENT

Surgical excision of the entire septum is required in symptomatic patients or women with an obstructed hemivagina due to the risk of infection and endometriosis from retrograde menses.

VAGINAL AGENESIS

- Vaginal agenesis, which is the result of *agenesis* or hypoplasia of the müllerian duct system, is also known as müllerian aplasia or Mayer-Rokitansky-Küster-Hauser (MRKH) syndrome.
- It is a rare disorder with the incidence of 1 per 4000–10,000 females. The underlying etiology remains unknown.
- Cervical and uterine agenesis is usually found in these patients as well; however, 7–10% of women with MRKH have a uterus with functional endometrium, which is obstructed.
- A normal female karyotype and functional ovaries are present. Extragenital anomalies often accompany MRKH. Urologic anomalies being the most common (25–40% of the cases), followed by skeletal abnormalities of spine and limbs (12–15%). Eighth nerve

deafness and cardiac defects also have been found in association with MRKH.
- The external genitalia appear normal and a vaginal dimple or pouch is usually present, as the lower third of the vagina is derived from the urogenital sinus.
- Ultrasound examination should be performed to assess the kidneys and confirm the presence of ovaries and the absence of a uterus. If uterus is present MRI can help determine whether it has functional endometrium.
- Vaginal agenesis is the second most common cause of primary amenorrhea, the first one being gonadal dysgenesis.
- It is important to differentiate MRKH from *androgen insensitivity syndrome (AIS)* (formerly known as testicular feminization), which is also characterized by a short or absent vagina, absent cervix and uterus secondary to the presence of müllerian inhibiting substance. Because of insensitivity to androgens and increased estrogen production, these patients develop female body habitus and external genitalia. They lack pubic and axillary hair. The karyotype is 46,XY and serum testosterone is in the normal male range. Because of female phenotype these individuals are often raised as females. Gonads in patients with AIS have a high rate of malignant degeneration (dysgerminoma being the most common malignancy) and should be removed after pubertal development is completed and adult height is reached. Vaginal dilators are used to create a functional vagina.

TREATMENT

- Two treatment approaches exist: nonoperative and surgical. A nonoperative approach to creaing a functional vagina uses vaginal dilators.
  ◦ *Frank procedure*: Graduated hard dilators with progressive increase in size are placed against vaginal dimple and enough pressure to produce a mild discomfort is applied to progressively invaginate the mucosa. Dilators are pressed inward and downward (line of normal vaginal axis). Starting with the smallest dilator the procedure should be performed two to three times per day for 30–60 min each session, preferably after a warm bath. The procedure might take months to a year to be effective depending on patient's compliance and motivation; however, 80% success rate had been reported.
  ◦ *Ingram procedure*: This procedure is a modification of Frank method for creating vagina via progressive dilation. Graduated dilators are used in the same way; however, Ingram procedure uses a patient's own trunk weight to apply pressure while sitting on

a bicycle seat mounted on a stool and allows for other productive tasks to be performed during the dilation. Through this technique 86% of patients were able to create vaginas, which allowed for satisfactory intercourse.
- A review including 334 patients who underwent dilator therapy reported 86% were able to achieve satisfactory intercourse.
- Alternatively, repetitive coitus can also create a functional vagina.
- At present, there is no consensus on the ideal surgical method for creation of a functional vagina. Surgical procedures should be considered only if a woman failed to achieve a functional vagina using dilators. The most common surgical procedures include the following:
  ◦ *Abbe-Wharton-McIndoe vaginoplasty*: This procedure consists of a split-thickness skin graft taken from the buttocks. Graft is placed over a mold dermal side out. A transverse incision is made at the vaginal dimple and a cavity is dissected to the level of peritoneum. The mold with skin graft over it is inserted into the cavity and labia minora is secured around the stent to prevent expulsion. The mold is left inside for 7 days which patient must spend on strict bed rest. After first postoperative week, the mold is removed and a dilator is worn continually for 3 months to prevent contraction of the graft. The dilator is removed during defecation, urination, and intercourse, which can be initiated 3 weeks postoperatively. For the next 6 months, patients must wear the dilator nightly unless they engage in regular intercourse; 83% of patients reported satisfactory intercourse.
  ◦ *Williams vaginoplasty*: This technique creates a vaginal pouch from the skin of labia majora. A U-shaped incision is made inferior to labia majora, full-thickness skin flaps are created. First, the edges of the inner layer are brought together followed by suturing the outer layers in the midline; thus, a new "vaginal pouch" is created. The axis of neovagina is different than normal vaginal axis; however, satisfactory intercourse can be achieved. The advantage of Williams vaginoplasty is decreased risk of fistula formation given that pelvic structures are not entered during operation. This procedure is especially useful in patients with previously failed vaginoplasty or after radical pelvic surgery or irradiation. Vaginal dilators must be used for 1 month following Williams procedure.
  ◦ *Pratt sigmoid vaginoplasty*: This procedure requires laparotomy and uses a segment of sigmoid colon for creation of neovagina. A vascular pedicle of the bowel loop is preserved; the distal end is pulled

through to the introitus and the proximal end closed to create a blind pouch. The end-to-end reanastomosis reestablishes continuity of colon. No postoperative dilation is necessary. A disadvantage of Pratt sigmoid vaginoplasty is chronic discharge from mucus secreted by colonic cells.

AGENESIS OF THE LOWER VAGINA

- The lower vagina is replaced by fibrous tissue in cases of abnormal development of the sinovaginal bulbs or vaginal plate.
- The müllerian ducts and gonads are intact; therefore, ovaries, uterus, cervix, and upper vagina are normal in these patients.
- The most common presentation is primary amenorrhea with cyclic pelvic pain.
- On physical examination, a vaginal dimple is noted.

TREATMENT

- The dissection through the fibrous tissue is carried out till normal vaginal mucosa is encountered. A "pull-through" of upper vaginal tissue reestablishes a normal vagina.
- By distending upper vagina, a large hematocolpos increases the amount of tissue available for surgical procedure.

ANOMALIES OF THE CERVIX

- Most anomalies include duplication, which is the result of *fusion* defect, or *agenesis* of the cervix. Hypoplasia can also occur.
- In cases of cervical agenesis, the upper vagina does not develop as well. These patients present with primary amenorrhea, cyclic or chronic pelvic pain, and sometimes abdominal mass secondary to the uterine distention.
- Occasionally, large cysts can develop within the cervical stroma from the microscopic remnants of the mesometanephric ducts. When large, these cysts can cause dyspareunia.

TREATMENT

- Symptoms develop secondary to the obstruction of the menstrual blood egress; therefore, medications to suppress menstruation until pregnancy is desired can be used.

- Surgical options include creation of an endocervical tract and vagina using skin and mucosal grafts or hysterectomy for patients with uteri and cervical agenesis. Excising the cyst and marsupializing its base can treat symptomatic cervical cysts.

ANOMALIES OF THE UTERUS

- The American Fertility Society in 1988 produced a standard form for classification of müllerian defects, which is a descriptive form with focus on vertical fusion defects.
- The true incidence is hard to determine because a lot of these patients are asymptomatic; however, uterine anomalies may negatively impact a woman's obstetric outcomes. The incidence among women with recurrent first trimester miscarriage is 5–10%, 25% of women with second trimester miscarriages or preterm deliveries have a uterine anomaly. Septate (33.6%) and arcuate (32.8%) uteri are the most common uterine malformations observed.
- Diagnostic laparoscopy has been largely replaced by the imaging studies in the evaluation of uterine anomalies. The main available imaging modalities include: ultrasonography (US), hysterosalpingography (HSG), and MRI. MRI is considered a gold standard and is superior to other modalities secondary to its ability to differentiate between endometrium, myometrium, and fibrous tissue.
- In regards to reproductive impact of uterine malformations, the highest rate of live birth is observed with arcuate uteri (83%), followed by bicornuate and septate uteri (62%). In women with unicornuate and didelphys uteri this rate drops off to 37–40%. In all these abnormalities, early miscarriages (25–38%) and preterm deliveries (25–47%) are common.

SEPTATE/ARCUATE UTERUS

- A septate uterus develops from a defect in *canalization*. Such uteri have a normal external surface and two endometrial cavities.
- The extent of resorption of the midline septum between the two müllerian ducts determines the length of the remaining septum.
- An arcuate uterus has a small midline septum and a minimal fundal indentation. A total failure in resorption results in a longitudinal vaginal septum.
- The risk of recurrent miscarriage is proportional to the length of the septa; however, the rate of live birth is 60% if septum is left untreated.
- Urinary tract anomalies are found in 15% of cases.

- The method of choice for correction of the uterine septa is hysteroscopic resection.

UNICORNUATE UTERUS

- The unicornuate uterus results from a defect in *fusion*. Also a failure in the development of one of the müllerian ducts can be accountable for this anomaly. The cavity on the side of the developed müllerian duct is usually normal, with a fallopian tube and cervix, while the anomalous side can have various configurations.
- Partial development of the duct will result in the formation of a rudimentary horn. Occasionally, such horns will contain functional endometrium, if the obstruction is also present, patients will develop cyclic or chronic pelvic pain. Risk of infertility, endometriosis, premature labor, and malpresentations are higher in these women.
- The obstructed horn must be surgically excised in a symptomatic patient.
- Contralateral renal agenesis is invariably noted with obstructive müllerian defects.

BICORNUATE UTERUS

- A bicornuate uterus has an indented fundus which is the result of *partial fusion* of the müllerian ducts. The degree of separation of the uterine horns varies from complete to minimal.
- Most pregnancy outcomes are normal but pregnancy loss, preterm labor, or malpresentation (especially breech presentation) can occur. In those cases, surgical treatment, which involves unification of the uterine cavities through a laparotomy, is indicated.
- Three reunification procedures exist:
  - *Jones metroplasty*: The Jones procedure refers to a wedge resection of the portion of the uterine fundus containing the septum. A triangular incision forming a wedge in the anterior-posterior plane of the uterus is made. Vasopressin or tourniquet, placed through an avascular space in the broad ligament and tied at the junction of the lower uterine segment and the cervix and around infundibular pelvic ligaments, should be used to reduce uterine bleeding. The wedge is then incised until the common uterine cavity is found and the septum is totally removed. Reconstruction of the uterus begins at the lower portion of the cavity. The anterior and then posterior walls are closed in either a continuous or interrupted fashion. The first layer should include the endometrium and a small amount of myometrium.

The knot should be tied so that it remains in the uterine cavity. The second closure layer is begun inferiorly and performed with interrupted sutures that include the remainder of the myometrium. The final layer incorporates the remainder of the myometrium and serosa.
  - *Tompkins metroplasty*: The uterus is incised in the midline anterior-posterior plane until the uterine cavity is reached. The septa are then excised from the two cavities using sharp dissection, and the uterus is closed as in the Jones procedure. The benefit of this technique is that the resultant uterine cavity is larger than with wedge resection because no portion of the uterine fundus is removed.
  - *Strassman metroplasty*: This procedure consists of wedge resection of the medial aspect of each uterine horn and subsequent unification of the two cavities. The resultant cavity is similar to one achieved with Jones metroplasty.

UTERUS DIDELPHYS

- Uterine didelphys is another example of *fusion* defect. The two müllerian ducts produce duplication of the uterus and cervix. Occasionally, duplication of the vulva, bladder, urethra, vagina, and anus occurs as well.
- Majority of the patients are asymptomatic; however, uterus didelphys is frequently accompanied by vaginal septum, which can cause dyspareunia and interference with vaginal delivery. The resection of the septum is indicated in these cases.
- A hemivagina can be obstructed, in which case cyclic pain can occur. Treatment involves resection of the wall of the obstructed hemivagina and creation of a single vaginal vault. Rarely bilateral obstruction is found in patients presenting with primary amenorrhea.

DISORDERS OF EMBRYONIC CELLS

VAGINAL CYSTS

- Lateral or posterior vaginal wall cysts arise from müllerian remnants. They can also represent epidermal inclusion cyst or Gartner's duct cysts.
- Differential diagnosis of anterior vaginal wall masses includes:
  - Epidermal inclusion cysts
  - Cystocele
  - Ectopic ureter
  - Urethral prolapse
  - Urethral diverticulum

- Most cysts are asymptomatic but when large can cause difficulty with tampon insertion or intercourse. Symptomatic cysts can be excised or marsupialized.

DIETHYLSTILBESTROL-INDUCED DEFECTS

- Diethylstilbestrol (DES) is a synthetic estrogen used from 1949 to 1971 to treat recurrent first trimester miscarriages.
- Uterine anomalies, associated with DES exposure, include:
  - T-shaped uterine cavity
  - Hypoplastic uterus
  - Midfundal constrictions
  - Filling defects
  - Endometrial cavity adhesions
- Associated vaginal abnormalities predominantly consist of
  - Vaginal adenosis
  - Vaginal ridges
  - Transverse septa
- Cervical anomalies include:
  - Hypoplasia
  - Presence of hoods, collars, or pseudopolyps
- These patients are also at increased risk of clear cell carcinoma of the vagina and cervix.
- Term pregnancy rate in DES exposed patients is 64%, these patients are at increased risk of ectopic pregnancy (4%) and preterm delivery (12%). Weekly cervical examinations are recommended starting at 12 weeks to detect early cervical shortening and dilatation and assess need for cerclage.

BIBLIOGRAPHY

Acien P. Incidence of Mullerian defects in fertile and infertile women. *Hum Reprod.* 1997;12(7):1372–1376.

ACOG Committee Opinion. Number 274. Nonsurgical diagnosis and management of vaginal agenesis. *Obstet Gynecol.* 2002;100:213.

D'Alberton A, Santi F. Formation of neovagina by coitus. *Obstet Gynecol.* 1972;40:763.

Emans SJ, Laufer MR, Goldstein DP, et al. *Pediatric and Adolescent Gynecology.* 5th ed. Philadelphia, PA: Lippincott Williams & Wilkins; Chap. 10; 2005:334.

Frank RT. The formation of artificial vagina without operation. *Am J Obstet Gynecol.* 1938;35:1053.

Gearhart JP. Exstrophy, epispadias, and other bladder anomalies. In: Walsh PC, Retik AB, Vaughan ED, eds. *Campbell's Urology.* 8th ed. Philadelphia, PA: WB Saunders; 2002:2136.

Ingram JM. The bicycle seat stool in the treatment of vaginal agenesis and stenosis: a preliminary report. *Am J Obstet Gynecol.* 1981;140:867.

Kaufman RH, Adam E, Hatch EE, et al. Continued follow-up of pregnancy outcomes in diethylstilbestrol-exposed offspring. *Obstet Gynecol.* 2000;96(4):483–489.

Lin PC, Bhatnagar KP, Nettleton S, et al. Female genital anomalies affecting reproduction. *Fertil Steril.* 2002;78(5):899–915.

Marshall VF, Muecke EC. Variations in exstrophy of the bladder. *J Urol.* 1962;88:766.

Raga F, Bauset C, Remohi J, et al. Reproductive impact of congenital Mullerian anomalies. *Hum Reprod.* 1997;12(10):2277–2281.

Roberts CP, Haber MJ, Rock JA, et al. Vaginal creation for mullerian agenesis. *Am J Obstet Gynecol.* 2001;185(6):1349–1352.

Rock JA, Azziz R. Genital anomalies in childhood. *Clin Obstet Gynecol.* 1987;30(3):682–696.

Romero R. *Prenatal Diagnosis of Congenital Anomalies.* East Norwalk, CT: Appleton and Lange; 1988:220.

Salvatore CA, Lodovicci O. Vaginal agenesis: an analysis of ninety cases. *Acta Obstet Gynecol Scand.* 1978;57(1):89–94.

The American Fertility Society. The American Fertility Society classifications of adnexal adhesions, distal tubal occlusion, tubal occlusion secondary to tubal ligations, tubal pregnancies, müllerian anomalies, and intrauterine adhesions. *Fertil Steril.* 1988;49:944.

Web site: www.youngwomenshealth.org/McIndoe

Williams EA. Congenital absence of the vagina-a simple operation for its relief. *J Obstet Gynaecol Br Commonw.* 1964;71:511.

QUESTIONS

1. A 34-year-old $G_2P_0A_1$ woman at 16 weeks presents to your office for obstetric care. Her gynecologic history is significant for bicornuate uterus. Her first pregnancy resulted in first trimester miscarriage. This anomaly is a result of
   (A) resorption defect
   (B) canalization defect
   (C) agenesis
   (D) migration defect
   (E) fusion defect

2. A 16-year-old girl presents to your office for evaluation of primary amenorrhea. She reports cyclic pelvic and low abdominal pain, which is getting progressively worse. On physical examination, she appears appropriately grown, has Tanner V breasts, normal external genitalia, and there is no visible mass at the introitus. You perform a rectovaginal examination and palpate a mass above your finger. What is the most likely abnormality in this patient?
   (A) imperforate hymen
   (B) bicornuate uterus
   (C) longitudinal vaginal septum
   (D) transverse vaginal septum
   (E) Gartner's duct cyst

3. In your further evaluation of the patient presented in Question number 2, you order an imaging study. What is the most likely anomaly to coexist with her condition?
   (A) ipsilateral renal agenesis
   (B) contralateral renal agenesis
   (C) ovarian agenesis
   (D) coarctation of the aorta
   (E) uterine septum

4. A 34-year-old woman comes to your office for consultation. She states that she has just learned that her mother took DES while pregnant with her. She heard that DES exposure increases your risk of some cancers. She would like to know what cancer is she at any increased risk for?
   (A) renal cell carcinoma
   (B) clear cell carcinoma of the vagina
   (C) endometrial cancer
   (D) breast cancer
   (E) sarcoma of the uterus

5. A 27-year-old $G_3P_0A_3$ woman presents for preconceptual counseling. Her previous pregnancies all resulted in miscarriages. She and her husband had undergone an extensive evaluation for recurrent pregnancy losses, which was significant for findings of bicornuate uterus. The rest of the evaluation was completely normal. The surgical treatment option that you discuss with the patient is
   (A) hysteroscopic metroplasty
   (B) abdominal metroplasty
   (C) laparoscopic metroplasty
   (D) laparoscopically assisted vaginal metroplasty
   (E) vaginal metroplasty

6. A 17-year-old girl presents for the evaluation of primary amenorrhea. She is of normal stature and her examination reveals presence of secondary sexual characteristics as well as normal external genitalia. On vaginal examination, only a small pouch is noted. Pelvic US reveals presence of ovaries bilaterally, a small uterine horn, absence of uterine cervix, and a horseshoe kidney. The karyotype is 46,XX. The most likely diagnosis is
   (A) MRKH syndrome
   (B) agenesis of the lower vagina
   (C) McCune-Albright syndrome
   (D) imperforate hymen
   (E) transverse vaginal septum

ANSWERS

1. *(E)*. A bicornuate uterus refers to a uterus with indented fundus. This anomaly results from the defect in fusion of the müllerian ducts. Depending on the degree of fusion failure, the separation of uterine horns can range from minimal to complete. The causes of müllerian defects are polygenic and multifactorial. The karyotype of these patients is usually normal. The majority of pregnancies in women with bicornuate uteri will result in term birth. Obstetrical complications, such as pregnancy loss, preterm labor, or malpresentations, do occur in these patients with a slightly higher frequency than general population. Agenesis results in a complete absence of the structure. Defects of canalization would produce anomalies such as imperforate hymen or vaginal septum. Defect of migration of the undifferentiated germ cells from the yolk sac to the gonadal ridge, where they are required for development of the ovaries, would result in gonadal dysgenesis.

2. *(D)*. A transverse vaginal septum is the result of the failure of canalization of the urogenital sinus and müllerian ducts. The incidence is approximately 1 in 30,000 to 1 in 80,000 women. The septum has been noted at various levels in the vagina with the following distribution: 45% in the upper vagina, 35–40% in the middle, and 15–20% in the lower vagina. Primary amenorrhea is a common presentation, accompanied by cyclical pain secondary to expanding hematocolpos. Hematocolpos can often be palpated on the rectovaginal examination as a mass. Ultrasound or MRI is integral in defining the exact location and thickness of the septum. Bulging at the introitus, caused by hematocolpos, which is commonly seen in cases of imperforate hymen, will likely not be present on the examination secondary to the thickness of the septum. Patients with longitudinal vaginal septum may complain of dyspareunia or difficulty with tampon insertion. Cyclic pain and palpable mass on the bimanual examination can be noted if an obstructed hemivagina from a complete longitudinal septum is present; however, these patients will still menstruate. Gartner's duct cysts present as vaginal masses on the posterior or lateral walls of the vagina. Most cysts are asymptomatic but when large can cause difficulty with tampon insertion or intercourse. These cysts are not associated with amenorrhea or cyclic pain.

3. *(A)*. Renal anomalies are found in 20–30% of women with müllerian defects. These include renal duplication, solitary kidney, hydronephrosis, anomalous position or shape of the kidney. Therefore, all women with müllerian defects should undergo a radiologic renal investigation, such as an intravenous pyelogram or renal ultrasound. Obstructive müllerian defects, such as obstructed noncommunicating uterine horn, obstructed uterine hemicavity,

and vaginal septum, are associated with ipsilateral renal agenesis. In addition, upper urinary tract anomalies such as horseshoe kidney, duplication of the collecting system, pelvic kidney, and ectopically located ureteral orifices have all been noted at increased frequency. Gonadal development is independent of the müllerian system and normal ovaries are usually present in patients with the defects of the müllerian ducts or urogenital sinus. The karyotype of these patients is also usually normal; therefore, coarctation of the aorta, which is associated with Turner's syndrome, will not be the most likely associated anomaly.

4. *(B)*. DES is a nonsteroidal estrogen first synthesized in 1938. It became an established intervention for prevention of miscarriage, premature birth, and other pregnancy problems. Uterine anomalies, associated with DES exposure, include: T-shaped uterine cavity, hypoplastic uterus, midfundal constrictions, filling defects, and endometrial cavity adhesions. Associated vaginal abnormalities predominantly consist of vaginal adenosis, vaginal ridges, and transverse septa. Cervical anomalies include hypoplasia, presence of hoods, collars, or pseudopolyps. Women exposed to DES *in utero* have a 40-fold increase in risk of clear cell adenocarcinoma of the vagina and cervix compared to unexposed women. There is no firm evidence to link DES exposure *in utero* with increased risk of breast cancer. DES exposure has not been associated with increased risk of renal cell carcinoma or uterine cancers. Pelvic irradiation increases risk of uterine sarcomas and unopposed estrogen is a risk factor for endometrial adenocarcinoma.

5. *(B)*. Surgical management of the bicornuate uterus requires a laparotomy. Two abdominal procedures exist: Jones metroplasty and Tompkins metroplasty. The Jones procedure involves a wedge resection of the portion of the uterine fundus between the two uterine horns followed by anastomosis. The advantage of the Tompkins metroplasty is that no uterine tissue is removed. The uterine fundus is incised transversely and the cavities are unified. The benefit of this technique is that the resultant uterine cavity is larger than with wedge resection. Repair of bicornuate uteri has been reported to reduce the rate of miscarriage from 84 to 12%. Hysteroscopic metroplasty is the method of choice for repair of uterine septum. There are no laparoscopic or vaginal procedures described at this time for the correction of bicornuate uterus. Cesarean delivery will be required after abdominal metroplasty.

6. *(A)*. Vaginal agenesis is also known as müllerian aplasia or MRKH syndrome. It is a rare disorder with the incidence of 1 per 4000–10,000 females. The underlying etiology remains unknown. Cervical and uterine agenesis is usually found in these patients as well; however, 7–10% of women with MRKH have a uterus with functional endometrium, which is obstructed. A normal female karyotype and functional ovaries are present. Extragenital anomalies, involving urologic, skeletal, or cardiac systems, often accompany MRKH. Vaginal agenesis is the second most common cause of primary amenorrhea, the first one being gonadal dysgenesis. The external genitalia appear normal and a vaginal dimple or pouch is usually present, as the lower third of the vagina is derived from the urogenital sinus. Ultrasound examination should be performed to assess the kidneys and confirm the presence of ovaries and the absence of a uterus. If uterus is present, MRI can help determine whether it has functional endometrium. In cases of agenesis of the lower vagina, it is replaced by fibrous tissue. This anomaly is the result of abnormal development of the sinovaginal bulbs or vaginal plate. The müllerian ducts and gonads are intact; therefore, ovaries, uterus, cervix, and upper vagina are normal in these patients. Patients with McCune-Albright syndrome usually present with symptoms of precocious puberty. This syndrome is due to mutations in the gene encoding the alpha subunit of the G protein, resulting in activation of the signal-transduction pathway generating cyclic adenosine monophosphate (cAMP). Other characteristics associated with this syndrome are café au lait spots, polyostotic fibrous dysplasia, and multinodular goiter. An imperforate hymen is one of the most common obstructive congenital anomalies in females. Together with transverse vaginal septum, it results from müllerian canalization defect. Imperforate hymen or transverse vaginal septum is not commonly associated with uterine or cervical agenesis/hypoplasia.

37 MEDICINES USED IN UROGYNECOLOGY

Sam Siddighi and Sandy Chuan

INTRODUCTION

- The pharmaceutical industry spends billions ($33.2 in 2003) of dollars on research and development of drugs alone.
- The United States is the most rigorous country in the world when it comes to drug approval.
  - It takes an average of 10–15 years for an experimental drug to go from the laboratory to the patient.
  - It costs a drug company $802 million to get one new drug from the lab to a patient.
  - Only 5 out of 5000 new compounds make it to human testing.
  - Of the 5, only one will receive approval by the Food and Drug Administration (FDA).
- It is important to understand the drug development and approval process:
  - Preclinical → Clinical (Phases I–III) → FDA approval of New Drug Application (NDA) → Phase IV
    - Preclinical: Conduct lab and animal studies to see effect on the targeted tissue and safety. Once this is successful, a company files an Investigational New Drug Application (IND) to the FDA. If the FDA does not disapprove it in 1 month, then the IND is effective.
    - Clinical trials: Phase I—20–100 health volunteers to see its safety, duration of action, metabolism, and excretion.
    - Clinical trials: Phase II—controlled trial of 100–500 volunteers to assess drug's effectiveness.
    - Clinical trials: Phase III—1000–5000 patients in clinics and hospitals are given drug, then efficacy and safety is monitored.
    - NDA is filed with the FDA after all three phases are completed. The NDA can be >100,000 pages and takes an average of 16.9 months to approve.
    - Phase IV: FDA-approved drug is available to physicians for prescription. The drug company has to give periodic update reports to the FDA about their drug. Long-term effects are evaluated in Phase IV, and on occasion, a drug can be withdrawn if long-term adverse effects become apparent.
- A survey by the Pharmaceutical Research and Manufacturers of America in 2004 revealed that 67 new drugs for Obstetric/Gynecologic (48) or Kidney/Urologic (19) conditions are either in clinical trials or awaiting approval by the FDA. This is second only to new drugs in the pipeline for treatment of cancer (71).
- In this chapter, we will discuss drugs utilized for the management of overactive bladder (OAB), urinary urgency incontinence (UUI), stress urinary incontinence (SUI), and mixed incontinence. We will not only discuss commonly prescribed oral agents but also intravesical (instillation of medications and injection with Botulinum toxin), rectal, transdermal, and intravaginal agents. However, let us first review basic physiologic and pharmacologic principles relevant to Urogynecology.
- Drugs utilized for the management of interstitial cystitis will be discussed in Chap. 26, Interstitial Cystitis, Urethral Syndrome, and Sensory Urgency-Frequency Syndrome.
- Estrogen therapy will be discussed in Chap. 34, The Effect of Estrogen and SERMs on the Lower Urinary Tract and Pelvic Floor.

BASIC PHYSIOLOGY AND PHARMACOLOGY REVIEW

- Based on positron emission tomography (PET) scan and other studies, the pontine reticular formation (PRF) and the preoptic area of the hypothalamus are active during micturition.
- Efferent: Sympathetic and parasympathetic systems directly control micturition by sending their lower

motor neurons to synapse onto ganglia, detrusor muscle, or internal urethral sphincter. Sensory (afferent) information is also received from the periphery and transmitted to the spinal cord.

- ○ Efferent—parasympathetic (pelvic nerve: most important for detrusor contraction): presynaptic neurons of S2-S4 (intermediolateral column of spinal cord) → ganglia near bladder → postsynaptic neurons release acetylcholine (Ach) which binds *muscarinic receptors* (subtype M_3) on the detrusor smooth muscle → bladder contraction
  - ○ Efferent—sympathetic (hypogastric and pelvic nerves) → presynaptic neurons of T10-L2 pass through paravertebral chain (via pelvic nerve) or go to inferior mesenteric and hypogastric ganglia (via hypogastric nerve) → (1) detrusor wall relaxation and urethral sphincter contraction and (2) synapse with parasympathetic fibers at the level of the spinal cord or ganglia to inhibit them by releasing norepinephrine (NE)
  - ○ Afferent—most of the sensory information from bladder and internal urethral sphincter reaches the spinal cord via pelvic nerve and dorsal root ganglia (although some information also goes through hypogastric nerve afferents)
  - ○ Afferent—sensory information from the striated urethral sphincter reaches spinal cord via pudendal nerve
- Muscarinic Ach receptors
  - ○ Five subtypes have been identified by messenger ribonucleic acid (mRNA) blotting techniques
  - ○ M_1 → *brain* > spinal cord > salivary gland
    - Cognition ↓ = sedation, delirium, amnesia? hallucination?
    - Salivary gland
  - ○ M_2 → *heart* > brainstem, cerebellum > > gastrointestinal (GI), bladder
    - SA node and contractility → heart rate ↑
  - ○ M_3 → *exocrine glands*, bladder > GI wall smooth muscle and sphincters
    - Dry mouth (salivary gland) > lacrimation ↓ > sweating ↓
    - Slow peristalsis → constipation
  - ○ M_4 → inhibitory prejunctional muscarinic receptor in guinea pig bladder
  - ○ M_5 → ciliary muscle of eye
    - Visual accommodation ↓ = cycloplegia
- M_2 and M_3 receptors are found in the human bladder
  - ○ Role of M_2 in the human bladder is unclear; its activation may lead to contraction during certain disease states (e.g., neurogenic bladder)
  - ○ In animal model, binding of ligand to M_2 receptors → G_i protein → cyclic adenosine monophosphate (cAMP) ↓ → bladder relaxation
  - ○ Role of M_3 in human bladder is to cause detrusor muscle contraction:

- Binding of ligand to M_3 receptors → G_q protein → +Phospholipase C (PLC) → Dilacylglycerol (DAG) + IP3 ↑ → Ca^{2+} from sarcoplasmic reticulum → detrusor contraction which allows normal micturition to occur
- Muscarinic receptor antagonists, or commonly called *antimuscarinic* drugs, are extremely useful in the management of OAB and UUI.
- α_1-Adrenergic receptors are located in the bladder neck and proximal urethra. Activation of these receptors leads to bladder outlet closure and can be useful for the treatment of SUI.
- Although theoretically, β_2-adrenergic receptors are found on the detrusor wall and contribute to bladder relaxation, there is weak or inconsistent evidence to support the use of β-agonists (e.g., terbutaline, salbutamol, and clenbuterol) to treat OAB and UUI.
- β-Adrenergic receptors, calcium channel receptors, and potassium channel receptors and their agonists or antagonist will not be discussed in this chapter because currently, they play a limited role in the management of SUI, OAB, and UUI.

PHARMACOLOGIC TREATMENT OF OAB AND UUI

- Pharmacologic treatment of OAB and UUI should be an adjunct to other therapies as many patients discontinue its use months-years after initiation of treatment even though most have not been "cured" by them.
- Data for the majority of medications discussed in this chapter are Level I (i.e., prospective, randomized, and controlled clinical trials).
- However, no study is perfect. The following are common pitfalls: short follow-up, small number of patients (low Power), variable outcome measures (see below), study populations are not always representative of many everyday patients (e.g., studies in elderly only, in multiple sclerosis [MS] patient only, and so forth).
- Efficacy
  - ○ Patients with OAB and UUI have involuntary bladder contractions, episodes of urinary leakage, and lack the ability to store large urine volumes inside the bladder. Therefore, the following outcome measures have been studied in order to measure the efficacy of these medications:
    - Number of leakage episodes (aka episodes of incontinence)
    - Frequency of voids (micturition frequency = number of voids in a 24-hour period)
    - Urge symptoms (frequency and severity)
    - Bladder capacity (total or maximum cystometric capacity measured by cystometrogram [CMG])

- Amplitude of bladder contractions (measured by CMG)
- Bladder compliance ($\Delta V/\Delta P_{det}$)
- Overall subjective improvement (change in quality of life [QoL])
  - Although some drugs used for OAB and UUI may show statistically significant changes on CMG, this does not necessarily mean that clinical improvement is experienced by the patient. Therefore, subjective and QoL measures are very important.
  - There is a high placebo effect (some studies 40%) in most studies that use pills or capsules to treat OAB of UUI. Therefore, the drug being studied must do much better than placebo to be clinically significant.
- Tolerability
  - All medications have adverse effects.
  - Many of the drugs utilized for the treatment OAB and UUI are nonselective for the subtypes of muscarinic receptors therefore they may activate receptors in areas of the body that are not desired.
    - Dry mouth (M_3 and M_1)
    - Constipation (M_3)
    - Blurry vision (M_5)
    - Cognitive impairment and drowsiness (M_1)
    - Tachycardia (M_2)
  - Selective muscarinic receptor agonists also have adverse effects, but to a lesser degree than the nonselective muscarinic agonists.
  - Other adverse effects can include but are not limited to headache, drowsiness, dizziness, dysphagia, stomach ulcers, and diarrhea (yes, not a typo!), increased intraocular pressure, blurry vision.
  - Sometimes the adverse effect is so pronounced that patients withdraw from clinical studies or discontinue using the prescribed medication.
  - For OAB/UUI medications, dry mouth is the most common early, adverse effect, and one that can lead to discontinuation.
  - However, the patient should be told that tolerance to dry mouth does develop with time and there are things the patient can do to overcome this problem (e.g., sour candy to increase salivation).
  - Adverse effects on cognition are important in the elderly as they are more prone to delirium and altered sensorium.
- Contraindications
  - Uncontrolled narrow-angle glaucoma
    - Glaucoma is the no. 2 cause of blindness in the United States (no. 1 is cataracts).
    - Two types of glaucoma exist: open angle and narrow angle.
    - Most patients will have open angle which is usually asymptomatic.
    - Narrow angle is symptomatic (eye pain, blurry vision, rainbow-colored halos, nausea, and vomiting)
    - Narrow angle results because iris apposes the trabecular meshwork hence blocking drainage of aqueous humor → rise in intraocular pressure above normal range (normal = 10–21 mmHg).
    - Currently, mainstays of treatment for narrow-angle glaucoma are prostaglandin analog eye drops, laser trabeculoplasty (microscopic holes into iris to allow drainage), and surgery (hole in sclera or tube implantation).
  - Significant cardiac arrhythmias
  - Urinary retention
  - Gastric retention
  - Myasthenia gravis
  - Caution with renal and hepatic patients

ANTICHOLINERGIC MEDICINES

- Oxybutynin (Ditropan [ALZA Pharmaceuticals])—Level I evidence
  - Has been available for more than 30 years and some consider it the gold standard for treatment of OAB and UUI
  - Compound is a tertiary amine that is well absorbed
  - High first-pass metabolism (biologic availability = 6%)
  - $t_{1/2}$ = 2 hours
  - PO oxybutynin exerts its intended action as well as its adverse effects through the active metabolite, N-desthyloxybutynin
  - Mechanisms of action
    - Nonselective antimuscarinic → M_1 and $M_3 >> M_2$; is primary mechanism of action
    - Direct smooth muscle relaxation (antispasmodic) → may involve blockage of Ca^{2+} channels
    - Local anesthetic properties → important only for intravesical infusion
    - Antihistamine properties
  - Available in immediate release (IR: 2.5–5-mg tid) and extended release (ER or XL: 5–30-mg qd), syrup (1 tsp = 5 mg), and transdermal system (TDS) (the patch comes in 3.9 mg biw [twice weekly])
  - Ten milligrams of XL per day costs $100.41 per month; twice weekly of TDS costs $96.59

Note: If a drug name is not accompanied by ER or XL, then it is an immediate release form.
  - Oxybutynin has high efficacy for treatment of OAB and UUI (incontinence episodes ↓ up to 70%, frequency ↓ 33%, subjective improvement = 74%)
  - In the elderly:
    - It may be less efficacious in the elderly.
    - Dry mouth and cognitive impairment can be pronounced in the elderly (2.5-mg tid may decrease this side effect).

○ Oxybutynin XL improves drug tolerability and patient compliance

■ Oxybutynin XL uses OROS system: core 1 (osmotic agent) + core 2 (surrounds core 1; contain oxybutynin) + semipermeable membrane (surrounds core 2) → osmotic agent is hydrated as pill goes down GI tract → it expands and pushes oxybutynin out of semipermeable membrane (in effect, more drug is released in distal small intestine and colon) → less marked blood concentration fluctuations (peak → trough) and reduced first-pass metabolism which results in lower but still therapeutic drug concentrations

■ Oxybutynin IR versus oxybutynin XL → similar efficacy and less dry mouth in XL group

■ Oxybutynin XL versus tolterodine IR → oxybutynin XL more effective but dry mouth was similar between groups

■ Oxybutynin ER (XL) versus tolterodine ER (LA) → oxybutynin is slightly more effective (72% vs. 67% respectively), but tolterodine has less dry mouth (29.7% vs. 22.3%, respectively)

○ Oxybutynin transdermal delivery system (TDS) [Oxytrol]

■ Oxybutynin TDS versus tolterodine ER → one study showed similar efficacy, less dry mouth in TDS group but more application-site pruritus in TDS group (which is the most frequent reason for discontinuation of TDS)

○ Rectal oxybutynin is possible and has less adverse effects

○ Oxybutynin vaginal ring and *S*-oxybutynin are in the pipeline

○ Intravesical oxybutynin has anesthetic properties and is efficacious but may have less than optimal tolerability

■ In one study, dry mouth, flushing, and recurring infections still led to discontinuation in many patients

■ In children, cognitive impairment is still an issue

○ As a rule of thumb, pharmacologic treatments combined with behavioral treatments are better than either one by itself

■ Oxybutynin versus oxybutynin + bladder retraining → combination is more effective

• Tolterodine (Detrol [Pharmacia & Upjohn])—Level I evidence

○ Compound is a tertiary amine which is absorbed rapidly

○ Low lipid solubility → ↓ propensity to cross blood-brain barrier (BBB) (but is too small to see on electroencephalogram [EEG])

○ $t_{1/2}$ = 2–3 hours

○ Active metabolite is similar to parent compound in many respects (same half-life, same pharmacologic profile)

○ Mechanism of action: nonselective antimuscarinic (competitive antagonist) → in animal model, salivary M_3 > bladder M_3

○ Available in IR: 1–2-mg bid and LA (or ER): 4-mg qd

○ Detrol 2-mg bid costs $115.34 per month; Detrol LA 4-mg costs $100.04 per month

○ Tolterodine has high efficacy for treatment of OAB and UUI (incontinence episodes ↓ 46%)

○ Tolterodine ER was introduced to improve tolerability and compliance

■ Detrol LA uses OROS system (as described above) for ER formulations and to maintain non-fluctuating blood levels of the drug

■ Tolterodine IR versus tolterodine ER → similar efficacy but less dry mouth in ER group

○ Which is better, tolterodine or oxybutynin?

■ Tolterodine IR versus oxybutynin IR → similar efficacy but Tolterodine is better tolerated (especially less dry mouth)

■ Tolterodine IR versus oxybutynin XL → oxybutynin is more effective but dry mouth was similar between groups

■ Oxybutynin ER (XL) versus tolterodine ER (LA) → oxybutynin slightly more effective (72% vs. 67%, respectively), but Tolterodine has less dry mouth (29.7% vs. 22.3%, respectively)

• Trospium (Sanctura [Indevus Pharmaceuticals])—Level I evidence

○ A quaternary ammonium compound → does not cross BBB (but is too small to see on EEG)

○ Low serum protein binding

○ $t_{1/2}$ = 20 hours

○ Low biologic availability = 5%

○ Is minimally metabolized by liver enzymes (good for patients already on multiple medications)

○ May be more potent than oxybutynin and tolterodine

○ Mechanism of action: nonselective antimuscarinic which blocks detrusor smooth muscle receptors as well as receptors in the ganglia

○ Is available for oral intake: 20-mg bid; $89.33 per month

○ Is efficacious for the treatment of OAB and UUI

○ Trospium versus oxybutynin:

■ Trospium versus oxybutynin IR → one Level I study showed similar efficacy but Trospium had lower adverse effects and withdrawal from the study

○ Trospium versus tolterodine:

■ Trospium versus tolterodine IR → one Level I study showed Trospium may be more effective but adverse effects were similar

• Darifenacin (Enablex [Novartis Pharmaceuticals])—Level I evidence

○ Compound is a tertiary amine

○ Long half-life

○ Mechanism of action: an M_3-selective antimuscurinic (antagonist)

- Theoretically, darifenacin should cause less dry mouth (M_1), no effect on cognition (M_1), no effect on heart rate (M_2), no effect on visual accommodation (M_5)
- In reality, no effects on cognition and heart rate have been appreciated in Phase II trials
- In animal studies, more selective for bladder M_3 than salivary gland M_3

○ Is available for oral intake: 7.5-mg or 15-mg qd (is immediate release); costs $95.76 per month

○ Phase III data are only available in abstract form to the scientific community

○ Phase II data: darifenacin versus oxybutynin:

- Darifenacin IR versus oxybutynin IR → small ($n = 25$) study showed had similar efficacy but darifenacin had less dry mouth

• Solefenacin (Vesicare [GlaxoSmithKline])—Level I evidence

○ Compound YM-905
○ Long half-life
○ High potency
○ Mechanism of action: an M_3-selective antimuscurinic (antagonist)
○ Is available in 5-mg or 10-mg qd (is extended release); costs $101.16 per month
○ Although Solefenacin is approved by the FDA for OAB, only Phase II data are available to the scientific community in published form while Phase III data are available in presentation form

- Phase II: solefenacin versus tolterodine IR → solefenacin reduced frequency of voids more than tolterodine and had less dry mouth than tolterodine
- Phase III: solefenacin versus tolterodine IR → both are effective but solefenacin had slightly better efficacy; dry mouth was similar between the groups

• Propiverine—Level I evidence

○ Rapidly absorbed
○ High first pass
○ Several active metabolites (properties poorly characterized thus far; need to be studied)
○ Mechanism: (1) antimuscarinic and (2) Ca^{2+} channel antagonist
○ Propiverine is effective for the treatment of OAB and UUI (micturitions ↓, bladder capacity ↑, incontinence episodes ↓, subjective improvement)
○ Available in 15-mg tid
○ Propiverine versus oxybutynin:

- Propiverine IR versus oxybutynin IR → similar efficacy but propiverine had less dry mouth

• Atropine (aka D-, L-hyoscyamine, Levsin [Shartz Pharma, Inc], Cytospaz [PolyMedica Pharmaceuticals]—Level II evidence

○ It is the prototype of all antimuscarinic agents and is supported by good quality studies (Level II), therefore it will be briefly mentioned here
○ Derived from the plant *Atropa belladonna* (first proposed for use in OAB/UUI in 1936)
○ Today it is rarely used for OAB/UUI, though it continues to be used in the lab, because of systemic adverse effects

- Sublingual form may have fewer adverse effects

○ Intravesical form may be effective for OAB without adverse effects

• Propantheline (Pro-Banthine [Roberts Pharmaceutical Corp.]—Level II evidence

○ Quaternary ammonium compound
○ Nonselective antimuscarinic
○ Two small studies showed at high dosages (15-, 30-, or 60-mg qid), propantheline may be effective for OAB and UUI
○ However, a larger, randomized study of propantheline IR versus oxybutynin IR found no difference between propantheline and placebo

OTHER MEDICINES FOR OAB

• Baclofen

○ A gamma-aminobutyric acid receptor agonist (GABA agonist) in spinal cord

- Baclofen inhibits motor neurons and interneurons in the spinal cord

○ Effective (Level II) for neurogenic detrusor overactivity (e.g., MS)

• Botulinum toxin (aka Botox, Myoblock)

○ Protein produced by anaerobic bacteria during fermentation
○ Eight subtypes of botulinum toxin have been discovered
○ Botulinum toxin type A (Botox) and Botulinum toxin type B (Myoblock) are approved by FDA
○ Mechanism: blocks release of Ach by cholinergic nerves terminals at the neuromuscular junction → muscle paralysis and muscle atrophy
○ Has been used for disorder of muscle spasticity, wrinkles, migraine, chronic pain, bladder outlet obstruction (from sphincter spasticity), and detrusor sphincter dyssynergia (by injecting striated urethral sphincter muscles)
○ Intravesical injection: cystoscopy-assisted injections of Botox into multiple areas of bladder wall have been effective for patients with neurogenic detrusor overactivity (bladder capacity ↑, voiding pressure ↓)

○ Magnetic resonance imaging (MRI)-guided or EMG-guided injection is also possible
○ Minimal complications of UTI and transient urinary retention (and does not cross BBB)
○ Maximal effects 10–14 days after injection
○ Disadvantages: (1) costly and (2) requires repeat injections every 5.3 months (small duration of effect 3–9 months)
○ A comparison study is necessary: botox versus oxybutynin or tolterodine versus combination

PHARMACOLOGIC TREATMENT OF NOCTURIA AND NOCTURNAL ENURESIS (BED-WETTING)

- Desmopressin (aka DDAVP or 1-desamino-8-D-arginine vasopressin)—Level I evidence
  ○ A synthetic analog of vasopressin that has antidiuretic effects (antidiuretic hormone [ADH]) but lacks vasopressor effects
  ○ Nocturnal surge of ADH may be necessary to prevent high urine production during the night
  ○ Oral form, bioavailability is low (1%) while intranasal form has high bioavailability (2–10%)
  ○ Is available in intranasal preparation: 10–40-μg qhs (for children); oral form is also available but 10× greater dose (200–400 μg) is required because of lower bioavailability
  ○ Is highly effective for treatment of nocturnal enuresis in children
  ○ Also effective for treatment of adult nocturia (number and frequency of nocturnal voids ↓, nocturnal urine volume ↓, uninterrupted sleeping hours ↑)
  ○ Adverse effects
    ▪ Hyponatremia → rare but serious; send a Chem-7 periodically
    ▪ Dizziness, headache, mood changes, edema may occur uncommonly
- Imipramine → is used for nocturnal enuresis and nocturia (see below)
- Antimuscarinic drugs → although ER form of antimuscarinics is often used by clinicians for nocturnal enuresis and nocturia, there are few studies conducted to demonstrate the effectiveness of antimuscarinic agents for nocturia and nocturnal enuresis

PHARMACOLOGIC TREATMENT OF SUI

- Nonselective α-adrenergic receptor agonists—Levels II–III evidence (depends on drug type)
  ○ Phenylpropanolamine (aka norephdrine)
    ▪ It not only binds α_1-adrenergic and β-adrenergic receptors, but also enhances release of NE by presynaptic neurons

▪ Phenylpropanolamine can be effective in patients with mild SUI (MUCP ↑, leakage episodes ↓, improved symptoms of SUI), but is no longer marketed in United States because of recent adverse effects
▪ Estrogen may enhance the sensitivity and number of α-adrenergic receptors at proximal urethra and bladder neck: conflicting studies but, phenylpropanolamine ± estriol/estradiol versus phenylpropanolamine alone → combination seems more effective (subjective improvement in SUI symptoms, MUCP ↑, leakage episodes ↓)
▪ Adverse effects
  • Cardiac arrhythmias → phenylpropanolamine is no longer marketed in the United States for SUI; however, it is a component of all over-the-counter diet pills or appetite suppressants (e.g., Ornade and Dexatrim contain 75 mg of phenylpropanolamine in each tablet)
  • Hypertension
  • Insomnia
  • Headache
  • Tremor
  • Anxiety
  • Stroke (in women also taking appetite suppressants)
- Duloxetine—Level I evidence
  ○ Is currently FDA approved for treatment of major depression and diabetic neuropathic pain in the United States and is awaiting approval for SUI; already used in Europe for SUI
  ○ A selective reuptake inhibitor of both NE and 5-hydroxytryptamine (5-HT) (aka SNRI)
    ▪ Normal pathway: brainstem → Onuf's nucleus (sacral spinal cord) → to striated urethral sphincter via pudendal nerve
    ▪ Brainstem neurons release NE and 5-HT onto Onuf's nucleus to mediate their message
    ▪ NE and 5-HT are normally taken back (reuptake) by nerve terminal that released them → striated urethral sphincter contraction ↓
    ▪ By blocking reuptake of NE and 5-HT, Duloxetine increases the concentration of these neurotransmitters at Onuf's nucleus → striated urethral sphincter contraction ↑
  ○ Is effective at higher doses for treatment of SUI
    ▪ Incontinence frequency ↓ by ≥ 50% in most patients taking 40-mg bid dose
    ▪ Similar benefit even for severe SUI
    ▪ Improved Qol scores after only 4 weeks (one-third were "much better" or "very much better")
    ▪ Increases bladder capacity and time between voids (OAB/UUI has not been evaluated for Duloxetine)
    ▪ Twenty percent of patients with SUI cancelled surgery after 2 months on Duloxetine

- Adverse effects
  - Nausea
    - No. 1 adverse effect which leads to discontinuation in 15%
    - Incidence of nausea (23%) is similar to incidence of nausea in patients who take SSRIs for depression
    - It may help to take Duloxetine with food ± antiemetic
  - Fatigue, somnolence, dry mouth, constipation, insomnia also occurred

PHARMACOLOGIC TREATMENT OF MIXED INCONTINENCE

- Tricyclic antidepressants—Level II evidence
  - Imipramine (Tofranil); Doxepin (Sinequan)
  - Proposed mechanisms of action:
    - Minimal anticholinergic effect on detrusor (but does have systemic anticholinergic effects)
    - Block reuptake of 5-HT and NE
    - α-Adrenergic receptor activity (bladder neck and proximal urethra)
    - Direct antispasmodic effect on detrusor?
    - Local anesthetic effect on detrusor?
  - Available in 25–75-mg qhs-bid
  - May be effective for OAB/UUI and mixed incontinence; Level I evidence is needed
  - Has ADH properties → may benefit some patients with nocturnal enuresis
  - Adverse effects (must be used with caution, if at all, in elderly)
    - Orthostatic hypotension → may lead to falls and hip fracture
    - Sedation and drowsiness → may lead to falls
    - Confusion
    - Dysphoric reaction
    - Prolongation of QT_c interval → ventricular arrhythmias

PHARMACOLOGIC TREATMENT OF URINARY RETENTION AND VOIDING DYSFUNCTION

- Most of the agents used to treat urinary retention (α-adrenergic antagonists [prazosin, terazosin, tamsulosin, doxazosin, alfuzosin], muscarinic receptor agonists [bethanechol, carbachol], and cholinesterase inhibitors [distigmine] are based on case series) (Level IV)
- Bethanechol alone does not improve urinary retention
- One study shows that phenoxybenzamine (an α-adrenergic antagonist) *may* decrease postoperative urinary retention time

- Phenoxybenzamine + bethanechol → improvement in voiding
- Oral diazepam taken qhs starting the night before surgery up until spontaneous voiding occurs postoperatively has been shown to reduce time to spontaneous void by 2 days

MEDICATIONS THAT MAY BE USED IN THE FUTURE

- Selective α-adrenergic receptor agonists for SUI are in research and development
  - $α_{1A}$-Adrenergic receptor agonists (e.g., ABT-866) → found in bladder neck and proximal urethra
  - $α_{1B}$-Adrenergic and $α_{1C}$-adrenergic → found in blood vessels
- Intravaginal and intravesical oxybutynin for OAB/UUI are in the pipeline
- Vanilloids receptor agonists (Level III)
  - Capsaicin, an ingredient found in red hot chili peppers, binds vanilloids receptors on afferent neurons (sensory) innervating the detrusor and urethra
  - Capsaicin binds sensory neurons and initially excites them then overwhelms them → leading to blockade of sensory input from detrusor and urethra to the spinal cord
  - Intravesical capsaicin for patients with neurogenic detrusor overactivity has been effective
  - Resiniferatoxin, compound derived from a cactus-like plant *Euphorbia*, is 1000 times more potent than capsaicin. Currently in experimentation

BIBLIOGRAPHY

Altenbach RJ, Khilevich A, Meyer MD, et al. *N*-[3-(1H-imidazol-4-ylmethyl)-phenyl] ethanesulfonamie (ABT-866), a novel alpha(1)-adrenoceptor ligand with an enhanced in vitro and in vivo profile relative to phenylpropanolamine and midodrine. *J Med Chem.* 2002;45:4395–4397.

Dmochowski RR, Davila GW, Zinner NR, et al. Efficacy and safety of transdermal oxybutynin in patients with urge and mixed urinary incontinence. *J Urol.* 2002;168:580–586.

Klausner AP, Steers WD. Research frontiers in the treatment of urinary incontinence. In: Weber A, ed. *Clinical Obstetrics and Gynecology—Incontinence 2004.* Philadelphia, PA: Lippincott William & Wilkins; 2004:104–113.

Newgreen DT, Anderson CWP, Carter AJ, et al. Darifenacin: a novel bladder-selective agent for urge incontinence. *Neurourol Urodyn.* 1995;14:95.

Norton PA, Zinner NR, Yalcin I, et al. Duloxetine versus placebo in the treatment of stress urinary incontinence. *Am J Obstet Gynecol.* 2002;187:40–48.

Pharmaceutical Manufactores Association (www.phrma.org).

Phelan MW, Franks M, Somogyi GR, et al. Botulinum toxin urethral sphincter injection to restore bladder emptying in men and women with voiding dysfunction. *J Urol.* 2001;165:1107—1110.

Schurch B, Stohreer M, Dramer G, et al. Botulinum-A toxin urethral sphincter injection to restore bladder emptying in men and women with voiding dysfunction. *J Urol.* 2000;164:692–697.

Yamaguchi O, Shisda K, Tamura K, et al. Evaluation of mRNAs encoding muscarinic receptor subtypes in human detrusor muscle. *J Urol.* 1996;156:1208.

2004 Survey Medicines in Development for Women (a report by the pharmaceutical companies). Odyssey Pharmaceuticals, Inc. and Indevus Pharmaceuticals, Inc. OISA-57053 (3/05).

QUESTIONS

1. A 58-year-old gravida 3, para 3 presents to your office complaining of loss of urine when she strains. She denies loss of urine with key turning or from the sound of running water. She has no medical problems except for her bladder. During multichannel cystometry, you note several detrusor contractions which are stronger than 20 cm of water and which produce urgency. At her maximum cystometric capacity (300 mL), she demonstrates a detrusor contraction. She has loss of urine with valsalva at both 150 and 300 mL in the supine position. The next *best* step in management of this patient is _____.
   - (A) Periurethral bulking agent
   - (B) Tension-free vaginal tape sling (TVT)
   - (C) Imipramine
   - (D) Duloxetine
   - (E) Nifedipine

2. A 60-year-old patient with OAB was increased to oxybutynin extended release 10 mg per day. She presents to you because although the oxybutynin has worked well for her urge urinary incontinence, the dry mouth side effect of the drug is annoying. Upon review of her past medical history, you notice that she also has arthritis and cataracts. She says she drinks eight to nine glasses of fluids every day. She takes a 20-minute walk each night. She drinks one glass of red wine with dinner every night. A conservative management at this point would be to _____.

   - (A) Discontinue oxybutynin
   - (B) Decrease dose to 5 mg
   - (C) Increase fluid intake
   - (D) Suck on sour candy
   - (E) Stop drinking wine

QUESTIONS 3 AND 4

Match the statement below with the drug/agent which best describes it above. Each answer may be used once, more than once, or not at all.
   - (A) Botulinum toxin
   - (B) Oxybutynin
   - (C) Tolterodine
   - (D) Solefenacin
   - (E) Darifenacin
   - (F) Trospium
   - (G) Imipramine
   - (H) Phenylpropanolamine
   - (I) Desmopressin
   - (J) Baclofen
   - (K) Atropine
   - (L) Propantheline

3. Effective for OAB. It is hydrophilic and less likely to cross the blood-brain barrier

4. Is available in an intranasal form which is highly effective in children

ANSWERS

1. *(C).* In a patient with mixed urinary incontinence, it is best to treat conservatively first since a large percentage will have worsening or continuation of urgency and urge incontinence symptoms after surgery. The treatment of choice for mixed incontinence is imipramine because it has both anticholinergic as well as α-adrenergic properties. Duloxetine is effective for stress incontinence (off label) and it has not yet been approved by the FDA for this purpose. Nifedipine is a calcium channel blocker which theoretically blocks the influx of calcium required for detrusor contraction. It is not as effective for OAB as the anticholinergics mentioned in this chapter.

2. *(D).* Discontinuing oxybutynin is not a conservative step and the patient seems to be benefiting from it. Decreasing the dose may reduce its effectiveness as she was increased to 10 mg. She is already taking the recommended daily fluid intake (six to eight glasses per day). Stopping red wine each night

probably will not help her with her dry mouth and one glass of red wine is not harmful and may have beneficial effects for her heart. Sour candy will increase salivation in patients with dry mouth. This keeps the mouth moist. Be sure to encourage the patient to brush her teeth every night so that she does not develop dental cavities.

ANSWERS 3 AND 4

3. *(F)*, 4. *(I)*. Desmopressin is a synthetic analog of vasopressin that has antidiuretic effects (ADH) but lacks vasopressor effects. A nocturnal surge of ADH may be necessary to prevent high urine production during the night. It is available in two forms: oral form, bioavailability is low (1%) while intranasal form has high bioavailability (2–10%). The intranasal preparation (10–40 µg qhs) is highly effective for children. The oral form is also available but 10x greater dose (200–400 µg) is required because of lower bioavailability. Trospium is a quaternary ammonium compound (thus hydrophilic and lipophobic) and thus does not cross the blood brain barrier. This may prove to be useful in the elderly who may be on multiple medications and who are more susceptible to cognitive impairment with anticholinergics.

38 PREOPERATIVE ISSUES IN PELVIC SURGERY

Christopher M. Rooney,
Steven D. Kleeman, and Sam Siddighi

OVERVIEW

- Operative risk is a function of the patient's baseline medical status as well as any alteration in the patient's baseline medical condition as a result of the procedure.
- As the population ages, the gynecologist can expect the number of women seeking elective gynecologic procedures to increase dramatically over the next decade. As a corollary, the increase in the percentage of postmenopausal patients will lead to a subsequent increase in the conditions of urinary incontinence and pelvic organ prolapse for a multitude of reasons.
- A careful preoperative assessment results in fewer postoperative complications as well as a reduction in the number of elective procedures placed on delay secondary to medical conditions.

HISTORY

For urogynecologic history, see Chap. 5, Evaluation of Pelvic Organ Prolapse (POP) and Chap. 6, Evaluation of Urinary Incontinence in the Office and Indications for Referral to a Specialist.

- All preoperative evaluations should begin with a detailed history of the patient's complaint as well as their current medical status
  - Medical history
    - Cardiac
      - Hypertension (controlled, uncontrolled)
      - Stroke or transient ischemic attacks
      - Coronary artery disease
        - History of coronary artery bypass or stents
      - Valvular heart disease
        - Need for prophylactic antibiotics
      - Congestive heart failure
      - Myocardial infarction (MI)
      - Arrhythmia
        - Atrial fibrillation (anticoagulation status)
      - Peripheral vascular disease
    - Respiratory
      - Asthma
      - Chronic obstructive pulmonary disease (COPD)
      - Pneumonia
      - Emphysema
      - Pulmonary embolus (PE)
    - Endocrine
      - Diabetes mellitus
      - Adrenal insufficiency
        - Cushing's, Addison's disease
      - Hyperthyroidism, hypothyroidism
    - Renal
      - Cystic kidney disease
      - Congenital anomalies
        - Double ureter, renal agenesis
      - Acute or chronic renal insufficiency
    - Liver
      - Hepatitis
      - Cirrhosis
    - Gastrointestinal
      - Peptic ulcer disease
      - Gastroesophageal reflux
      - Esophageal varices
      - Small bowel obstruction
    - Hematology/oncology
      - Anemia
        - Iron deficiency, nutritional, chronic disease
      - Thrombophilia
        - Deep venous thrombosis (DVT)
        - PE
      - Malignancy
      - Coagulation disorder
        - Von Willebrand's disease, factor deficiency

- ○ Surgical history
  - ▪ Previous hysterectomy, vaginal repair, retropubic procedure or cesarean sections
    - • Important when considering route of repair
  - ▪ Previous bowel surgery (i.e., colectomy), laparotomy with lysis of adhesions or history of ruptured appendix
    - • May indicate severe pelvic scarring or adhesions
      - ○ May guide physician when considering route of repair
- ○ Medications
  - ▪ See Table 38-1
- ○ Social
  - ▪ Alcohol consumption
    - • Possible withdrawal symptoms postoperatively
  - ▪ Tobacco use
  - ▪ Compromised respiratory function postoperatively
- ○ Drug use

PHYSICAL EXAMINATION

- A thorough physical examination is essential in the evaluation of the preoperative patient
  - ○ General examination
    - ▪ Skin
      - • Ecchymoses, tenting of the skin
    - ▪ Auscultation of the heart
      - • Evidence of cardiomyopathy or murmurs
    - ▪ Auscultation of the lungs
      - • Wheezing or poor inspiratory effort
    - ▪ Abdominal examination
      - • Pain, hepatosplenomegaly, renal artery bruits
      - • Previous surgical scars
    - ▪ Extremities
      - • Evidence of peripheral edema or vascular insufficiency
    - ▪ Auscultation of the neck for carotid bruits
    - ▪ Mental status examination
  - ○ Urogynecologic examination (see Chaps. 5 and 6)

PREOPERATIVE TESTING

- See Table 38-2 for recommended preoperative testing.

THE GYNECOLOGIC PATIENT WITH CARDIAC DISEASE

- Cardiovascular disease is the leading cause of death among women

TABLE 38-1   **Perioperative Medication Management**

	DISCONTINUE PRIOR TO SURGERY	CONTINUE THE DAY OF SURGERY	DISCONTINUE THE DAY OF SURGERY
NSAIDs	48 h		
Aspirin	7 days		
Warfarin	4 days		
Plavix	7 days		
Ticlid	14 days		
Herbals	7 days		
Nonvitamin supplements	7 days		
MAOIs	21 days		
Antihypertensives		X	
Cardiac meds		X	
Antidepressants		X	
Birth control pills		X	
Thyroid meds		X	
Eye drops		X	
Antireflux meds		X	
Narcotics		X	
Antiseizure meds		X	
Asthma meds		X	
Steroids		X	
Statins		X	
Vitamins			X
Topical meds			X
Oral hypoglycemic meds			X
Insulin			X
Diuretics			X

SOURCE: Adapted from Yamada SD, Sweitzer B, McHale MT. Preoperative assessment for gynecologic surgery. *Contemp Ob Gyn.* 2005;50–57.

TABLE 38-2 Recommended Preoperative Testing

	CBC	PT/PTT	T&S	HCG	ELECTROLYTES	BUN/Cr	GLUCOSE	AST/ALK PHOS	ECG	CXR	UA
Alcohol abuse	X	X						X			
Anemia	X								X		
Bleeding disorder (personal or family history)	X	X						X			
Cardiovascular disease	X					X			X		
Cerebrovascular disease					X		X		X		
Diabetes					X	X	X		X		
Hepatitis		X			X	X	X	X	X		
Intracranial disease	X				X	X	X		X		
Liver disease	X	X				X	X	X	X		
Malignancy	X	X							X		
Malnutrition	X	X			X	X			X		
Obesity	X					X	X		X		
Peripheral vascular disease	X					X	X		X		
Poor exercise tolerance	X										
Possible pregnancy				X							
Pulmonary disease	X				X				X	X	
Renal disease	X					X			X	X	
Rheumatoid arthritis	X								X	X	
Sleep apnea	X								X	X	
Smoking history (>40 pack years)	X										
Suspected UTI						X			X		X
Systemic lupus erythematosus									X	X	
Radiation therapy	X										
Use of anticoagulants	X	X									
Use of digoxin					X	X			X		
Use of diuretics					X	X					
Use of steroids					X	X	X				
Anticipate significant blood loss	X		X								
Procedure with radiographic dye	X					X					

SOURCE: Adapted from Yamada SD, Sweitzer B, McHale MT. Preoperative assessment for gynecologic surgery. *Contemp Ob Gyn.* 2005;50–57. Template developed by the University of Chicago Department of Anesthesia Preoperative Medicine Clinic.

- One of the most common predictors for postoperative complications
- Preoperative risk stratification remains one of the premier tools available
  - Goldman's criteria (see Table 38-3)
    - Class I (0–5 points): 0.9% risk of serious cardiac event or death
    - Class II (6–12 points): 1.7% risk
    - Class III (13–35 points): 16.0% risk
    - Class IV (>26 points): 63.6% risk
  - Metabolic equivalent levels (METs)
    - Metabolic equivalent units are a useful way to express a patient's functional status
    - Risk of serious cardiac event or death is increased in patients unable to meet a 4-MET demand during normal daily activity (see Table 38-4)
  - Low-risk patients: recommend noninvasive testing (exercise stress test vs. pharmacological stress test with subsequent echocardiogram [ECG])
    - Advanced age
    - Abnormal ECG
    - Low functional capacity
    - History of stroke
    - Uncontrolled hypertension
  - Intermediate risk: recommend noninvasive testing (exercise stress test vs. pharmacological stress test with subsequent ECG) with subsequent coronary angiography based on findings
    - Mild angina pectoris
    - Prior MI

TABLE 38-3   Computation of the Cardiac Risk Index

CRITERIA	POINTS
History	
Age > 70 years	5
MI < 6 months	10
Physical examination	
S_3 gallop or jugular venous distention	11
Aortic valvular stenosis	3
ECG	
Rhythm other than sinus or PACs	7
>5 PVCs/min	7
General status	
PO_2 < 60 or PCO_2 > 50	3
K < 3.0 or HCO_3 < 20 meq/L	
BUN > 50 or Cr > 3.0 mg/dL	
Abnormal SGOT or chronic liver disease	
Bedridden	
Operation	
Intraperitoneal, intrathoracic, or aortic operation	3
Emergency operation	4
Total	Possible 53 points

SOURCE: Goldman L, Caldera DL, Nussbaum SR, et al. Multifactorial index of cardiac risk in noncardiac surgical procedures. *N Engl J Med.* 1977;297:26. Used with permission of the Massachusetts Medical Society.

TABLE 38-4   Estimated Energy Requirements for Various Activities

1 MET	Can you take care of yourself?
	Eat, dress, or use the toilet?
	Walk indoors around the house?
	Walk a block or two on level ground at 2–3 mph?
4 METs	Do light work around the house like dusting or washing dishes?
	Climb a flight of stairs or walk up a hill?
	Walk on level ground at 4 mph?
	Run a short distance?
	Do heavy work around the house like scrubbing floors or lifting or moving heavy furniture?
	Participate in moderate recreational activities like golf, bowling, dancing, doubles tennis, or throwing a baseball or football?
Greater than 10 METs	Participate in strenuous sports like swimming, singles tennis, football, basketball, or skiing?

SOURCE: Adapted from the Duke Activity Status Index and American Heart Association (AHA) Exercise Standards. Used with permission of Lippincott Williams & Wilkins.

- The optimal timing of surgical procedures following acute MI is 4–6 months
  - Compensated congestive heart failure
  - Diabetes mellitus
  - Renal insufficiency
  - High-risk patients: recommend delay of surgery until invasive testing (coronary angiography) is performed
    - Unstable coronary syndromes
    - Decompensated congestive heart failure
    - Significant arrhythmias
    - Severe valvular disease

GYNECOLOGIC PATIENT WITH PULMONARY DISEASE

- Pulmonary disease accounts for a significant percentage of postoperative morbidity.
- Routine testing is not indicated unless the patient has significant underlying respiratory disease, e.g., a history of smoking or is symptomatic.
  - Chest x-rays may be useful in screening prior to surgical intervention.
  - Pulmonary function testing is recommended in the face of significant underlying disease.
    - Forced expiratory volume at 1s (FEV_1) < 30% predicted have a significant risk of respiratory insufficiency.
      - Pulmonary function should be optimized or nonsurgical solutions sought.

GYNECOLOGIC PATIENT WITH RENAL DISEASE

- Preoperative testing in a patient with known renal insufficiency should include a baseline ECG, baseline creatinine, and baseline complete blood count.
- Metabolic abnormalities should be corrected prior to surgical intervention.
- Postoperative fluid and electrolyte status must be monitored judiciously.

GYNECOLOGIC PATIENT WITH ENDOCRINE DISORDERS

- Diabetes mellitus
  - Assessment of glycemic control
    - Fasting and postprandial blood glucose
    - Hemoglobin A1C
      - Indicator of long-term glycemic control
  - Assessment of serum electrolytes
  - Routine baseline ECG
  - Evaluation for diabetic complications
    - Retinopathy
    - Nephropathy
    - Peripheral vascular disease
    - Peripheral neuropathy
  - Management of pharmacological agents
    - Insulin
      - Long-acting agents (Ultralente) should be held preoperatively in favor of shorter-acting preparations (neutral protamine Hagedorn [NPH] or Lente).
    - Oral hypoglycemics should be held preoperatively.
  - Postoperative management
    - Frequent blood glucose testing (every 4–6 h).
    - Sliding scale insulin coverage with short-acting agents until the patient is tolerating oral feeds.
    - Oral hypoglycemic agents should be held until the patient is tolerating oral intake.
- Thyroid disorders
  - Routine testing is not necessary unless the patient is symptomatic or noncompliant with medications.
  - Surgery should be delayed until a euthyroid state is achieved.
- Adrenal insufficiency
  - Patients with a history of steroid use may require supplemental steroids secondary to the surgical stress response.
    - Patients taking 5 mg of prednisone daily for at least 2 weeks are considered at risk of adrenal insufficiency.
    - Supplemental doses are still considered controversial, but most authors would suggest hydrocortisone 100 mg IV daily for 2 days postoperatively as prophylaxis following a major surgical procedure.

TABLE 38-5   Child-Pugh Scoring System*

	POINTS		
	1	2	3
Encephalopathy	None	Stage I or II	Stage III or IV
Ascites	Absent	Slight (controlled with diuretics)	Moderate despite diuretic treatment
Bilirubin (mg/dL)	<2	2–3	>3
Albumin (g/L)	>3.5	2.8–3.5	<2.8
PT (prolonged seconds)	<4	4–6	>6
INR	<1.7	1.7–2.3	>2.3

ABBREVIATIONS: PT, prothrombin time; INR, International normalized ratio.
*Class A = 5–6 points; class B = 7–9 points; class C = 10–15 points.
SOURCE: Weintraub SL, Wang Y, Hunt JP, et al. *Principles of Preoperative and Operative Surgery. Sabiston Textbook of Surgery.* 17th ed. Philadelphia, PA: WB Saunders; 2004:221–239. Used with permission of Elsevier.

GYNECOLOGIC PATIENT WITH HEPATIC DISEASE

- Preoperative evaluation should include a liver function panel as well as serum electrolytes to assess nutritional status.
  - Elevated transaminases may be indicative of an acute or chronic process.
    - Alcohol-related hepatitis is suggested by an aspartate aminotransferase (AST)/alanine aminotransferase (ALT) ratio of greater than 2.
  - Elective surgery should be delayed in patients with elevated transaminases until normalization.
  - Patients with cirrhosis can have their risk stratified using the Child-Pugh classification (see Table 38-5)
    - Child's class A: 10% mortality rate
    - Child's class B: 31% mortality rate
    - Child's class C: 76% mortality rate

GYNECOLOGIC PATIENT WITH HEMATOLOGIC DISORDERS

- Anemia is the most common laboratory finding in the preoperative patient
  - Iron deficiency anemia
    - Most common form of anemia, affecting 20% of women
    - Diagnosis
      - Low serum iron
      - Low levels of serum ferritin
      - Elevated total iron binding capacity (TIBC)
  - Anemia of chronic disease
  - Macrocytic anemia
    - Folate deficiency
    - Vitamin B_{12} deficiency

- May present with neurological symptoms (posterior column)
  ◦ Preoperative transfusion should be reserved for patients with significant anemia (hemoglobin < 6 g/dL) or for patients with significant cardiac risk
    ▪ Recombinant human erythropoietin (Epoetin alpha)
      • Stimulates red blood cell production if used preoperatively
        ◦ Equivalent of one unit of blood is produced 1 week following administration
        ◦ Equivalent of five units of blood is produced 4 weeks following administration
      • May decrease the need for allogenic blood transfusion postoperatively
        ◦ Significantly more costly than allogenic transfusion
- Thrombophilias
  ◦ Inherited disorders
    ▪ Rarest and most thrombogenic
      • Homozygous for factor V Leiden mutation
      • Homozygous for prothrombin gene mutation (G20210A)
      • Autosomal dominant for antithrombin III deficiency (#1 in thrombogenicity)
    ▪ Most common and least thrombogenic
      • Homozygosity for Type 1 plasminogen activator inhibitor (PAI-1) gene
      • Methyltetrahydrofolate reductase gene (MTHFR)
        ◦ Common cause of hyperhomocysteinemia
    ▪ Relatively common and relatively thrombogenic
      • Heterozygous for factor V Leiden mutation (most common thrombophilia)
      • Heterozygous for prothrombin gene mutation (G20210A)
      • Autosomal-dominant deficiency of protein C
      • Autosomal-dominant deficiency of protein S
  ◦ Acquired disorders
    ▪ Antiphospholipid antibody syndrome
- Venothromboembolic (VTE) disorders
  ◦ Prophylaxis
    ▪ Patients should be assessed preoperatively as to their risk of developing VTE disorder and receive appropriate prophylaxis
      • Virchow's triad
        ◦ Hypercoagulable state
        ◦ Venous stasis
        ◦ Endothelial damage
      • Low risk
        ◦ Age ≤ 40 and surgery < 30 min
      • Moderate risk
        ◦ Age ≥ 40 and surgery of any duration
        ◦ No other risk factors

- High risk
  ◦ Age > 40 with risk factors
    ▪ Prior DVT/PE
    ▪ Infection
    ▪ Malignancy
    ▪ Varicose veins
    ▪ Estrogen therapy
    ▪ Prolonged surgery
    ▪ Obesity
- Low risk
  • No prophylaxis needed assuming early ambulation
- Moderate risk
  • Compression stockings
  • Pneumatic compression boots—must be one and plugged-in prior to induction of anesthesia!
  • Low dose unfractionated heparin (5000 units subcutaneously every 8 h postoperatively)
    ◦ Preoperative dose 2 h prior to surgery
    ◦ Postoperative dose beginning at 12 h
  • Low dose low molecular weight heparin daily
    ◦ Enoxaparin (Lovenox) 40 mg daily beginning at 12 h postoperatively
    ◦ Dalteparin (Fragmin) 2500 units daily beginning at 12 h postoperatively
- High risk
  • Pneumatic compression boots with
    ◦ Low dose unfractionated heparin (5000 units subcutaneously every 8 h postoperatively)
      ▪ Preoperative dose 2 h prior to surgery
      ▪ Postoperative dose beginning at 12 h
    ◦ Low dose low molecular weight heparin daily
      ▪ Enoxaparin (Lovenox) 40 mg daily beginning evening before surgery
      ▪ Dalteparin (Fragmin) 5000 units daily beginning evening before surgery
  • Consideration of inferior vena cava filter
◦ Chronic anticoagulation therapy
  ▪ Patients may require preoperative reversal of chronic anticoagulant agents.
    • Warfarin (Coumadin) should be discontinued 4 days prior to scheduled procedure.
      ◦ Patient may receive preoperative unfractionated heparin or low molecular weight heparin.
    • Ticlopidine (Ticlid) should be discontinued 14 days prior to surgery.
    • Clopidogrel (Plavix) should be discontinued 7 days prior to surgery.
    • Aspirin should be discontinued 7 days prior to surgery.
      ◦ Nonsteroidal anti-inflammatory drugs (NSAIDs) should be discontinued 48 h prior to scheduled procedures secondary to antiplatelet properties.

- Recommendations to reduce surgical wound infections
  - ○ Reschedule elective surgery if patient has a concomitant infection (e.g., urinary tract infection [UTI], pneumonia).
  - ○ Minimize smoking in smokers (wound healing).
  - ○ Lose weight before surgery for obese patients (technical difficulties and wound healing).
  - ○ Keeping blood sugar < 200 in diabetics may help.
  - ○ Antiseptic showering before surgery reduces skin bacterial count (especially chlorhexidine); standard soap just removes debris.
  - ○ Antibiotic prophylaxis
    - ▪ Most urogynecologic procedures are considered clean-contaminated.
  - ○ Genitourinary tract is entered
    - ▪ Patients undergoing clean-contaminated procedures should be treated with a single dose of a broad-spectrum antibiotic, such as cefazolin or metronidazole (other acceptable antibiotics are cefotetan, cefoxitin, ceftriaxone, ampicillin, mezlocillin, Zosyn, and tinidazole), 1–2 h prior to incision. The goal is to achieve maximal concentration of antibiotic before skin incision.
    - ▪ An additional dose of antibiotic should be given if the procedure time exceeds two half-lives of antibiotic (usually 3 h for pelvic surgery).
    - ▪ Additional dose should also be given if blood loss exceeds 1500 mL.
  - ○ Why are antibiotic concentrations reduced?
    - ▪ Do not maintain antibiotic prophylaxis more than a few hours after surgery is finished (no benefit and resistance ↑).
  - ○ Hair removal
    - ▪ Electrical clipper is better than razor blade shaving.
    - ▪ Shaving just before operation is better than at-home shaving > 24 h before surgery.
  - ○ Prepping the surgical field
    - ▪ Povidone-iodine solution
      - • Postulated that iodine results in the destruction of bacterial cellular structures
    - ▪ Chlorhexidine gluconate
      - • Causes destruction of bacterial cell membranes
    - ▪ Povidone-iodine solution versus chlorhexidine gluconate
      - • Chlorhexidine gluconate is more effective than povidone-iodine solution in reducing bacterial cell counts during vaginal surgery
  - ○ Surgeon should scrub up to elbows for 2 min (no benefit to scrubbing 10 min); surgeon should keep fingernails short and clean underneath.
  - ○ Washing hands traditionally (chlorhexidine or povidone-iodine solution) is equal to washing with new aqueous alcohol solution. Some experts recommend that if alcohol solution is used the first scrub of the day should be done traditionally.
  - ○ Prevent hypothermia during surgery with body warmer (vasoconstriction → reduced tissue perfusion of oxygen and immune cells → infection).
  - ○ Good surgical technique is important
    - ▪ Keep good hemostasis
    - ▪ Minimize tissue trauma
    - ▪ Eliminate dead space
    - ▪ When suturing, tie knots to approximate rather than strangulate tissue
    - ▪ Cut permanent suture short
- Mechanical bowel prep
  - ○ If injury to the large or small intestine is anticipated or part of the procedure (i.e., repair of rectovaginal fistula), a mechanical preparation should be used.
    - ▪ Ultimate goal is to lavage the lower intestinal tract and reduce bacterial colony counts.
  - ○ Examples
    - ▪ Golytely
      - • Polyethylene glycol, sodium sulfate, sodium bicarbonate, sodium chloride, potassium chloride
    - ▪ Nulytely
      - • Polyethylene glycol, sodium bicarbonate, sodium chloride, potassium chloride
    - ▪ Magnesium citrate
    - ▪ Fleet enemas (especially for posterior repair or sphincter repair)
- Miscellaneous considerations
  - ○ Fluids and electrolytes
    - ▪ Anatomy of body fluids
      - • Total body water = 60% of total body weight
        - ○ Total extracellular volume = 20%
          - ▪ Plasma = 5%
          - ▪ Interstitial fluid = 15%
        - ○ Total intracellular volume = 40%
    - ▪ Normal exchange
      - • Normal individual consumes 2000–2500 mL of water per day
      - • Daily water losses
        - ○ 250 mL in stool
        - ○ 800–1500 mL in urine
        - ○ 600 mL insensible loss
      - • Salt gain and losses
        - ○ Normal individual takes in 50–90 meq of sodium chloride per day
        - ○ Normal individual takes in 50–100 meq of potassium per day
    - ▪ Daily requirements
      - • Based on the "mythical" 70 kg male/female
        - ○ Sodium (Na$^+$)
          - ▪ 1–2 meq/kg/day

TABLE 38-6   Composition of Parenteral Fluids

SOLUTIONS	CATIONS				ANIONS	
	Na⁺	K⁺	Ca²⁺	MG²⁺	Cl⁻	HCO₃⁻
Extracellular fluid	142	4	5	3	103	27
Lactated Ringer's solution	130	4	3	—	109	28 (lactate)
0.9% NaCl	154	—	—	—	154	—
0.45% NaCl	77	—	—	—	77	—
D₅W	—	—	—	—	—	—
3% NaCl	513	—	—	—	513	—

- ◦ Potassium (K⁺)
  - ▪ 0.5–1.0 meq/kg/day
- ▪ Composition of parenteral fluids (see Table 38-6)
- ▪ The ideal maintenance fluid
  - • D51/2 NS with 20 meq KCl/L at 125 cc/h
  - • Based on the "mythical" 70 kg male/female
    - ◦ Requires 140 meq Na⁺ per day (2 meq/kg/day ×70 kg)
    - ◦ Requires 70 meq K⁺ per day (1 meq/kg/day ×70 kg)
  - • Lactated Ringer's solution
    - ◦ Lacks glucose
    - ◦ Poor supply of potassium
  - • 0.9% NaCl
    - ◦ Supplies 154 meq Na⁺/L
    - ◦ No K⁺
    - ◦ No glucose
  - • 0.45% NaCl
    - ◦ Supplies 77 meq Na⁺/L
    - ◦ No K⁺
    - ◦ No glucose
  - • D5 0.45% NaCl with 20 meq KCl/L
    - ◦ Supplies 77 meq Na⁺/L
    - ◦ Supplies 20 meq K⁺/L
    - ◦ Supplies glucose load
  - • Rate
    - ◦ Why 125 cc/h?
      - ▪ Based on an 8 h nursing shift
      - ▪ Average individual requires almost 3 L of fluid per day
      - ▪ With a rate of 125 cc/h, an individual will receive
        - • 250 cc in 2 h
        - • 500 cc in 4 h
        - • 1000 cc in 8 h
        - • 3000 cc in 24 h

BIBLIOGRAPHY

Basil JB. *Water, Electrolyte, and Acid-Base Metabolism. TeLinde's Operative Gynecology.* 9th ed. Philadelphia, PA: Lippincott Williams and Wilkins; 2003:163–194.

Culligan PJ, Kubik K, Murphy M, et al. A randomized trial that compared povidone iodine and chlorhexidine as antiseptics for vaginal hysterectomy. *Am J Obstet Gynecol.* 2005;192: 422–425.

DiRocco JD, Lucio AP, Weiss CA. The evidence-based way to prevent wound infections. Are some CDC recommendations more equal than others? *OBG Manage.* 2005;22–32.

Eagle KA, Berger PB, Antman EM, et al. ACC/AHA guideline update for perioperative cardiovascular evaluation for noncardiac surgery—executive summary. *Circulation.* 2002;105: 1257–1267.

Walters MD. *Evaluation of Urinary Incontinence: History, Physical Examination and Office Tests. Urogynecology and Reconstructive Pelvic Surgery.* 2nd ed. St. Louis, MO: Mosby; 1999:45–53.

Weintraub SL, Wang Y, Hunt JP, et al. *Principles of Preoperative and Operative Surgery. Sabiston Textbook of Surgery.* 17th ed. Philadelphia, PA: WB Saunders; 2004:221–239.

Yamada SD, Sweitzer B, McHale MT. Preoperative assessment for gynecologic surgery. *Contemp Ob Gyn.* 2005;50–57.

QUESTIONS

1. You have scheduled a 36-year-old patient for an elective synthetic midurethral sling for a diagnosis of urodynamic stress incontinence. The patient's past medical history is significant for a DVT in her left lower extremity 1 year ago following the delivery of her child that led to the development of a PE. The patient is on chronic anticoagulation with Warfarin, and is compliant with an International normalized ratio (INR) of 2.1. The best way to manage this patient's anticoagulation preoperatively is ____.

   (A) instruct the patient to continue taking the Warfarin until the day of surgery due to her risk of developing a VTE event

   (B) instruct the patient to discontinue taking the Warfarin 14 days prior to surgery secondary to the risk of excessive operative blood loss

   (C) instruct the patient to stop taking the Warfarin 4 days prior to surgery, and manage the patient preoperatively with heparin subcutaneously

(D) instruct the patient to discontinue taking the Warfarin 7 days prior to surgery secondary to the risk of excessive operative blood loss

2. A 58-year-old postmenopausal woman presents to your office for evaluation of urinary incontinence. The past medical history is significant for ulcerative colitis managed by a hemicolectomy. Past surgical history is also significant for exploratory laparotomies × 2 for bowel obstructions and pelvic adhesions. Examination reveals a well-supported, fixed uterus with no evidence of pelvic organ prolapse. Multichannel urodynamic testing reveals the sign of urodynamic stress incontinence with Valsalva leak point pressures of 75 and 82 cm H_2O at maximum cystometric capacity. Of the following, the most appropriate treatment of this patient's incontinence based on history is ____.

(A) abdominal-guided retropubic synthetic midurethral sling

(B) transobturator synthetic midurethral sling

(C) vaginal-guided retropubic synthetic midurethral sling

(D) periurethral bulking agent

(E) incontinence pessary

3. You have been asked to evaluate a 73-year-old postmenopausal woman with a complete procidentia. Physical examination confirms a complete procidentia with complete eversion of the anterior and posterior vaginal walls. Past medical history is significant for COPD and several episodes of pneumonia requiring hospitalization. The patient has a 40 pack year history of smoking. You have asked her to see a pulmonologist for surgical clearance. Pulmonary function tests are performed. Which of the following values for the FEV_1 would be considered a relative contraindication to elective surgery under general anesthesia?

(A) 90%

(B) 50%

(C) 30%

(D) 70%

(E) 80%

4. You receive a call from your patient's daughter 2 weeks before elective surgery for pelvic organ prolapse. She is concerned about her mother's blood sugar and would like to know how to manage her mother's medications before surgery. Your patient is 67 years old and has insulin-dependent diabetes mellitus. She has been successfully controlled with an Ultralente preparation twice daily. Her hemoglobin A1C is 5.0. The best advice to the daughter is ____.

(A) the patient will need to continue taking her Ultralente insulin until surgery, including her morning dose

(B) the patient will need to stop taking her Ultralente insulin 1 week before surgery

(C) the patient will need to stop taking her Ultralente insulin the night before surgery at which point she will be managed with a shorter-acting agent

(D) the patient will need to continue taking her Ultralente insulin and continue oral intake until surgery

5. You are preparing to perform a LeForte colpocleisis on an 89-year-old woman with a complete procidentia. Other than a history of rheumatoid arthritis, the patient is in good health. Her rheumatoid arthritis has been managed with weekly methotrexate and 5 mg prednisone daily for the last 20 years. The patient has never undergone surgery. The best management is ____.

(A) hydrocortisone 100 mg intravenously prior to surgery

(B) no steroids are necessary

(C) prednisone 5 mg orally prior to surgery

(C) hydrocortisone 100 mg intravenously prior to surgery and

(D) a single postoperative dose of hydrocortisone 100 mg intravenously

ANSWERS

1. *(C)*. The appropriate management of this patient's anticoagulation involves cessation of the Warfarin 4 days prior to surgery. Perioperatively, the patient's anticoagulation can be managed with heparin or enoxaparin subcutaneously. These subcutaneous regimens should be discontinued at least 12 h prior to the scheduled procedure. Continuing the Warfarin until day of surgery would place this patient at unnecessary risk of excessive intraoperative bleeding or postoperative hematoma formation. Complete cessation of Warfarin 7–14 days prior to surgery would place this patient at undue risk of developing a VTE disorder.

2. *(B)*. This patient has had multiple abdominal surgeries and has a documented history of pelvic adhesions. Examination reveals a fixed uterus which is suggestive of adhesive disease and pelvic scarring. The risk of bowel injury during a synthetic retropubic midurethral sling is approximately 1%. Although a rare complication, a history of pelvic adhesions and scarring could possibly increase the rate of bowel

injury. An incontinence pessary is not an appropriate management option in this patient. Periurethral bulking agents are a consideration, but would not be first-line therapy. A transobturator synthetic midurethral sling is the most appropriate treatment for this woman's stress incontinence. The transobturator approach avoids the space of Retzius, therefore, minimizing the possibility of bowel injury.

3. *(C)*. This patient has multiple pulmonary risk factors including COPD, extensive smoking history, as well as a history of pneumonia. Pulmonary function testing is an appropriate test in the preoperative work up of this patient. The FEV_1 is very telling of the patient's respiratory status. A $FEV_1 \leq 30\%$ of predicted is associated with a high risk of postoperative complications including respiratory insufficiency. A nonsurgical solution should be sought in a patient with a $FEV_1 \leq 30\%$. If surgery must be performed, consideration should be given to regional or local anesthesia.

4. *(C)*. The best way to manage the insulin-dependent diabetic perioperatively is to discontinue long-acting preparations, like Ultralente and insulin lispro, in favor of shorter-acting agents, like Humulin and NovoLog. The patient will still need to be NPO (nothing by mouth) prior to surgery, so choice D is an inappropriate answer. In addition, cessation of all insulin regimens 1 week prior to surgery places the patient at risk of unnecessary hyperglycemic complications.

5. *(D)*. This patient is on chronic steroids for rheumatoid arthritis. Patients who are on prednisone 5 mg daily for at least 2 weeks prior to surgery are at risk of complications related to adrenal insufficiency. Prevention of adrenal insufficiency in the adrenal suppressed patient remains a controversial topic. However, most authors would agree that a preoperative and postoperative dose of intravenous hydrocortisone is an appropriate management scheme.

39 POTPOURRI: VULVOVAGINAL AND URETHRAL DISORDERS

Sam Siddighi and Tricia Lin Kam

- The American Board of Obstetricians and Gynecologists (ABOG) and the American Board of Urologists (ABU) list as one of their requirements for the graduating fellow in Female Pelvic Medicine and Reconstructive Surgery (FPMRS) → a knowledge of "nonurologic, irritative conditions."
- In this chapter, we will briefly review selected nonurologic, irritative conditions of the vulva, vagina, and urethra.
- With the advent of Viagra and media influence to stay sexually active into the later years, sexually transmitted diseases (STDs), especially herpes, have risen rapidly in the elderly population.
- Additionally, herpes, chlamydia, and gonorrhea can involve the urinary tract as they may cause symptoms of urinary tract infection (UTI).
- Atrophic vaginitis is also a source of irritative problems in postmenopausal patients.
- Conditions such as urethral prolapse and urethral caruncle have not been discussed anywhere else in this book, so these will be discussed in this chapter first.
- There are also a few common differential diagnoses for a condition that a urogynecologist may encounter, urethral diverticula. These will also be reviewed in this chapter.
- Urethral diverticula, interstitial cystitis, chronic pelvic pain, and vulvar vestibulitis will not be discussed in this chapter as they are reviewed elsewhere in this book.

URETHRAL ABNORMALITIES

- **Urethral prolapse**
  - Appears as a beefy protruding mass (color: pink/red, violet, black) in the area of the external urethral orifice
  - May be large (up to 5 cm in width)
  - It is a circumferential eversion of urethral mucosa (mucosa turned inside-out) on the very distal portion of the urethra with the external urethral orifice within the prolapse center (doughnut hole)
  - Asymptomatic or symptoms of bleeding, frequency, urgency
  - Risk factors: children 8–12, postmenopausal women, estrogen deficiency, increased intraabdominal pressure, Blacks > Whites
  - Differential diagnosis: caruncle, condyloma, polyp, cyst, cancer, ureterocele
  - Treatment: estrogen cream and sometimes cryotherapy or local excision
- **Urethral caruncle**
  - Small red mass arising from the posterior lip of external urethral meatus
  - Asymptomatic or symptoms of bleeding, frequency, urgency, or pain
  - Symptoms also if it becomes superinfected
  - Risk factors: age 40–80, postmenopausal, multiparity
  - Differential diagnosis: urethral prolapse, pseudo-caruncle (diffuse small growths as a result of previous

trichomonas or candida infection which can arise from any portion of the ureteral meatus; pseudocaruncles are more difficult to treat than caruncles)
  - Evaluation: culture for candida, gonorrhea, chlamydia, and wet mount to rule out trichomonas infection
  - Treatment only if symptomatic: estrogen cream, excision, or laser if needed (careful to avoid urethral stenosis if attempting surgery)

IMPORTANT MASSES IN THE DIFFERENTIAL DIAGNOSIS OF URETHRAL DIVERTICULA

- Skene's duct cyst
  - Mass arising from anterior lateral vaginal introitus
  - Skene's glands are the largest of paraurethral glands surrounding distal urethral; they usually secrete into the urethra
  - Excretory urography (voiding cystourethrogram [VCUG]) or urethrocystoscopy may be needed to distinguish between Skene's duct cyst and urethral diverticulum
  - Treatment: (1) in children → partial excision with marsupialization of cyst wall and (2) in adults → total excision
- Bartholin's gland cyst
  - Pair of glands at 5 and 7 o'clock just inside the entrance of the vagina which produce nonessential secretions
  - Normally, the glands are not palpable
  - Bartholin's duct opens into area between hymen and labia minora
  - Mechanism of cyst formation: inflammation or trauma → duct obstruction → fluid secretion against closed duct causes cyst formation
  - Culture of Bartholin's cyst is usually sterile (80%) or polymicrobial (20%)
  - Most Bartholin's gland cysts are asymptomatic but some patients may have dyspareunia and pain with walking
  - Secondary infection can occur and can rapidly (within 2–3 days) turn into a Bartholin's abscess
  - Treatment: (1) asymptomatic + age < 40 years → observation, (2) symptomatic cyst or abscess → marsupialization or Word catheter insertion × 4–6 weeks, (3) antibiotics are not needed unless there is cellulitis, (4) recurrent abscess or enlargement + age > 40 years → excision of Bartholin's gland (bloody operation!)
- Epithelial inclusion cyst (aka vaginal wall inclusion cyst)
  - No. 1 most common cystic mass found in the vagina
  - Usually is distal one-third of the vagina
  - Usually arising from lateral or posterior vaginal walls
  - Risk factor: birth trauma or previous surgery
  - Contain greasy, yellow substance
  - Most are asymptomatic or can cause pain or dyspareunia
  - Treatment: surgical excision
- Fibroma
  - No. 1 most common benign solid tumor of the vulva
  - Anterior vulva in the midline (can be near the clitoris)
  - Mobile and firm in consistency
  - Usually asymptomatic but can cause discomfort
  - Treatment: observation or wide excision (if symptomatic)

NONUROLOGIC CONDITIONS OF THE VULVA

- Many nonurologic conditions of the vulva can be categorized into the following six groups: red, white, and dark lesions, ulcers, small tumors, and large tumors. A discussion of all of these lesions and tumors is beyond the scope of this book. Specific lesions or tumors have been chosen from Table 39-1 for review based on relevance and prevalence.
- Candida, lichen sclerosus, squamous hyperplasia, herpes simplex, and condyloma acuminata will be reviewed. Bartholin's gland cyst and fibromas have already been discussed earlier in this chapter.
- Nonurologic irritative conditions also include vaginal and urethral infections such as trichomonas, chlamydia, and gonorrhea. Similarly, atrophic vaginitis is a source of irritative problems in postmenopausal patients. These conditions will be discussed as well.

CANDIDA

- Symptoms and signs: discharge, pruritus, dysuria, vulvar erythema, and irritation
- This is usually found in premenopausal urogynecology patients
- Risk factors: recent antibiotic use, diabetes mellitus (DM), sexual intercourse, nonbreathable and tight clothing, suppressed immunity
- Speculum examination reveals cottage-cheese appearing vaginal discharge but this may not be true for other *Candida* species *Torulopsis glabrata* and *Candida tropicalis* (normal vaginal pH < 4.5)
- Microscopic examination with KOH may reveal hyphae or pseudohypha ± budding yeast, but it absence does not rule out candida vaginitis

TABLE 39-1 Lesions, Ulcers, Tumors

RED LESIONS	WHITE LESIONS	DARK LESIONS	ULCERS	SMALL TUMORS	LARGE TUMORS
Candida	Lichen sclerosus	Nevi	Herpes simplex	Condyloma acuminata	Bartholin's gland Cyst/abscess
Seborrheic dermatitis	Squamous cell hyperplasia	Seborrheic keratosis	Syphilis	Molluscum contagiosum	Edema
Carcinoma in situ	Carcinoma in situ	Lentigo	Granuloma inguinale	Herpes vesicles	Hematoma
Invasive cancer	Vitiligo	Melanoma	Lymphogranuloma venereum	Carcinoma in situ	Invasive squamous carcinoma
Paget's disease	Albinism	Lice	Chancroid	Epidermal cyst	Varicosities
Tinea cruris	Leukoderma	Histiocytoma	Crohn's disease	Hemangioma	Hernia
Tinea versicolor	Intertrigo		Hidradenitis suppurativa	Mucous cyst	Fibroma
Erythrasma	Radiation reaction		Behcet's disease	Hidradenoma	Lipoma
Folliculitis			Tuberculosis	Accessory breast tissue	Giant condyloma
Psoriasis			Invasive cancer	Endometriosis	Verrucous carcinoma
Contact dermatitis			Ecthyma	Mesonephric duct cyst	
Scabies				Neurofibroma	
Lichen planus				Acrochordon	
Lichen simplex chronicus				Fox-Fordyce disease	
				Syringoma	

- One may also culture on Nickerson's media or Sabouraud's if there is uncertainty of diagnosis or recurrence
- Usually caused by *Candida albicans,* but *T. glabrata* is also a possible cause
- For recurrent vaginitis → rule out human immunodeficiency virus (HIV) and DM; consider fungal culture for resistant species, *C. tropicalis* or *T. glabrata;* is she taking chronic antibiotic therapy? Treat the male partner?
- Treatment
  ○ Topical and suppository antifungals for 3–7 days (available over the counter); PO fluconazole 150 mg × 1 day
  ○ Treatment of recurrent infections: 1% gentian violet painting, boric acid suppositories, oral nystatin, and oral ketoconazole (200-mg bid × 5 days then 100 mg × 6 months; use caution in patients with liver disorders and liver function tests (LFTs) may need to be monitored for prolonged treatment regimens)

TRICHOMONAS

- Symptoms and signs: profuse, malodorous, green-gray, frothy vaginal discharge, pruritus, irritation, dysuria, and possible punctuate "strawberry" hemorrhages on cervix
- This may be found in premenopausal urogynecology patients because the unestrogenized vagina is relatively resistant to trichomonas

- Microscopic examination of wet mount will reveal many white blood cells (WBCs) and motile flagellated protozoan, usually found at the edge of the smear and pH > 5
- If pap smear reveals trichomonas, then a wet mount should be done
- Caused by *Trichomonas vaginalis*
- It is an STD so the partner needs to be treated also
- Treatment: metronidazole 500-mg bid × 7 days or 250-mg tid × 7 days, or single dose of 2 g (be careful to avoid alcohol with metronidazole as it may cause a disulfiram or Antabuse reaction since it inhibits metabolism of ethanol); an alternative treatment is topical clotrimazole but this is less effective

GENITAL HERPES SIMPLEX

- Symptoms and signs: asymptomatic, *symptoms of UTI and urinary retention,* prodrome of itching, tingling, burning, or hypesthesia followed by cluster of clear, fluid-filled vesicles on an erythematous base on different areas of the vulva
- Caused by a double-stranded DNA virus
- ≈90% of herpes simplex virus (HSV)-2 have a predilection (aka tropism) for genital cells versus 10% for HSV-1
- HSV is not curable; therapy only decreases viral shedding, duration of symptoms, and time to healing; HSV can become latent with periodic recurrences
- It can be autoinoculated (self-infection of the eye from contaminated fingers)

- HSV is an STD but can also be spread by close contact with unintact epithelium (e.g., wrestling)
- Twenty-five percent of the infection is acquired from an asymptomatic carrier who is shedding virus; nevertheless, the highest viral shedding occurs when symptoms and lesions are present
- Diagnosis: viral culture has >90% sensitivity if obtained from vesicles (rather than crusted lesion)
- Treatment: acyclovir 200-mg PO 5× per day × 5–10 days (longer duration of treatment for primary herpes (i.e., 10 days); topical is not as effective as oral; famciclovir 250-mg tid or valacyclovir 1000-mg bid × 5–10 days (this dosing has better compliance)
- Local measures are also helpful (sitz baths and topical anesthetic)
- Suppression prophylaxis: if ≥6 recurrences per year then give acyclovir 400-mg bid or 200-mg tid for up to 5 years; it can decrease recurrences by 75%; famciclovir 250-mg bid or 500-mg qd; valacyclovir 500-mg bid or 1000-mg qd

CONDYLOMA ACUMINATA

- Symptoms and sings: usually asymptomatic, can cause irritation depending on size and location; wart-like projections from skin of vulva, vagina, perineum, and anus
- Caused by double-stranded DNA virus, human papilloma virus (HPV) subtypes 6 and 11 (other subtypes, for example, 16 and 18 are cause of cervical cancer)
- About 50–75% of sexually active women will have HPV some time in their lifetime
- It is an STD
- Diagnosis by visual inspection also by koilocytes on pap smear
- Treatment
  - Patient-applied → imiquimod cream 3× per week at bedtime and wash off in the morning (may be used for 4 months)
  - Provider-applied → podophyllin resin (10–25%), bi or trichloroacetic acid (80%), cryotherapy, laser, surgical excision

CHLAMYDIA

- Symptoms and signs: asymptomatic, vaginal discharge, symptoms of UTI
- This condition may be found in premenopausal urogynecology patients
- Microscopic examination reveals many WBCs but no clue cells, pseudohypha, or flagellated organisms
- Diagnosis:

  - Chlamydia culture of endocervix using cotton swabs on plastic shaft (rather than wooden shafts which can be toxic to *Chlamydia*). This method is preferred for test of cure.
  - New technique: sampling of first-stream urine for DNA probe testing using ligase chain reaction to amplify specific DNA sequences is 95% sensitive.
    - Why first-stream urine? Because the external urethral meatus contains both cervical and vaginal secretions.
    - This method is more comfortable and obviates pelvic examination.
    - Sample can also be tested for *Neisseria gonorrhea* also.
  - Other tests: fluorescent antibody and Chlamydiazyme testing are also available.
- Chlamydia is an STD so the partner needs to be treated as well
- Treatment: doxycycline 100-mg bid × 7 days; single dose azithromycin 1 g; erythromycin base 500-mg qid × 7 days for pregnant patients; ofloxacin 300-mg bid × 7 days (also used for gonorrhea)

GONORRHEA

- Symptoms: asymptomatic, mucopurulent cervical discharge, symptoms of UTI, symptoms of pelvic inflammatory disease (PID) (lower abdomen pain, fever, anorexia), pharyngitis, arthritis (in disseminated gonococcal infection)
- Diagnosis: culture on Thayer-Martin, Gram stain (gram-negative diplococci in polymorpho nucleocyte (PMNs)), DNA probe testing using ligase chain reaction (as described above)
- Treatment: cefixime 400-mg or ceftriaxone 125-mg intramuscular (IM) but because there is a high rate of coinfection, antibiotics to treat chlamydia should also be given; alternative regimen: ofloxacin, spectinomycin 2 g in penicillin-allergic patient

ATROPHIC VAGINITIS

- Symptoms and signs: dyspareunia, burning, vaginal discharge, odor, and irritation
- Decrease in estrogen → thinning of epithelium and structures in the vulva atrophy → glycogen ↓ and pH ↑ (>4.5)
- Risk factors: postmenopausal and breast-feeding women
- Diagnosis: pale, white appearance + wet mount of vagina → predominantly parabasal cells (absence of superficial cells)
- Treatment: local vaginal estrogen cream every night for 2 weeks then 1–2 per week with apparent change seen in 3–4 months

LICHEN SCLEROSUS VERSUS SQUAMOUS CELL HYPERPLASIA

- Symptoms and signs: pruritus, burning, irritation, chronic soreness, white or pale, smooth surface of vulva and anus which may encircle these structures to form a "figure 8" ; in advanced cases can lead to phimosis of clitoris and narrowing of the introitus
- Lichen sclerosus is in a category which was formerly called vulvar dystrophy; this includes squamous cell hyperplasia (aka hyperplastic dystrophy)
  - Squamous hyperplasia can be found in 30% of women with lichen sclerosus
  - On inspection, the skin appears thickened and raised (like elephant skin)
  - Biopsy reveals: (1) acellular, thickened surface area of keratin and (2) widening and lengthening of rete pegs (acanthosis)
- Lichen sclerosus is a slowly developing, chronic vulvar, or perineal lesion of unknown etiology (it may occur on other part of body like neck, shoulder, axilla also)
- Koebner phenomenon → trauma or friction to normal skin areas induces lichen sclerosus
- Risk factor: most patients >50 years (also can occur in children, especially after trauma induced by sexual molestation)
- These patients have ≤ 5% risk of intraepithelial carcinoma
- Diagnosis by biopsy: (1) epithelial thinning, (2) flattening of rete pegs, (3) cytoplasmic vacuolization of basal layers, and (4) monocytes in the subdermal layer
- Treatment of lichen sclerosus → areas with ulcer, thickening, fissuring must be biopsied before treatment; topical clobetasol ointment 0.05% or halobetasol propionate 0.05% is applied qd or bid × 2–3 weeks then tapered (topical testosterone cream is not effective); surgery may be necessary if vaginal introitus is stenosed or clitoris is buried

BIBLIOGRAPHY

Bracco GL, Carli P, Sonni L, et al. Clinical and histological effects of topical treatments of vulval lichen sclerosus: a critical evaluation. *J Reprod Med.* 1993;38:37–40.

Emans SJH, Laufer MR, Goldstein DP. *Pediatric and Adolescent Gynecology.* 4th ed. Philadelphia, PA: Lippincott-Raven; 1998: 75–90.

Friedrich EG. *Vulvar Diseases.* Philadelphia, PA: W.B. Saunders; 1976:98–214.

Kaufman RH, et al. *Benign Diseases of the Vulva and Vagina.* 4th ed. St. Louis, MO: Mosby; 1994.

Meffert JJ, Davis BM, Grimwood RE. Lichen sclerosus. *J Am Acad Dermatol.* 1995;32:393–416.

Mroczkowski TF, Martin DH. Genital ulcer disease. *Dermatol Clin.* 1994;12:753–764.

Schmid GP. Approach to the patient with genital ulcer disease. *Med Clin North Am.* 1990;74:1559–1572.

Sobel JD. Vaginitis. *N Engl J Med.* 1997;337:1896–1903.

QUESTIONS

QUESTIONS 1–5

Match the word or statement below with the word that best describes it above. Each answer may be used once, more than once, or not at all.

   (A) Lichen sclerosus
   (B) Squamous cell hyperplasia
   (C) Atrophic vaginitis
   (D) Gonorrhea
   (E) Chlamydia
   (F) Condyloma acuminata
   (G) Herpes simplex II
   (H) Trichomonas
   (I) Candida
   (J) Urethral prolapse
   (K) Pseudocaruncle
   (L) Skene's duct cyst
   (M) Inclusion cyst
   (N) Fibroma
   (O) Lipoma

1. In addition to being acquired sexually, _____ may be acquired through certain contact sports
2. Nontender, cystic mass on the distal posterior vaginal wall
3. Diffuse small growths which result because of previous trichomonas or candida infection. The growths may arise from any portion of the external urethral meatus
4. An 8-year-old African American child with a 2 cm mass at the urethral orifice
5. Formerly called hyperplastic dystrophy

ANSWERS

ANSWERS 1–5

   1. *(G),* 2. *(M),* 3. *(K),* 4. *(J),* 5. *(B).* Herpes simplex can be acquired through contact sports

such as wrestling. A vaginal inclusion cyst is usually located posterior or lateral on the distal vaginal wall. Pseudocaruncles are diffuse small growths which may result because of previous candida or trichomonas infections. They are differentiated from urethral caruncles in that they are usually multiple and may be located anywhere on the urethral meatus whereas caruncles are usually on the posterior lip of the external urethral meatus. Urethral prolapse may occur in children ages 8–12. It is a circumferential eversion of urethral mucosa (mucosa turned inside-out) on the distal portion of the urethra. Squamous cell hyperplasia was formerly known as hyperplastic dystrophy.

40 ABSORPTIVE PRODUCTS (PANTILINERS, PADS, AND UNDERGARMENTS) AND BLADDER CATHETERS AND URETERAL STENTS IN USE TODAY

Sam Siddighi

ABSORPTIVE PRODUCTS

- Today, absorptive products are a billion dollar industry in the United States.
- There are several reasons why they are so popular
  - Women's embarrassment, discomfort, or fear of seeing a physician.
  - Denial of the problem.
  - False belief that incontinence is part of the normal aging process.
  - False belief that there is no adequate treatment for incontinence.
  - Women may prefer not to be treated for incontinence by a physician.
  - Women may prefer to use absorptive products as they may be less hassle.
  - Caregiver may prefer these products for impaired, terminally ill patients, or those with skin wounds.
  - Rarely, women's medical condition may not be adequately corrected or correctable with medical and/or surgical therapies.

- Even celebrities like June Allyson (who is on the American Urogynecologic Society [AUGS] Web site) has made it her mission to raise awareness of pelvic floor disorders which afflict so many people.
- These products are usually found in department stores (e.g., Wal-Mart, K-Mart, and Target), drug stores, and supermarkets.
- They are usually found in proximity to female absorptive products (e.g., tampons and pads) but are distinctly separated from them.
- These products are not only used in nursing homes, but also in residential and retirement homes.
- Even young, active women may use these products for stress urinary incontinence (SUI) with certain activities (e.g., tennis and jogging).
- Absorptive products are not meant to replace toileting or proper diagnosis and treatment by medical personnel.
- The following are some of the commonly encountered absorptive products on the market today:
  - Assurance (Tyco Healthcare, [Kings of Prussia, PA]) → 1800-262-0042
  - Depend (Kimberly-Clark, [Neenah, WI]) → 1800-558-6423; www.depend.com
  - Options (Tyco Healthcare, [Kings of Prussia, PA]) → 1800-262-0042
  - Serenity (SCA Personal Care, [Bowling Green, KY]) → www.serenity.com
  - Poise (Kimberly-Clark, [Neenah, WI]) → 1800-262-0042
- The above products have various sizes, shapes, absorbencies, flexibilities, softness, discreetness, breathabilities, odor prevention ability, and ease of use.
- Pantiliners, pads, and underwear (regular, fitted, belted shields, underwear inserts for additional protection) are available.
- The ideal product should be
  - Inexpensive
  - Accessible (found in ordinary stores and markets)
  - Absorbent (max = 10–12 oz → heavy = 8 oz → med-light = 4–5 oz → liner = 2 oz)
  - Prevents odor (deodorants are also available)
  - Protects skin
  - Stay quiet with activity (i.e., discreet)
  - Inconspicuous
  - Soft and comfortable
  - Fit snugly
  - Easy to use
  - Breathable
- Reusable products may be preferred by certain women based on their living situation, financial ability, or convenience to caregivers.
- It is important to keep the skin clean, dry, and moisturized prior to contact with these products.

- Certain products may contain powder (e.g., sodium polyacrylate) within the absorptive layer which absorbs urine and then turns into gel. This is not felt as wetness by the active women.
- For patients with severe (large amounts of) incontinence, a rubber or vinyl underpants may be added over the absorptive product in order to contain urine.
- Chlorophyllin copper tablets taken orally may help decrease odor from urine.
- More information about incontinence products and education can be found at the Web sites mentioned earlier and at the following:
  ○ National Association of Continence: 1800 bladder
  ○ www.incontinent.com
  ○ June Allyson Foundation

BLADDER CATHETERS

- Basic concepts in urinary drainage
  ○ If a catheter is not needed then do not use it as it is associated with morbidity and problems (e.g., infection, irritation to epithelium, discomfort, and restricts ambulation).
  ○ Intermittent self-catheterization (ISC) is preferable to an indwelling catheter (either transurethral or suprapubic).
  ○ Prevention of overdistention by catheterization is very important because even one episode of bladder stretching beyond intrinsic elastic limit (>1000 mL) may (1) delay return to normal voiding, (2) place excessive tension on suture lines, (3) cause decreased blood flow and promote anoxia of the urothelium, which may increase stasis and predispose to urinary tract infections (UTIs).
  ○ Bladder training by clamping the catheter without voiding attempts does not decrease time to normal voiding and may inadvertently lead to an overdistention episode.
  ○ The narrower the diameter of the catheter (high Fr #), the higher the chance for blood clots and particulate occlusion.
  ○ Always leave the drainage bag below the level of the bladder to promote pressure gradient, which allows urine drainage into the bag rather than away from it.
  ○ Prophylactic antibiotics are not helpful for preventing bacterial colonization of the catheter-bag system
    - Bacterial colonization rate = 5–10%/day.
    - ≈50% with indwelling catheter will develop UTI by day 5.
    - ≈50% of patients who perform clean, ISC have asymptomatic bacteriuria.
    - 100% of patients with long-term indwelling catheters have asymptomatic bacteriuria → and 100% will develop UTI with time if catheter is left

in place → 10% of elderly with indwelling catheters will develop sepsis → disseminated intravascular coagulation (DIC), acute respiratory distress syndrome (ARDS), shock.
  ○ Prophylactic antibiotics are not useful for prevention of cystitis in someone with an indwelling catheter.
  ○ The most important concept for prevention of UTI with indwelling catheters is their removal as soon as possible rather than antibiotic prophylaxis because with time all patients with indwelling catheters will develop a UTI.
  ○ To lower the risk of infection in someone with an indwelling catheter one must
    - Ensure sterile technique during insertion of catheter.
    - Provide continuous attention and care to patients with indwelling catheters.
    - If an indwelling transurethral catheter is needed longer than anticipated, change the catheter with a new one every few days or preferably, insert a suprapubic catheter.
  ○ Asymptomatic bacteriuria which develops with catheterization does not need antibiotic treatment.
  ○ Although urine cultures may show colonization, antibiotic treatment is not necessary unless the patient has symptoms of UTI, systemic infection, or sepsis.
  ○ Some indications for catheterization are
    - Urinary retention
    - Voiding dysfunction
    - Areflexic bladder
    - Postoperative state (especially after surgery for SUI or pelvic organ prolapse [POP])
- Catheter anatomy and common names
  ○ Two ends + body: urine influx end or tip (e.g., in bladder), urine efflux end (e.g., connected to collection bag), and long, hollow cylindrical tube (*body*).
  ○ Efflux end may have access port(s) with its/their respective channels within the catheter for (1) saline-inflatable balloon, (2) infusion of medications or liquids. Note: For ureteral catheters → both influx and efflux end may be bent into "J" configuration to prevent catheter migration.
  ○ Influx end may be bent (J-shape), coiled, or contain inflatable balloon to prevent migration and movement of catheter.
  ○ Ureter catheters are made of silicone, polyurethane, C-Flex (Concept Polymer Technology), Silitek (Medical Engineering Corp.).
  ○ Bladder catheters are made of latex, rubber, or silicone.
  ○ Catheters are also coated to minimize irritation to epithelium, lower chance of it serving as a nidus for stone formation, improve patient comfort.

- ◦ Catheters come in different diameter (8–16 Fr), lengths, shapes, number of access ports, and size of balloon.
- ◦ The following are the names of available catheters: Foley, Malecot, Rutner (Cook), Pigtail (Cook), Stamey (Cook), Dover-Ingram (Kendall Healthcare), Argyle-Ingra (Sherwood Med Co.), Trocha Fix (Rusch Inc.), Robertson (Mentor), Bonanno (Becton-Dickinson), Self-Cath (Cook or Mentor), Sof-Flex, Cystocath (Dow Corning Corp.), Suprapubic introducer/Foley/collection bag set (C.R. Bard).
- Bladder catheters: transurethral
  - ◦ Self-retaining catheters were introduced by Malecot in 1892.
  - ◦ Frederic Foley introduced balloon catheter in 1927.
  - ◦ Ideal size for women's urethra → diameter = 14–16 Fr; balloon = 5–10 cc.
    - ▪ Larger diameter → are more uncomfortable, irritate epithelium, prevent drainage of periurethral glands, interfere with blood flow in area.
    - ▪ Smaller diameter → may leak around catheter.
  - ◦ Disadvantages: (1) infection risk, (2) discomfort (periurethral and balloon irritation of trigone) → discomfort may be reduced by securing catheter to patient so it does not scrape or pull.
  - ◦ Use of antiseptic solutions and antimicrobial irrigations does not prevent bacteriuria after insertion of indwelling transurethral catheter.
  - ◦ O'Leary and O'Leary mini-catheter (1970) → pediatric feeding tube into bladder then taped or sewn to skin. Advantages: (1) less irritation to urethra, (2) voiding trials by clamping tube and allowing patient to avoid around catheter.
- Bladder catheters: suprapubic
  - ◦ First published account in Switzerland (1556) by Pierre Franco.
  - ◦ Three placement techniques have been described using the catheters mentioned earlier (e.g., Pigtail, Cystocath, Malecot, and Foley):
    1. Open insertion: Bladder is filled → catheter with introducer pushed through skin, muscle, fascia, bladder dome → catheter pushed over needle guide while guide is removed → catheter balloon is inflated (if present) → catheter is sutured on skin.
    2. Blind closed insertion: Patient in Trendelenburg → fill bladder transurethrally to > 400 mL → clean skin → trocar inserted < 3 cm above pubic bone and aimed toward pubic symphysis (30°) and inserted into bladder → catheter is put into bladder through trocar and trocar is removed → catheter is sutured to skin.
       - ▪ This technique is quick but is blind; therefore, keep the following technical hints in mind: (1) patient should be in Trendelenburg position to reduce any possibility of bowel trapped between bladder and abdominal wall, (2) be cautious in patients with previous incisions in the suprapubic area, (3) bladder should be full, (4) trocar should be inserted at an angle, (5) avoid too deep insertion of trocar as you may hit bladder base structures (e.g., ureteral orifices).
    3. Closed insertion using transurethral sound: A hollow male urethral sound, uterine packing forceps, Robertson catheter introducer, or Lowsley retractor is placed into bladder transurethrally and directed toward suprapubic skin → the retractor or sound is tented up and a skin puncture is made, then sound is perforated through bladder wall and out through the skin → the catheter is sutured to sound and the sound is pulled back out through the urethra (which also pulls the catheter) → the sound and catheter are disconnected → the catheter is pulled back into the bladder by pulling on its suprapubic end → catheter balloon may now be inflated (if present).
  - ◦ Indications
    - ▪ After significant dissection around bladder and urethra
    - ▪ When prolonged urinary retention is anticipated
    - ▪ Patients who need ISC but cannot perform it because of obesity or disability
    - ▪ Some experts will use suprapubic catheter after any anti-incontinence surgery
  - ◦ Advantages of suprapubic over transurethral catheters
    - ▪ Lower bacteriuria (lower rate of UTI)
    - ▪ No urethritis
    - ▪ Possible shorter time to normal voiding after surgery
    - ▪ Easier for nursing staff
    - ▪ Patients are more comfortable
    - ▪ Assists in ambulation
    - ▪ Repeated urethral catheterization is unnecessary for voiding trials
  - ◦ Disadvantages of suprapubic catheters (in general)
    - ▪ Infection
    - ▪ Leakage of urine around catheter
    - ▪ Invasive insertion may be associated with morbidities (bowel injury, skin cellulites, hematuria, and blood clots in bladder)
    - ▪ Catheter breaking, clotting, kinking, or calcification (less likely with larger catheters, e.g., 14–16 Fr and urine acidification with vitamin C 9000 mg/day)
    - ▪ Decreases bladder capacity with long-term use
    - ▪ May leave a small scar after removal
- Bladder catheters: ISC
  - ◦ Concept of clean, ISC was introduced in 1972 by Lapides.

- Use short plastic or rubber catheters and containers to measure urine.
- Should be done every 3–4 h but this may be more or less frequent depending on the postvoid residual (PVR) volume. For example, if PVR is high, then ISC should be done more frequently.
- Catheter does not need to be sterile and infection is usually not a problem. Therefore, prophylactic antibiotics are not needed.
  - Study of children with neurogenic bladders who required clean ISC → 10 years follow-up: 90% free of kidney infection
  - Essentially no difference in infection rate of clean versus sterile catheterization
- Risk versus benefit argument: Advantages of preventing overdistention of bladder (and its associated morbidities) outweighs the risks of infection.
- Requirements for ISC
  - Education and training of patient is necessary.
    - Catheterize often enough to keep volume of bladder < 300 mL.
    - Teach anatomy: Urethral orifice is below the clitoris and above the vaginal orifice.
    - Spread labia with index and fourth finger and use middle finger to locate urethra then insert lubricated catheter into urethral to drain.
    - Always try to void first → then do ISC → if PVR is ever < 20% of total voided then ISC can be stopped.
  - The patient has to be motivated to do this on her own.
    - The idea of ISC has to be introduced to the patient in a nonnegative fashion:
      - "By using ISC you will avoid undergoing surgery."
      - "By using ISC you will be able to maintain normal kidney function."
      - "By using ISC you can walk around freely without having a cumbersome tube and bag."
    - Manual dexterity and mental capacity is important requirement for ISC (i.e., demented, quadriplegic patients are not candidates for ISC).

URETERAL CATHETERS (AKA STENTS)

- Concept first introduced in Germany in 1875 by Gustav Simon.
- First manufactured catheter by Joaquin Albarran, a Cuban surgeon living in France in 1900.
- Characteristics of an ideal stent
  - Prevents migration (upward or downward)
  - Easy to insert (retrograde, antegrade, or open techniques)
  - Easily removed/changed by endoscopy
  - Radiopaque
  - Biologically inert
  - Chemically stable
  - Resists encrustation
  - High flow
  - Reasonable price
- Stents come in different diameters, lengths, shapes, textures, and compositions. The following is a list of some of the available stents:
  - Double-J
  - Double-Pigtail
  - Towers Peripheral
  - Multi-Flo Silitek ESWL (extracorporeal shockwave lithotripsy)
  - Silitek
  - Tract Finder
  - Ureteral stone displacement or ureteral anesthetic lubricant stent
  - Single-J Urinary Diversion
  - Fistula Set
  - Injection
- Double-J stent is the most popular of all stents. It was introduced by Finney in 1978. It is cystoscopically inserted silicone ureteral catheter with J configuration at both ends which prevent it from migrating.
- Double-Pigtail stents are also widely used. These are usually made of polyurethane (Sof-Flex) or C-Flex. The Pigtails are better than the Js for prevention of migration.
- Indications for insertion
  - After inadvertent injury to ureter(s) during surgery
  - Purposeful surgery of the ureters (ureteroureterostomy, ureteroneocystostomy, ureteroenteral diversions, ureterotomy, ureterolysis, ureteroscopy)
  - To bypass fistulas (ureterovaginal, ureteroenteral, ureterocutaneous)
  - Ureteral obstruction (kidney or ureteral stones, stricture tumor)
  - Prior to ESWL
  - To help normalize blood urea nitrogen/creatinine (BUN/Cr, e.g., patient with cervical cancer and bilateral ureteral encroachment)
  - To prevent stenosis, fibrosis, kinking, obstruction of ureter(s)
  - To aid in identification of the ureters during surgery
- Determination of stent length is important.
  - Appropriate length is determined by intravenous urogram or retrograde pyelogram. Measure directly from the film then reduce by 10% (correction for magnification) + 1 cm.
  - The length of double-J or double-Pigtail is only along the straight segment.

○ The double-Pigtail coils have diameter = 1.4 cm which adds 6 cm (× 2) when straightened out.
- Complications
  ○ Patient discomfort: pain (flank, suprapubic), dysuria, frequency, hematuria; these are all reversible within 3–4 days after removal of stent.
  ○ Long-term complications
    ▪ Migration (double-Pigtails prevent migration; polyurethane composition has better memory and thus least migration potential)
    ▪ Vesicoureteral reflux (VUR) (may cause increased intrarenal pressure; VUR is reason why side holes are drilled into the stents → refluxing urine can escape from side holes)
    ▪ Infection (frank infection happens in the setting of stent obstruction; although colonization can occur [i.e., positive urine culture], antibiotics are not necessary unless patient is symptomatic; some experts recommend low-dose prophylaxis)
    ▪ Encrustation and stone formation
    ▪ Ureteral erosion and necrosis (to reduce this, change stent more frequently)
    ▪ Ureteral fistula

EXTERNAL OR VAGINAL URINARY DRAINAGE DEVICES

- Several types of drainage devices exist: (1) rubber funnel connected to drainage tube, (2) diaphragm with drainage pore connected to drainage tube, (3) form-fitting cup connected to drainage tube.
- These are held in place by a strap, adhesive, suction, or form-fitting mechanism.
- May be placed in the vagina and connected to drainage tube-bag system.
- Disadvantage: urinary leakage around device.
- Advantage: avoids invasive catheter with its associated morbidities.
- Indication: genitourinary fistula (± continuous incontinence).

BIBLIOGRAPHY

Hodgkinson CP, Hodari AA. Trocar suprapubic cystostomy for postoperative bladder drainage in the female. *Am J Obstet Gynecol.* 1966;96:773–781.
Hurt GW. Urinary drainage devices. In: Hurt GW, ed. *The Masters' Techniques in Urogynecologic Surgery.* 2nd ed. Philadelphia, PA: Lippincott William & Wilkins; 2000;187–191.
Lapides J, Diokno AC, Silber SJ, et al. Clean intermittent self-catheterization in the treatment of urinary tract disease. *J Urol.* 1972;107:458–461.
O'Leary JL, O'Leary JA. The mini-catheter: a reliable indwelling catheter substitute. *Obstet Gynecol.* 1970;36:141–143.
Saltzman B. Ureteral stents: indications, variations, and complications. *Urol Clin North Am.* 1988;15:481–491.
Summitt RL Jr., Stovall TG, Bran DF. Prospective comparison of indwelling bladder catheter drainage versus no catheter drainage after vaginal hysterectomy. *Am J Obstet Gynecol.* 1994;170:1815–1818.
www.augs.org
www.depend.com
www.incontinent.com

QUESTIONS

1. In patient who used absorptive products, _____ may help reduce odor associated with urine.
   (A) vinyl underpants
   (B) double pantiliners
   (C) chlorophyllin copper tablets
   (D) vinegar
2. When calculating the length of stent, the following is a TRUE statement:
   (A) Add 12 cm to the total to account for a double-Pigtail stents.
   (B) Subtract 10% from the length measured on film.
   (C) Add 10% minus 1 cm from the length measured on film.
   (D) Add 6 cm to the total for a double-J stent.
3. A patient who has a stent in place MUST _____.
   (A) receive prophylactic antibiotics
   (B) acidify her urine with acidic foods
   (C) have stent changed frequently if long-term
   (D) receive an anticholinergic to prevent detrusor irritability

ANSWERS

1. *(C).* Chlorophyllin copper tablets taken orally may help decrease odor from urine. Vinyl underpants are useful for large volume leaks.
2. *(A).* Since the diameter of the Pigtail is 1.4 cm this adds 6 cm to each end of the stent. Thus, the total

length of the stent will be +12 cm. The measurement obtained from the film should be decreased by 10% since film is magnified and 1 cm should be added to the new value obtained.

3. *(C)*. Prophylactic antibiotics are not a "MUST." In fact, many surgeons do not recommend these. Anticholinergic medication may be used when indicated. Acidification of urine is not absolutely necessary. It is important to change the stent often in someone who will require it for long periods of time in order to prevent encrustation, erosion, necrosis, or stone formation.

41 URINARY DIVERSION (RESERVOIRS, POUCHES, AND CONDUITS)

Dobie Giles

INTRODUCTION

- The native bladder is a low-pressure, high-volume storage device that holds urine until a socially acceptable time to void. A bladder damaged or diseased secondary to gynecologic or bladder cancer, may need to be replaced. The bladder may also become nonfunctional due to disease processes such as detrusor overactivity, interstitial cystitis, or neurogenic bladder.
- The first urinary diversion was reported over 150 years ago and since then modifications and new surgical techniques have been developed. The most appropriate technique depends not only on the disease process but also on the desired outcome. The patient's expectations, mobility, and life expectancy are important in the selection. For example, if the patient is frail and immobile, then a continent diversion that relies on regular catheterization may not be the best choice. Regardless of type of technique, the main goal of a urinary diversion is to preserve renal function.
- There are three different ways to surgically divert the lower urinary system. The ureters are either implanted into intact bowel (ureterosigmoidostomy), into partially excluded segments of bowel (conduits and reservoirs), or into a new bladder (orthotopic). Some techniques allow the patient to remain continent (ureterosigmoidostomy, reservoirs, and orthotopics) and void when

they desire, while other techniques require the patient to wear an external collection device (conduits).

INCONTINENT DIVERSIONS

ILEAL CONDUIT

- Creates a continuation of the ureters to the abdominal wall and relies on an external device to collect urine.
- First described by Seiffert in 1935. Modified by Bricker in the 1950s, this is one of the technically easier diversions and is associated with the fewest complications.
- A 10–15 cm segment of ileum located approximately 10–15 cm proximal to the ileocecal valve is isolated. The remaining ileum is reapproximated with an ileoileostomy and the mesentery defect closed. The proximal end of the ileal conduit is closed. The ureters are mobilized and the left ureter is brought under the mesentery to the right side. The ureters are attached to the proximal end of the ileal conduit. The distal end of the conduit is brought to the anterior abdominal wall to form a stoma in the right lower quadrant.
- There are several techniques to attach the ureters to the conduit: end of ureters to side of bowel (Bricker), tunneling the ureters into the bowel so that the tunnel acts as an anti-incontinence mechanism (Leadbetter), and joining the ureters to each other and then attaching the anastomosis to the end of the bowel (Wallace).
- If the ileum is damaged from previous surgery or radiation, or too technically difficult to reach, then the jejunum can be used as a substitute. A 10–15 cm segment is taken at approximately 20 cm distal to the ligament of Treitz. The jejunal defect is repaired and the conduit is made in a similar fashion to an ileal conduit. The stoma is usually formed in the left upper quadrant.
- Hyperkalemic, hyponatremic metabolic acidosis is the possible complication.

LARGE BOWEL CONDUIT

- The large bowel offers another alternative if ileum is unavailable. The colon is very mobile and has a lower risk of stomal stenosis than the ileum, but absorbs more chloride and excretes more bicarbonate. Therefore, there is an increased risk of hyperchloremic acidosis. The different segments of the bowel each have their own advantage.
- The ileocecal segment is ideal when ureters are very short. The stoma is in the right upper quadrant.
- Transverse colon is an alternative for people with extensive pelvic radiation because this area is usually

out of the radiation field. The stoma is developed in the upper quadrant.

- Sigmoid colon is an alternative for people who undergo an exenteration. The sigmoid is mobilized utilizing the line of Toldt. The conduit is placed lateral to the bowel and the stoma is in the left lower quadrant.

CONTRAINDICATIONS AND COMPLICATIONS OF CONDUITS

- Contraindications to conduit diversion include severe renal disease secondary to long-term obstruction, severe hepatic disease, and bowel dysfunction.
- The length of the conduit is important because if too short, the blood supply is compromised, and if too long, the absorption of electrolytes increases resulting in more metabolic disorders.
- The most common complication is a metabolic acidosis which can be managed with oral alkalotic agents.
- Prior to surgery, an enterostomal nurse can help facilitate optimal ostomy site.
- Stents are removed after a week and imaging studies obtained to verify the integrity of the anastomosis.

CONTINENT DIVERSIONS (RECTAL DIVERSIONS)

URETEROSIGMOIDOSTOMY

- First described by Simon in 1852 and involved implanting the ureters into the intact sigmoid
- Continence achieved by utilizing the anal sphincter mechanism
- Electrolyte abnormalities, such as hyperchloremic acidosis, due to reabsorption
- Renal function eventually becomes compromised due to increased pressure transmitted from the intact bowel back through the ureters

MAINZ POUCH II

- Modification of the classic ureterosigmoidostomy.
- A reservoir is created from the rectosigmoid. The rectosigmoid is opened 10 cm distal and 10 cm proximal to the rectosigmoid junction. The medial margins are brought together in a side-to-side anastomosis. The ureters are mobilized and the left ureter is brought under the mesentery to the right side. The ureters are implanted into the posterior side of the rectosigmoid;

the pouch is closed and attached to the sacrum. Stents placed into the ureters are brought out of the anus.
- The pouch achieves a low pressure system because detubularization of the rectosigmoid disorganizes the peristaltic movements that lead to complications typically seen by the classical ureterosigmoidostomy.
- Hyperchloremic acidosis is seen but can be treated with oral alkalizing agents.

CUTANEOUS DIVERSIONS (URINARY RESERVOIRS)

- An internal storage system developed from an isolated segment of bowel that relies on regular intermittent catheterization.
- The Indiana pouch, Mainz, Miami, and Studer are also internal continent reservoirs which are simpler to construct than the Kock pouch but they also hold a smaller volume of urine.

KOCK ILEAL RESERVOIR

- Developed in 1982 to better mimic the natural urinary system. Results in a continent low pressure, high capacity reservoir with a built-in antireflux mechanism.
- A 78 cm segment of the small bowel is isolated 15 cm from the cecum. The segment is marked into four smaller subsegments measuring 17, 22, 22, and 17 cm. The remaining ileum is reapproximated with an ileoileostomy and the mesentery defect closed. The ureters are mobilized. The isolated ileal segment is brought together so that it resembles a T with the middle composed of the two 22 cm segments. The 22 cm segments are opened and sutured to each other to form the reservoir. The proximal 17 cm segment is formed into an afferent continence nipple complex containing an intussuscepted valve to which the ureters are attached. The distal 17 cm segment becomes the efferent continence nipple complex with another intussuscepted valve and is brought to the abdominal wall.
- The efferent nipple complex is catheterized through the abdominal wall every 2 hours initially, and eventually every 6 hours.
- Higher rate of nocturnal incontinence when compared to other diversions.

RIGHT COLON RESERVOIR

- Developed from a segment of bowel that consists of the distal 12 cm of the ileum through to the right half of the transverse colon.

- The colon segment is detubularized and used as the reservoir in which the ureters are implanted.
- The ileal segment is made into an anti-incontinence mechanism and brought to the abdominal wall.
- The reservoir must be catheterized every 4–6 hours.

MITROFANOFF RESERVOIR

- The ascending colon is isolated and detubularized except for the lower 5 cm of the cecum. The ureters are implanted into the reservoir.
- The appendix is embedded into the submucosa of the cecum to act as an anti-incontinence mechanism and then attached to abdominal wall.

BLADDER RECONSTRUCTION (ORTHOTOPIC BLADDERS)

- The goal is to create a storage system that has a sufficient storage capacity, a pressure < 40 cm H_2O, and connects to the native urethra to maintain voluntary volition.
- There is no standardization of techniques and various segments of the bowel have been used. The ileum is the most common.

KOCK ILEAL BLADDER

- Functions as an acontractile substitute for the detrusor.
- A 60 cm segment of ileum is isolated approximately 20–25 cm from cecum. The remaining ileum is reapproximated with an ileoileostomy and the mesentery defect closed. Two 22 cm segments are brought together and closed to form the reservoir. The ureters are implanted into the remaining 14 cm ileal segment. An opening is made in the lowest aspect of the newly formed reservoir and this is attached to the native urethra.
- Nocturnal incontinence is seen.

COLONIC NEOBLADDER (MAINZ POUCH)

- Utilizes 15 cm of cecum, 10–15 cm of ascending colon, and two loops of ileum (each 10—15 cm). The antimesentery sides of the ileal loops are opened and a side-to-side anastomosis is performed.
- The cecum is detubularized and attached to the ileal segments. The ureters are implanted and an opening is made in the inferior portion of cecum and attached to the urethra. The pouch is closed.
- Advantageous because of its larger storage size.

COMPLICATIONS OF ORTHOTOPIC BLADDERS

- May rupture if not adequately catheterized.
- Long recovery time and may take months for the neobladder to mature.
- Comparatively, the conduit is easier, quicker, and the patient goes home sooner.

BIBLIOGRAPHY

Carr LK, Webster GD. Conduit urinary diversion. In: *Glen's Urologic Surgery*. 5th ed. Philadelphia, PA: Lippincott Williams & Wilkins; 1998.

Danuser H, Studer UE. Orthotopic urinary diversion using an ileal low-pressure reservoir with an afferent tubular segment. In: *Glen's Urologic Surgery*. 5th ed. Philadelphia, PA: Lippincott Williams & Wilkins; 1998.

Fisch M, Hohenfellner R. Ureterosigmoidostomy and the Mainz Pouch II. In: *Glen's Urologic Surgery*. 5th ed. Philadelphia, PA: Lippincott Williams & Wilkins; 1998.

Freeman JA. Kock Pouch continent urinary diversion. In: *Glen's Urologic Surgery*. 5th ed. Philadelphia, PA: Lippincott Williams & Wilkins; 1998.

Hautmann RE. Orthotopic bladder substitution in the male and female. In: Oesterling JE, Richie J, eds. *Urologic Oncology*; 1997:341–354.

Hautmann RE. Urinary diversion: ileal conduit to neobladder. *J Urol.* 2003;169:834–842.

Hovey RM, Carroll PR. Noncontinent urinary diversion. In: Oesterling JE, Richie J, eds. *Urologic Oncology*; 1997: 323–335.

Lockhart JL. Right colon reservoir. In: *Glen's Urologic Surgery*. 5th ed. Philadelphia, PA: Lippincott Williams & Wilkins; 1998.

McDougal WS. Continent urinary diversion. In: Oesterling JE, Richie J, eds. *Urologic Oncology*; 1997:336–340.

Morrow CP, Curtin JP. Surgery on the urinary tract. In: *Gynecologic Cancer Surgery*. Philadelphia, PA: Churchill Livingstone; 1996:269–322.

Riedmiller H, Gerharz EW. Mitrofanoff continent urinary diversion. In: *Glen's Urologic Surgery*. 5th ed. Philadelphia, PA: Lippincott Williams & Wilkins; 1998.

Schultz-Lampel D, Thuroff JW. Orthotopic urinary diversion using a colonic segment. In: *Glen's Urologic Surgery*. 5th ed. Philadelphia, PA: Lippincott Williams & Wilkins; 1998.

Stein JP, Skinner DG. Orthotopic bladder replacement in women. In: *Glen's Urologic Surgery*. 5th ed. Philadelphia, PA: Lippincott Williams & Wilkins; 1998.

Yong SM, Dublin N, et al. Urinary diversion and bladder reconstruction/replacement using intestinal segments for intractable incontinence or following cystectomy. Cochrane Incontinence Group. July 15, 2004.

QUESTIONS

QUESTIONS 1–3

Match the sentence below with the best word that describes it above.

   (A) Kock ileal bladder
   (B) Kock ileal reservoir
   (C) Mainz pouch
   (D) Ileal conduit

1. Ureters attached to low-pressure rectosigmoid system; urination occurs through the anus
2. Ureters are attached to a ileal reservoir which is in turn attached to the native urethra; urination occurs through the urethra
3. Ureters are attached to an ileal reservoir which is in turn connected to the skin and has a pseudo-sphincter at its end; urination occurs by catheterization through the skin
4. The main difference between a pouch and a conduit is
   (A) Segment of intestine utilized
   (B) Risk of renal tubular acidosis
   (C) Ability to maintain continence
   (D) Site of ureteral attachment
5. One of the complications of urinary diversion systems is _____.
   (A) Normal anion gap, metabolic acidosis
   (B) Wide anion gap, metabolic acidosis
   (C) Metabolic alkalosis
   (D) Hypokalemic, hypochloremic acidosis

ANSWERS

1. *(C)*.
2. *(A)*.
3. *(B)*.
4. *(C)*. Urinary diversions are categorized as follows: the ureters are either implanted into intact bowel (ureterosigmoidostomy), into partially excluded segments of bowel (conduits and reservoirs), or into a new bladder (orthotopic). Some techniques allow the patient to remain continent (ureterosigmoidostomy,

reservoirs, and orthotopics) and void when they desire, while other techniques require the patient to wear an external collection device (conduits).
5. *(A)*. Urinary diversion systems result in metabolic acidosis (hyperkalemic, hyperchloremic) with a normal anion gap. Wide anion gap metabolic acidosis is caused by renal failure or toxins (diabetic ketoacids, alcohol, methanol, salicylates). Causes of metabolic alkalosis include vomiting, nasogastric (NG) tube, diuretics, milk-alkali syndrome, and Bartter syndrome.

42 UROLITHIASIS
Jessica Bracken

EPIDEMIOLOGY

• Several factors influence the production of urinary tract stones and therefore, the prevalence of renal stones varies per population studied. It is estimated that stone disease will affect between 2 and 15% of the population during their lifetime. Temperature, diet, sunlight exposure, age, sex, and metabolic abnormalities are some of the factors found to influence stone formation. The rate of urolithiasis increases with age with the highest incidence in the fourth to sixth decades. It has four times greater predilection for men than women. It is more common in Caucasians and Asians than in African Americans or Native Americans.

ETIOLOGY

• Eighty percent of stones are calcium stones (including calcium oxalate and calcium phosphate). Stones can also be comprised of uric acid, struvite (magnesium ammonium phosphate), and cystine, xanthine, triamterene, silicate, and indinavir. It is possible for a patient to have more than one stone type concomitantly.
• Stones form from soluble ionic materials that become supersaturated in the urine and begin a process of nucleation in which the free ions associate into microscopic particles. This crystallization is pH and ion concentration dependent. Crystallization can occur with or without interaction with renal tubule cells. There are inhibitors (i.e., citrate, magnesium, and pyrophosphate) to crystal growth and aggregation. When these are deficient, stone formation can occur.

SYMPTOMS

- *Pain* may radiate from the costovertebral angle to the groin, labia, or scrotum. The amount of pain experienced is not reliable to stone size. Small stones may cause intense pain, while large stones may cause a dull pain.
- *Renal colic* is a sudden onset of severe flank pain in which no position is comfortable for the patient. The stone is causing obstruction and distention of the urinary tract or it may be causing the ureter to spasm.
- *Nausea and vomiting* may be present. It is important that IV hydration be given to prevent dehydration. A person may have to be admitted to the hospital for persistent nausea and vomiting.
- *Hematuria*, either gross or microscopic, is usually present. The lack of either does not rule out a stone.
- *Fever, tachycardia, hypotension, and cutaneous vasodilatation* can be signs of urosepsis which is a medical emergency. A retrograde catheter should be inserted or a percutaneous nephrostomy tube should be placed to allow the kidney to drain to decrease chances of renal damage.

RISK FACTORS

- Obesity and hypertension
- Diet
  - High animal protein intake
  - Low fluid intake
  - Low calcium intake
  - High salt intake
- Hot climate
- Sedentary occupation
- Family history
- Medications

EVALUATION

- *Differential diagnoses* should include appendicitis, ectopic pregnancy, diverticular disease, bowel obstruction, mesenteric ischemia, biliary stones, abdominal aortic aneurysm, pyelonephritis, muscular skeletal causes, and so on.
- *History* should elicit information specifically about the pain, including the onset, the character, whether or not the pain radiates, and activities that worsen or lessen the pain. It should be asked whether the patient has urinary symptoms, hematuria, nausea, or vomiting. Also inquire about a personal history of stones or a family history of stone disease. One should consider lithiasis in a patient who has frequent urinary tract infections (UTIs) not improved with antibiotics.
- *Stone composition* is important to explore. This determines which treatment plan will be used to remove the stone and decrease the chances of recurrent stones. Stones can be analyzed with roentgen crystallography or infrared spectroscopy. If possible, all patients should have a stone analyzed.
- *Diseases* can increase the risk of a patient getting a stone by altering metabolic balances. It is important to elicit a past medical history to rule out a cause of stone formation. Altered intestinal function as seen in Crohn's disease, small bowel resection, jejuno-ileal bypass, or other conditions causing malabsorption of fatty acids can lead to hyperoxaluria. Hypercalcemic conditions, seen in hyperparathyroidism, hyperthyroid, sarcoidosis, and immobilization states increase the risk of stone formation. Renal tubular acidosis (RTA) is known to increase stone formation as well.
- *Medications* used to treat other diseases in the body can alter ion concentrations or urinary pH leading to increased formation of stones. Some medications have low solubility in urine and become stones themselves. These include indinavir, triamterene, sulfadiazine, and silicate.
- *Diet* modifications can sometimes reduce the rate of urolithiasis. Limiting the amount of animal protein intake can reduce calcium oxalate stone formation. Decreasing products high in oxalate (i.e., chocolate and nuts) can lower urinary oxalate levels. Limiting dairy intake to the dietary recommended amounts of calcium helps to avoid increased urinary calcium and the ion-activity products of calcium oxalate and calcium pyrophosphate. Adequate daily hydration patterns need to be addressed as well.
- *Blood analysis* can be useful when examining a patient for metabolic abnormalities. Serum or plasma concentration of calcium may indicate a hypercalcemic condition. When calcium levels exceed 2.6 mmol/L a parathyroid hormone level should be drawn. Serum creatinine can be used to examine renal function. Elevated serum urate levels may indicate abnormal purine metabolism.
- Urine analysis
  - Randomly collected urine is useful for establishing bacteriuria, microscopic evaluation for crystals after centrifugation, and determining cystinuria with the nitroprusside test.
  - 24-hour collections are useful for assessing the number of variables excreted in the urine that affect the levels of supersaturation and or ion-activity products on the salts. Encourage compliance with a 24-h collection as the results are important. Also, patients may subconsciously change their eating/drinking habits when they are collecting the sample.

RADIOLOGICAL IMAGING

- *Noncontrast spiral computed tomography* (CT) is the gold standard imaging technique. It has 97–100% sensitivity and 92–100% specificity. It is less expensive than an intravenous pyelogram (IVP). The results are rapid; 4 min versus 62 min for an IVP. It includes images of the peritoneal and retroperitoneal structures and can identify nongenitourinary disease. No contrast is needed. On CT, a phlebolith can be mistaken for a distal urethral calculus. All types of stones can be identified on CT, but not readily differentiated into what specific type. Disadvantages include its cost and radiation exposure.

- *IVP* is a study that images the upper genitourinary tract anatomy. A preliminary scout film of the abdomen is obtained followed by an intravenous injection of iodine-containing contrast. A number of x-rays are taken as the kidneys rapidly excrete the contrast medium. An IVP has the ability to visualize a bifid collecting system and nephrolithiasis. Extra osseous calcifications will show on the radiograph as well. Limitations to an IVP can occur with an inadequate bowel prep, ileus, or swallowed air.

- *Tomography* uses x-ray imaging of a particular plane in the body. Structures in the kidney can be viewed when obscured in other radiographic views by bone or feces. Tomograms are not useful in morbidly obese patients.

- *Kidney, ureter, and bladder (KUB)/ultrasonography* in combination are about as effective as an IVP. If an area of uncertainty is seen on a KUB, the ultrasound is directed to that position. The sonogram is operator dependent. A sonogram can appreciate a stone not visualized on IVP. Ultrasound minus the KUB is also the modality of choice for a woman who is pregnant.

STONE VARIETIES

- *Calcium stones* make up about 80% of urolithiasis. Calculi form because of elevated urinary calcium, urinary uric acid, urinary oxalate, or decreased urinary citrate. There can be solitary defects, but more often they appear in combination.
  - *Absorptive hypercalciuric nephrolithiasis* is due to increased absorption of calcium from the small bowel, mainly the jejunum. The increased serum calcium load is filtered through the glomerulus. This suppresses parathyroid hormone levels and decreases tubular reabsorption of calcium leading to hypercalciuria. There are three types of hypercalciuric nephrolithiasis.
    - *Type 1* represents 15% of calcareous calculi. This form is independent of dietary intake of calcium. Treatment is with cellulose phosphate taken with meals. It binds to the calcium in bowel so that it cannot be absorbed. It is contraindicated in postmenopausal women and in children experiencing active growth. Hydrochlorothiazide (HCTZ) is an alternate treatment to cellulose phosphate. It decreases renal excretion of calcium and the excess calcium is placed into bones. It is useful for 3–5 years until the bone reaches its storage capacity.
    - *Type 2* is dependent on calcium intake and is fairly common. Calcium excretion is normal on a calcium-restricted diet of 400–600 mg/day.
    - *Type 3* is due to a renal phosphate leak. This type represents about 5% of stones. A decreased serum phosphate leads to an increase production of 1,25-dihydroxyvitamin D. This stimulates increased absorption of phosphate and calcium from the small bowel, which eventually leads to increased renal excretion into the urine. Phosphate supplements are taken three times a day to inhibit vitamin D synthesis.
  - *Resorptive hypercalciuric nephrolithiasis* results from primary hyperparathyroidism. Hypercalcemia is the most consistent sign. Parathyroid hormone affects calcium and phosphorus by increasing serum calcium and decreasing urinary calcium. It exerts the opposite affect on phosphorus by increasing the urinary phosphorus and decreasing serum phosphorus. The hypercalcemic state is stressful to the kidneys and ultimately damages them. The kidney eventually cannot acidify the urine. Treatment results from surgical removal of the adenoma.
  - *Renal-induced hypercalciuric nephrolithiasis* is secondary to an intrinsic renal tubular defect in calcium excretion. Excessive calcium excretion occurs in the urine decreasing serum calcium levels. This in turn stimulates the parathyroid to release hormone and mobilize calcium from the bone and increase calcium absorption from the gut. The calcium is filtered to the kidney and the kidney excretes it into the urine and the cycle continues. Lab studies will show elevated fasting urine calcium, normal serum calcium, and elevated parathyroid hormone. Treatment is with HCTZ and it exerts a long-term effect by decreasing circulating blood volume to the glomerulus. This stimulates the proximal tubules to absorb calcium and other constituents and leads to increased absorption at the distal tubule. This will correct the hyperparathyroid state.
  - *Hyperuricosuric calcium nephrolithiasis* involves one of two mechanisms. There may be too much intake of purines in the diet or there is an endogenous uric acid

production. Both of these lead to increased urinary monosodium urates. These monosodium urates absorb and adsorb urinary stone inhibitors and facilitate heterogenous nucleation. Treatment can be with decreased purine intake or with allopurinol. Allopurinol inhibits production of uric acid and decreases renal excretion of uric acid. If a patient cannot tolerate allopurinol then potassium citrate is an option.

○ *Hyperoxaluric calcium nephrolithiasis* is caused by increased urinary oxalate levels rarely associated with excessive dietary intake. It usually results from inflammatory bowel syndrome (IBS) or chronic diarrhea states and severe dehydration. Malabsorption in the gut results in excess intraluminal fat and bile. Calcium binds to this fat and therefore is less available to bind to oxalate. Oxalate is readily absorbed and is excreted in the urine. Stones do not form just because of hyperoxaluria. Other factors must be present including dehydration, decreased excretion of inhibitors, and increased acidosis and protein malabsorption. Treatment involves calcium supplements with meals to bind to the free oxalate.

○ *Hypocitraturic calcium nephrolithiasis* occurs when reduced citrate is excreted into the urine. Citrate is an inhibitor of urinary stone formation. It complexes with calcium decreasing the ionic calcium concentration which in turn decreases crystallization. Citrate also inhibits agglomeration, nucleation, and crystal growth of calcium oxalate. Citrate excretion is decreased when the metabolic demands of the mitochondria in renal cells increases, during fasting, metabolic acidosis, gluconeogenesis, and hypokalemia. Citrate can also be consumed by bacteria if a UTI is present. Hypocitraturic calcium nephrolithiasis is often seen in RTA Type 1. It can also be seen with thiazide treatment and chronic diarrhea. It is treated with potassium citrate supplementation two to three times per day.

○ *Uric acid stones* characterize less than 5% of urolithiasis. Uric acid stones typically appear in men. They usually are not from hyperuricemia, but secondary to dehydration and excessive dietary intake of purines. They are commonly found in patients with gout, myeloproliferative disorders, and those treated with cytotoxic drugs. It can be differentiated from hyperuricosuric calcium nephrolithiasis when the urine pH is found to be less than 5.5. Treating uric acid stones with allopurinol can decrease uric acid excretion. Alkalinization of the urine by maintaining a urine pH of greater than 6 allows the urate ion to remain soluble and will dissolve the stones of less than 1 cm diameter. With good compliance, this can take about a month to accomplish. Progress can be followed with a KUB film.

• *Cystine stones* represent 1–2% of urolithiasis. The stones result from metabolic abnormalities leading to increased absorption of dibasic amino acids including cystine, ornithine, lysine, and arginine from the mucosal surface of the small bowel and renal tubules. Cystine is the only amino acid of the four listed that can produce stones when supersaturated. The genetic defect has been mapped to chromosomes 2 and 19. It is autosomal recessive with homozygous and heterozygous forms. Normally, cystine is filtered and then reabsorbed in the proximal tubules, but in affected individuals, reabsorption of cystine is impaired. The stone burden can be single, multiple, or staghorn.

• The diagnosis should be suspected in a person with a history of childhood stones, recurrent episodes of lithiasis, a family history of stones, or amber-colored calculi.

• On radiographs, the stones appear opaque, smooth edged, with a ground glass appearance. Hexagonal crystals in the urine are diagnostic. A positive cyanide nitroprusside urine test suggests excess cystine excretion and a quantitation of cystine excretion should be done in a 24-h urine collection.

• Management of cystinuria includes adequately hydrating oneself to maintain a urinary specific gravity of 1.010. Also, the incidence of stones is reduced if one consumes only a moderate amount of protein and less than 2 g of sodium per day. Urine alkalinization (pH 6.5–7) can be attempted with sodium bicarbonate or potassium citrate. This is monitored with pH paper and is very challenging. Thiol derivatives are chelating agents which bind to cystine and help dissolve existing stones and help to prevent recurrences. These include D-penicillamine, α-mercaptopropionylglycine (α-MPG), bucillamine, and captopril.

• *Struvite stones* make up about 15–20% of renal lithiasis. They occur more often in women. The stones are composed of magnesium, ammonium, and phosphate (MAP) and are synonymous with infectious stones. They are associated with urea-splitting organisms such as *Proteus*, *Klebsiella*, *Staphylococcus*, *Pseudomonas*, and *Serratia*. The bacteria produce high amounts of ammonia that elevate the pH allowing precipitation of MAP crystals.

• Urine cultures will not always identify the organisms mentioned earlier. If a person has persistent UTI without resolution with appropriate antibiotics, then struvite stones should be suspected.

• Struvite stones are usually staghorn shaped. A KUB, ultrasound, and CT can visualize struvite stones.

Antibiotics may slow stone growth and decrease infectious symptoms. Acetohydroxamic acid inhibits bacteria urease, but side effects limit its use. Stone removal is therapeutic and can be done by shock wave lithotripsy, percutaneous nephrolithotomy, ureteroscopy, a combination of the three, or by open surgery.

TREATMENT OF UROLITHIASIS

- *Observation* can be a good option for some stones. Most calculi pass on their own. If a stone is 5 mm or less, it has a 50% chance of spontaneous passage. When a stone is 6 mm or greater, the chance of successful passing is less than 5%. Of course, it all depends on the size and shape of the stone and where it is located. Proximal stones are less likely to pass spontaneously than distal ureteral stones. A stone may take up to 6 weeks to pass. Narcotics may be necessary for pain control and additional nonsteroidal anti-inflammatory drugs (NSAIDs) are said to be helpful. A patient should be admitted for intractable pain, severe nausea and vomiting that could lead to dehydration, or any signs or symptoms of urosepsis.
- Extracorporeal shock wave lithotripsy (ESWL)
  - ESWL uses energy to create shock waves. A coupling mechanism is used to transfer the energy from outside to inside the body. Fluoroscopy or ultrasonography is used to locate the position of the stone so that the shock waves can be directly focused. The focused waves will fragment the stones by forces that cause erosion and shattering. Double-J stents may be placed which do not facilitate stone passage but ensure kidney drainage. Proper patient positioning is important for successful fragmentation.
  - Radiographic or ultrasonographic imaging is performed earlier to locate the stone. Stone type analysis prior to ESWL can be useful as some stones are not easy to fragment. Also, it should be determined that the distal urinary tract below the stone is not obstructed.
  - Stones greater than 2 cm may be more easily removed by percutaneous approach rather than repeated shock wave treatments.
  - ESWL is contraindicated in pregnant women, women of childbearing age, patients with bleeding disorders, and those with large abdominal aortic aneurysms. It is not recommended for obese patients.
  - ESWL can be performed with intravenous analgesia and sedation.
  - It is normal to have ecchymosis at the entry site of the shock waves. Gross hematuria always occurs.

Patients should ambulate and maintain adequate fluid intake postoperatively.
  - Follow-up ultrasound and KUB should be performed 2 weeks postoperatively and a 3-month follow-up KUB should be obtained as well. Inadequate fragmentation can occur as well as painful passage of the offending calculi pieces or obstruction from fragments. Silent hydronephrosis should be ruled out.
- Ureteroscopic stone extraction
  - Stone extraction of proximal and midureteral stones can be accomplished with flexible and rigid ureteroscopes with high success rates of 66–100%. Balloon dilators can be used to help the stone pass and a basket can be attached to the ureteroscope to aid in catching the stone. Not all stones readily pass and may need fragmentation. Several methods of fragmentation can be done through the ureteroscope including, electrohydraulic lithotripsy, ultrasonic probes, laser energy, electromechanical impactors, and pneumatic systems.
  - Complications range from 5 to 30% most commonly being ureteral injury.
- Percutaneous nephrolithotomy
  - Percutaneous nephrolithotomy is a reliable modality of stone removal for stones greater than 2.5 cm in size, impacted stones, stones that fill the intrarenal space (i.e., staghorn), or stones that could not be removed by alternative methods listed earlier. It is useful for patients who have anatomical abnormalities where passing an ureteroscope would not be safe. Using fluoroscopy or ultrasound, a needle puncture is directed into the posterior inferior calyx. Tract dilation is performed. Patience must be employed. If the stone is not removed completely, the procedure can be followed up with methods described earlier. It is comparable in success to open surgery and offers a shorter hospital stay, quicker rate of recovery with earlier return to work, and overall less expensive.
- Open stone surgery
  - Open stone surgery is a relatively uncommon procedure today. All other stone removal procedures are compared to it because open procedures are the "gold standard" in stone removal. However, because of the morbidity of the incision and the successfulness of less invasive techniques, open stone removal is usually only performed when the other medical and surgical approaches have failed.

BIBLIOGRAPHY

Kenney PJ. CT evaluation of urinary lithiasis. *Radiol Clin North Am.* 2003;41:979–999.

Matlaga BR, Assimos DG. Urologic manifestation of nonuro-logic disease urolithiasis. *Urol Clin North Am*. 2003;31:91–99.

Menon M, Resnick M. Urinary lithiasis: etiology, diagnosis and medical management. In: Campbell MF, ed. *Campbell's Urology*. 8th ed. Philadelphia, PA: WB Saunders; 2002:3229–3305.

Segura JW, Preminger GM, Assimos DG, et al. Ureteral Stones Clinical Guidelines Panel summary report on the management of ureteral calculi. *J Urol*. 1997;158(5):1915–1921.

Shekarriz B, Stoller ML. Cystinuria and other noncalcareous calculi. *Endocrinol Metab Clin North Am*. 2002;31:951–977.

Stoller ML, Bolton DM. Urinary stone disease. In: Tanagho EA, McAninch JW, eds. *Smith's General Urology*. 15th ed. New York, NY: McGraw-Hill; 2000:291–320.

Tiselius H. Medical evaluation of nephrolithiasis. *Endocrinol Metab Clin North Am*. 2002;31:1031–1050.

Wasserstein AG. Nephrolithiasis. *Am J Kidney Dis*. 2005; 45(2):422–428.

Worster A, Preyra I, Weaver B, et al. The accuracy of noncontrast helical computed tomography versus intravenous pyelography in the diagnosis of suspected acute urolithiasis: a meta-analysis. *Ann Emerg Med*. 2002;40(3):280–286.

QUESTIONS

1. A 52-year-old female presents to the emergency room with complaints of right-sided pain. She ranks the pain 8/10. She states that she was at work and suddenly experienced throbbing pain. She took two Tylenol with no relief. She denies prior urinary complaints, fevers, or hematuria. You notice that she is in acute distress, leaning forward, and holding her side. A microscopic view of her spun urine reveals hexagonal crystals. A CT scan revealed a 4-mm stone at the uretero-vesical junction. What would be the next best treatment for this patient?

   (A) Encourage adequate fluid hydration, recommend decreased calcium intake in the diet, prescribe allopurinol, and strain urine for a stone.

   (B) Encourage adequate fluid hydration, recommend minimal protein intake and low sodium diet, prescribe α-MPG, and strain urine for a stone.

   (C) Encourage adequate fluid hydration, strain urine for a stone, and have the patient return in 6 weeks for follow up.

   (D) Prescribe a cephalosporin and schedule the patient for an ESWL procedure.

2. A 33-year-old G_3P_2 at 23 and 4/7 weeks' gestation presents to triage with complaints of left flank pain. Vitals are T 99.3, P 98, R 20, and BP 128/82. She rates her pain as 10/10 and states this feels "exactly like the pain I had before 6 years ago when I had a kidney stone." Her urinalysis (UA) shows specific gravity of 1.025, negative protein, negative glucose, 1+ ketones, 1+ blood, negative nitrites, and 1+ leukocyte esterase. You establish that the patient is stable and would like to have imaging done for evaluation. You order a

   (A) CT scan

   (B) KUB film

   (C) Ultrasound

   (D) IVP

3. A 44-year-old patient is diagnosed with a calcium stone. Metabolic workup reveals elevated fasting calcium in the urine, normal serum calcium, and increased parathyroid hormone levels. The most likely diagnosis is

   (A) absorptive hypercalciuric nephrolithiasis

   (B) resorptive hypercalciuric nephrolithiasis

   (C) renal-induced hypercalciuric nephrolithiasis

   (D) hyperuricosuric calcium nephrolithiasis

   (E) hyperoxaluric calcium nephrolithiasis

ANSWERS

1. *(B)*. The patient has hexagonal crystals in her urine which is diagnostic of cystine stones. Cystine stones are due to a genetic metabolic defect and therefore, diet modifications and medications are necessary to prevent stones. No procedure is necessary at this time as the stone only measures 4 mm and is in the distal ureter; therefore, chances are it will pass on its own. Choice A is treatment for uric acid stones. Choice C does not offer any preventative plan for future stones. Antibiotics would not be appropriate in this situation as suggested in choice D.

2. *(C)*. Choice A is incorrect because of radiation exposure to a patient who is pregnant. A KUB or IVP can be done (as a one shot IVP) for a pregnant patient if ultrasound is negative and clinical suspicion is high for a stone, but it would not be the first treatment. Choice C is correct because there is no radiation exposure during an ultrasound. Ultrasound can detect roughly 60% of stones.

3. *(C)*. Choice A, metabolic workup would reveal elevated urinary calcium, elevated serum calcium, and normal parathyroid hormone. Choice B results in decreased urinary calcium, elevated serum calcium,

and elevated parathyroid levels. Choice D results in elevated levels of uric acid in the urine. Choice E is incorrect because one would find elevated oxalate in the urine.

43 MICROSCOPIC HEMATURIA

Sandra J. Bosman

HEMATURIA

- Potentially originating from any site along the urinary tract, hematuria is a common condition where blood is present in the urine, which ranges from microscopic amounts to gross, visible bleeding; it may be the sole symptom of a serious underlying condition, such as a urologic malignancy.
- A minimum of 1 mL of blood per 1 L of urine may cause gross red or brown discoloration of the urine.
- Gross hematuria ranges broadly in etiology, and always requires a prompt, thorough evaluation as there is a greater chance of malignancy occurring in women with gross hematuria as opposed to microscopic hematuria.
- Red urine may be caused by clinical scenarios other than hematuria, such as hemoglobinuria or methoglobinuria, medications (e.g., Rifampin, Phenytoin, Ibuprofen, Levodopa, Nitrofurantoin, and Sulfamethoxazole), beets and berries in susceptible patients, artificial food coloring, or infection with *Serratia marcescens*.

MICROSCOPIC HEMATURIA

- Microscopic hematuria is often an incidental finding on urinalysis.
- Although definitions vary slightly, it is defined as greater than two to three red blood cells per high-powered field of centrifuged urinary sediment.
- Situations such as sexual intercourse, vigorous exercise, mild trauma, or menstrual contamination may cause blood to be detected in the urine of healthy patients.
- Because there is no established "cut-off" level below which an underlying lesion may be excluded (the degree of hematuria is not directly correlated to the

seriousness of the underlying pathology as malignancy may cause only intermittent bleeding), it must be considered serious until proven otherwise.

COMMON METHODS OF DETECTION

- Urine Dipstick
  - One of the most widely used and cost-effective methods for evaluating urine is urine dipstick.
  - The oxidative properties of hemoglobin promote reaction with the *chromagen* present on the cellulose dipstick when placed in the urine specimen. The dipstick produces varying shades of green which correlate to the amount of hemoglobin in the urine.
    - A negative test excludes hematuria (sensitivity is 91–100%); it detects 1–2 RBCs/hpf. Specificity is 65–99%.
    - *False positives* may be caused by free hemoglobin or myoglobin, oxidizing contamination (bacterial peroxidases, hypochlorite, povidone-iodine), antiseptic solutions, menstrual contamination, instrumentation, or dehydration causing high urine specific gravity.
    - *False negatives* may be caused by reducing agents (e.g., vitamin C), acidic pH (less than 5.1), or prolonged exposure of the dipstick to air.
- Urine Microscopy
  - Urine microscopy is another popular urine evaluation method, and is the gold standard.
  - Various protocols exist for urine preparation. For best results, freshly voided, midstream, clean-catch urine without instrumentation should be used. The urine should be centrifuged, resuspended, and examined under a high power objective (400×).
    - Red cell casts (pathognomonic for glomerular disease), cells with irregular outer cell membranes (dysmorphic cells), proteinuria (greater than 500 mg/day), and cells with multiple, variable membrane protrusions (acanthocytes) suggest a glomerular source of bleeding.
    - Normal appearing (isomorphic) red blood cells and clumped erythrocytes suggest a nonglomerular or lower urinary tract source of bleeding.

EPIDEMIOLOGY AND ETIOLOGY

- Epidemiology
  - Increasing with age, female gender, and repeat testing, 2–13% of the population has microscopic

TABLE 43-1 Etiologies of Microscopic Hematuria—Examples by Location

GLOMERULAR ORIGIN	NONGLOMERULAR ORIGIN—UPPER URINARY TRACT	NONGLOMERULAR—LOWER URINARY TRACT ORIGIN	MISCELLANEOUS ORIGINS
IgA nephropathy (Berger's disease)*	Nephrolithiasis* Renal cell or transitional cell cancer*,†	Urinary tract infection*	Exercise-induced hematuria
Thin basement membrane disease (benign familial hematuria)*	Pyelonephritis	Malignancy (transitional cell cancer)*,†	Excessive anticoagulation (usually warfarin)
Hereditary nephritis (Alport's syndrome)*	Polycystic kidney disease or medullary sponge kidney (familial)	Bladder stone or foreign body*	Factitious
Glomerulonephritis (postinfectious, membranoproliferative, rapidly progressive)	Interstitial nephritis (can be caused by allopurinol, captopril, cephalosporins or penicillins, thiazides)	Benign polyps and tumors Condyloma acuminatum	Genitourinary trauma
Focal glomerulosclerosis	Renal infarction	Hemorrhagic cystitis (can be caused by radiation cyclophosphamide, ifosfamide, methicillin, mitotane)	Abdominal aortic aneurysm†
Lupus nephritis	Renal vein thrombosis	*Schistosoma haematobium* in North Africans	Coagulopathy (thrombocytopenia, hemophilia, von Willebrand's disease, DIC, fibrinolysis)
Goodpasture's syndrome	Papillary necrosis		Sickle-cell trait or disease
Loin-pain hematuria	Arteriovenous malformation		Lymphoma†
Loin-pain hematuria syndrome	Amyloidosis		Multiple myeloma†
Vasculitis (polyarteritis nodosa, Wegner's granulomatosis)	Metabolic (hypercalciuria, hyperuricosuria)		Indwelling catheter
Hemolytic-uremic syndrome	Ureteral stricture and hydronephrosis		Radiation therapy
			Infection (genitourinary tuberculosis, CMV, or mononucleosis)
			Wilms' tumors in children
			Idiopathic*

ABBREVIATIONS: CMV, cytomegalovirus; *DIC, disseminated intravascular coagulation.*
*Common etiologies.
†Life-threatening etiologies.

hematuria, which is responsible for 6% of referrals to urologists.

○ Of patients with confirmed hematuria, 2–20% have disease with significant morbidity: Approximately 2.5–5% of cases are caused by urologic malignancy, most commonly bladder cancer.

• Etiology
• The etiologies of microscopic hematuria range widely with respect to associated morbidity and mortality. The list below gives risk factors for significant disease and Table 43-1 lists possible etiologies.

RISK FACTORS FOR SIGNIFICANT DISEASE

• Age greater than 40 years
• Analgesic abuse (e.g., Phenacetin)
• Aristolochic acid (found in some herbal weight loss preparations)
• Cigarette smoking
• Cyclophosphamide (Cytoxan)
• Dietary nitrites and nitrates (used in processed meats and cheeses as a preservative)
• Irritative voiding
• Male gender
• Occupational exposure (benzene, aromatic amines, leather dye, rubber manufacturing, aniline dyes)
• Pelvic irradiation
• Previous history of urologic disease
• Urinary tract infection (recurrent or chronic)

HISTORY AND PHYSICAL EXAMINATION

• A thorough history and physical examination are pivotal in narrowing the broad differential diagnosis for microscopic hematuria.
• Especially important are risk factors for significant disease (see list), such as the age and sex of the patient, occupational or radiation exposures, social

history (especially smoking history), and medication history. Do any findings suggest a particular diagnosis?

RADIOLOGIC EVALUATION OF THE UPPER URINARY TRACT

- Imaging of the upper urinary tract identifies sources of bleeding, such as renal cell cancer, transitional cell cancer, urolithiasis, or cystic disease.
- However, for lesions located inside the bladder, all imaging modalities are limited in their use.
- Commonly used imaging methods include intravenous pyelography, ultrasound, and computed tomography (CT) scan (see Chap. 12).
- Magnetic resonance imaging (MRI) also provides excellent imaging, but its use is limited by availability and relatively higher cost. (see Chap. 12).
- Other imaging modalities include ureteroscopy with biopsy and angiography.

EVALUATION OF THE LOWER URINARY TRACT

- Cytology
  - Cytological examination detects exfoliated malignant cells in the urine with a sensitivity of only 40–50%, which can be improved with early-morning, barbotaged (bladder wash obtained during cystoscopy), or consecutive specimens: The sensitivity is greater for higher grade cancer of the bladder.
  - Carcinoma in situ may be detected with cytology before it is visualized with cystoscopy; nevertheless, *a negative test does not rule out malignancy.*
- Tumor Markers
  - Further investigation is needed to determine the efficacy of tumor markers as a screening test as their role in detection of malignancy is uncertain.
  - Examples include BTA Stat and Trak (Bladder Tumor Antigen), NMP22 (Nuclear Matrix Protein), and telomerase.
  - BTA Stat and NMP22 are Food and Drug Administration (FDA) approved. Most studies have been conducted in the detection of papillary cancer, although some studies have been conducted in the detection of high-grade carcinoma in situ.
- Cystoscopy
  - A small camera inserted into the bladder allows direct visualization of the bladder mucosa and urethra. Cystoscopy can be performed in the office under local anesthesia (see Chap. 11).

- Common findings include bladder stones and tumors.

SUGGESTED STEPS TO FOLLOW IN EVALUATION

Steps to follow in evaluation have been provided in Fig. 43-1.

CONCLUSION

- General screening of the population for microscopic hematuria is not recommended at this time by the U.S. Preventative Task Force and Canadian Task Force on Periodic Health Examination.
- The American Urologic Association's best practice policy states that complete evaluation should be performed on patients with microscopic hematuria who are older than 40 or younger patients if risk factors for disease are present.
- The value of the hematuria workup should be weighted against the cost and morbidity of testing. Does early detection of the disease improve survival or decrease treatment costs?
  - In about 10–35% of cases, no etiology is discovered after complete evaluation.
  - If initial evaluation is negative, urologic malignancy is diagnosed in 1–3% of patients within 3 years.
  - With negative radiologic and cystoscopic evaluation, about 50% of patients will have hematuria due to immunoglobulin A (IgA) nephropathy, hereditary nephritis, or thin basement membrane disease.

BIBLIOGRAPHY

Cohen RA, Brown RS. Microscopic hematuria. *N Engl J Med.* 2003;348:2330–2338.

Messing EM, Young TB, Hunt VB, et al. Urinary tract cancers found by homescreening with hematuria dipsticks in healthy men over 50 years of age. *Cancer.* 1989;64:2361–2367.

Restrepo NC, Carey PO. Evaluating hematuria in adults. *Am Fam Physician.* 1989;40:149–156.

Rose BD, Fletcher RH. Evaluation of hematuria in adults. *Up to Date 2004*; Volume 12: Number 3 (www.uptodate.com).

Thaller TR, Wang LP. Evaluation of asymptomatic microscopic hematuria in adults. *Am Fam Physician.* 1999;60:1143–1152.

Weber AM. Hematuria. In: *Office Urogynecology-Practical Pathways in Obstetrics and Gynecology.* New York: McGraw-Hill Company; 2004 :157–169.

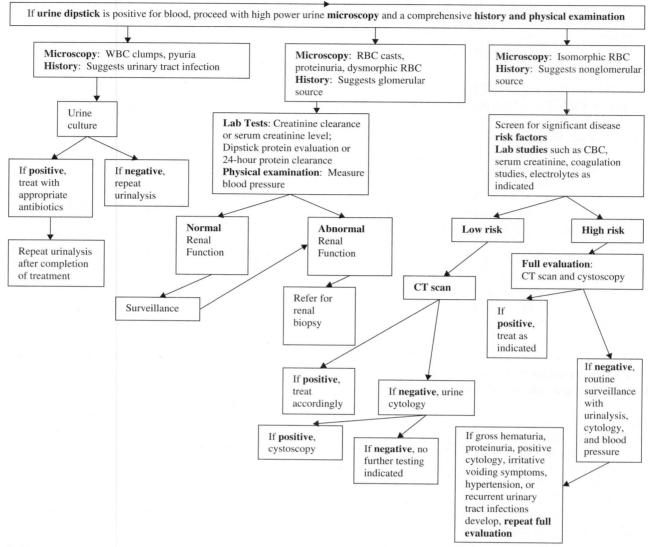

FIG. 43-1 Suggested steps to follow in evaluation of cystoscopy.

Woolhandler S, Pels RJ, Bor DH, et al. Dipstick urinalysis screening of asymptomatic adults for urinary tract disorders. I. Hematuria and proteinuria. *JAMA*. 1989;262:1214–1219.

Yun EJ, Meng MV, Carroll PR. Evaluation of the patient with hematuria. *Med Clin N Am*. 2004;88:329–343.

QUESTIONS

1. A 33-year-old female is found to have asymptomatic, microscopic hematuria. On physical examination, palpation of her abdomen reveals moderately enlarged kidneys. She has a family history of renal cysts. The best initial imaging modality to evaluate her upper urinary tract would be which of the following?

(A) Intravenous pyelography

(B) Ultrasound

(C) CT scan

(D) Kidney, ureter, and bladder (KUB)

(E) MRI

2. A 62-year-old female presents with microscopic hematuria on routine evaluation. She currently reports some mild dysuria and urinary incontinence when coughing or straining. She is postmenopausal and not taking hormone replacement. Eight months ago, she had a mild cerebrovascular accident (CVA) due to embolus and is currently anticoagulated with

warfarin (lab studies show that she is in the therapeutic range). The next best step in management of this patient is which of the following?

(A) Observation

(B) Discontinue her warfarin

(C) Reevaluate the patient in 3 months

(D) Cystoscopy

(E) Complete evaluation should be undertaken including CT scan and urine cytology

3. A 54-year-old obese woman with type 2 diabetes mellitus presents with a urine dipstick positive for blood, confirmed by microscopy. Her diabetes is controlled with diet and Metformin; she had a hysterectomy 10 years ago for large fibroids. She has a 15 pack year history of smoking, but quit 7 years ago when she was diagnosed with diabetes. The next most appropriate step in evaluation of this patient for malignancy is which of the following?

(A) Routine repeat urine dipsticks

(B) CT scan

(C) Urine culture

(D) Discontinue Metformin

(E) Urine cytology

4. A 32-year-old nulligravid woman presents to the physician with worsening dysmenorrhea. She has a tampon in place, and after thoroughly cleansing the perineum, a urine sample is obtained which is positive for blood on dipstick and microscopy. She returns 2 weeks later for reevaluation, and the dipstick is negative for blood. She returns again during her next menstrual cycle, and her urine is again positive for blood. The most likely etiology of her hematuria is which of the following?

(A) Menstrual contamination of the urine sample

(B) Endometriosis of the urinary tract

(C) Nephrolithiasis

(D) Transitional cell carcinoma

(E) Urinary tract infection

5. A 62-year-old postmenopausal female, not currently taking hormone replacement therapy, was noted to have hematuria on dipstick evaluation, which was confirmed by microscopy. She recently finished a course of Cefotetan for an infection. She routinely takes Captopril and Furosemide to treat her hypertension. What is the most likely cause of her hematuria?

(A) Interstitial nephritis

(B) Papillary necrosis

(C) Hemorrhagic cystitis

(D) Urolithiasis

(E) Loin-pain syndrome

ANSWERS

1. *(B)* See Table 43-2 for explanation. Answer D is incorrect because a pain x-ray may not detect a renal cyst. Answer E is incorrect because MRI may provide good imaging, but is cost and availability prohibitive.

2. *(E).* Anticoagulation, if kept within the therapeutic range, does not usually cause hematuria in of itself; nevertheless, it may uncover serious underlying

TABLE 43-2 Comparison of the Common Initial Imaging Modalities for Microscopic Hematuria

IMAGING MODALITY	DESCRIPTION/MECHANISM	STRENGTHS	WEAKNESSES
(A) Intravenous pyelography (also known as excretory urography or IV urography)	Study of choice for many years Contrast material injected into an arm vein and a series of x-rays taken at timed intervals	Visualize entire upper urinary system Use is continued because of standardized protocols, efficacy, and lower cost	Limited sensitivity for lesions less than 3 cm Limited use in pregnant women (radiation exposure)
(B) Ultrasonography (the correct answer is B).	High-frequency sound pulses transmitted from the probe, reflected from tissue planes, and detected by the probe. Distances are calculated by computer to created 2-D images	Safe for pregnant patients and those with increased risk of contrast reaction Test of choice if renal cyst suspected Least expensive	Limited sensitivity for subtle mucosal abnormalities Collecting system and ureteral anatomy better with IVP and CT
(C) CT scan	Becoming the study of choice Series of x-ray pulses through the region of interest, where a computer integrates the "slices" into images	More sensitive and specific than IVP and U/S	Risks associated with IV contrast and radiation (less safe for pregnant women) Highest cost

ABBREVIATIONS: IV, intravenous; IVP, intravenous pyelogram; U/S, ultrasound.

pathology earlier. Therefore, a full evaluation of the urinary system is warranted including imaging of the upper urinary system with CT scan, urine cytology, and/or cystoscopy. Answer A is incorrect because as stated above, complete evaluation is warranted because malignancy may be present. Answer B is incorrect because her warfarin should not be the cause of the hematuria because she is within the therapeutic range, and would be at increased risk for repeat embolus if warfarin is discontinued. Answer C in is incorrect because, as stated above, complete evaluation for malignancy is indicated at this time. Answer D is incorrect. Although cystoscopy is part of a complete work-up, it does not evaluate the kidneys and ureters.

3. *(D)*. Metformin (Glucophage) usage may precipitate lactic acidosis and acute renal failure when used with contrast, as it is primarily renally excreted. Its use should be discontinued 48 hours prior to and following contrast infusion, and renal function should be evaluated before reinitiating Metformin. Answer A is incorrect because she has significant risk factors for urologic disease, and should undergo a full evaluation. Answer B is incorrect. Although a CT scan is appropriate, Metformin must be discontinued beforehand by this patient to minimize the potential complications. Contrast nephropathy has been reported in previously healthy patients, but usually occurs in patients with preexisting renal disease and previous reaction to contrast (strongest two risk factors). Other risk factors are cardiac decompensation, history of allergy or asthma, dehydration, or diabetes mellitus. To minimize the risk of IV contrast reaction, preprocedure hydration, evaluation of renal function, oral *N*-acetylcysteine, a selective dopamine agonist (e.g., Fenoldopam), and a low osmolar, nonionic contrast agent (e.g., Iopromide) should be used. Death from conventional contrast material occurs in 1–7/100,000 infusions. Answer C is incorrect, because it is not part of the evaluation for malignancy and the patient does not have any irritative voiding symptoms. Answer E is incorrect, because she should undergo complete evaluation rather than cytology alone.

4. *(B)*. Hematuria occurring during or shortly after menstruation is correlated with the infrequent finding of endometriosis of the urinary tract. Answer A is incorrect. Although menstrual contamination of

TABLE 43-3   Mechanisms By Which Selected Drugs May Cause Hematuria

(A) Interstitial nephritis	Allopurinol, captopril, cephalosporins, ciprofloxacin, furosemide, NSAIDs, olsalazine, omeprazole, penicillins, pentobarbital, phenylbutazone, rifampin, silver sulfadiazine, thiazides, trimethoprim-sulfamethoxazole
(B) Papillary necrosis	Acetylsalicylic acid, ibuprofen, indomethacin, naproxen, phenacetin phenylbutazone
(C) Hemorrhagic cystitis (see below)	Cyclophosphamide, ifosfamide, methicillin, mitotane
(D) Urolithiasis	Carbonic anhydrase inhibitors, dichlorphenamide, indinavir, mirtazapine, ritonavir, triamterene
(E) Loin-pain syndrome	Oral contraceptives

ABBREVIATION: NSAIDs, nonsteroidal anti-inflammatory drugs.

urine samples is a common reason to have a false-positive dipstick reading for blood, in this case it is unlikely because precautions have been taken to avoid this complication as tampon placement followed by thorough cleansing of the perineum is recommended if a urine specimen must be taken while a woman is menstruating. Answer C is incorrect because her history is inconsistent with nephrolithiasis; unilateral flank pain with possible radiation to groin and the patient unable to remain still would be more consistent with nephrolithiasis. Answer D is incorrect because her young age makes malignancy unlikely, also, other historical clues pointing toward malignancy are weight loss, anorexia, or fatigue or gross, painless hematuria. Answer E is incorrect. Urinary frequency, urgency, dysuria, or pyuria would suggest a urinary tract infection.

5. *(A)*. See Table 43-3. Cyclophosphamide and ifosfamide are associated with hemorrhagic cystitis; these agents metabolize to produce the intermediate acrolein, which irritates the bladder lining (usually within the first couple of weeks of treatment). Hemorrhagic cystitis can be difficult to treat, therefore, prevention is pivotal. Three commonly used preventative techniques include Mesna, a detoxifying agent that acts in the kidney; hyperhydration with furosemide; and continuous bladder irrigation with distilled water or normal saline. Other treatments include formalin, phenol, prostaglandin, alum, E-aminocaproic acid, or hyperbaric oxygen.

44 CONSTIPATION

Jeffrey S. Hardesty

DEFINITION

- A perception of abnormal bowel movements that include at least one of these four symptoms:
  1. Infrequent defecation (<3 stools per week)
  2. Excessive straining with defecation
  3. Passage of hard stools
  4. Feeling of incomplete evacuation

PREVALENCE

- Results of surveys vary depending on how constipation is defined but a study of self-reported bowel habits in the United States revealed that 21% of women and 8% of men suffer from these symptoms.

RISK FACTORS

- Advancing age
  - Occurs in up to 33% of the U.S. population above 65.
  - Problem further aggravated by physical immobility or inadequate toileting arrangements which make responding to defecatory signals difficult leading to fecal retention, megarectum, diminished rectal sensation, and fecal impaction.
- Low socioeconomic status
- Sedentary lifestyle
- Increasing number of medications being taken
  - Irrespective of listed side effect profile
  - One of the most common causes for constipation in the elderly and most easily correctable cause
- Inadequate intake of fluids, calories, or dietary fiber

- Female gender
  - Elevated levels of progesterone may be responsible for the gender bias.
    - Constipation is more common during pregnancy.
    - Delayed colonic transit has been reported during the luteal phase.

PHYSIOLOGY OF THE COLON

- The colon's primary functions are as follows:
  - Conversion of the ileal effluent into formed stool by extracting water and electrolytes
    - One liter of liquid chyme is changed to 200 g of solid feces daily
  - Fermentation of carbohydrate residues with digestive bacteria to allow for nutrient breakdown and absorption
  - Transportation and storage of stool to its distal segments until defecation is socially conducive
- Colon is embryologically, anatomically, and functionally divided into three regions.
  - Right colon (from ileocecal valve to hepatic flexure) serves as a reservoir for fermenting, mixing, and slowly transporting digestive residues.
    - Fecal chyme is churned by rhythmic, segmental, and retrograde contractions that retard fecal passage in this region.
    - Intermittent orthograde contractions occur that propel the more solid contents forward.
  - Left colon (from hepatic flexure to sigmoid) serves as a conduit for solidifying and more rapidly transporting feces.
    - Rhythmic orthograde contractions occur regularly in this region allowing for forward movement of solid stool and absorption of fluid and electrolytes from the liquid component.
  - Rectosigmoid region serves as a storage site for solid feces until elimination is convenient.
- Colon has unique aspects compared to the rest of the gastrointestinal (GI) tract that aid in accomplishing its functions.

○ Colon does not have a continuous outer layer of longitudinal muscle. Instead its external muscle is organized into three flat bands called tenia coli.

▪ Contractions of the tenia coli cause the colon to open and close like an accordion.

○ Segmental contractions of the inner circular muscle divide the colon into haustrations.

▪ Frequency of segmental contractions is dependent on regional basal electric rhythm (BER).

▪ BER frequency increases from rostral to caudal allowing for slower fecal transport (and more time for fermentation and absorption) within the right colon than the left.

○ Vasoactive intestinal polypeptide (VIP) is a hormone that functions as a neurotransmitter in enteric neurons as well as in the central nervous system (CNS) and urogenital systems.

▪ VIP modulates intestinal peristalsis as well as relaxation of the tenia coli and internal anal sphincter (IAS).

▪ Elevated levels of VIP such as in patients with VIPoma cause watery diarrhea, hypokalemia, and achlorhydria.

▪ Decreasing levels of VIP within the muscularis of the colon has been documented in patients with constipation and acquired megacolon.

○ Cholinergic innervation (parasympathetic) stimulates and modulates mechanical activity of the colon.

○ Sympathetic innervation inhibits colonic motility.

PHYSIOLOGY OF DEFECATION

For detailed review, also see Chap. 20, Fecal Incontinence.

• The mechanisms that allow for the storage and timely elimination of stool from the rectum involve a complex synergy between the autonomic and voluntary neuromuscular systems.

• In the storage phase, rectal continence is assisted by tonic contraction of the involuntary IAS, as well as the acute anorectal angulation caused by contraction of the sling-like levator ani (LA) muscles.

○ IAS receives parasympathetic innervation via sacral nerves (S2–S4).

○ LA receive voluntary innervation via the pudendal nerve.

• In response to rectal distention, parasympathetic nerve reflexes cause the IAS to relax.

○ If defecation is not desired, voluntary mediated contraction of the external anal sphincter (EAS) and LA muscles prevent passage of stool until the IAS tone returns.

○ If defecation is desired, voluntary mediated relaxation of the EAS and LA muscles allows straightening of the anorectal angle.

○ Further, perineal descent is facilitated by assuming a sitting or squatting position.

○ Passage of stool then occurs when a Valsalva maneuver is accompanied by a rectal contraction.

ETIOLOGY OF CONSTIPATION

• Constipation can occur for a large variety of reasons as any disease process that affects the structure, muscles, or nerves of the colorectal unit may cause a dysfunction in fecal transit time or of defecation.

• Impairment of large intestine transit can occur because of structural abnormalities, lifestyle problems, metabolic or endocrine disorders, neurological disorders, myopathic conditions, toxins or drugs, and idiopathic, functional disorders of the colon (see Tables 44-1 and 44-2).

• In the absence of alarm symptoms, the vast majority of patients with a complaint of constipation have an

TABLE 44-1 Possible Causes of Constipation in Adults

Structural abnormalities	Metabolic and endocrine disorders
Colonic stricture	
Intraabdominal adhesions	Pregnancy
Diverticular disease	Diabetes mellitus
Effects of radiation or ischemia	Thyroid disorders
Colon neoplasms	Hypopituitarism
Megacolon and megarectum	Hyperparathyroidism
Ogilvie's syndrome	Hypercalcemia
Cathartic colon	Hypokalemia
Fecal impaction	Porphyria
Anorectal disease	Pheochromocytoma
Anal fissure	Glucagonoma
Thrombosed hemorrhoids	
Perirectal abscess	**Neurological disorders**
	Hypoganglionosis
Lifestyle problems	Hirschsprung disease
	Chagas disease
Dehydration	Irritant laxative induced
Inadequate fiber intake	Multiple sclerosis
Inadequate toileting arrangements	Parkinson's disease
Inadequate exercise	Cerebrovascular accident
Autonomic neuropathy	Spinal cord injury
Prior pelvic surgery with disruption of parasympathetics	
Trauma to nervi erigentes	
Myopathic conditions	
Myotonic dystrophy	
Dermatomyositis	
Amyloidosis	
Ceroidosis	
Scleroderma	
Functional or idiopathic disorders	
Colonic inertia	
Rectal outlet obstruction	
Anismus	
Rectocele	
Rectal prolapse or intussusception	
Excessive perineal descent	
Constipation predominate IBS	

TABLE 44-2   Drugs That Constipate

Analgesics

Opiates and nonopiates
Anticholinergics

Antidepressants

Antihistamines
Antioveractive bladder drugs
Antiparkinsonian drugs
Antipsychotics
Antispasmodics
Neuroleptic agents

Antihypertensives

Calcium channel blockers
Clonidine

Cationcontaining agents

Aluminum
  Antacids
    Sucralfate
Barium sulfate
Calcium
  Antacids
    Supplements
Iron supplements

---

idiopathic, functional disorder affecting the colon or anorectum.
  ○ Alarm symptoms include abdominal pain, fever, hematochezia (occult or overt), unintended weight loss, or recent change in bowel habits.
• Consensus criteria for diagnosing functional constipation have been developed by an international panel of experts (Rome II Criteria).
  ○ Patient must report two or more of the following symptoms for at least 12 weeks in the past 12 months:
    ▪ Fewer than three bowel movements per week
    ▪ Greater than one-fourth of defecation associated with hard stool, sensation of incomplete evacuation, sensation of anorectal obstruction, or manual maneuvers required to facilitate defecation
    ▪ Insufficient criteria for irritable bowel syndrome (IBS)
• Functional or idiopathic constipation can be categorized into three subtypes depending on colonic transit and rectosphincteric studies.
  ○ Colonic inertia or slow-transit constipation is characterized by a prolonged delay in the transit of radiopaque markers through the proximal colon.
    ▪ Histological studies have shown decreased numbers of interstitial cells of Cajal, abnormalities in the enteric nerve ganglia, as well as abnormalities of the contractile properties of the colonic smooth muscle in these patients.
    ▪ Colonic inertia patients may also have esophageal dysmotility, delayed transit through the small bowel, and a high incidence of urinary bladder dysfunction.
      ▪ Arbuthnot Lane disease is a severe form of slow-transit constipation that almost exclusively affects young women. Reduced numbers of neurons in the colonic myenteric plexus are found on histology examinations. Since the neurological disorder is limited to the colon in these patients subtotal colectomy with ileorectal anastomosis can be dramatically beneficial.
  ○ Rectal outlet obstruction (aka dyschezia or spastic pelvic floor syndrome) is characterized by disability in emptying stool from the rectum. The radiopaque transit markers progress normally through the colon but stagnate in the rectum. Two recognizable causes for this type of constipation are as follows:
    ▪ Anismus or rectosphincteric dyssynergia is diagnosed when a patient is unable to relax the LA and EAS muscles when attempting to defecate. This results in impaired evacuation of the rectum. This may be learned behavior if the patient had an anal fissure and attempts at emptying a large stool were painful. It has also been linked with sexual abuse and psychiatric disorders. Treatment with biofeedback and counseling is usually beneficial.
    ▪ Pelvic floor relaxation with rectocele, excessive perineal descent, rectal prolapse, or intussusception can impede or obstruct stool passage. Patients report the need to manually assist defecation or perform vaginal splinting. Surgery to repair the rectal support abnormality is usually beneficial although underlying nerve or rectal muscle damage may inhibit regaining normal function.
  ○ Constipation with normal colonic transit is characterized by a group of patients with complaints of infrequent defecation yet are found to have no delay in passing radiopaque markers.
    ▪ 30% of patients who consult a physician for constipation have normal colonic transit.
    ▪ Almost all of these patients are women.
    ▪ Since the patients do not have abdominal pain they cannot be classified as having the constipation form of IBS yet their psychological profiles are similar. They often exhibit evidence of psychosocial distress. A high fibre diet coupled with an exercise and stress reduction programs is often beneficial.

EVALUATION OF CONSTIPATION

• History
  ○ Onset and duration of symptoms are important features.
    ▪ Recent change in bowel habits necessitates a workup for organic disorders.

- Complaints of many years duration are usually caused by functional or idiopathic disorders.
  ○ Nature of the symptoms is important to categorize the type of bowel dysfunction.
    - Are the complaints related to decreased frequency of stools, excessive straining, hard stools, or incomplete evacuation?
    - Decreased frequency suggests colonic inertia, neuropathy, or drug side effects.
    - Excessive straining, persistent rectal fullness, or the need for manual assisting defecation suggests rectal outlet obstruction.
    - Presence of abdominal pain or bloating along with constipation suggests IBS.
    - A stool diary can provide helpful information.
  ○ Are alarm symptoms such as fever, weight loss, or bloody stools present? These symptoms require a more extensive workup than functional symptoms alone.
  ○ Inquiries about toilet habits including time of day and duration of use are necessary.
  ○ Dietary habits and amounts of fluid intake and daily exercise are important features.
  ○ Questions about emotional distress and depression may establish contributing factors to the problem.
  ○ Inquiries about the patient's past obstetrical, medical, and surgical history may be contributory.
  ○ Complete review of both prescription and nonprescription medicines being taken and use of laxatives is essential.
  ○ Family history of GI disorders and parental views of "normal" bowel habits and need for laxatives are helpful.
- Physical examination
  ○ A search for non-GI diseases that can cause or worsen constipation should be done.
    - Diabetic neuropathy changes
    - Hyporeflexia, skin hair loss, or other signs of hypothyroidism
    - Paresis from spinal cord injuries or strokes
    - Evidence of autonomic disorders
  ○ Abdominal examination is an essential part of the physical findings.
    - A palpable mass suggests malignancy.
    - Distended bowel loops may be present in colonic inertia or megacolon.
    - Scars from previous surgeries should be noted.
  ○ Pertinent anorectal and perineal examination findings include the following:
    - Atrophy of gluteal or pelvic muscles
    - Abnormal location of the anal orifice
    - Presence of hemorrhoids or anal fissure
    - Perineal sensation and reflex contraction of anal canal after pin prick (anal wink)

- Digital rectal examination may reveal a rectal mass, fecal impaction, stenosis of the anal canal, hematochezia, and provide assessment of the tone and strength of the anal sphincter
- Gaping of the anal orifice following withdrawal of the examining finger suggests denervation of the EAS
- Examination done with the patient straining may detect presence of a rectocele, rectal prolapse, disorders of perineal descent, or signs of rectosphincteric dyssynergia
- Rectosphincteric dyssynergia is present when during a digital rectal examination the patient is asked to expel the examiner's finger and there is lack of posterior descent of the LA and perineum muscles as well as failure of the EAS to relax
- Diagnostic studies
  ○ Screening tests include complete blood count (CBC), Chem panel, glucose, calcium, and thyroid-stimulating hormone/thyroxine (TSH/T_4).
  ○ For suspicious cases, serum protein electrophoresis, urine porphyrins, parathyroid hormone, and cortisol levels can be done.
  ○ Flexible sigmoidoscopy should be done in patients aged 45 or older.
    - Lesions that occlude or narrow the rectosigmoid area can be seen.
    - Estimation of bowel diameter and displacement by rectocele can be determined.
    - Brown-black pigmented lesions called melanosis coli that result from long-term anthraquinone laxative use can be seen.
  ○ In patients with alarm symptoms, colonoscopy or barium enema radiography should be done to look for structural abnormalities such as neoplasms, diverticular disease, polyps, or megacolon.
- Studies of colonic and anorectal function
  ○ Tests of colonic motility and rectosphincteric function are usually reserved for patients with severe symptoms who have failed conservative therapeutic measures and have had structural abnormalities ruled out by colonoscopy or barium enema.
    - This group with intractable, functional constipation makes up only 1% of the total population of patients with constipation.
  ○ Colonic transit study is useful in patients with intractable constipation whose major complaint is infrequent defecation.
    - Patient swallows a single Sitz-Mark capsule (Konsyl Pharmaceuticals, Ft. Worth, TX) containing 24 radiopaque markers on day 1 followed by a single abdominal radiograph 5 days later (day 6 to 120 hours).

- Normal colonic transit time is about 35 h while transit times of >72 hours are significantly abnormal.
- If less than five markers are present then normal transit is diagnosed.
- If more than five markers are present then slow transit or colonic inertia is diagnosed.
- If more than five markers remain in the rectosigmoid area with near normal transit markers in the rest of the colon then rectal outlet obstruction is diagnosed.
- Balloon expulsion test provides an assessment of defecation ability.
  - A fecom (silicone-filled stool-like device) or Foley catheter (inflated with 50 mL of water) is inserted into the patient's rectum. After instructing the patient to expel the device without manual assistance the attendant starts a stopwatch and leaves the room.
  - Normal subjects expel the stool-like device within 1 min. Rectal outlet obstruction is diagnosed when the patient is unable to expel the device within 3 min.
- Defecography is a radiographic study of defecation that is helpful in patients who complain of excessive straining or who must use digital manipulation to facilitate evacuation.
  - Study involves instillation of 150 mL of barium paste of stool consistency into the rectum followed by fluoroscopic assessment of rectal evacuation while the patient sits on a specially designed commode.
  - Study allows for evaluation of anorectal angle at rest and with attempted defecation. In the presence of rectosphincteric dyssynergia the anorectal angle fails to open.
  - Anatomical abnormalities such as rectoceles and intussusceptions may also be diagnosed as the patient strains to defecate.
- Anorectal manometry provides an assessment of pressure within the rectum and anosphincteric region as well as information regarding rectal sensation, rectal compliance, and ability to relax the IAS during attempted expulsion of the apparatus.
  - Various types of devices including open-tipped perfused catheters, direct pressure transducers, or air-filled balloons are commercially available to perform these studies.
  - In normal subjects there is a reflex relaxation of the IAS when a balloon is distended in the rectum. In patients with Hirschsprung disease this reflex is absent.
  - Rectal compliance can be measured by sequentially inflating a balloon in the rectum and measuring pressures at each level of distention.

- Patients with megarectum have little sensation as their highly compliant rectum is distended, whereas patients with the constipation form of IBS have low compliance and tolerate rectal distention poorly.
- Anismus is diagnosed, if the anosphincteric pressure remains high during attempts at defecation.
- Dynamic pelvic MRI is emerging as a potentially valuable tool to evaluate anorectal function and anatomy in patients with pelvic outlet obstruction or dyssynergic defecation.

TREATMENT OF CHRONIC CONSTIPATION

- General principles
  - Although most patients with chronic constipation have an idiopathic or functional disorder of the bowels, a search for a secondary cause for the symptoms should be undertaken by performing the routine testing previously mentioned.
  - Drug side effects are the most common cause of constipation in the elderly. Drugs exert this effect by altering colonic motility, interfering with intrinsic colonic reflexes, over-dehydrating the stools, or by reducing the patient's awareness for stooling.
  - Timed toilet training is inexpensive, effective, and should be tried in all patients with constipation.
    - Consists of having patients attempt a bowel movement at least twice a day usually within 30 min after a meal to take advantage of the gastrocolic reflex.
    - Patients should push at a level of 5–7 out of 10 when attempting to defecate and strain no more than 5 min.
- Dietary modifications
  - An increase in fluid intake to 1500 mL/day may help.
  - Many patients claim improvement in their symptoms by drinking a warm, caffeinated beverage such as coffee or tea each morning.
  - An increase in dietary fiber to 20–30 g/day is the first line of therapy.
    - Fruits, vegetables, and bran cereals/bran powder are excellent sources of dietary fiber.
    - Fiber supplements such as methylcellulose and psyllium are derived from vegetable matter and are available over-the-counter (OTC). Polycarbophil is a synthetic fiber that may be less gas producing.
- Pharmacological therapy (see Table 44-3)
  - The regular use of laxatives (with the exception of bulk-forming fiber) should be avoided if possible.
  - If general measures and fiber supplementation fails then a daily dose of an osmotic laxative is the next

TABLE 44-3   Oral Agents for the Treatment of Chronic Constipation

LAXATIVES	DOSAGE	ONSET OF ACTION (h)	SITE AND MECHANISM OF ACTION
Osmotic laxatives			
Lactulose (Cephulac)	15–30 mL/day	24–48	Colon; nonabsorbable sugar
Sorbitol 70%	15–30 mL/day	24–48	Colon; nonabsorbable sugar
Polyethylene glycol (MiraLax)	17 g in 8 oz fluid/day	48–96	GI tract, hyperosmolar nonabsorbable
Magnesium hydroxide (Milk of Magnesia)	30 mL/day	$1/_2$–3	Colon, saline osmotic, also increases peristalsis
Sodium phosphate (Fleet phospho-soda)	20–30 mL/day	$1/_2$–3	Colon, saline osmotic
Emollient laxatives			
Mineral oil (Agoral)	15–45 mL/day	24–72	GI tract, softens stool
Docusate (Colace)	100–400 mg/day	24–72	GI tract, detergent stool softener
Stimulant laxatives			
Bisacodyl (Dulcolax)	5–15 mg/day	6–10	Colon, increases motility and fluid content
Castor oil (Purge)	15–30 mL/day	4–8	Colon, increases motility and fluid content
Cascara	325 mg/day	6–10	Ileum and colon, increases fluid and electrolyte content
Prokinetic drugs			
Colchicine	0.6 mg tid	24–48	Colon, increases motility and fluid content
Misoprostol (Cytotec)	100–200 µg tid	12–24	Colon, increases motility
Tegaserod (Zelnorm)	6 mg bid	24–48	GI tract, serotonin agonist
Naloxone (Narcan)	2 mg tid	12–24	Colon, binds to opioid receptors, increases motility

line of therapy as they have minimal risks even with long-term usage.
- Saline laxatives are the next line of therapy if the above fails.
  - Hypermagnesemia may result in patients with impaired renal function.
- Emollient laxatives are given to promote stool softening.
  - Caution for use of mineral oil in patients with esophageal dysmotility or dysphagia as lipid pneumonitis can occur with aspiration.
  - Since mineral oil interferes with absorption of the fat soluble vitamins it should be given between meals.
- Stimulant laxatives are given if all of the above fail. Concern about damage to the enteric nervous system with development of cathartic colon with long-term usage exists.
  - Phenolphthalein was reclassified by Food and Drug Administration (FDA) as "not generally recognized as safe or effective" in 1997 when a study showed an increase of neoplasms in rodents given this agent.
- Prokinetic agents are drugs that stimulate intestinal motility.
  - Metoclopramide has been used to treat upper GI motility disorder but has little effect on the colon and is not helpful in treatment of constipation.
  - Cisapride had been shown to enhance colonic motility but was withdrawn by the FDA due to the risk of cardiac toxicity.
  - Cholinergic agents that are currently available have not been generally effective for constipation.

- Colchicine has been shown in limited studies to be effective in treatment of refractory constipation.
- Misoprostol has been shown to be effective for some patients with slow-transit constipation.
- Tegaserod (and other 5-HT$_4$ agonists) stimulates intestinal motility by enhancing enteric cholinergic transmission. It is approved in United States for treatment of constipation predominant form of IBS.
- Naloxone is an opioid receptor antagonist that may improve intestinal motility by inhibiting the effect of either endogenous or exogenous opioids on the bowel.
- Biofeedback therapy
  - For patients with dyssynergic defecation, biofeedback with neuromuscular conditioning gives symptomatic improvement in 60–80%.
    - Patients are initially taught diaphragmatic breathing techniques so that improved abdominal pushing efforts can be achieved.
    - Using a visual or auditory feedback signal from the electromyography (EMG) reading of the EAS patients are then taught to relax the pelvic floor in synchrony with their pushing efforts during simulated defecation.
    - Manometric techniques to improve impaired rectal sensation provide additional therapeutic benefits.
- Surgical interventions
  - Except in cases of documented structural abnormalities, surgery should be considered as a last resort for patients with chronic constipation.
  - Rectosphincteric dyssynergia

- Injection of botulinum toxin into the EAS or LA muscles in patients with anismus and dyssynergic defecation has shown some benefits.
- Myectomy or posterior division of the LA muscles has not been found to be beneficial and may cause fecal incontinence.
  - Rectal intussusception and prolapse
    - Abdominal rectopexy with partial resection and reanastomosis of the sigmoid is successful in relieving intussusception but may not relieve the constipation.
    - An endorectal pull-through technique with transanal resection of the prolapsed segment of rectum through a dilated anus followed by a sigmoid-anal anastomosis can effectively treat the prolapse but may not relieve the constipation.
  - Rectocele
    - Because these are commonly found in nonconstipated subjects, care must be taken in advising patients about the expected benefit of repair if their only symptom is constipation.
    - Patients who report improvement in defecation with vaginal splinting are expected to get the most benefit from surgical repair of the rectocele.
  - Colonic inertia
    - Refractory patients who have failed aggressive medical therapy and have incapacitating symptoms may have dramatic benefit from colectomy with ileorectal anastomosis.
    - Motility studies of the upper GI tract must be done preoperatively to ensure that the problem is confined to the colon and that a generalized neuromuscular dysfunction of the gut is not present.
    - Segmental resection of the colon often produces unsatisfactory results in these patients and is associated with a high rate of anastomotic leaks.
  - Hirschsprung disease
    - Surgical resection of the aganglionic segment of colon is the treatment of choice for all forms of this disease.
    - In patients with ultrashort-segment disease a relaxing incision into the IAS and portion of the rectal smooth muscle (anal myotomy) may be all that is necessary to achieve successful results.

TREATMENT OF ACUTE CONSTIPATION IN ADULTS

- Can occur in response to acute surgical or medical illness, medications, and ingestion of toxins, dietary changes, or travel.

  - Therapies previously described for chronic constipation may be insufficient to achieve prompt defecation in acute cases.
  - Therapies used for relief of acute constipation must not be given in cases of bowel obstruction or fecal impaction.
- Osmotic laxatives
  - These agents exert an osmotic effect to increase intraluminal water content.
  - Produce results within 3 hours and are less likely to cause intestinal cramps than stimulant laxatives.
  - Magnesium citrate: 150–300 mL orally.
  - Magnesium hydroxide (Milk of Magnesia): 30 mL (2400 mg) orally.
  - Magnesium sulfate (Epsom salts): 10–30 g orally.
  - Sodium phosphate (Fleet): 20–45 mL (15–30 g) orally.
  - Polyethylene glycol (Golytely): 240 mL orally every 10 min until 1–4 L is consumed.
  - Glycerin suppository: 3 g rectal suppository.
- Stimulant laxatives
  - These agents stimulate intestinal secretions and colonic motility.
    - Defecation usually results within 60 minutes of rectal administration and within 8 hours of oral ingestion.
    - May cause diarrhea and painful intestinal cramps.
    - For short-term use only as they may result in loss of normal colonic neuromuscular function (cathartic colon).
  - Bisacodyl (Dulcolax): 10 mg rectal suppository or 10–15 mg orally.
  - Cascara: 4–8 mL of aromatic fluid extract or 325 mg tablet orally.
  - Castor oil (Purge): 15–30 mL or 30–60 mL of emulsified castor oil orally.
- Enemas
  - Often best to treat severe acute constipation with an enema first before giving laxatives.
  - Work within a few minutes.
  - Sodium phosphate (Fleet): one adult enema per rectum.
  - Tap water: 500–1000 mL per rectum.
  - Saline: 120–240 mL per rectum.
  - Mineral oil retention: 120 mL per rectum.

Bibliography

Anti M, Pignataro G, Armuzzi A, et al. Water supplementation enhances the effect of high fiber diet on stool frequency and laxative consumption in adult patients with functional constipation. *Hepatogastroenterology.* 1998;45:727.

Bassotti G, Chistolini F, Sietchiping-Nzepa F, et al. Biofeedback for pelvic floor dysfunction in constipation. *BMJ.* 2004;328(7436): 393–396.

Burkitt DP, Walker ARP, Painter NS. Effect of dietary fiber on stool and transit times and its role in the causation of disease. *Lancet.* 1972;2:1408.

Corazziaria E, Badiali D, Bazzocchi G, et al. Long term efficacy, safety and tolerability of low daily doses of isosmotic polyethylene glycol balanced solution (PMF-100) in treatment of functional chronic constipation. *Gut.* 2000;46: 522.

Douglas J. Constipation overview: evaluation and management [Review]. *Curr Womens Health Rep.* 2002;2(4):280–284.

Dukas S, Willett WC, Giovannucci EL, et al. Association between physical activity, fiber intake, and other lifestyle variables and constipation in a study of women. *Am J Gastroenterol.* 2003;98(8):1990–1996.

Gamss JS. Motility disorders in the elderly. In: Gelb AM, ed. *Clinical Gastroenterology in the Elderly.* New York: Marcell Dekker; 1996;115–132.

He CL, Burgart L, Wang L, et al. Decreased interstitial cells of Cajal volume in patients with slow transit constipation. *Gastroenterology.* 2000;30:176.

Higgins J, Johanson JF. Epidemiology of constipation in North America: a systematic review. *Am J Gastroenterol.* 2004;99(4): 750–759.

Hinds JP, Stoney B, Wald A. Does gender or the menstrual cycle affect colonic transit? *Am J Gastroenterol.* 1989;84:123.

Joo JS, Agachan F, Wolff B, et al. Initial North American experience with botulinum toxin for treatment of anismus. *Dis Colon Rectum.* 1996;39:1107–1111.

Kearney DJ. Approach to the patient with gastrointestinal disorders. In: Friedman SL, McQuaid KR, Grendehl JH, eds. *Current Diagnosis and Treatment in Gastroenterology.* 2nd ed. New York: Lange Medical Books; 2003;20–26.

Knowles CH, Scott SM, Lunniss PJ, et al. Outcome of colectomy for slow transit constipation. *Ann Surg.* 1999;230: 627.

Knowles CH, Scott SM, Rayner C, et al. Idiopathic slow transit constipation: an almost exclusively female disorder. *Dis Colon Rectum.* 2003;46(12):1706–1717.

Koch TR, Carney JA, Go VL, et al. Idiopathic chronic constipation is associated with decreased vasoactive intestinal peptide. *Gastroenterology.* 1990;98:1219–1225.

Lembo A, Camiileri M. Chronic constipation. *N Engl J Med.* 2003;349(14):1360–1368.

Locke GR III, Pemberton JH, Phillips SF, et al. American Gastroenterological Association Medical position statement: guidelines on constipation. *Gastroenterology.* 2000;119: 1761–1778.

Muller-Lissner S. What has happened to the cathartic colon? *Gut.* 1996;39:486.

Prather CM, Camilleri M, Zinsmeister AR, et al. Tegaserod accelerates orocecal transit in patients with constipation-predominant irritable bowel syndrome. *Gastroenterology.* 2000;118(3): 463–468.

Ramkumar D, Rao S. Chronic constipation: systematic review. *Am J Gastroenterol.* 2005;100:936–971.

Rao SSC. Constipation: evaluation and treatment. *Gastroenterol Clin North Am.* 2003;32:659–683.

Roy AJ, Emmanuel AV, Storrie JB, et al. Behavioral treatment (biofeedback) for constipation following hysterectomy. *Br J Surg.* 2000;87(3):100–105.

Sloots CE, Meulen AJ, Felt-Bersma FJ, et al. Rectocele repair improves evacuation and proleptic complaints independent of anorectal function and colonic transit time. *Int J Colorectal Dis.* 2003;18(4):342–348.

Talley NJ. Management of chronic constipation. *Rev Gastroenterol Disord.* 2004;4(1):18–24.

Verne GN, Davis RH, Robinson ME, et al. Treatment of chronic constipation with colchicine: randomized, double-blind, placebo controlled, cross over trial. *Am J Gastroenterol.* 2003;98(5):1112–1116.

Wald A. Approach to the patient with constipation. In: Yamada T, Alpers DH, Owyang C, et al., eds. *Textbook of Gastroenterology.* 4th ed. Philadelphia, PA: Lippincott Williams and Wilkins; 2003;894–910.

Waldron D, Bowes KL, Kingma YJ, et al. Colonic and anorectal motility in young women with severe idiopathic constipation. *Gastroenterology.* 1988;95:1388.

Wofford SA, Verne GN. Approach to patients with refractory constipation. *Curr Gastroenterol Rep.* 2000;2:389.

QUESTIONS

1. A 63-year-old $G_8P_7A_1$ diabetic female had total vaginal hysterectomy/bilateral salpingoopherectomy (TVH/BSO)/high uterosacral ligament colposuspension/anterior and posterior colporrhaphy (A&P repair) done 2 days ago for uterovaginal prolapse. She is to be discharged home today, but first wants relief of pelvic pressure and left flank pain. She attributes pain symptoms to her constipation. Being an excellent junior resident wanting to impress your senior who did the surgery, you order

   (A) magnesium hydroxide (Milk of Magnesia): 30 mL PO now

   (B) tap water enema: 750 mL per rectum now

   (C) acute abdominal x-ray series STAT

   (D) serum glucose, electrolytes with blood urea nitrogen/creatinine (BUN/Cr), and bladder scan STAT

2. A 34-year-old $G_2P_0A_2$ complains of chronic abdominal pain, intermittent bloating, and infrequent stooling. Her symptoms have worsened since her second spontaneous abortion 3 months ago. The most likely cause for her constipation is

   (A) colonic inertia

   (B) megarectum

(C) constipation-predominant IBS

(D) rectosphincteric dyssynergia

3. A 40-year-old $G_3P_2A_1$ presents to your office with complaints of chronic constipation despite adding fiber supplements to her diet. Physical examination is normal except for a moderate rectocele. The best way to determine if the rectocele is contributing to her constipation is

(A) barium enema x-ray series

(B) defecography

(C) anorectal manometry

(D) colon transit study

ANSWERS

1. *(D).* Choice A may be the correct answer for most patients with postoperative constipation symptoms, but in light of the potential renal insufficiency from Kimmelstiel-Wilson disease and potential ligation of left ureter causing her left flank pain, ingestion of magnesium is contraindicated at this time. Choice B may be able to correct her constipation, but could also potentially break down the posterior colporrhaphy so is not advisable. Choice C may give some information about feces in the colon, but does not help with determining if she has left ureteral obstruction or urinary retention which are the more likely cause of her symptoms than is constipation. Choice D will answer the most important questions about the cause of her left flank pain and pelvic pressure. Constipation is seldom an emergency and there are more potentially serious causes of her symptoms that need evaluation first.

2. *(C).* Colonic inertia or slow-transit constipation does not usually cause pain and bloating unless it is severe. Psychosocial problems are not associated with this type of constipation. Megarectum occurs when there is an overly compliant rectum with loss of rectal sensation causing chronically worsening distention of the rectum with constipated stool. It is not associated with abdominal pain or bloating. Constipation-predominant IBS fits her history and symptoms best. Episodes of psychosocial stress or anxiety can cause the symptoms to worsen. Rectosphincteric dyssynergia causes inappropriately long time spent straining to defecate. It does not usually cause abdominal pain or bloating. It can be associated with psychosocial stress reaction, however.

3. *(B).* Barium enema x-ray series is chiefly used to look for structural abnormalities of the colon and does not provide much information about rectal outlet obstruction related to rectocele. Defecography is the best way to evaluate if feces are being trapped in the rectocele pouch. If the patient is asked to perform vaginal splinting during the study and is then able to defecate easily the rectocele is most certainly contributing to her constipation problem. Anorectal manometry measures pressures within the anus and rectum but gives very little information concerning functional obstruction caused by a rectocele. Colon transit study may help somewhat if the radiopaque markers are found stagnating in the rectum but does not conclusively prove that the rectocele is responsible for the rectal outlet obstruction.

45 MULTIPLE SCLEROSIS

Fatta B. Nahab

INTRODUCTION

- Multiple sclerosis (MS) is a chronic autoimmune disease of the central nervous system (CNS), which leads to myelin destruction in discrete areas (called lesions) over time. A clinical diagnosis of MS requires the dissemination of CNS lesions in space and time.
- Onset is typically between 20 and 40 years of age in 70% of people with twice as many women affected as men. Approximately 10% of cases occur in the pediatric population, while 20% may occur in older age groups.
- The cause of MS is not known, though susceptibility to developing MS seems genetically determined with an environmental trigger.
- The genetic susceptibilities are not entirely known though individuals that are positive for the human leukocyte antigen (HLA) DR2 allele appear to be more susceptible.
- Environmental factors provide additional interesting risk factors for MS, with the number of hours of sunlight being inversely related to disease prevalence. This may explain the geographic variation in MS prevalence, with those populations at highest risk (>30/100,000) being at higher latitudes such as Northern and Central Europe and those populations at lowest risk (<5/100,000) residing in the African continent, Asia, the Caribbean, Mexico, and northern South America.

SUBTYPES

- Four main subtypes of MS exist to describe the disease course and also convey prognostic and therapeutic value: Relapsing-remitting (RRMS), relapsing-remitting with secondary progression (SPMS), primary progressive (PPMS), and progressive relapsing (PRMS).
- RRMS is the most common subtype (80–85% of all MS patients) characterized by obvious attacks (called exacerbations or relapses) lasting for days to weeks followed by complete or near-complete remission. As RRMS progresses, 50% of cases within 10 years and 90% of cases within 25 years will go on to become SPMS, evident by continued disease disability with less exacerbations and remissions.
- PPMS makes up about 10–15% of all cases and has a slowly progressive course without obvious exacerbations.
- PRMS are an even smaller minority with less than 5% of all MS patients having slow but continuous progression with superimposed relapses.

PATHOPHYSIOLOGY

- The pathogenesis of MS appears to be an organ-specific autoimmune attack causing injury to myelin, damage to its cell of origin (the oligodendrocyte), as well as damage to the underlying axon.
- MS is characterized by a combination of demyelination (more common in RRMS) and axonal damage (primary pathology in PPMS) to brain and spinal cord white matter structures.
- The areas most susceptible to injury include tissues bordering the lateral ventricles and fourth ventricle, periaqueductal tissue, the corpus callosum, the optic nerves/chiasm/tracts, and spinal cord structures such as the anterior and dorsal columns.
- Damage to myelin and the underlying axon occurs as a result of activated T cells in the peripheral blood crossing the blood-brain barrier, entering the CNS, and secreting immune mediators such as cytokines and chemokines. Activated T cells appear to be specific to myelin basic protein (MBP) or other myelin proteins. What initiates this T-cell activation is unknown, though hypotheses of molecular mimicry from underlying viral infection have been suggested.
- More recent work suggests four main patterns of pathology, two of which are primarily inflammatory and spare oligodendrocytes, and two of which lead to oligodendrocyte death. The more inflammatory pathologies may be the underlying mechanisms leading to RRMS, which

is primarily demyelinating, while oligodendrocyte death may underlie the pathology of other MS subtypes, which tend to have more axonal damage.

DIAGNOSTIC STUDIES

- A revised criteria (called the McDonald Criteria) for the diagnosis of MS was published in 2001 by a panel of experts and continues to be the basis for making a diagnosis. It is important to note that cerebrospinal fluid (CSF) studies are no longer mandatory, compared with past recommendations.
- It is important to understand what constitutes an "attack" or exacerbation when making the diagnosis or deciding on treatment. Based on the International Panel on MS diagnosis recommendations, an attack is a neurologic disturbance which lasts for at least 24 hours. An attack may include any of the following: optic neuritis, disturbance of extraocular muscle function (e.g., internuclear ophthalmoplegia or third nerve palsy), trigeminal neuralgia, dysarthria, dysphagia, focal weakness, cerebellar ataxia, or neurogenic bladder among others. Note: Nonspecific sensory symptoms such as tingling and numbness in isolation should be excluded as an attack since these symptoms are habitually present and variable in the areas involved (Table 45-1).

TREATMENT

- No prevention or cure for MS is currently available.
- Treatment paradigms center on two main purposes: providing faster resolution of symptoms during an acute attack *and* minimizing long-term disability from MS progression.
- Treatment of acute MS exacerbations: Recommendations by the American Academy of Neurology regarding the management of optic neuritis in MS are commonly generalized to include any type of exacerbation. These guidelines recommend the use of intravenous methylprednisolone, which has been shown in studies to be superior to oral prednisone, to decrease recovery time following an attack, and increase the time to next relapse.
- Disease-modifying drugs for MS: In addition to treating acute attacks, patients now have an additional category of medications which aim to minimize the number of attacks. Interferon β-based agents (Avonex, Betaseron, Rebif) and glatiramer acetate (Copaxone) have been shown to decrease the rate of relapse. Such a reduction

TABLE 45-1   McDonald Criteria for the diagnosis of Multiple Sclerosis

CLINICAL PRESENTATION	ADDITIONAL DATA NEEDED FOR MS DIAGNOSIS
Two or more attacks; objective clinical evidence of two or more lesions	None*
Two or more attacks; objective clinical evidence of one lesion	Dissemination in space demonstrated by MRI, or Two or more MRI lesions consistent with MS plus positive CSF,† or Await further clinical attack implicating a different site
One attack; objective clinical evidence of two or more lesions	Dissemination in time demonstrated by MRI, or Second clinical attack
One attack; objective clinical evidence of one lesion (clinically isolated syndrome)	Dissemination in space demonstrated by MRI, or Two or more MRI lesions consistent with MS plus positive CSF† And Dissemination in time, demonstrated by MRI, or Second clinical attack
Insidious neurological progression suggestive of MS	Positive CSF, and dissemination in space, demonstrated by (1) Nine or more T2 lesions in brain, or (2) Two or more lesions in spinal cord, or (3) Four to eight brain lesions plus one spinal cord lesion; or Abnormal visual evoked potentials, and MRI demonstrating four to eight brain lesions, or fewer than four brain lesions plus one spinal cord lesion; or Dissemination in time demonstrated by MRI; or Continued progression for 1 year

ABBREVIATION: MRI, magnetic resonance imaging.
*Brain MRI is recommended to exclude other etiologies.
†Positive CSF defined as oligoclonal bands different from those in serum, or raised immunoglobulin G (IgG) index.

in relapse rate could in theory minimize long-term disability, though studies to date have not conclusively shown any delay in progression of disability. Serious side effects can occur with these agents and it is important to review this information before starting any such medication.

PROGNOSIS

• In patients with RRMS, SPMS, and PRMS, the frequency of relapses is about 0.5 relapses per patient per year.
• Relapse frequency is highest in young patients and during the early stages of MS.
• Poor prognostic variables include the following:
  ◦ Older age at disease onset (>40 years)
  ◦ Presentation with prominent motor, cerebellar, and/or sphincter dysfunction
  ◦ Frequent relapses during the early years of MS
  ◦ Short interval between first relapses
  ◦ Incomplete remissions
  ◦ Rapid progression of disability
  ◦ A diagnosis of PPMS or rapid time of conversion from RRMS to SPMS
• Rates of disability are highly variable between patients and various subtypes. However, population data suggest

that the median time to impaired ambulation (requiring an assistive device such as a cane or walker) is approximately 15–20 years.
• MS impact upon life expectancy has been reported as a reduction of 4–14 years depending on the study, with 50% of patients eventually dying from medical complications of the disease.

IMPACT ON PREGNANCY

• Based on a large multicenter prospective observational study, the yearly rate of MS relapse was 0.7 ± 0.9 prior to pregnancy, with a dramatic reduction to 0.2 ± 1.0 relapses/year during the first trimester, and a postpartum increase to 1.2 ± 2.0 relapses/year prior to returning to baseline within several months. Despite the variation in relapse rates, the overall rate of disability was unaffected by pregnancy.
• The Pregnancy in Multiple Sclerosis (PRIMS) study also found no additional risk of relapse or disability associated with epidural analgesia or breastfeeding.
• Overall, MS does not seem to have any significant negative impact on pregnancy, childbirth, or the fetus.
• The safety profiles of Avonex, Betaseron, Copaxone, and Rebif are not entirely known in pregnancy. Avonex,

Betaseron, and Rebif have a Pregnancy Category C rating with possible abortifacient effects in animal studies at doses above those recommended in humans. Copaxone has a Pregnancy Category B rating with no adequate trials in pregnant women. It is not known whether any of these agents are excreted in breast milk. Methylprednisolone has a Pregnancy Category B rating. Women with RRMS planning a pregnancy should be informed about the potential teratogenicity of the various agents and should be advised to discontinue using any immunomodulator agent during the pregnancy, noting the risk of relapse is much lower. Due to the increased postpartum risk of relapse, it is, however, recommended that the immunomodulator agent be restarted soon after delivery.

- Should a woman experience an MS relapse during pregnancy, it would be acceptable to treat with a short course of methylprednisolone to shorten the exacerbation.

UROGYNECOLOGIC ISSUES IN MULTIPLE SCLEROSIS

- Bladder dysfunction is a common and early symptom complaint in all subtypes of MS. Symptoms of urgency, frequency, or urinary incontinence may suggest a hyper-reflexic bladder, while symptoms of bladder fullness, a feeling of incomplete emptying, or hesitancy suggest a flaccid bladder causing retention.
- With a high incidence of bladder dysfunction, it is important that anytime a patient reports such symptoms or even other unrelated symptoms of MS that they be evaluated for a urinary tract infection (UTI). An MS relapse can be mimicked by any infection which can exacerbate symptoms from an old relapse. A simple urinalysis should be performed anytime bladder dysfunction is suspected or the patient reports new symptoms, which could be attributed to a relapse. Frequent UTIs may require further urologic evaluation.
- Symptoms of bladder hyper-reflexia can be treated with anticholinergics such as oxybutynin, propantheline, or imipramine.
- The extent of bladder flaccidity should be assessed with ultrasound to measure postvoid residual volume. Residuals in excess of 15 mL are abnormal, with patients having residuals >100 mL requiring intermittent self-catheterization. Symptoms can be minimized with the use of bethanechol. Chronic indwelling catheters should be avoided to minimize the risk of infection.
- Detrusor-sphincter dyssynergia (DSD) may occur following the interruption of spinal cord pathways involved in micturition. In this disorder, bladder hyper-reflexia along with incoordination of the detrusor-

sphincter reflex leads to the simultaneous contraction of the external urethral sphincter and bladder causing problems such as vesicoureteral reflux and exacerbating underlying incontinence. DSD is diagnosed by cystometrography and can be treated with anticholinergics, alpha-1 blockers, and/or intermittent catheterization.

BIBLIOGRAPHY

Beck RW. The optic neuritis treatment trial: three-year follow-up results. *Arch Ophthalmol*. 1995;113:136–137.

Bronnum-Hansen H. Survival in disseminated sclerosis in Denmark. A nation-wide study of the period 1948–1986. *Ugeskr Laeger*. 1995;157:7131–7135.

Confavreux C, Hutchinson M, Hours MM, et al. Rate of pregnancy-related relapse in multiple sclerosis. *N Engl J Med*. 1998;330:285–291.

Confavreux C, Vukusic S, Adeleine P, et al. Pregnancy and multiple sclerosis (the PRIMS study): two-year results [abstract]. *Neurology*. 2001;56:A197.

Kaufman DI, et al. Practice parameter: the role of corticosteroids in the management of acute monosymptomatic optic neuritis. Report of the quality standards subcommittee of the American Academy of Neurology. June 2001.

Litwiller SE, Frohman EM, Zimmern PE. Multiple sclerosis and the urologist [Review]. *J Urol*. 1999;161(3):743–757.

McDonald WI, Compston A, Edan G, et al. Recommended diagnostic criteria for multiple sclerosis: guidelines from the International Panel on the Diagnosis of Multiple Sclerosis. *Ann Neurol*. 2001;50:121–127.

O'Connor P. Key issues in the diagnosis and treatment of multiple sclerosis, an overview. *Neurology*. 2002;59(Suppl. 3):S1–33.

Refer to Physicians' Desk Reference for up-to-date information.

Sadovnick AD, Ebers GC, Wilson RW, et al. Life expectancy in patients attending multiple sclerosis clinics. *Neurology*. 1992;42:991–994.

Weinshenker BG, Bass B, Rice GP, et al. The natural history of multiple sclerosis: a geographically based study. I. Clinical course and disability. *Brain*. 1989;112:133–146.

Weinshenker BG, Bass B, Rice GP, et al. The natural history of multiple sclerosis: a geographically based study. II. Predictive value of the early clinical course. *Brain*. 1989;112: 1419–1428.

QUESTIONS

1. Which of the following MS symptoms is not indicative of an acute MS exacerbation?
   (A) Two-day onset of urinary retention
   (B) Six-hour onset of monocular blurred vision

(C) One-day onset of bilateral arm paresthesias

(D) Three-day history of left-sided weakness

(E) Twelve-hour onset of diplopia

2. A confirmatory diagnosis of MS requires the following:

(A) CSF oligoclonal bands and a brain MRI showing one MS plaque

(B) An attack consistent with MS with brain MRI showing 10 MS plaques

(C) An attack consistent with MS with CSF oligoclonal bands

(D) No definite history of attacks, but brain MRI showing three plaques and CSF oligoclonal bands

(E) Two confirmed attacks consistent with MS over a 1-year period

3. Which of the following agents is recommended for treating the symptoms of bladder spasticity?

(A) Terazosin

(B) Oxybutynin

(C) Bethanechol

(D) 4-Aminopyridine

(E) Amantadine

4. A 35-year-old woman presents to your office with an acute attack of right optic neuritis. The agent you would start to minimize the duration of the relapse is

(A) Methylprednisolone

(B) Prednisone

(C) Glatiramer acetate

(D) Interferon β-1a

(E) Mitoxantrone

5. A 42-year-old G3P3 woman with a 12-year history of relapsing-remitting MS presents with symptoms of overflow incontinence. A postvoid residual of 65 mL is found by ultrasound. Which of the following medications can be used to minimize symptoms:

(A) Propantheline

(B) Terazosin

(C) Imipramine

(D) Oxybutynin

(E) Bethanechol

ANSWERS

1. *(C)*. Acute onset of urinary retention (especially in a young patient), monocular blindness or blurred vision (optic neuritis), focal weakness (from brain or spinal cord MS plaques), and new-onset diplopia (most commonly an internuclear ophthalmoplegia from an MS plaque in the medial longitudinal fasciculus) are all suggestive of a new MS exacerbation. With new symptoms of shorter duration, it is necessary to follow the patient for at least 24 hours for confirmation of a true relapse. Symptoms such as paresthesias or dysesthesias are nonspecific, waxing and waning, and do not qualify alone as signs of MS relapse.

Anytime a new relapse is suspected, it is important to ensure that symptoms are not simply from an acute infection (most commonly UTI), which has exacerbated symptoms associated with old MS plaques. With the high rate of bladder dysfunction in MS, the frequency of UTIs is higher than the population, with some individuals requiring chronic prophylactic antibiotics. If no infection is found, a 5-day course of intravenous methylprednisolone is indicated to shorten the duration of relapse.

2. *(E)*. The basic guideline for making a diagnosis of MS requires the occurrence of lesions over space and time. The clinician must establish the presence of MS by history and/or data (plaques on brain or spinal cord MRI, oligoclonal bands in CSF, prolonged visual evoked potentials with a history of optic neuritis) in addition to showing a temporal course of relapses at least 1 month apart. Choices A–C provide data suggestive of a demyelinating etiology such as MS without showing temporal course of relapse. Choice D could be suggestive of a more insidious demyelinating disease such as primary progressive MS, but has too few brain lesions on MRI to make a confirmatory diagnosis. Choice E provides a history of two relapses separated by a period of 1 year, which is adequate to make a diagnosis of relapsing-remitting MS.

3. *(B)*. Symptoms in MS patients suggestive of bladder spasticity include urinary urgency, frequency, or incontinence. Treatment is directed at minimizing spasticity by using anticholinergic agents (oxybutynin, propantheline, imipramine), or GABAergic agents such as baclofen and the benzodiazepines. Alpha-1 blockers such as terazosin are useful for the treatment of DSD and the associated abnormal external urethral sphincter contraction. Bethanechol is useful in the treatment of a flaccid bladder by stimulating the parasympathetic nervous system to increase detrusor tone. 4-Aminopyridine is a potassium channel blocker, which has been found in MS patients to improve temperature sensitivity. Amantadine is an antiviral agent, which may work to inhibit NMDA receptors. Amantadine is commonly used in MS patients for relief of fatigue.

4. *(A)*. Current guidelines recommend the use of intravenous methylprednisolone in doses of 500–1000 mg daily for 5 days for the treatment of an MS relapse. In comparative trials, prednisone was not found to be as effective as methylprednisolone for reducing recovery time and increasing time to next relapse. Glatiramer acetate and interferon β-1a are both disease-modifying injectable drugs which have been shown to modestly decrease the number of relapses over time. These agents are not indicated for the acute treatment of an MS exacerbation. Mitoxantrone is a chemotherapeutic agent which has been found to reduce relapse rate and disease progression in patients with primary and secondary progressive MS. Mitoxantrone causes DNA cross-linking and strand breaks, interferes with RNA synthesis, and DNA repair. Long-term therapy is limited due to cardiotoxicity in large cumulative doses.

5. *(E)*. This woman with symptoms of overflow incontinence underwent ultrasonography to measure her postvoid residual. Although the residual is abnormal, this patient is not likely to require intermittent self-catheterization at this time. Propantheline, imipramine, and oxybutynin are all anticholinergic agents which are used in the setting of bladder spasticity to minimize abnormal contractions. Alpha-1 adrenergic blockers such as Terazosin work to block sympathetic outflow to smooth muscle fibers in the bladder neck, which can limit urine outflow. Bethanechol is recommended in mild-to-moderate bladder flaccidity in order to stimulate parasympathetic outflow to the bladder. This leads to increased tone of the detrusor urinae muscle, which can produce contractions sufficient to initiate urination and optimize bladder emptying.

46 PSYCHOLOGICAL ISSUES RELATED TO INCONTINENCE AND PELVIC ORGAN PROLAPSE
Elizabeth Dameff

BACKGROUND

- The prevalence of urinary incontinence in women living in the ambulatory American community ranges from 10 to 40%.

- There is less information about fecal incontinence than urinary incontinence, but it appears to have an even greater stigma and shame associated with it.
- This disease not only affects these women physically, but also psychosocially.
- Many of these women also suffer from depression, anxiety, sexual dysfunction, and social isolation.
- The literature is inconsistent in demonstrating whether urge or stress incontinence is associated with more psychological issues.

EARLY DEVELOPMENT

- At 2 years of age, children begin to realize that they can control when and what they eat, when they sleep, and when they urinate and defecate.
- This is an important stage of development and gives them a sense of independence.
- Later in life many elderly adults develop incontinence and lose this sense of independence and control.
- This can have implications on their emotional and mental well-being.

INFORMING HEALTHCARE PROVIDERS

- Although urinary incontinence appears to be a prevalent problem in the elderly population, fewer than half of them report their symptoms to their healthcare provider.
- There are a variety of reasons for not consulting their healthcare provider.
  ○ Embarrassment
  ○ Not having enough information about treatment options
  ○ Low expectations from the treatment options available
  ○ The ease of purchasing absorbent products
- It is important as a healthcare provider to question not only about urinary incontinence, but also how it affects the patient's quality of life.

PSYCHOLOGICAL IMPLICATIONS OF URINARY AND FECAL INCONTINENCE

- The symptoms associated with urinary incontinence have implications on the activities of daily life, social relationships, and self-esteem.
- Many experience increased levels of anxiety and depression.
- Others harbor feelings of embarrassment, shame, disgust, anger, apathy, guilt, denial, indignity, and feeling of abandonment.

- Some believe that life is not worth living because of their urinary symptoms.
- Many often feel isolated from family and friends.
  ○ Others withdraw from all social contact.
  ○ It may restrict their normal activities (e.g., shopping, traveling, chores, and hobbies).
  ○ Some remain at home to be near the toilet to avoid loss of urine and or feces in public.
- There can be negative effects on sexuality and spousal relationships.
  ○ Many patients with incontinence are elderly females who at their age already have vaginal atrophy and lack of lubrication. The incontinence is an added inconvenience for sexual intercourse.
  ○ Urinary incontinence during penetration is more common with stress urinary incontinence.
  ○ Urinary incontinence during orgasm is more common with urge incontinence.
  ○ There is frequently dyspareunia in patients with urethral diverticula.
  ○ There may be a fear of fecal incontinence during intercourse.
  ○ Some patients who never enjoyed sexual intercourse use the incontinence as an excuse to avoid intercourse.
- There is often a burden on the caregiver.
  ○ Institutionalization of the elderly frequently occurs once bowel and/or bladder control is compromised.
  ○ There is the potential for abuse and neglect.
  ○ The family may develop economic worries associated with the incontinence.
  ○ The family sometimes has impaired intrapersonal relationships because of association with the incontinent member.
- Even healthcare professionals may develop negative feelings toward the patient with incontinence due to feelings of extra care and responsibility.

RESEARCH OF PSYCHOSOCIAL SYMPTOMS AND URINARY INCONTINENCE

- There have been a variety of studies done on women with urinary incontinence and its psychosocial impact.
- Chiverton et al. (1996) found a strong relationship between depression and low self-esteem with urinary incontinence.
  ○ The incidence of depression in the general population was approximately 6%.
  ○ The incidence of depression of the subjects with urinary incontinence was 22%.
- Berglund et al. (1994) found a higher level of somatic and psychic anxiety in incontinent patients when compared with controls.

- One study found a 50% increase in the risk of symptoms of anxiety associated with those with urinary incontinence.
- Fonda et al. (1995) found statistically significant improvements in the subjective quality of life measures (which included depression, social isolation, and embarrassment) after treatment of urinary incontinence.
- Rosenzweig et al. (1991) found that sleep disturbances and tension significantly improved after therapy for urinary incontinence.

NEUROLOGICAL DIFFERENTIAL DIAGNOSIS OF INCONTINENCE

- There are transient causes of incontinence (DIAPPERS) as well as neurological and psychiatric diseases that are associated with incontinence.
  ○ Delirium may present with transient incontinence.
  ○ Multi-infarct dementia is sometimes associated with incontinence.
  ○ Normal pressure hydrocephalus is a triad consisting of cognitive impairment, gait disturbance, and urinary incontinence.
  ○ Seizures frequently result in incontinence.

PSYCHIATRIC DIFFERENTIAL DIAGNOSES ASSOCIATED WITH INCONTINENCE

- It is important to properly diagnose these patients' psychological disorders in order to offer them the most effective treatment.
- The most common psychological disorders that frequently coexist with urinary incontinence are depression and anxiety (based on retrospective studies).
- Personality inventory questionnaires showed higher anxiety scores in incontinent woman than in controls.

DIFFERENTIAL DIAGNOSIS OF DEPRESSION

- *Major depressive disorder*: DSM-IV criteria is five of the following nine symptoms that present daily for at least 2 weeks:
  ○ Depressed mood most of the day, particularly in the morning
  ○ Markedly diminished pleasure in almost all activities nearly everyday (anhedonia)
  ○ Significant weight loss or gain
  ○ Insomnia or hypersomnia
  ○ Psychomotor agitation or retardation

- Fatigue or loss of energy
- Feelings of worthlessness or guilt
- Impaired concentration, indecisiveness
- Recurrent thoughts of death or suicide
- *Minor depression*: Two to four of the nine depressive symptoms that present daily for at least 2 weeks.
- *Dysthymia*: Classified by anhedonia, low self-esteem, and low energy present for two consecutive years.
- *Grief and bereavement*: A normal response to the loss of a close relationship that normally resolves within 13 months of the loss. These patients frequently show symptoms of depression; however, the difference being that most of these symptoms will resolve within approximately 13 months of the loss.

DIFFERENTIAL DIAGNOSIS OF ANXIETY

- *Generalized anxiety disorder*: Excessive anxiety and worry about a number of activities that occurs more days than not for at least 6 months, that are out of proportion to the likelihood or impact of feared events.
- The anxiety and worry are associated with at least three of the following symptoms:
  - Restlessness or feeling keyed up or on edge
  - Being easily fatigued
  - Difficulty concentrating or mind going blank
  - Irritability
  - Muscle tension
  - Sleep disturbances
- *Panic attacks*: A discrete period of intense fear in which at least four of the following symptoms develop abruptly and peak within 10 min:
  - *Cardiopulmonary symptoms*: chest pain, shortness of breath, or palpitations
  - *Neurological symptoms*: trembling, paresthesias, or feeling dizzy
  - *Psychiatric symptoms*: derealization, fear of loosing control, or fear of dying
  - *Autonomic symptoms*: sweating, or chills or hot flashes
  - *Gastrointestinal symptoms*: feeling of choking, nausea, or abdominal distress
- *Social phobia*: A fear of social situations in which the person fears that he or she will act in a way that will be humiliating or embarrassing. Exposure to this social situation produces an immediate anxiety response, which may present as a panic attack. The avoidance or distress in the feared social situation interferes significantly with the person's normal routine or relationships with others.
- *Somatization disorder*: History of many physical complaints beginning before the age of 30 that happen over several years and results in the seeking of treatment.

- All of the following are present at any time during the course of the illness:
  - Four pain symptoms
  - Two gastrointestinal tract symptoms
  - One pseudoneurological symptom
  - One sexual symptom

TREATMENT FOR DEPRESSION

- There is evidence showing that treating urge incontinence by bladder retraining improved the psychiatric symptoms associated with incontinence, regardless of the actual response of the bladder to the treatment.
- It appears as if treating the incontinence improves quality of life for many patients. However, we must also consider treating the depression and anxiety that may accompany the incontinence.
- There are a variety of treatment options for depression
  - Pharmacological options
    - *Selective serotonin reuptake inhibitors (SSRIs)*: Most recent medication class that is used most commonly since they have the least amount of serious side effects.
      - Paroxetine (Paxil)
      - Fluoxetine (Prozac)
      - Sertraline (Zoloft)
      - Citalopram (Celexa)
      - Escitalopram (Lexapro)
  - *Tricyclic antidepressants (TCAs)*: Should be used with caution in the elderly since side effects include orthostatic hypotension and confusion. However, this class may improve certain types of incontinence.
    - Amitriptyline (Elavil)
    - Desipramine (Norpramin)
    - Doxepin (Adapin, Sinequan)
    - Imipramine (Tofranil)
    - Nortriptyline (Pamelor)
  - *Monoamine oxidase (MAO) inhibitors*: Not first-line medication due to severe hypertension if ingestion of tyramine-containing foods (certain cheeses, wine, and beer) and their drug/drug interactions.
    - Phenelzine (Nardil)
    - Tranylcypromine (Parnate)
  - Psychotherapy
    - Behavior therapy
    - Cognitive-behavioral therapy
    - Interpersonal therapy

TREATMENT FOR ANXIETY

- Pharmacological options
  - Benzodiazepines
    - Alprazolam (Xanax)

- Clonazepam (Klonopin)
- Diazepam (Valium)
- Lorazepam (Ativan)
- Oxazepam (Serax)
  - Antidepressants (SSRIs, TCAs, and MAO inhibitors)
- Psychotherapy
  - Behavioral therapy
  - Cognitive-behavioral therapy
  - Applied relaxation therapy

BIBLIOGRAPHY

Chiverton CA, Wells TJ, Brink CA. Psychological factors associated with urinary incontinence. *Clin Nurse Spec.* 1996;10(5):229–233.

Dugan E, Cohen SJ, Bland DR, et al. The association of depressive symptoms and urinary incontinence among older adults. *J Am Ger Soc.* 2000;48(4):413–416.

Fonda D, Woodward M, D'Astoli M. Sustained improvement of subjective quality of life in older community-dwelling people after treatment of urinary incontinence. *Age Ageing.* 1995;24:283–286.

Fricchione G. Clinical practice. Generalized anxiety disorder. *N Engl J Med.* 2004;351:675.

Kapczinski F, Lima MS, Souza JS, et al. Antidepressants for generalized anxiety disorder. *Cochrane Database Syst Rev.* 2003;(2):CD004592.

Miner PB Jr. Economic and personal impact of fecal and urinary incontinence. *Gastroenterology.* 2004;126(1):S8–S13.

Mulrow CD, Williams JW Jr, Chiquette E, et al. Efficacy of newer medications for treating depression in primary care patients. *Am J Med.* 2000;108:54.

Rosenzweig BA, Hischke D, Thomas S, et al. Stress incontinence in women: psychological status before and after treatment. *J Reprod Med.* 1991;36(12):835–838.

Snow V, Lascher S, Mottur-Pilson C. Pharmacologic treatment of acute major depression and dysthymia. *Ann Intern Med.* 2000;132:738.

Williams JW Jr, Mulrow CD, Chiquette E, et al. A systematic review of newer pharmacotherapies for depression in adults: evidence report summary. *Ann Intern Med.* 2000;132:743.

QUESTIONS

1. A 79-year-old female, whose only medical problem is mild dementia, has been having increased episodes of not being able to make it in time to the restroom without urinating on herself. She also has occasional loss of her urine when she coughs. Due to the above occurrences she is feeling not only frustrated, but also very sad. She does not eat as much as she used to, has difficulty sleeping, and feels constantly fatigued. Which of the following medications might help the above urinary symptoms as well as her psychiatric disturbance?
   (A) fluoxetine (Prozac)
   (B) amitriptyline (Elavil)
   (C) nefazodone (Serzone)
   (D) sertraline (Zoloft)
   (E) paroxetine (Paxil)

2. A 74-year-old female with a history of mixed urinary incontinence presents to your office for an evaluation. She feels distressed because every time she goes into a crowded grocery store, she feels her hears "start racing." She also starts sweating, feels nauseous, and has shortness of breath. For the past 6 months her daughter must do the grocery shopping, since the patient does not want to leave the house. Which of the following medical conditions does the patient most likely have?
   (A) generalized anxiety disorder
   (B) somatization disorder
   (C) social anxiety manifested by panic attacks
   (D) a cardiac arrhythmia

3. Since the birth of her fourth child 18 months ago, a 45-year-old female has struggled with losing her urine while coughing, laughing, and with excessive exercise. It is interfering in so much of her daily activities that she does not want to leave her house. She rarely sleeps through the night, constantly feels tired, has lost approximately 20 lb in the past year, feels worthless, and finds it difficult to concentrate. Which of the following psychiatric diagnosis does she have?
   (A) major depressive disorder
   (B) postpartum depression
   (C) dysthymia
   (D) grief and bereavement
   (E) minor depression

4. Which of the following is a transient cause of urinary incontinence?
   (A) normal pressure hydrocephalus
   (B) delirium
   (C) multi-infarct dementia
   (D) seizure
   (E) urinary incontinence due to the aging process

5. A 68-year-old patient with a history of stress incontinence and newly diagnosed major depression will be taking a trip to France this summer for a tour of French wineries. Which medication is associated

with a serious side effect that could be life threatening to the patient?

(A) phenelzine

(B) paroxetine

(C) amitriptyline

(D) sertraline

ANSWERS

1. *(B)*. Fluoxetine (choice A) is an SSRI. This classification of medications can help with both depression and anxiety, however, does not improve the symptoms of urinary incontinence. Amitriptyline (choice B) is a TCA. This classification of medications will likely improve her symptoms of depression. TCAs are also anticholinergic medications that may cause urinary retention, which may actually improve her urge incontinence symptoms. However, this classification of medications must be used with caution in the elderly since it may cause confusion and/or orthostatic hypotension. Nefazodone (choice C) is a MAO inhibitor. This classification of medications is very rarely used in the United States due to the risk of serious side effects, the most serious being hypertensive crisis. Urinary retention is not one of the side effects. Sertraline (choice D), like fluoxetine, is an SSRI. It may help the depression but not the incontinence. Paroxetine (choice E), like fluoxetine and sertraline, is also an SSRI.

2. *(C)*. The patient's symptoms only occur in public places and she has cardiopulmonary symptoms (shortness of breath and heart palpitations), autonomic symptoms (sweating), and gastrointestinal symptoms (nausea). Generalized anxiety disorder (choice A) is a diagnosis based on anxiety occurring on more days than not for at least 6 months; however, it is not only situational anxiety. Somatization disorder (choice B) includes a history of many physical complaints that occur over several years, but it usually presents before the age of 30 and is not situational. Cardiac arrhythmia (choice D) is possible, but unlikely, since the palpitations are situational and since she has noncardiac symptoms, such as sweating and nausea.

3. *(A)*. The patient has five of the nine symptoms that have been present for well over 2 weeks. Her symptoms include: insomnia, fatigue, weight loss, feelings of worthlessness, and impaired concentration. Postpartum depression (choice B) usually resolves within a few weeks. Dysthymia (choice C) is classified by anhedonia, low self-esteem, and low energy. The symptoms have to be present for 2 years to meet the diagnostic criteria. The patient has only had her symptoms for 18 months. Patients with grief and bereavement (choice D) do show signs of depression; however, this is usually after a traumatic life event (such as a death or serious illness). Also these symptoms will resolve within approximately 13 months of the event. Minor depression (choice E) only needs two to four of the nine depressive symptoms.

4. *(B)*. People with delirium sometimes also have episodes of urinary or fecal incontinence; however, this usually resolves when the delirium passes. Normal pressure hydrocephalus (choice A) is a triad of gait disturbance, cognitive impairment, and urinary incontinence. The urinary incontinence usually does not resolve without treatment. Multi-infarct dementia (choice C) affects many elderly patients. Urinary incontinence is not always associated with this disease, but when it occurs, it usually does not resolve without treatment. During seizures (choice D), bowel or bladder function may be compromised. Although the prevalence of urinary incontinence increases with age, it is not a part of the normal aging process (choice E).

5. *(A)*. Phenelzine is a MAO inhibitor, which may have severe hypertension when ingesting tyramine. This is one of the earlier classes of antidepressants but is not used as much due to its severe side effects. Paroxetine (choice B) is an SSRI that does not have interactions with tyramine and can safely be used in this patient. Amitriptyline (choice C) is a TCA that can be used in this patient. Sertraline (choice D) is also an SSRI that can be used in this patient.

47 DYSPAREUNIA AND CHRONIC PELVIC PAIN OF URINARY TRACT ORIGIN

Elaine Hart and Sam Siddighi

INTRODUCTION

• Chronic pelvic pain (CPP) and dyspareunia are diagnostic and therapeutic challenges.
  ◦ They both have a long differential diagnosis

- Patients can be difficult.
- It can be frustrating for the physician (especially specialists).
- They require extra time and effort to evaluate.
- They can be refractory to treatment.
- CPP may be best dealt with by the primary care physician and referrals should be made for complex cases.
- Dyspareunia requires a detailed physical examination and attention to certain anatomic areas.
- In this chapter, we will mainly discuss dyspareunia and CPP of urinary tract origin. We will also briefly discuss pelvic floor muscle and abdominal wall pain, which are often associated.
- Interstitial cystitis (IC) is also described from a different perspective in Chap. 26, Interstitial Cystitis, Urethral Syndrome, and Sensory Urgency-Frequency Syndrome.

EVALUATION OF DYSPAREUNIA AND CPP

- A thorough history and a gentle examination can be therapeutic and revealing.
- It is crucial to perform the physical examination from the most comfortable to the least comfortable evaluation. Save the most uncomfortable part of the examination for last.
- A full history and physical examination (H&P) is described in Chap. 5, Evaluation of Pelvic Organ Prolapse (POP) and Chap. 6, Evaluation of Urinary Incontinence in the Office and Indications for Referral to a Specialist. The following are some *highlights* of the H&P for dyspareunia and CPP:
  - History
    - Sexual history (see Chap. 49, Female Sexual Dysfunction)
    - Abuse history
    - Concurrent medical condition(s)
    - Depression
  - Physical examination
    - Try to duplicate pain by palpation
    - Map the location of pain on an anatomic drawing
    - Order in which the examination should be performed:
      - Abdominal wall → vulva → perineum → vagina → pelvic floor → → urethra → bimanual → rectovaginal → speculum (Table 47-1)
- Selected studies are appropriate to rule out (r/o) other conditions that can mimic CPP.
  - **Complete blood count** (CBC), erythrocyte sedimentation rate (ESR) (rule out infection, chronic PID)
  - Urinalysis (UA), urine culture and sensitivity (UC&S)
  - Gonorrhea and Chlamydia (rule out acute PID)
  - Ultrasound (especially if pelvic examination was difficult or unrevealing)
  - Sigmoidoscopy (especially change in bowel habits)

DIFFERENTIAL DIAGNOSIS DYSPAREUNIA AND CHRONIC PELVIC PAIN

- Note: The **bold** diagnoses below are common while the *italicized* ones are rare.
  - Gynecologic origin
    - **Endometriosis**
    - Vulvar vestibulitis (aka vulvodynia)
    - **Vaginismus**
    - **Atrophic vaginitis**
    - *Lichen sclerosus*
    - PID
    - Dysmenorrhea
    - **Adenomyosis**
    - Pelvic adhesions
    - Large leiomyomas
    - *Ovarian remnant syndrome*
  - Gastrointestinal origin
    - Irritable bowel syndrome
    - Chronic constipation
    - Inflammatory bowel disease
  - Musculoskeletal origin
    - *Separation of symphysis pubis*
    - *Osteitis pubis*
    - Abdominal wall scar (even if they look completely innocent)
    - **Abnormal muscle activity** (**myofascial pain**; trigger points)
      - Pelvic floor tension myalgia (aka coccygodynia)
      - Obturator internus
      - Rectus abdominis (usually at insertion of muscle into pubic bone)
      - Quadratum lumborum
  - Urinary tract origin
    - **IC**
    - Urinary tract infection (UTI)
    - Overactive bladder
    - Urethral syndrome
    - *Stones*
    - *Urethral diverticula*
    - *Tumor*
  - Other causes
    - Fibromyalgia
    - *Scar neuroma (episiotomy, obstetric laceration, posthysterectomy cuff)*
    - *Pudendal nerve neuralgia (existence is controversial)*
    - Referred pain from hip or low back

TABLE 47-1 Diagnosis and Management of Pelvic Pain

ANATOMIC AREA	EXAMINATION	DIAGNOSIS	COMMENTS	MANAGEMENT
Abdominal wall	Straight leg test	Abdominal wall trigger points	Have patient tighten abdominal muscles by flexing straight leg at hip or doing a "crunchie." If pain is elicited during these maneuvers then diagnosis is abdominal wall myalgia rather than intraperitoneal pathology	Injection of local anesthetic/steroid combination into trigger point, physical therapy
Vulva	Observe, palpate	Lichen sclerosus, Lichen planus, Bartholin's gland		Lichen (clobetasol or fluocinonide topical), ± dilators
Vulva (between hymen and Hart's line)	Cotton swab	Vulvar vestibulitis		Antidepressants, surgical removal of vestibular skin
Perineum	Palpate episiotomy or obstetrical laceration scar	Scar neuroma	May have pain on initial penetration, severe tenderness in scar	Injection with local anesthetic/steroid, surgical removal of scar
Vagina	Palpate and perform 1-finger pelvic examination	Vaginismus, vaginitis, vaginal cuff scar	Pain, tightness, spasm of bulbocavernosusm.	Vaginismus (gradual dilation, lubrication, see Chap. 49, Female Sexual Dysfunction), vaginitis (treat accordingly), vaginal cuff scar (treated same way as scar neuroma [above])
Pelvic floor	1-finger massage of pelvic floor lateral to sacrum	Pelvic floor tension myalgia	Massage will reproduce patient's symptoms; Kegel will make symptoms worse	Reverse Kegel, heat, pillows, injections (see full description below)
Bladder and urethra	Palpate bladder, milk urethra	IC, urethral diverticulum		IC described in detail in this chapter; Urethral Diverticula (see Chap. 28)
Bimanual examination	Two fingers in vagina and opposite hand on abdomen	Cervical, uterine (e.g., adenomyosis), adnexal, and bladder pathology	BME is a routine part of the annual gynecologic examination	
Rectovaginal examination	Uterosacral ligaments nodularity, rectovaginal septum, cul-de-sac scarring, foreign bodies	Endometriosis, PID, previous urethral sling or colpopexy mesh		Endometriosis, oral contraceptive pill (OCP), medroxyprogesterone acetate (MPA), leuprolide, lapararoscopic fulguration, hysterectomy), PID (antibiotics, hysterectomy), sling or mesh removal
Speculum examination	Observation	Atrophy, discharge, lesions	Speculum examination is largest and least comfortable part of pelvic examination	Local estrogen cream, antibiotics, antifungal, antiviral,surgical excision?

ABBREVIATIONS: BME, Board of Medical Examiners; PID, pelvic inflammatory disease.

CONCEPTS IN PAIN MANAGEMENT

- A primary painful insult may create a secondary or tertiary pain response that lingers even after primary insult is removed. Why? Secondary and tertiary pain is created by the central nervous system (similar to phantom limb phenomenon).
  - For example, a simple UTI → chronic suprapubic pain
  - In IC patients, previously innocent bladder filling → now perceived as painful
- Sometimes patients develop bad behaviors to cope with their pain. These behaviors can lead to development of new pain.
  - Dysuria or urgency → chronic contraction of pelvic floor muscles → abnormal muscle activity and dyspareunia
- Sensory pain disorders are affected by cyclic hormone fluctuations. Therefore, a CPP patient can have flares around time of menses.
- Chronic pain states are best treated with a combination of therapies (physical therapy, behavioral therapy, analgesics, other oral agents, injection, psychological support, and so forth).

PREVALENCE OF CHRONIC PELVIC PAIN

- Defined as pain in the pelvis lasting at least 6 months.
- One in seven women will experience this.
- One-third of women have CPP sometime in their lifetime.
- Nine to fifteen million women in the United States have CPP.
- Fifteen percent of adult women seek treatment for this.
- Five to ten percent of laparoscopies and 10% of hysterectomies are done for this.
- Twelve percent of gynecologic operative referrals are for this.
- No gynecologic pathology found in approximately 60% of laparoscopies performed for CPP.
- May have direct cost of $880 million dollars in the United States.
- Majority of women with CPP are premenopausal.

PAIN RELATED TO ABNORMAL MUSCLE ACTIVITY

- Pelvic floor tension myalgia or coccygodynia is an involuntary spasm of the pelvic floor muscles.
- Patient may experience the following:
  - Pelvic pressure and fullness
  - Aching pain in pelvis
  - Pain worsened by sex
  - Pain worsened by sitting for long periods
  - Pain worsened by bowel movements
- Treatment may involve several things.
  - It can be treated with physical therapy by a trained pelvic floor physical therapist (may take 3 months of weekly visits)
    - Mobilization of scars
    - Desensitization
    - Deep heat with ultrasound
    - Increase range of motion, stretching, and relaxation of levator ani and perineal muscles (i.e., opposite of Kegel)
  - Horseshoe-shaped pillow to sit on → redistributes pressure from body weight away from pelvic and perineal muscles
  - Painful trigger points should be identified, massaged, injected with steroid + local anesthetic combinations
- Avoid pelvic floor muscle exercises (Kegel) as they may worsen symptoms.
- Often patients with IC will also have tenderness of abdominal wall, pelvic floor, and hip girdle musculature.
- This may be because of lowering of pain thresholds.
- Many of the pain syndromes are associated with each other. For example fibromyalgia and vulvodynia are both associated with IC.

HAVE HIGH INDEX OF SUSPICION FOR INTERSTITIAL CYSTITIS WHEN WOMEN SEEK GYNECOLOGIC CARE

- Women with CPP are more likely to consult a gynecologist than any other specialty.
- Two most common reasons women seek care are abnormal bleeding and pelvic pain.
- In patients presenting with cyclic or noncyclic CPP or with urinary frequency and urgency, suspect IC.
- Many patients with overactive bladder have sensory urgency that does not respond to anticholinergic agents which may point to a potential diagnosis of IC.
- Patients with recurrent UTIs may not be infected but instead be having IC symptom flares only.
- Premenstrual pain or dysmenorrhea; 18% of women with IC experienced fluctuations of symptoms during the menstrual cycle.
- Dyspareunia and/or pain surrounding intercourse is a common symptom of IC.
- History or a suspicion of endometriosis.

INTERSTITIAL CYSTITIS AS A CAUSE OF CHRONIC PELVIC PAIN

- In the majority of patients, neither the patient nor the physician recognizes the bladder as the source of symptoms.
- One in four to five women have CPP of bladder origin.
- Studies show that endometriosis, UTI, and vulvodynia may actually be IC.
- IC can mimic symptoms of other causes of CPP.
- Pathogenesis is unknown; thought to be multifactorial.

DEFINITION OF INTERSTITIAL CYSTITIS

- Progressive disorder characterized by intermittent or persistent pelvic or perineal pain with or without urinary frequency, urgency, or nocturia in the absence of other identified pathology such as infection or bladder cancer.

SYMPTOMS OF INTERSTITIAL CYSTITIS

- Pain can be perceived in the vagina, perineal area, inguinal region, labia, lower abdomen, lower back, or medial aspect of the thighs.
- Pain may or may not worsen with bladder filling or emptying; may just remain the same.
- Usually very volume sensitive.
- Most women report an increase in pelvic pain 1 week before menses.
- Some have dysmenorrhea.
- Pain also common in both men and women before, during, or after sexual intimacy.
- During flares, patients may experience stress-urge incontinence and/or a slow urinary stream.
- Can void up to 60 times per day and up to 12 times per night (high-frequency and low-voided volumes are characteristic).
- Patients with IC on average void 16.5 times per day compared to normal healthy women who void 6.5 times per day.
- Symptoms may be exacerbated by particular foods or beverages, stress, or allergic conditions.
- Can be chronic and debilitating if severe.

PREVALENCE OF INTERSTITIAL CYSTITIS

- According to the World Health Organization: IC can occur in women or men, in any age or race including children or the elderly.

- Majority are White premenopausal females.
- Median age at diagnosis is 42–46.
- In 1994, the Nurses health study identified 52 cases per 100,000 and in 1995, 67 per 100,000.
- Greater than 100,000 Americans have the severe form.
- One to two million of Americans have a mild form.
- Far more common than previously thought.

DIAGNOSIS OF INTERSTITIAL CYSTITIS

- No single definitive test that conclusively confirms diagnosis of IC.
- Difficult to diagnose and treat and is often overlooked as a cause of CPP.
- Also greatly underestimated.
- High rate of comorbidity with diseases such as endometriosis and vulvodynia.
- Ability to masquerade as other diseases such as UTI or endometriosis leading to frequent misdiagnosis.
- First manifestation of the disease is usually in the thirties, diagnosis made in forties, although flare cycle may have begun in teenage years and been misdiagnosed as UTIs.
- Usually 5–7 years before diagnosis is established.
- On average, a patient will visit eight clinicians before a diagnosis is reached.
- Important to obtain both sexual and urinary history.
- UA and culture can r/o UTI.
- Cytology can r/o bladder cancer.
- Voiding log; eight or more voids in 24 hours consistent with IC.
- Pelvic pain and urgency/frequency (PUF) is a questionnaire that helps with the diagnosis.
- IC symptom index and problem index; questionnaire designed to measure lower urinary tract symptoms in patients with IC.

PELVIC PAIN AND URGENCY/FREQUENCY

- Simple patient symptom questionnaire.
- Identifies patients early on with a bladder component to their CPP.
- 8-Question symptom scale that assists in the differential diagnosis; only takes 5 minutes to complete.
- Focuses on pain and urologic symptoms characteristic of IC including symptoms associated with sexual intercourse and how much the patient is bothered by the symptoms.
- Score of greater than or equal to 15 out of a maximum of 35 is a definite sign of bladder as source of CPP.

- Bladder etiology as a cause of CPP can be ruled out for a score of <3.
- Recent study suggests that any patient scoring 5 or greater has a 57% chance of having IC.
- Patients with a score of 5–9 are in a median range and are then candidates for a potassium sensitivity test (PST).

PHYSICAL EXAMINATION

- May have anterior vaginal wall/bladder base tenderness, pelvic floor spasm, rectal spasm, or suprapubic tenderness.
- Gently palpating the bladder and urethra underneath the anterior vaginal wall may reproduce the symptoms of IC.
- PE can r/o vaginitis, vulvodynia, urethral diverticula, pelvic floor dysfunction, and uterovaginal prolapse.
- IC can not only coexist with any of the above but can also cause them.

POTASSIUM SENSITIVITY TEST

- Highly specific test enabling the physician to recognize a bladder-origin problem in symptomatic patients with IC.
- Minimally invasive office-based procedure.
- Measures the epithelial permeability of the bladder.
- Healthy patients do not respond with pain/urgency to bladder instillation of H_2O or KCl; sensitivity to potassium is an abnormal state.
- Positive test is highly suggestive of IC; definitive sign that CPP has a bladder component.
- False positives are extremely rare.
- Also positive in radiation cystitis and acute bacterial cystitis.
- About 70–90% of patients with IC have a positive PST.
- Recent studies demonstrated that 81–85% of gynecology patients who present with CPP have a positive PST despite other initial diagnosis.
- Negative PST does not r/o IC.
- Involves very slow introduction of 40 mL of room temperature sterile water into the bladder through a thin catheter over a 2–3-minute period.
- Establishes a baseline of pain perception and urgency upon bladder filling using a 0–5 point scale; 5 being the most severe pain.
- Water is left in the bladder for 5 minutes, then emptied, then 40 mL of KCl is instilled and patient is asked to reevaluate the level of pain and/or urgency.

- If no immediate reaction, solution can be held in the bladder for up to 5 minutes.
- Any increase of greater than or equal to 2 points over baseline for pain or urgency is a positive PST as long as the water causes no pain.
- Rapid recovery time in minutes but can cause immediate discomfort and flare-ups of the disease but symptoms usually subside within minutes.

CYSTOSCOPY

- Should be performed routinely on any patient with microscopic or gross hematuria.
- Can be performed in the office or operating room with a rigid or flexible cystoscope.
- Not required to diagnose IC.
- Most patients with IC have no lesions visible upon routine inspection of the bladder.
- May have the presence of diffuse petechial hemorrhages called glomerulations or Hunner's ulcer/patch, with distension and redistension of the bladder.
- Petechial hemorrhages can be present in normal women.
- May also have fibrosis.
- Glomerulations occur in the presence of pelvic pain, urgency, frequency with or without nocturia.
- Maximum bladder capacity can be assessed under anesthesia.
- Small bladder capacity supports diagnosis of IC.
- Maximum bladder capacity is inversely proportional to presence of Hunner's patch.
- In summary, cystoscopy is not as useful as history for the diagnosis of IC.
- <1% of patients will have disease with the classic sign of Hunner's ulcers visualized.

CORRELATION OF PUF SCALE AND PST

- Studies have demonstrated a strong correlation between these two diagnostic modalities.
- Ninety-one percent of patients with PUF > 20 have a positive PST as do 74% of patients with a PUF score of 10–14 and 55% of patients with PUF score >5.
- Eighty-four percent of patients with a score of 15 or greater on the PUF scale will have a positive PST.
- Control patients generally have low PUF scores <2% and 0% positive PST results.
- High correlation between these may enable clinicians to minimize use of the PST for patients with lower PUF for diagnostic purposes.

WHY IC IS SO EASY TO MISDIAGNOSE

- Even though the pain of IC originates in the bladder, it may be perceived in several other pelvic locations such as the lower abdomen, lower back, vagina, vulva, labial, urethral, and inguinal area.
- Substance P can be transmitted along C fibers to peritoneal cavity or vestibule.
- Close relationship of dyspareunia and IC possibly due to close proximity of bladder to vagina or the common embryologic endodermal derivation of the vestibule and bladder trigone.

PRINCIPLES OF TREATING INTERSTITIAL CYSTITIS

- Treat epithelium, allergies, and neural upregulation.
- For young patients with a short disease duration, treatment usually is necessary for 6–8 weeks to 4–6 months.
- Patients with long-standing disease usually require much longer treatment.
- Often best to treat for 1.5 months for every year that patient has had IC.
- IC can usually be effectively managed using a multimodal approach with Pentosyn Polysulfate sodium (PPS) as the basis of treatment.

TREATMENT OF INTERSTITIAL CYSTITIS

- PPS orally (100 mg tid) or per bladder instillation.
- Bladder instillation with dimethyl sulfoxide (DMSO).
- Intravesical administration of heparin sulfate or PPS although not FDA approved.
- Flares can be treated with instillation of an anesthetic therapeutic relief solution of heparin or PPS combined with sodium bicarbonate or lidocaine.
- Antihistamines such as hydroxyzine (25 mg qhs) can alleviate nocturia and aid sleeping and help patients with allergic flares.
- Analgesics; nonsteroidal anti-inflammatory drug (NSAIDs) may release histamine, thus, should be used with caution as they may exacerbate IC.
- Antispasmodics such as hyoscyamine sulfate.
- Tricyclic antidepressants such as amitriptyline (10–25 mg qd/bid) may help with neuropathic pain.
- Anticholinergics may help patients with severe urgency and frequency.
- Antiepileptic agents such as gabapentin (100–500 mg tid).
- Hormone therapy such as gonadotropin releasing hormone (GnRH) analogues with add-back or oral contraceptive pills even if standard therapies for IC have failed.

NONPHARMACOLOGIC TREATMENT OF INTERSTITIAL CYSTITIS

- Bladder training to gradually increase the interval in between voiding to 3–4 hours.
- Physical therapy to teach pelvic floor relaxation exercises and biofeedback to relax the pelvic floor muscles.
- Dietary changes such as eliminating caffeine, spices, foods high in acidity, and artificial sweeteners.
- Smoking cessation as nicotine appears to exacerbate the symptoms.
- Warm sitz bath, heating pads, or ice packs especially after coitus.
- Psychological counseling to deal with the chronic pain and quality-of-life issues can improve response rates.
- Sacral neuromodulation may be helpful for some patients.

PENTOSYN POLYSULFATE SODIUM

- PPS was approved by the FDA in 1996.
- Effective and safe oral treatment for pain and urgency symptoms.
- Specifically targets and repairs the damaged urothelium.
- Plant derived, cross-linked, semisynthetic polysaccharide with a xylan backbone.
- Heparin-like compound similar to the glycosaminoglycans (GAG) produced in the urinary epithelium.
- Acts primarily by replenishing a defective GAG layer, buffering to control cell permeability, and prevent irritating solutes from affecting epithelial cells.
- FDA recommended dose is 100 mg three times a day.
- In early disease, relief may occur in 6–8 weeks, but 2–4 months is usually required for pain relief in the majority of patients.
- Minimum of 3–6 months of treatment necessary for oral PPS to exert its effect, repair the defect, and provide relief.

DIMETHYL SULFOXIDE

- Was the only FDA-approved treatment from 1978 until 1996.
- Bladder instillation with DMSO is an intravesical therapeutic option.

- Invasive but moderately effective and safe; increases bladder capacity for most patients.
- Antiinflammatory analgesic with muscle-relaxing properties.
- Mechanism underlying efficacy unknown but it appears to increase reflex firing of pelvic nerve efferent axons and increase bladder capacity.
- Also increases neuronal expression of the immediate early gene c-fos in specific spinal cord regions.
- Releases nitric oxide from afferent neurons and inhibits mast cell secretion.
- Administered and retained in the bladder for 15 minutes in the outpatient setting once per week or every other week for 6–8 weeks.
- Response usually evident within 3–4 weeks of a 6–8-week cycle.
- Affords patients partial but rarely complete remission; majority of patients require additional treatment courses.

OTHER INTRAVESICAL AGENTS

- Heparin sulfate, hyaluronic acid (HA), botulinum toxin, capsaicin, and resiniferatoxin (RTX) have been used or are under investigation for management of IC.
- Heparin, a natural bladder epithelium protects the bladder against bacterial invasion by an antiadherence action component.
- Heparin can be used as both monotherapy or in combination therapy; reduces bladder irritative symptoms by correcting the mucosal defect.
- Heparin may offer greater symptom relief than DMSO as it may have a greater dose-dependent effect on blocking adenosine triphosphate (ATP).
- Heparin is administered intravesically 10,000 units in 10 mL of sterile water three times per week for 3 months with remission in over 50% of patients, and remission is maintained if therapy is continued for 3–9 months.
- HA, available in Canada and some European countries is thought to temporarily replace the defective mucosal lining of the bladder.
- RTX also is not yet available in the United States; similar to capsaicin, it works by desensitizing sensory nerve fibers in the bladder.

CYSTOSCOPY WITH HYDRODISTENTION UNDER ANESTHESIA

- Can be useful for initial treatment or for worsening symptoms.
- After 2–4 weeks, improves symptoms in 30–60% of patients.

- Study in European Urology showed good but transient results in least severe forms of the disease; 37.7– 60% at 6 months and 21.9–43.3% at 1 year in two series.
- This study found that the results were better for patients with a bladder capacity of greater than or equal to 150 cc during cystometry before distension.
- Usually have a temporary period after initiating therapy when symptoms worsen before experiencing improvement in symptoms.
- Rare risk of small ureteral tears and bladder perforation.

SURGERY

- Used only as a last resort.
- Hunner's ulcers can be resected or burned with electricity or laser fulguration.
- Performed under general anesthesia through the urethra.
- Symptoms often initially improve; however, pain and ulcers usually recur within 1–2 years.
- Bladder augmentation enlarges the bladder by attaching a small portion of bowel to the bladder; decreases voiding frequency but does not necessarily decrease pain and may lead to incontinence.
- IC-related pain may remain or return in the bowel used to augment the bladder.
- Total or subtotal cystectomy; definitive treatment for severe forms of the disease refractory to conservative therapy.

BIBLIOGRAPHY

Burkman RT. Chronic pelvic pain of bladder origin, epidemiology, pathogenesis and quality of life. *J Reprod Med.* 2004;49:225–229.

Clemons JL, Arya LA, Meyers DL. Diagnosing interstitial cystitis in women with chronic pelvic pain. *Obstet Gynecol.* 2002;100:337–341.

Dell JR, Parsons CL. Multimodal therapy for interstitial cystitis. *J Reprod Med.* 2004;49:243–252.

Gaunt G, Good A, Stanhope CR. Vestibulectomy for vulvar vestibulitis. *J Reprod Med.* 2003; 48(8): 591–595

Glemain P, Reviere C, Lenormand L, et al. Prolonged hydrodistention of the bladder for symptomatic treatment of interstitial cystitis: efficacy at 6 months and 1 year. *Eur Urol.* 2002;41:79–84.

Lentz GM, Bavendam T, Stenchever MA, et al. Hormonal manipulation in women with chronic, cyclic irritable bladder symptoms and pelvic pain. *Am J Obstet Gynecol.* 2002; 186:1268–1273.

Mishell DR. Chronic pelvic pain in women, focus on the bladder. *J Reprod Med.* 2004;49:223–224.

Parson CL. Diagnosing chronic pelvic pain of bladder origin. *J Reprod Med.* 2004;49:235–242.

Parsons CL, Bullen M, Kahn BS, et al. Gynecologic presentation of interstitial cystitis as detected by intravesical potassium sensitivity. *Obstet Gynecol.* 2001;98:127–132.

Parsons CL, Dell J, Edward J, et al. Increased prevalence of interstitial cystitis: previously unrecognized urologic and gynecologic cases identified using a new symptom questionnaire and intravesical potassium sensitivity. *Urology.* 2002;60:573–578.

Sand PK. Chronic pain syndromes of gynecologic origin. *J Reprod Med.* 2004;49:230—234.

Sinaki M, Merritt JL, Stillwell GK. Tension myalgia of the pelvic floor. *Mayo Clin Proc.* 1977;52(11):717–722.

Slocumb J. Neurological factors in chronic pelvic pain: trigger points and the abdominal pelvic pain syndrome. *Am J Obstet Gynecol.* 1984;149(5):536–543.

QUESTIONS

1. The most common reasons that women seek care from a gynecologist are
   (A) Pelvic pain
   (B) Urinary incontinence and pelvic pain
   (C) Pelvic pain and abnormal bleeding
   (D) Abnormal bleeding and incontinence

2. Symptoms of IC include all but
   (A) Can void up to 60 times per day
   (B) Is always worse with a full bladder
   (C) Pain common before, during, or after sexual intimacy
   (D) Pain may be perceived in vagina, perineum, labia, lower back, lower abdomen, or medial aspect of the thighs

3. The most reliable way to diagnose IC is
   (A) Cystoscopy with hydrodistension
   (B) IC symptom index and problem index questionnaire
   (C) PUF questionnaire
   (D) Pelvic examination
   (E) PST

4. Pharmacologic treatment for IC may include all but
   (A) Anticholinergics
   (B) PPS
   (C) Narcotics
   (D) Bladder instillation of DMSO or heparin
   (E) Antidepressants such as amitriptyline

5. Facts about the pelvic pain and urgency/frequency questionnaire do not include
   (A) 8-Question symptom scale
   (B) Takes approximately 30 minutes to complete
   (C) Focuses on pain and urologic symptoms characteristic of IC
   (D) A score of ≥15/35 is a definite sign of bladder cause for CPP
   (E) Patients scoring in the median range of 5–9 are candidates for a PST

6. Theories of IC include all but
   (A) Unusual microbes or bacterium not detectable through routine urinalysis (UA)
   (B) Increased levels of neuropeptide substance P
   (C) Significant lower levels of glycoproteins GPS1
   (D) Relative lack of blood flow in the bladder
   (E) All of the above

ANSWERS

1. *(C).* All of these are reasons that women seek care from a gynecologist but the two most common reasons are pelvic pain and abnormal bleeding.

2. *(B).* The pain may or may not be worse with a full bladder but is often volume sensitive. Patients with IC void on average 16.5 times per day compared to normal healthy women who void on average 6.5 times per day. They can void up to 60 times per day and up to 12 times/night. In both men and women, pain is common before, during, and after sexual intercourse. Since substance P can be transmitted along C fibers to the peritoneal cavity or vestibule, pain from IC may be perceived in the vagina, perineum, labia, lower back, lower abdomen, or medial aspect of the thighs.

3. *(C).* The best way to diagnose IC is with the PUF questionnaire. Cystoscopy with hydrodistension is not very useful for diagnosing IC as <1% of patients with IC will have disease with the classic sign of Hunner's ulcers and petechial hemorrhages can also be present in normal women. The IC symptom index and problem index is another type of questionnaire. Pelvic examination can help reproduce symptoms of IC and can help r/o vaginitis, vulvodynia, urethral diverticula, pelvic floor dysfunction, and uterovaginal prolapse. The PST is a minimally invasive office procedure to diagnose IC in patients that have a median range score on the PUF questionnaire.

4. *(C).* Narcotics are not the best treatment for IC as it is a chronic disease. The most promising current treatment is PPS. Anticholinergics, bladder instillation of DMSO or heparin, and antidepressants are also used.

5. *(B)*. The PUF questionnaire takes only 5 minutes to complete. It is an 8-question symptom scale that focuses on pain and urologic symptoms characteristic of IC. A score of ≥15/35 is a definite sign of bladder cause for CPP and bladder etiology can be ruled out for a score of <3. A patient with a score in the median range of 5–9 should be further tested with a PST.

6. *(E)*. These are all possible theories about the cause of IC.

48 FEMALE SEXUALITY AND "NORMAL" SEXUAL FUNCTION[1]

Sam Siddighi and Rachel N. Pauls

RECENT EVENTS IN THE EVOLUTION OF SEXUALITY

• Kinsey Report (1948)—Dr. Alfred Kinsey published *Sexual Behavior* in the human male (and female in 1953). Extremely controversial, the report changed the view of sexuality to one that is more open and accepting. For example, the report said that people indulge in more sexual activities than they claim. It was also highly criticized for (1) proclaiming that 10–47% of Americans have homosexual tendencies and (2) data found in Chap. 5, Evaluation of Pelvic Organ Prolapse (POP), which were based on experiments on children aged 5 months to 14 years (their ability and speed to orgasm).

• Privately owned automobiles (1950s)—Vacation by car; adolescents borrowing family car for dating; and relocation to big cities.

• Playboy (1953)—Hugh Marston Hefner's graduate school paper on freedom and sex laws in the United States and subsequent publishing of the revolutionary and eventually mainstream men's magazine.

• The Pill (1960)—Development of the birth control pill is a product of a woman's right activist, Margaret Sanger, who spent almost 40 years fighting for the right of a woman to control her own body and sexual freedom.

• Mid-1960s, many consider beginning of the "sexual revolution"—antithesis to the sexual repression prevalent in the 1950s and before.

[1]Caution: This chapter contains explicit material!

• *Human Sexual Response* (1966)—Doctors William Masters and Virginia Johnson's best-selling publication based on special instruments and motion pictures of men and women who voluntarily engaged in sexual activity.

• Miniskirt (1966)—Mary Quant introduced it to the world. It is, perhaps, a symbol of women's new confidence and embracing of sexuality.

• Stonewall Riots (1969)—On Friday, June 27, 1969, New York City police raided the Stonewall Inn in Greenwich Village. Over the next few days, gays and lesbians gathered outside to protest by holding hands, singing, and dancing. The following month, the Gay Liberation Front was formed.

• *The Joy of Sex* (1972)—Alex Comfort's best seller which unlike previous works, did not assume that couples engaging in sex were married and did not make assumptions of proper mating rituals.

• Internet (1990s)—In 1995, the Carnegie Mellon Institute released a report of online pornography which they found was widespread, profitable, and geared mostly toward men. Today women make up almost a quarter of people who use sexual chat rooms and visit sexual Web sites.

• The Blue Pill or Viagra (1998)—Approved by the Food and Drug Administration (FDA) on March 27, its name implies vitality and rhymes with Niagara connoting force and endurance. The pill which increases blood flow to genitalia of men (questionable effect on women) has changed sexual dynamics in many age groups, especially those > 40 years of age.

HUMAN SEXUAL RESPONSE

• Traditional, linear sexual response phases (Masters and Johnson, and in 1974 Kaplan added *Desire* phase)

• Proximation (desire), preparation (arousal), consummation (arousal, plateau, and orgasm)
  ◦ Desire → arousal → plateau → orgasm (multiple possible) → resolution.
  ◦ Synonymous terms: desire = appetite = libido; arousal = excitement; orgasm = climax; resolution = refractory period.
  ◦ Desire: Sexual yearning and fantasy may be absent initially in a relationship. Complaints of problems with desire may be the first presentation of problems with relationships, depression, or previous sexual failures.
  ◦ Sexual stimuli are extremely important in the sexual response.

• Nonlinear, circular sexual response cycle (R. Basson)
  ◦ Emotional intimacy →allows response to sexual stimuli → arousal → desire → satisfaction → emotional intimacy.

○ Arousal is modulated by the woman's emotional response.
○ Spontaneous desire augments entire cycle at several points.
○ Spontaneous desire is common early in a relationship and is influenced by the menstrual cycle.
• Difference in libido between men and women: Men are more goal-oriented, driven by fantasy, more urgent, and focused on act of intercourse and orgasm while women are driven by desire for intimacy, more receptive, and more distractable

SEXUAL ANATOMY, PHYSIOLOGY, AND BIOCHIEMISTRY

• Brain imaging demonstrates activity in orbital frontal, anterior cingulate, medial preoptic, anterior hypothalamic, and rostral anterior cingulate (especially emotional stimulus) during arousal.
• The temporal lobe and basal ganglia may be involved in inhibition of arousal.
• Congestion of the vulva involves blood in corporal tissue of clitoris and crus × 2, vestibular bulb × 2, and blood in the spongiosal tissue surrounding the urethra.
• Congestion involves engorgement (tumescence) rather than erection (rigidity): Unlike in men, trapping of venous blood in the corporal tissue does not occur during congestion because of lack of the compressive middle layer between the tunica albuginea and erectile tissue. Instead, blood pools as a result of persistent and constant inflow and outflow of blood.
• Genital congestion may augment arousal. Congestion which occurs in response to visual sexual stimuli may not be noticed by women; may be unwanted; or may provoke negative feelings.
• Lubrication: Secretions are not from a gland. Arterial dilation causes inflow of blood → increase blood in submucosa of vagina (engorgement) → increase interstitial fluid (transudate) → diffusion of drops into lumen of vagina (see Chap. 1, Anatomy Relevant to Female Reconstructive Pelvic Surgery: Part I, for anatomy of the vagina). Lubrication also contains secretions from uterine and cervical glands.
• The sensation of wetness (lubrication) may not be arousing to women.
• Bartholin's glands may add moisture during intercourse, but do not contribute significantly to vaginal lubrication.
• The clitoris is made up to three parts (glands, corpus, and paired crura): glands + corpus = 2–4 cm and crura = 9–11 cm.
• The clitoris may contain as many as twice the number of nerve endings as the male penis. More research is needed.

• Prepuce is portion of labia minora that covers the clitoris like a hood.
• Penile movement during intercourse causes movement of the labia minora which puts traction on the prepuce and thus stimulates the clitoris.
• Genital arousal is complex and is a result of both sympathetic and parasympathetic activity.
○ Autonomic innervation: (1) sympathetic—lateral gray column of spinal cord, T11–L2, fibers form hypogastric plexus, (2) parasympathetic—intermediolateral cell column of spinal cord, S2–S4, fiber form pelvic plexus.
○ Autonomic nerves go from pelvis through uterosacral and cardinal ligaments to supply vagina and clitoris.
○ Motor innervation: Anterior horn of spinal cord S2–S4 travels through pudendal nerve to innervate bulbocavernosus, ischiocavernosus, and superficial transverse perinei muscles.
○ Sensory innervation: Fibers from perineum and labia go through pudendal nerve to the spinal cord S2–S4 and ascends spinothalamic and spinoreticular pathways.
○ Sexual climax can be achieved as a spinal reflex.
• Arousal involves not only changes in the sexual organs (breast and genitals) but also changes in vital signs ($\uparrow$ HR, $\uparrow$ R, $\uparrow$ T, $\uparrow$ BP), increases in muscle tension, sweating, pupil dilation, and skin rash (see Table 48-1). All of these increase steadily throughout the sexual response and peak during orgasm.
• Many neurotransmitters are involved in the sexual response including nitric oxide (NO), vasoactive intestinal peptide (VIP), neuropeptide-Y, and substance-P. NO and VIP are probably the most important and both of these neurotransmitters are enhanced by estrogen.
• Phosphodiesterase-V has been isolated in human clitoris, vaginal smooth muscle, and vestibular bulb.

CHANGES IN SEXUALITY WITH PREGNANCY

• Overall frequency of sexual activity declines as pregnancy progresses due to
○ Physical discomfort
○ Possible change in libido
○ Fear of damaging the pregnancy or going into labor. Orgasm or prostaglandins inside semen may induce mild uterine contractions. This does not pose a threat to the pregnancy
○ Increased noncoital activities (holding, hugging, caressing, and massaging)
• One study showed frequency of sexual relations ↓↓ in first trimester (why? nausea, fatigue, sore breasts),

TABLE 48-1 Physiology of the Female Sexual Response

AREA	DESIRE (LASTS MIN-HRS)	PLATEAU (LASTS 30 SEC-3 MIN)	ORGASM (LASTS SECS)	RESOLUTION (WITH ORGASM LASTS 15 MIN; WITHOUT ORGASM LASTS UP TO 24 HRS)
Clitoris	Increased glans diameter, possible increase shaft size	Retraction: shaft withdraw into swollen prepuce	No change	Return to normal in 5-10 sec (full detumescence in 5-10 min)
Uterus	Ascends into false pelvis	Strong contractions	Strong contractions esp in pregnancy and masturbation	Slow return to normal position
Upper Vagina	Lubrication within 10-30 sec; balooning and lengthening of fornices	More ballooning	No change	Cervix descends into seminal pool in 3-4 min
Lower Vagina	Lubrication within 10-30 sec; dilation of lumen; congestion	Contracts lumen around penis which aids thrusting traction on clitoral shaft via labia and prepuce	8-12 contractions of levator ani, labia minor, and lower vagina at .75 sec intervals	If orgasm-congestion disappears; if no orgasm then congestion persists for 20-30 min
Labia Minora	Pink in nullipara; red in multipara; increase size 3x	More color; enlarged labia forms funnel into vagina	Contract with lower vagina	Return to resting in 5 min
Laba Majora	Nullipara: thins and flattens against perineum; multipara: congestion and edema 3x size	Nullipara: may now swells; multipara: more swelling	No change	Nullipara: to normal size in 1-2 min; multipara: to normal size 10-15 min
Skin	No change	Maybe flushing esp abdomen, breast, face, thighs (looks like rash)	No change	Disappearance of flush
Breast	Nipple erection; congestion; size of areola increases	Veins prominent; size increase 25%; areola enlarges and thickens giving appearance that nipples dissappeared	No change	Return to normal

↑second trimester (why? nausea and fatigue gone, and genitals more engorged), and ↓↓ third trimester (physical barrier of pregnancy, use of different positions).

- One study found decrease in orgasmic ability with pregnancy.
- Postpartum there is decrease in frequency of sexual activity (why? fatigue, new baby, healing episiotomy, blues, and so on).
- Sexual positions often change because of comfort (there are no scientific recommendations for particular sexual positions during pregnancy, but lay magazines do offer such advice).
- No need to restrict sexual activity during pregnancy except if the patient has
  ◦ Placenta previa
  ◦ Strong history of early-gestation premature labor
  ◦ Premature rupture of membrane
- May continue to use condoms during pregnancy (especially if one or both partners is not monogamous).
- May continue oral-genital sex. Should avoid blowing air into the vagina as there are case reports of air embolism.

CHANGES IN SEXUALITY WITH AGING

- 1999 Large Survey
  ◦ Majority (≥70%) of older (>45 years) males and females with partners had intercourse one to two times per week.
  ◦ Older females (>45 years) more likely to approve of oral sex and masturbation as opposed to their male counterparts.
- Age-based survey asking, "What would improve your sex life?" age 45–58: less stress and more free time; age 60–64: better health; age 60–74: better health for partner; age >75: a partner.
- Although the postmenopausal ovary continues to make androgens, the postmenopausal woman may have reduced levels of androgens compared to the premenopausal woman (up to 50% decreased).
- Genital atrophy (low estrogen, especially if < 50 pg/mL)
  ◦ Prolonged decreased estrogen → ↓ blood vessels (paleness).
  ◦ Thin epithelium (apoptosis), less dense muscles, and decreased elasticity of connective tissue change (apoptosis).
  ◦ ↓ lubrication (i.e., ↑ dryness and dyspareunia—is the most common sexual complaint in older women) and ↑ pH (vaginitis).
  ◦ Loss of vibration and pressure sensation.
  ◦ ↑ symptoms of dysuria, frequency, urgency, nocturia, and incontinence.

- Clitoral changes
  ◦ Decrease in clitoral perfusion and engorgement during desire phase.
  ◦ Shrinkage in size.
  ◦ Decrease in nerve fibers innervating cavernosal smooth muscle.
  ◦ Decline sensation of touch, vibration, cold.
- Decrease and/or delay in all physiological events described in Table 48-1 (desire—the second most common complaint in older women, lubrication, congestion, breast, skin, sensation, vaginal expansion, orgasm).
- On the other hand, some women have increased desire because of the higher proportion of androgen to estrogen ratio after menopause.
- Fewer or painful uterine contractions with orgasm.
- Besides improvement in the relationship, recommendations for improvement of physiological changes with aging: "use it or lose it," strength training, increase manual stimulation, masturbation, vibrator use, change sexual position and time of day, and educate about alternatives to genital-genital sex.
- Vaginal atrophy actually improves with frequent coitus and masturbation.
- Performance anxiety increases with age.
- Decline in quality of long-term relationship because of affairs (either emotional, physical, mental, or cyber sex), communication difficulties, power struggles, boredom, negative qualities of partner, and so on.
- Today some older women may be frustrated with their sexuality because (1) she has had diminishing sexual interest and activity but is being barraged with media messages of what is attractive, (2) to be sexually active in older age, (3) new demands for sex from formerly impotent, and possibly unintimate partner now treated by Viagra or surgery.
- Nevertheless, (1) assumption of decline in sexuality is welcomed by some, (2) as is new freedom from pregnancy, menstrual cycles, and taking care of children.

INTERESTING FACTS ABOUT SEX

- Human beings are the only animals that have sex not only for reproduction but also for pleasure. For example, humans have sex during periods when pregnancy is not possible: certain times during the menstrual cycle, menopause, and pregnancy.
- Overall frequency of sexual intercourse is seven times per month for men and six times per month for women.
- Frequency of orgasm during sex (1994 Large Survey with answer choice options as follows: "always, usually, sometimes, and rarely"):

CHAPTER 48 • FEMALE SEXUALITY AND "NORMAL" SEXUAL FUNCTION **319**

- Majority (75%) of men always achieve an orgasm.
- 42% of women usually and 29% of women always achieve an orgasm.
- As men age there is no change in orgasm potential (age 18: 70% always orgasm; age 30: 77% always orgasm; age 59: 72% always orgasm).
- As women age, there is an increase in orgasm potential (age 18: 39% usually orgasm; age 30: 41% usually orgasm; age 59: 47% usually orgasm).
- No change in orgasm potential of married, cohabiting, or noncohabiting men.
- On the other hand, women who cohabit and who are married are more likely to achieve orgasm.
- Most women are able to have an orgasm (but frequently through self-stimulation (manual or vibrator) and oral (cunnilingus) and/or manual stimulation by partner rather than by conventional intercourse which may not provide sufficient stimulation of the clitoris (e.g., missionary position).
- Stimuli that increase sympathetic tone initially (e.g., anxiety-provoking visual, ephedrine, exercise, and hyperventilation) and which are followed by erotic visual cues increase genital congestion.
- Female orgasm may have an evolutionary purpose; it may increase the chance of pregnancy. A woman who experiences orgasm likely to repeat the act (therefore increased sexual frequency). Additionally, rhythmic contractions of the uterus and dipping of the cervix into the seminal pool may help transport sperm into the uterus.
- Some believe the Bartholin's glands (aka greater vestibular gland) secretions' function is to emit an odoriferous fluid to attract the male (pheromone in nature).
- Based on MRI images taken during coitus
  - During copulation in the missionary position, the penis has the shape of a boomerang.
  - One-third of length of the penis consists of the root of the penis.
  - During rear-entry position, the penis preferentially contacts posterior vaginal wall and posterior fornix.
  - During missionary position, the penis preferentially contacts anterior vaginal wall and anterior portion of the cervix.
- The cervix is an insensitive structure, but pleasurable feelings can occur from its sudden movement (flicking) during intercourse or with devices such as Ben Wa Balls.
- Voluntary contraction of ischiocavernosi, bulbocavernosi, and superficial transverse perinea can intensify orgasm for both partners.
- Arnold Kegel claimed that stimulation of the levator ani (especially pubococcygeus), which are involved in contraction of the vagina, can induce orgasm.

- Human sexual practices include fellatio (Latin word fellare = to suck), cunnilingus (Latin words cunnus = vulva and lingere = licking), 69 (aka French translation, soiante-neut), nibbling, anal sex, multiple sexual positions (read *Kama Sutra Positions*), simultaneous stimulation of two or more highly sensitive areas, multiple simultaneous sexual partners, other variations and combinations of the above, and practices not mentioned.
- Sex aids (e.g., videos, audio tapes, written material, and pictures) or toys (e.g., vibrators, Ben Wa Balls, erotic lotions, French Ticklers, cock rings, and leather garments and accessories) may enhance pleasure during sexual activity. However, these are not readily accepted by all for various personal reasons. Use of sex aids and toys can be normal and a matter of individual preference.
- However, not everyone practices the aforementioned because of reservations: (1) either is not enjoyable, (2) felt to be unhygienic, (3) taboo, (4) not a true expression of femininity (or masculinity), (5) feelings of submissiveness or inferiority, (6) religious beliefs, and other personal reasons.
- Nongenital erogenous zones on a woman's body include but are not limited to: breast, buttocks, nape of neck, lips, ears, scalp, inner thighs, palms, and behind knees. (Note: Greek god of love Eros used words like erogenous and erotic.)
- Genital erogenous zones include: clitoris, mons, labia majora and minor, interlabial space, vestibular bulbs, hymen, vagina, crural fold, perineum, and others.
- Just knowing the location of these spots is not enough. It is important to ask your partner what she likes and how she likes. Communicate!!!!!
- Gräfenberg or G-spot—In 1950, Ernst Gräfenberg reported that digital stroking along the urethra can lead to a powerful climax. The G-spot is a small area approximately 4–5 cm inside the vagina on the anterior vaginal wall, along the urethra. Claimed to be the second most sensitive erogenous area in the female body (the first is the clitoris). Size of the G-spot varies; and some claim that it involves the entire anterior vaginal wall, including Halban's fascia (space between the bladder trigone and anterior vaginal wall which contains vascular tissue that may become engorged with arousal). The existence of the G-spot is controversial, but the following is considered supportive by some:
  - Immunohistochemistry shows more nerve fibers in distal vaginal wall.
  - The urethra is also a sexual organ as it is surrounded by tumescent tissue, corpus spongiosum.
- Female ejaculation—Claimed to be caused by G-spot stimulation. It is defined as the emission of abundant,

clear, odorless liquid from the urethra that is not urine or vaginal lubrication fluid. It may be periurethral gland in origin. The idea of female ejaculation is even more controversial as most women cannot achieve this.

BIBLIOGRAPHY

Altman AM, Ashner L. *Making Love The Way We Used To or Better: Secrets of Midlife Sexuality*. New York, NY: McGraw-Hill; 2002.

Alzate H, Londono ML. Vaginal erotic sensitivity. *J Sex Marital Ther.* 1984;10:49–56.

Andersen BL, Cyranowski JM. Women's sexuality: behaviors, responses, and individual differences. *J Consult Clin Psychol.* 1995;63:891–906.

Basson R. A model of women's sexual arousal. American College of Obestetrics and Gynecology (ACOG) Danvers, MA:ACOG Publication. *J Sex Marital Ther.* 2002;28:1–10.

Basson R. Sexuality and sexual disorders. In: *Clinical Updates in Women's Health Care* (ACOG). Spring; 2003;11(2):1–78.

Dennerstein L, Dudley E, Burger H. Are changes in sexual functioning during midlife due to aging or menopause? *Fertil Steril.* 2001;76:456–460.

Dennerstein L, Lehert P, Burger H, et al. Factors affecting sexual functioning women in the middle years. *Climacteric.* 1999;2:254–262.

Faix A, Lapray JF, Callede O, et al. Magnetic resonance imaging (MRI) of sexual intercourse: second experience in missionary position and initial experience in posterior position. *J Sex Marital Ther.* 2002;28(s):63–76.

Hilleges M, Falconer C, Ekman-Ordeberg G, et al. Innervation of the human vaginal mucosa as revealed by PGP 9.5 immuno-histocytochemistry. *Acta Anat (Basel).* 1995;153:119.

Kaplan HS. The new sex therapy: active treatment of sexual response revisited: understanding the multiorgasmic experience in women. *Arch Sex Behav.* 1991;20:527–540.

Karama S, Lecours AR, Leroux JM, et al. Areas of brain activation in males and females during viewing of erotic film excerpts. *Hum Brain Mapp.* 2002;16:1–13.

Krantz KE. Innervation of the human vulva and vagina. *Obstet Gynecol.* 1985;12:382–396.

Masters WH, Johnson VE. *Human Sexual Response*. Boston, MA: Little, Brown and Co.; 1966:141–168.

Masters WH, Johnson VE. *Human Sexual Inadequacy*. Boston, MA: Little, Brown and Co.; 1970.

Michael RT, Gagnon JH, Laumann EO, et al. *Sex in America: A Definitive Survey*. Boston, MA: Little, Brown and Co.; 1994.

Nusbaum MR, Gamble G, Skinner B, et al. The high prevalence of sexual concerns among women seeking routine gynecologic carfe. *J Fam Pract.* 2000;49:229–232.

Sarrel PM. Sexuality and menopause. *Obstet Gynecol.* 1990;74 (Suppl 4):26S–30S.

Solberg DA, Butler J, Wagner NN. Sexual behavior in pregnancy. *N Engl J Med.* 1973;288:1098–1103.

QUESTIONS

1. Rosemary Basson's theory of *Human Sexual Response* is different from that of Masters and Johnson's in that it is/claims that _____.
   (A) linear
   (B) men are focused on the act of intercourse
   (C) emotional intimacy is necessary for orgasm
   (D) arousal precedes desire
   (E) women are driven by fantasy
2. During the plateau phase of sexual response the _____.
   (A) uterus ascends in pelvis
   (B) vagina narrows and shortens
   (C) labia become pale
   (D) linear streaks form on the skin
   (E) nipple appears small

QUESTIONS 3–5

For the next three questions, match the statement or word below with the best word listed above. The answer choices may be used once, more than once, or not at all.
   (A) Vasocongestion
   (B) Rigidity
   (C) Erection
   (D) Pooling
   (E) Lubrication
   (F) Cingulate gyrus
   (G) Temporal lobe
   (H) Basal ganglia
   (I) Intermediolateral
   (J) Anterior horn
   (K) Spinothalamic
   (L) Lateral gray column
3. Engorgement (arousal phase).
4. Central nervous system area that "lights up" during sexual excitement.
5. Beads of transudate mixed with cervical gland secretions.
6. A vaginal photoplethysmograph is inserted inside a patient's vagina and minutes later, an erotic film is

shown. Of the following, which may increase values in the plethysmograph if received/performed prior to the showing of an erotic film?

(A) citric acid
(B) an apple
(C) slow deep breathing
(D) a picture of a dead, rotting, corpse
(E) a 2-min movie about basket weaving

ANSWERS

1. *(D).* Unlike Masters and Johnson's theory of the *Human Sexual Response* which is linear and where desire precedes arousal, Rosemary Basson's theory claims that sexual response is circular. Emotional intimacy is necessary because it allows the woman to respond to sexual stimuli which in turn allows her to become aroused. Although choice B is a correct statement, it was not part of Basson's theory. Choice E is incorrect because men (not women) are driven by fantasy while women are driven by the desire for emotional intimacy.

2. *(E).* During the plateau phase, the uterus contracts (it has already ascended during excitement phase). The vagina narrows (around penis) and lengthens (rather than shortens); Labia become more red. A skin rash may develop on thighs, chest, breast, abdomen, and face as a result of flushing (but not linear streaks). Finally, the areola enlarges and swells to the point that the nipples appear smaller.

ANSWERS 3–5

3. *(A),* 4. *(F),* 5. *(E).* Engorgement of genitalia during arousal phase is a result of vascular dilation and congestion. Pooling of blood rather than erection explains why women's genitalia become tumescent rather than rigid during arousal. The sensation of wetness is due to lubrication of the vagina which is due to (1) transudate (from vaginal submucosa vessels), (2) cervical glands, and (3) uterine glands.

6. *(D).* Any stimuli that increase sympathetic tone initially (e.g., anxiety-provoking visual like a dead rotting, corpse, ephedrine, exercise, and hyperventilation) which is then followed by an erotic film will increase genital congestion (measured by vaginal photoplethysmograph). Citric acid and an apple are unrelated to this question. Hyperventilation rather than slow deep breathing will increase sympathetic tone. A 2-min

movie about basket weaving does not increase sympathetic tone unless the patient is enamored with basket weaving.

49 FEMALE SEXUAL DYSFUNCTION
Rachel N. Pauls and Sam Siddighi

GENERAL

- Female Sexuality and Sexual Dysfunction is one of the newest fields in Female Pelvic Medicine and Reconstructive Surgery(FPM&RS).
- Quickly becoming an area of patient interest.
- However, good clinical data are lacking for both diagnosis and treatment.

DEFINITIONS

- World Health Organization: "the various ways in which an individual is unable to participate in a sexual relationship as he or she would wish."
- American Psychiatric Association (DSM-IV): "disturbances in sexual desire and in the psychophysiologic changes that characterize the sexual response cycle and cause marked distress and interpersonal difficulty."
- American Foundation for Urologic Disease 1988 established classification system for female sexual dysfunction (FSD) (Table 49-1). American Federation for Urologic Disease (AFUD) definitions state that disorders are diagnosed only if the women experience personal distress. Below are some clarifications of the above definitions of FSD listed in Table 49-1, commentary section, Clinical Updates in Women's Health Care (ACOG Spring 2003). Other details about each type of disorder are also included
  - Hypoactive sexual desire disorder (HASDD)—loss in sexual yearning or fantasizing should be unrelated to the normal lessening with relationship duration. Sexual desire may increase with time because of emotional intimacy in a relationship. Although almost anything can influence libido (sexual desire), the "brain is the most important sexual organ": knowledge, past experience, foreplay, afterplay, stress, personal well-being, hormones, and so forth.

TABLE 49-1 Classification of FSD

DISORDER	DEFINITION	POTENTIAL CAUSES
Hypoactive sexual desire disorder (HASDD)	Persistent recurring deficiency of sexual fantasies/thoughts, and/or receptivity to sexual activity, which causes personal distress	Menopause Aging Hormonal deficiency Interpersonal issues
Sexual aversion disorder	Persistent or recurring phobic aversion to, and avoidance of sexual contact with a sexual partner, which causes personal distress	Stress Psychological issues Expectation of negative outcome Sexual trauma
Female sexual arousal disorder (FSAD)	Persistent or recurring inability to attain or maintain sufficient sexual excitement causing personal distress	Menopause Surgery Diabetes Neurologic disease Vascular disorder Hypertension
FOD	Persistent or recurrent difficulty, delay in, or absence of attaining orgasm following sufficient sexual stimulation and arousal, which causes personal distress	Muscle weakness Hormonal deficiency Surgery Neurologic disease Lack of experience spectatoring/distractions Guilt Fear loss of control
Sexual pain disorders (i) Dyspareunia	Recurrent or persistent genital pain associated with sexual intercourse	Inadequate lubrication Atrophy
(ii) Vaginismus	Recurrent or persistent involuntary spasms of the musculature of the outer third of the vagina that interferes with vaginal penetration, and which causes personal distress	Infections Endometriosis Vestibulitis Cystitis Sexual trauma/abuse
(iii) Other sexual pain disorders	Recurrent or persistent genital pain induced by noncoital sexual stimulation	

SOURCE: Basson R, Berman J, Burnett A, et al. Report of the international consensus development conference on female sexual dysfunction: Definitions and classifications. J Urol. 2000;183:888–893.; Pauls RN, Kleeman SD, Karram MM. Female Sexual dysfunction: Principles of diagnosis and therapy. *Obstet Gynecol Surv.* 2005;60(3):196–205.

○ Female sexual arousal disorder—should distinguish between women with genital arousal dysfunction who are still aroused mentally by nongenital stimuli from those who are not aroused by any type of stimuli. Again, insufficient or ineffective communication and insufficient foreplay are important.

○ Female orgasmic disorder (FOD)—may coexist with arousal disorder. Usually, it is the intensity of orgasm rather than complete loss of it that is the cause of distress. Women with neurologic disorders or sudden premature loss of androgen production may experience this.

○ Dyspareunia—the movement and friction of intercourse may be impossible because of pain caused by penile entry. Vaginal examination is most important for diagnosis.

○ Vaginismus—muscular *spasm* has never been documented. Reflexive muscle tightening, fear of vaginal entry, and pain with its attempt are characteristics (perineal and levator muscle tightening on examination without cutaneous hypersensitivity or tenderness are key points of diagnosis).

• Above classifications may coexist (e.g., hypoactive sexual desire, sexual arousal disorder, and orgasmic disorder may exist simultaneously)

• Subtyped as lifelong versus acquired, generalized versus situational, and organic versus psychogenic or mixed

EPIDEMIOLOGY

• Somewhat controversial

• Estimates in clinic populations of 40–50%

• Population prevalence of 43–53% and increases with age

• Difficult as many studies include different definitions, or only evaluate particular age groups

- Several large surveys show relative distribution of sexual difficulties as follows: lack of desire or libido is the most common complaint in women
  - Lack of interest (desire) > difficulty with orgasm >> sex not pleasurable ≈ insufficient lubrication > dyspareunia > body image concerns > lack of information about sexual issues
- More FSD may be found in younger (<39 years), less educated, unmarried, and those who are in poor physical and emotional health

ETIOLOGY

- Hormonal:
  - Estrogens important in vaginal lubrication, libido, and orgasm
  - Estrogen replacement alone may not be enough to cure dysfunction
  - Role of androgens controversial: Androgen deficiency may be responsible for low libido (sexual desire), sexual receptivity (arousability), and pleasure. Additionally, it may cause fatigue and depression-like symptoms
    - Conditions with decreased androgen levels:
      - Bilateral salpingoophorectomy (BSO), chemo, gonadotropin-releasing hormone (GnRH) pulse changes, premature ovarian failure, oral
      - Estrogen, birth control pill (BCP), Addison's, hypopituitarism, hypothalamic
      - Amenorrhea, hyperprolactinemia, corticosteroid therapy, idiopathic
- Psychosocial:
  - Attraction to partner, intimacy and relationship, past experiences, level of knowledge, self-image, cultural convention, and expectations affect sexual function
  - Obstacles to sexual function: lack of communication, lack of nurturing environment, misguided perception of "normal," ineffective stimulation, daily stresses (e.g., residency), inability to relax, performance anxiety, physical discomfort, fear of pregnancy or infection
  - Psychiatric disorders such as depression or anxiety may lead to sexual dysfunction or may be concurrent with FSD. Depression is one of the most common causes of libidinal dysfunction/loss
  - Infertility, recurrent miscarriages, and menopause may also lead to FSD
  - Alcohol, smoking, and drugs may impair sexual function
- Medical and Surgical
  - Cardiovascular disease linked to arousal disorder
  - Neurologic disorders can affect arousal and orgasm
  - Gynecologic conditions such as endometriosis, fibroids, infections, atrophy, prolapse, and incontinence can impact on sexual function
  - Previous benign pelvic surgery may lead to sexual dysfunction
    - Hysterectomy ± oophorectomy—may lead to loss of uterine contractions with orgasm, decreased lubrication, shortened vagina, sexual function is similar in patients receiving total versus supracervical hysterectomy at 2 years
    - The overall sexual function usually improves after any type of hysterectomy in women
    - Burch + posterior colporrhaphy—postop dyspareunia
    - Posterior colporrhaphy + levator plication—vaginal stenosis and dyspareunia in 20–50%
    - Excessive trimming of vaginal mucosa during anterior or posterior colporrhaphy—dyspareunia or apareunia
  - Cancer (breast, colon, pelvic)
    - Breast cancer and mastectomy: percentage of women who *never* use female superior position increases 3×, breast stimulation decreases, ≈40% of partners do not view mastectomy scar in first 3 months after surgery, one-third of women do not resume intercourse 6 months after discharge from hospital
    - Pelvic (includes vulvar, vaginal, cervical, and endometrial)
    - Large change in sexuality after diagnosis of cancer because of change in appearance of genitals, damage to nerves, damage to anatomy, atrophy from radiation, ill-feeling after chemotherapy, change in psyche (loss of self-image, self-esteem, and so forth), fear of partner of hurting cancer patient
  - Medications often have sexual side effects (Table 49-2)
  - Partner's medical illness or frailty

EVALUATION

- History
  - Often the patient will not report sexual problems because
    - Fear that she is inadequate in some way
    - Fear that the question may lead the doctor to think less of her
    - Fear that doctor will be embarrassed and will not know what to do
    - Belief that there is no effective diagnosis or treatment
  - Often there are physician barriers to discussing sexual problems because
    - Lack of knowledge
    - Discomfort

TABLE 49-2 **Medications with sexual side effects (with example(s) and possible effect(s) in parentheses)**

Antihypertensives:
   Alpha blockers, beta blockers (e.g., propranolol—Δ libido), calcium channel blockers, diuretics (spironolactone—Δ libido), methyldopa (Δ libido), reserpine (Δ libido), clonidine
Chemotherapeutic agents (busulfan, cyclophosphamide)
Hormonally-active agents:
   Oral contraceptives, antiestrogens/estrogens/SERM, antiandrogen, spironolactone, cimetidine
Antidepressants:
   SSRI (fluoxetine—Δ orgasm), TCAs (e.g., imipramine—Δ orgasm while clomipramine—Δ both libido and orgasm), lithium
   MAO-I (isocarboxazid or phenelzine—Δ orgasm)
   Trazodone (*painful* clitoral tumescence)
   Anticholinergic agents, OTC meds, herbals, H$_2$ blockers (e.g., cimetidine—Δ libido, methazolamide for glaucoma Δ libido)
Antipsychotics—butyrophenones, phenothiazine
Carbamazepine, Phenytoin, Phenobarbital, Diazepam (Δ orgasm)
Amphetamines (Δ orgasm)
Narcotics (e.g., methadone, oxycodone—Δ orgasm)
Bromocriptine (*painful* clitoral tumescence)

ABBREVIATIONS: MAO, monoamine oxidase; OTC, over the counter; SERM, selective estrogen receptor modulator; SSRI, selective serotonin reuptake inhibitor.
Δ = *Change in* a function; either delayed, decreased, or lack of.
SOURCE: Mandal S, Goldstein I, Berman JR. Clinical evaluation of female sexual dysfunction: new diagnostic and treatment strategies. *Prim Psychiatry.* 2001;8(4):54–59; Montejo AL, Llorca G, Izquierdo JA. Incidence of sexual dysfunction associated with antidepressant agents: a prospective multicenter study of 1022 outpatients. *J Clin Psychiatry.* 2001;62(Suppl. 3):10–27.; Thomas DR. Medications and sexual function. *Clin Geriatr Med.* 2003;19(3):553–562.

- ▪ Own sexual issues
- ▪ Desire to avoid unpleasant or time-consuming issues (especially abuse or rape)
- ▪ Worry that patient may feel questions are too intimate
- ○ Nevertheless, patients are becoming more comfortable in seeking help from their physician, especially their gynecologist.
- ○ The simplest, most cost effective, and sensitive way to identify FSD is with an abbreviated interview consisting of three questions: (1) Are you sexually active? (2) Do you have any pain? (3) Do you have any sexual problems or questions?
- ○ You may also begin conversation with an open-ended statement that iterates the universality and frequency of sexual problems in the general population.
- ○ Scored tests such as Brief Index of Sexual Function for Women (BISF-W), Female Sexual Function Index, and Sexual Distress Scale are also available.
- ○ In your interview, be careful that your questions do not assume the gender or number of sexual partners. Use words like "partner" instead of "husband" and "sexual activity" instead of "intercourse."

- ○ If sexual problems are identified, perform complete medical history:
  - ▪ Past medical and surgical history
  - ▪ Gynecologic disorders (hypoestrogenism, prolapse, incontinence, fibroids, infections, endometriosis, ovaries in the cul-de-sac, pelvic pain, interstitial cystitis)
  - ▪ Psychiatric disorders-many forms of FSD may be the first indication of depression (use Beck Depression Inventory)
  - ▪ Medications
  - ▪ Obstetric history (forceps, tears, episiotomy)
  - ▪ History of pelvic trauma (motor vehicle collision, pelvic fracture)
  - ▪ History of sexual trauma or abuse
  - ▪ Social history including relationship factors, smoking, alcohol, or drug use
  - ▪ Sexual orientation
- ○ If there is pain, entry pain can be associated with dryness, atrophy, vulvar vestibulitis, whereas deep pain may be due to endometriosis or levator spasm (vaginismus)
- ○ Establish temporal relationship of symptoms (i.e., started after birth of child, surgery, or life stressor)
- ○ Impact of dysfunction on patient's quality of life
- ○ Must delineate principal nature of dysfunction: libido, arousal, orgasm, or pain
- • Physical
- ○ Neurologic examination: test sensation, motor strength in lower limbs, pelvic floor muscle strength/laxity (with a finger in vagina ask patient to contract pelvic floor muscles "as though they were stopping a stream of urine"). Graded 0-4
- ○ Assess external genitalia:
  - ▪ Look for signs of inflammation, atrophy, prolapse, episiotomy scars, or narrowing. May use a cotton swab to evaluate for vulvar erythema or vestibular pain (potential diagnosis of vulvar vestibulitis)
  - ▪ Sensory testing of the clitoris for women suspected of orgasmic disorder is best achieved by testing for cold rather than touch sensation (use cold water-based lubricant)
- ○ Assess internal genitalia: palpate for tenderness, masses, prolapse; assess levator muscles for spasm, pain; evaluate for infection or atrophy. Try to reproduce pain symptoms during examination
- • Laboratory testing
- ○ Can highlight a hormonal deficiency if suspected
  - ▪ Follicle-stimulating hormone (FSH) and luteinizing hormone (LH) to evaluate for potential menopause
    - • In perimenopause, follicular-phase estrogen are normal or somewhat increased
    - • Estrogen is preserved by elevated levels of follicular-phase FSH.

- In infertile women, elevated day 3 or early follicular-phase FSH is predictive of depletion of ovarian follicles and has poor prognosis for pregnancy
- Thyroid-stimulating hormone (TSH)
- Prolactin
- Dehydroepiandrosterone sulfate (DHEAS) ifadrenal androgen deficiency suspected
- *Normal* range for androgen levels in women has not been established, therefore, there is no consensus on the threshold that can be used to define androgen insufficiency
- Most assays are insensitive to low androgen levels
- Measure testosterone levels during middle of menstrual cycle and in the morning if possible since androgens are the highest then. May be measured in one of three ways:
  1. Total testosterone and sex hormone-binding globulin (SHBG)
  2. Total testosterone and free testosterone
  3. Free testosterone and SHBG
- Free testosterone most important because it binds receptors
- SHBG binds testosterone preferentially, but also binds estrogen
- SHBG ↑ by estrogen (or relative androgen deficiency) and SHBG ↓ by androgens
- Therefore, estrogen supplementation depletes free androgen
- Androgen levels in the lowest quartile + signs of androgen deficiency may be treated
- Consider complete blood count (CBC), liver function tests (LFTs), and cholesterol every month or two if anticipate need for medical therapy
- Other testing
  ○ Duplex Doppler ultrasound—peak systolic and end-diastolic blood velocity in clitoris, labia, and urethra
  ○ pH of vagina—measure of lubrication
  ○ Vaginal pressure catheters—measure of elasticity and compliance
  ○ Vaginal photoplethysmography—measure of vaginal vasocongestion

TREATMENT

- PLISSIT:
  ○ Permission—validate patient's feelings
  ○ Limited Information—educate about behavior, nature of problem, anatomy/physiology
  ○ Specific Suggestions—educate regarding sexual attitudes, expectations, and practices
  ○ Intensive Therapy—refer for couple therapy
    - Schedule more visits to establish trust and take an in-depth history

- Health education: encourage exercise, quality sleep, healthy diet, smoking cessation
- Encourage patient to familiarize herself with her anatomy and perform sensate focus exercises
  • Increase self-awareness by examining body and genitals with fingertips
  • Identify sensitive areas that produce pleasurable feelings
  • Manually stimulate pleasure-producing areas
  • Increase intensity and duration of stimulation and increase psychological stimulation by fantasizing
  • Once orgasm is achieved, masturbate with partner present in order to demonstrate effective and pleasurable techniques to him or her
  • Guide partner in manual stimulation through nonverbal communication
  • Once high level of arousal or orgasm is achieved, engage in intercourse
- Consider experimentation with different sexual practices, use of vibrators on or around the clitoris
- Modify medical causes, i.e., medication adjustments, treat infections, endometriosis
- Consider referral for individual or couple therapy if suspect relationship factor (lack of communication), intimacy problems or history of sexual trauma. Some counseling points to keep in mind are
  • Sex is not just intercourse
  • Leave each encounter feeling good as opposed to focusing on achievement of orgasm
  • Not having orgasm with each sexual encounter does not mean the experience was a failure
  • Both give and receive pleasure
  • Communicate, listen without criticizing
  • Say "yes" or "maybe" rather than "no"
  • Work on quality rather than quantity
  • Sex should not be work, it should be fun
  • Take your time and provide reassurance
- Pelvic muscle awareness and muscle strengthening exercises
- Topical lubricants (especially water-soluble like Astroglide or lubricating jelly can assist with arousal disorder and pain)
- Physical therapy may help with levator spasm and pelvic pain
- Dilators may help with vaginismus as a form of desensitization
  • Graduated dilators → increase size of dilator until largest can be accommodated
  • Insert dilator into the vagina deep enough to pass bulbocavernosus
  • Keep dilator in for 15 minutes, perform 2 × per week for 2 weeks

- Certain types of noncoital sexual pain may respond to low-dose tricyclic anti-depressants, venlafaxine, gabapentin, or valproic acid
- Disorder directed therapy
  - Somewhat controversial
  - SSRI for depression may be replaced with bupropion or nefazodone
  - Anxiolytics may be replaced by buspirone
  - Hormonal replacement:
    - Start with estrogen therapy if deficient—topical may be safest (e.g., vaginal estradiol ring—Estring, delivers low dose with negligible systemic absorption, and also may be useful in patients with breast cancer).
    - Androgen replacement to achieve superphysiologic levels of androgen is growing in popularity but therapies are largely "off label."
    - Superphisiologic levels of androgen may increase libido, frequency of sex, arousal, orgasm, feeling of well-being, energy, appetite, muscle mass, bone, and improve hot flushes, but can have serious side effects (early effects: irregular menses, ↓ high-density lipoprotein (HDL), ↑ cholesterol, acne, hirsutism; long-term irreversible effects: clitoral hypertrophy, male pattern baldness, voice changes).
    - Avoid in women with breast cancer as it may be converted to estrogen by aromatase enzyme.
    - The benefit of replacing of testosterone to midrange physiologic levels is unclear except in young females after bilateral salpingo-oophorectomy—BSO delivering 300 mcg/day via transdermal testosterone patch.
    - Dehydroepiandrosterone (DHEA) supplementation has unpredictable dosing and has unclear effects on libido (50 mg/day claimed to increase libido). It does, however, have a definite benefit on desire and receptivity in patients with Addison's disease.
    - DHEA may be added to regimen of estrogen + methyltestosterone in patients with androgen deficiency as needed in some clinics.
    - DHEA may also improve vaginal mucosal health, boost immune system, and improve bone mineral density. However, it ↓ HDL, ↑ cholesterol, changes glucose tolerance, increases central obesity, increase hirsutism, changes cortisol metabolism, and may be hepatotoxic and virilizing.
    - Androgens can be absorbed in form of gel (e.g., Androgel, testosterone propionate 1–2%, 3× per week), patch (e.g., Testoderm, 150 mcg patch × 2, 2× per week), orally (e.g., methyltestosterone or fluoxymesterone), injection (e.g., testosterone enanthate or cypionate), implanted pellet, and compound pharmacy-created hormone preparations with different strengths.
    - Each 150-mcg patch increases total serum testosterone by 25–30 ng/dL; 1 mg of testosterone gel 1% may increase serum testosterone by 7–8 ng/dL.
  - Other products (Sildenafil, Avlimil, Arginmax, Zestra, topical L-arginine, Chinese medicine, Tibolone, Eros therapy) may be useful for libido, arousal, and orgasm.
    - Sildenafil (Viagra)—phosphodiesterase-V inhibitor, which decreases catabolism of cyclic guanosine monophosphate (cGMP), a second messenger in NO-mediated smooth muscle relaxation. It has been used by women for treatment of decreased libido, arousal, decreased frequency of intercourse, and anorgasmia. It may be useful in postmenopausal women and women on SSRI. Overall, the studies in women have been conflicting. It is not approved by Food and Drug Administration (FDA) for women but is a Category B drug. One 50-mg tablet taken 1 hour before intercourse is the recommendation for men with impotence. Side effects are headache (33%), flushing, and dyspepsia. Several contraindications exist (e.g., nitrate use, history of coronary artery disease [CAD]). More high-quality research in women is needed.
    - Arginmax—L-arginine amino acid (precursor to NO-mediated smooth muscle relaxation) plus many other ingredients (ginseng, ginkgo, damiana, and so forth). The cream is supposed to increase blood flow to genitals (clitoral sensation), increase desire, and frequency of orgasm. Quality research is needed to establish safety and efficacy.
    - Zestra—massage oil containing many ingredients (evening primrose oil, alpha-tocopherol, extract of angelica, and so forth) applied to vulva before intercourse. Claimed to increase desire, arousal, sensation, orgasm in both normal as well as persons with FSD. Quality research is needed to establish safety and efficacy.
    - Avlimil—daily tablet containing many herbs and extracts, which the manufacturer claims increases desire, arousal, and orgasm. Quality research is needed to establish safety and efficacy.
    - Ginkgo biloba—Claimed to increase genital blood flow. Quality research is needed to establish safety and efficacy.
    - Epimedium (aka Horny goat weed, Yin Yang Huo; contains flavanoid, icariin) is a leafy plant that grows in high altitudes of China; the Chinese claim that it increases libido in both sexes and may treat erectile dysfunction in men. Quality research is needed to establish safety and efficacy.

- Tibolone is a SERM available in Canada. It has estrogen, progesterone, and androgen activity. It reduces vaginal atrophy, increases vasocongestion to visual erotic cues, increases desire, and arousability. It does not stimulate the endometrium or breast. No effect on coagulation or blood pressure. Positive effects on the heart. Possible use in the future for FSD.
- Eros therapy—not a medication; it is an FDA-approved handheld, battery operated vacuum suction that vibrates. It is placed over clitoral area and has been shown to increase blood flow to clitoris, vagina, and pelvis. It improves arousal, orgasm, and overall satisfaction.

CONCLUSION

- FSD multifactorial and prevalent
- Increasingly becoming part of gynecologic assessment
- History and physical, laboratory assessment crucial to establishing diagnosis and plan of treatment
- Patient education and behavioral modification are first line of therapy with psychological counseling when necessary
- Paraphilias such as fetishism, transvestism, pedophilia, masochism, sadism, exhibitionism, voyeurism, pyromania, and others were not discussed in this chapter.
- Work-up and treatment of pelvic pain and dyspareunia involves complex workup and therapy beyond scope of this chapter. See Chap. 47.

BIBLIOGRAPHY

Basson R, Berman J, Burnett A, et al. Report of the international consensus development conference on female sexual dysfunction: Definitions and classifications. *J Urol.* 2000;183:888–893.

Bergmark K, Avall-Lundqvist E, Dickman PW, et Al. Vaginal changes and sexuality in women with a history of cervical cancer. *N Eng J Med.* 1999;340:1383–1389.

Berman JB, Berman, L, Goldstein I: Female sexual dysfunction: incidence, pathophysiology, evaluation and treatment options. *Urology.* 1999;54:385–391.

Burger HG, Dudley EC, Cui J, et al. A prospective longitudinal study of serum testosterone, dehydroepiandrosterone sulfate, and sex hormone-binding globulin levels through the menopause transition. *J Clin Endocrinol Metab.* 2000;85:2832–2838.

Capone MA, Good RS, Westie KS, et al. Psychosocial rehabilitation of gynecologic oncology patients. *Arch Phys Med Rehab.* 1980;61:128–132.

Davis SR. Androgen treatment in women. *MJA.* 1999;170:545–549.

Frank D, Dornbush RL, Wester SK, et al. Mastectomy and sexual behavior: a pilot study. *Sex Disabil.* 1978;1:16–26.

Geiss IM, Umek WH, Dungl A, et al. Prevalence of female sexual dysfunction in gynecologic and urogynecologic patients according to the international consensus classification. *Urology.* 2003;62:514–518.

Laumann EO, Paik A, Rosen RC. Sexual dysfunction in the United States; prevalence and predictors. *JAMA.* 1999;281(6):537–544.

Mandal S, Goldstein I, Berman JR. Clinical evaluation of female sexual dysfunction: new diagnostic and treatment strategies. *Prim Psychiatry.* 2001;8(4):54–59.

Mercer CH, Fenton KA, Johnson AM, et al. Sexual function problems and help seeking behavior in Britain: national probability sample survey. *BMJ.* 2003;327:426–427.

Miller KK. Androgen deficiency in women. *J Clin Endocrinol Metab.* 2001;86:2395–2401.

Montejo AL, Llorca G, Izquierdo JA. Incidence of sexual dysfunction associated with antidepressant agents: a prospective multicenter study of 1022 outpatients. *J Clin Psychiatry.* 2001;62(Suppl. 3):10–27.

Nazareth I, Boynton P, King M. Problems with sexual function in people attending London general practitioners: cross sectional study. *BMJ.* 2003;327:423–426.

Pauls RN, Kleeman SD, Karram MM. Female Sexual dysfunction: Principles of diagnosis and therapy. *Obstet Gynecol Surv.* 2005;60(3):196–205.

Rosen RC, Taylor JF, Leiblum SR, et al. Prevalence of sexual dysfunction in women: results of a survey study of 329 women in an outpatient gynecologic clinic. *J Sex Marital Ther.* 1993;19:171–188.

Sarrel PM. Sexuality and menopause. *Obstet Gynecol.* 1990;75:26S–30S.

Semmons JP, Wagner G. Estrogen deprivation and vaginal function in postmenopausal women. *JAMA.* 1982;248(4):445–448.

Sherwin BB, Gelfand MM, Brender W. Androgen enhances sexual motivation in females: a perspective, crossover study of sex steroid administration in the surgical menopause. *Psychosom Med.* 1985;47:339–351.

Shifren JL, Braustein GD, Simon JA, et al. Transdermal testosterone treatment in women with impaired sexual function after oophorectomy. *N Engl J Med.* 2000;343:682–688.

Sipski ML, Alexander CJ, Rosen RC. Sexual response in women with spinal cord injuries: Implications for our understanding of the able-bodied. *J Sex Marital Ther.* 1999;25(1):11–22.

Smith RP. Sexual dysfunction. In: *Gynecology in Primary Care.* Baltimore, MD: Williams & Wilkins; 1997:517–536.

Thomas DR. Medications and sexual function. *Clin Geriatr Med.* 2003;19(3):553–562.

Witkin MH. Sex therapy and mastectomy. *J Sex Marital Ther.* 1975;1:290–304.

www.tlc.discovery.com
www.isswsh.org

QUESTIONS

1. The most important measurement when looking for androgen deficiency is _____.
   (A) DHEA
   (B) DHEAS
   (C) Total testosterone
   (D) SHBG
   (E) Free testosterone

2. A 40-year-old, gravida 2, para 2, reports loss of sexual desire after having a total abdominal hysterectomy and bilateral salpingo-ophorectomy for microinvasive cancer of the cervix several months ago. She is taking oral conjugated estrogen and progesterone. She is upset about her loss of sexuality. Caressing her breasts, nipples, and inner thighs which were previously erotic and arousing are not ineffective. Orgasms are less frequent and diminished. She reports no problems in her relationship and claims to communicate well with her partner. The Beck Depression Inventory is normal. The bimanual examination is also normal. The next best step in management of this patient is _____.
   (A) Progressive vaginal dilation
   (B) Fluoxetine
   (C) Couples therapy
   (D) Androgen therapy
   (E) Viagra

3. _____ is *not* one of the first-line therapies for FSD
   (A) Patient and partner education
   (B) Smoking cessation
   (C) Avlimil
   (D) Use of topical lubricants
   (E) Couples therapy

4. A 45-year-old, gravida 3, para 3, with recent history of radical hysterectomy complains of being unresponsive to genital stimulation even though she has desire to have sex. During intercourse, she does not experience wetness as she did before. She also complains of the inability to achieve orgasm as she used to before. She takes oral estrogen as well as testosterone. She also applies low-dose androgen cream to her genitalia. She finds her own lack of genital response to stimulation as very frustrating, especially since it is beginning to affect her relationship. Pelvic examination demonstrates a pink, rugated vaginal mucosa. A possible treatment for her problems may be _____.
   (A) Sildenafil
   (B) Estrogen cream
   (C) DHEA
   (D) Kegel exercises
   (E) Douching

5. Of the following, _____ is most likely to be associated with decreased libido.
   (A) Androgen excess
   (B) Dopamine excess
   (C) Prolactin excess
   (D) Unilateral oophorectomy
   (E) Polycystic ovary syndrome

ANSWERS

1. *(E)*. Free testosterone is reflective of the testosterone that is available to exert effects on the tissues. This measurement is determined using the total testosterone and SHBG levels. DHEA and DHEAS may also be helpful, especially if an adrenal insufficiency is suspected. TSH evaluates for a thyroid dysfunction, which may be a potential etiology for FSD, but does not provide any information regarding androgen levels.

2. *(D)*. When androgen levels are suddenly and prematurely reduced, desire to have sex and receptivity toward stimulation is decreased. Testosterone may also have effects on energy levels once normal sexual triggers are no longer effective and the outcome of sexual experience is unsatisfactory. Therefore, according to Dr. Basson's intimacy-based cycle, emotional intimacy decreases which again affects desire. You may prescribe 0.625-mg conjugated estrogen and 1.25-mg methyl testosterone. The patient must also be educated to bring back sexual behaviors and create atmospheres, in the past, used to encourage sexual closeness and activity. The woman should also be taught to focus on her feelings during sexual activity. Progressive vaginal dilators are effective for vaginismus. This patient has a normal pelvic examination. Fluoxetine is good for major depression but this patient has a normal Beck Depression Inventory. Couples therapy would be more helpful if there were signs of problems in the relationship. Viagra is not approved for treatment of decreased desire in women and is unlikely to be effective in this patient.

3. *(C)*. Avlimil is a new therapy for FSD that has been widely publicized. However, no placebo-controlled trials are published and safety and efficacy are unproven. Patient and partner education is the first step in establishing a treatment plan for FSD. Smoking cessation is an important lifestyle modification along

with decreasing alcohol and drug intake, encouraging physical fitness and rest. Couples therapy may be necessary if relationship problems or abuse are noted. Topical lubricants and moisturizers are helpful in treatment of arousal disorder and pain.

4. *(A)*. A radical hysterectomy involves removal of the upper vagina. This has the potential to damage autonomic nerves between the bladder and anterior vaginal wall, which are probably involved in vasodilation → congestion of vulva and vaginal → lubrication vagina and tingling vulva. Although, Sildenafil is not FDA approved for this purpose, theoretically a phosphodiesterase inhibitor may help increase blood flow to her genitalia. Estrogen cream would be useful if there were signs of atrophy. DHEA, an androgen, would not be helpful as this patient is already receiving testosterone. Kegel exercises and pelvic floor muscle awareness may be more helpful for someone with pelvic pain symptoms. Douching is unnecessary as it may change normal vaginal flora and may predispose her to vaginitis.

5. *(C)*. Conditions associated with lack of androgen, which is associated with low libido, are hyperprolactinemia, surgical menopause (bilateral and usually not unilateral), chemotherapy, GnRH pulse changes, premature ovarian failure, oral estrogen, BCP, Addison's, hypopituitarism, and hypothalamic amenorrhea. All of the other options listed do not affect libido negatively. Dopamine is a neurotransmitter associated with pleasure and positive sexual responses. Polycystic ovary syndrome (PCOS) has not been linked to low libido.

50 MATERIALS USED IN FEMALE PELVIC RECONSTRUCTIVE SURGERY (FPRS): GRAFTS, MESHES, AND SLING MATERIALS

Sam Siddighi

INTRODUCTION

- Materials used in surgery can be placed into two main categories: synthetic versus nonsynthetic (aka biological or organic).

- Biological materials consist of autologous (rectus fascia, fascia lata, vaginal wall), allograft or homologous (cadaveric fascia lata, cadaveric dermis [Hydrix or Repliform]), and xenografts or heterologous (porcine dermis [e.g., Pelvicol], porcine subintestinal mucosa [e.g., Symphasis], porcine pericardium [e.g., Veritas])—see Table 50-1.
- Basic definitions
  - Autologous: graft using one's own body tissues (e.g., autologous rectus fascia)
  - Homologous: graft using cadaveric tissue (e.g., cadaveric dermis)
  - Heterologous: graft using animal tissue (e.g., porcine intestinal submucosa)
  - Xenograft: graft from animal tissue
  - Allograft: graft from cadaveric source
- Synthetic materials consist of polypropylene (Marlex, Prolene, and most midurethral slings), polyester, expanded polytetrafluoroethylene (GORE-TEX), silastic band, multifilament polyethylene terephthalate (PETP;Mersilene)—see Table 50-2.
- Combination materials consist of synthetic + biological materials (e.g., Pelvitex, Apogee, Perigee, and Hybrid slings).
- The ideal graft or mesh material will have the following properties:
  - Inexpensive
  - Readily available
  - Decreases operating room (OR) time
  - Strong
  - Ideal amount of pliability, flexibility, and elasticity
    - For example: if sling material is too elastic → efficacy ↓ or
    - For example: if sling material is too inelastic → erosion rate ↑
  - Not too much mesh retraction
    - During healing and remodeling, the mesh can lose up to 30% of its surface area
  - Not rejected by host
  - Safe (i.e., infection risk, erosion risk, tissue inflammation and healing especially with synthetic mesh)
  - Not requiring additional incisions (e.g., to harvest biological graft) which can increase morbidity
- Relative contraindication to graft use
  - Immunocompromised patients (e.g., chronic steroids, human immunodeficiency virus [HIV], and cancer)
  - Patients with poor wound healing potential (e.g., long-standing diabetes mellitus [DM] and vitamin A deficiency)
  - Patients with poor tissue quality
- In treatment of stress urinary incontinence (SUI), the type of sling material probably does not significantly affect cure rates.

TABLE 50-1 Materials used today in FPMRS in the United States

NAME OF PRODUCT (TRADEMARK)	TYPE OF MATERIAL	PURPOSE IN FPMRS: POP VS SUI	SYNTHETIC MESH VS. BIOLOGICAL GRAFT (TYPE)
Rectus Abdominis	parietal fascia	SUI	Biological (autologous)
Rectus Abdominis	parietal fascia	SUI	Biological (homologous)
Fascia Lata	parietal fascia	SUI	Biological (autologous)
Fascia Lata	parietal fascia	SUI	Biological (homologous)
Vaginal Wall Patch	mucosa + submucosa	SUI	Biological (autologous)
Hydrix [Caldera]	cadaveric dermis	POP/SUI	Biological (homologous)
Repliform [Boston Scientific]	cadaveric dermis	POP**	Biological (homologous)
DermMatrix [Carbon Medical]	porcine dermis	POP	Biological (heterologous)
InteXen (Apogee/Perigee) [AMS]	porcine dermis	POP	Biological (heterologous)
InteDerm (Apogee/Perigee) [AMS]	cadaveric dermis	POP	Biological (homologous)
Fortaflex [Organogenesis Inc.]	porcine	POP	Biological (heterologous)
Pelvicol [CR Bard]	porcine dermis	POP	Biological (heterologous)
Pelvilace [CR Bard]	porcine dermis	SUI	Biological (heterologous)
Pelvisoft [CR Bard]	porcine dermis	POP	Biological (heterologous)
Symphasis [Cook]	porcine small intestine submucosa	POP	Biological (heterologous)
Strasis [Cook]	porcine small intestine submucosa	SUI	Biological (heterologous)
Veritas [Synovis]	bovine pericardium	POP/SUI	Biological (heterologous)
GORE-TEX [WL Gore & Associates Inc.]	multifilament expanded polytetrafuoroethylene	POP	Synthetic
Marlex	monofilament polypropylene	POP	Synthetic
ProLite [Atrium]	monofilament polypropylene	POP	Synthetic
Gynemesh PS [Ethicon]	monofilament polypropylene	POP	Synthetic
Mersilene [Ethicon]	multifilament polyehtylene terephthalate	POP	Synthetic
IntePro (used in Apogee/Perigee) [AMS]	polypropylene mesh	POP	Synthetic
Prolift (Ethicon)	monofilament polypropylene	POP	Synthetic
For Materials used in SUI (see Table 14)	monofilament polypropylene	SUI*	Synthetic

*The synthetic material used in sling procedures to correct SUI is some variation of polypropelene mesh tape. Biological materials and "hybrid" slings are also in use today (see Table 14-1)

NOTE: POP = Pelvic Organ Prolapse; SUI = stress urinary incontinence; AMS = American Medical Systems

TABLE 50-2 Tension free mid-urethral slings

TYPE OF SLING (MANUFACTURER)	MATERIAL	DIRECTION OF TROCAR INSERTION*	ADDITIONAL COMMENTS
Pubovaginal			
TVT (Ethicon [Gynecare])	Polypropylene	both directions	the original mid-urethral sling; knitted mesh (uniform elasticity), substantial data (>7 years, > 500,000 pts) on efficacy and complications of TVT, very low infection rate
IVS Tunneler (Tyco)	Polypropylene	vaginal	multifilament & knitted mesh, each filament diameter = 25 μm but as multifilament yarn diameter = 160 μm; "anterior" IVS used for SUI versus "posterior" IVS used for vaginal vault prolapse; data on efficacy and safety needed
SPARC (AMS)**	Polypropylene	suprapubic	absorbable tensioning sutures useful for readjustment of sling within 2 weeks of procedure, knitted mesh (uniform elasticity), more data is needed on efficacy
Pelvilace (C.R. Bard)	Pelvicol Implant (porcine acellular collagen matrix)	both directions	100% biological material (decrease erosion risk) which is advertised to be self- anchoring because of chevrons cut into material; minimizes risk of erosion and infection, more data is needed on efficacy
Uretex (C.R. Bard)	Polypropylene	both directions	knitted mesh (iso-elasticity) which doesn't curl or unravel with minimal force (5 lbs = 22N), mesh advertised as stronger than competitor because of its intricate knit design
Advantage (Boston Scientific)	Polypropylene	vaginal	via heat-sealing the suburethral portion of mesh is detangled; theoretically this reduces urethral irritation and mesh deformation during tensioning
Lynx (Boston Scientific)	Polypropylene	suprapubic	same mesh as Advantage, longer needle useful for morbid obese patients
Stratasis TF (Cook)	Porcine small intestine submucosa	both directions	same material as Symphasis [Cook], 100% biological material which minimizes risk of erosion and infection; serrated edges help it anchor to tissue (theoretically), more data is needed on efficacy
Sabre (Mentor)	Bioabsorbable polymer	both directions	sling absorbed in 14-18 months
BioArc (AMS)**	Polypropylene with intervening surgeon's choice material	both directions	a "hybrid" sling; knitted, non-woven mesh and surgeon's choice of graft in the suburethral area
T-Sling (Caldera)	Polypropylene/ Polydioxanone	vaginal, suprapubic, and transobturator	T-sling with Centrasorb= suburethral portion is entirely absorbable, trocars or introducers are re-usable instead of disposable
Transobturator			
Ob Tape (Mentor)	Polypropylene	outside-in	non-woven, non-knitted, heat-bonded mesh, low elasticity to help adjustment? (5% versus 20-30% for TVT), filament diameter = 50 μm; uses helical trocar/needle passers; lower efficacy at ≈ 11 mo compared to Monarch, higher inflammatory response than Monarch; erosion risk
Aris (Mentor)	Polypropylene	outside-in	low elasticity (7.5% instead of 30% for Monarch); more data needed
Monarch (AMS)**	Polypropylene	outside-in	woven mesh with uniform elasticity, filament diameter = 150 μm; mesh is slightly thicker and wider than some competitors; has tensioning suture that runs length of sling mesh; helical trocar/needle passers, good tissue in-growth and low inflammatory response at 3 mo.; most data for TOT
TVT-O (Gynecare)	Polypropylene	inside-out	woven mesh with uniform elasticity, helical trocar/needle passers
Obtryx (Boston Scientific)	Polypropylene	outside-in	same mesh as Advantage, 2 needle designs (Curved and Halo)
Uretex Transobturator "Uretex-TO" (C.R. Bard)	Polypropylene	outside-in	same macroporous, strong, woven mesh used with pubovaginal technique, helical needle passers
Pelvilace-TO (C.R. Bard)	Pelvicol Implant (porcine acellular collagen matrix)	outside-in	100% biological material (decrease erosion risk), also advertised as being self-anchoring; minimizes risk of erosion and infection; more data is needed
Bone Anchored			
Infast Ultra (AMS)**	xxx Prolene	vaginal	2 titanium screws attached to polypropylene suture which anchors biological graft or synthetic mesh underneath the urethra. The screws are driven into back of pubic symphysis with hand-held, battery operated driver. Anchorage to pubic bone carries a risk of osteitis pubis and osteomyelitis

** AMS = American Medical Systems

* both directions = vaginal and suprapubic insertion; vaginal = trocar begins in vaginal area and ends in abdominal area (ie vaginal → abdominal); suprapubic = trocar begins in abdominal area and ends in vaginal area (ie abdominal → vaginal); outside-in = helical passer begins lateral to folds (aka obturator → vaginal) of thigh and ends in vaginal area; inside-out = helical passer begins in the vagina and ends in the lateral folds (aka vaginal → obturator)

- Cure rates for fascial slings are very high (>90% at 4 years for hypermobile urethra [HMU], and ≈85% for intrinsic sphincter deficiency [ISD] at 4 years).
- Cure rates for synthetic slings are very high and are maintained at 10 years after surgery.
- Materials have been used to augment and repair pelvic organ prolapse (POP) because:
  ◦ ≈30% of women will fail primary prolapse repair (i.e., recurrent prolapse).
    ▪ Failure rate of anterior wall repair may be greater than that of posterior repair (≈30% vs. ≈20%).
    ▪ Some experts believe that one of the reasons for recurrence of POP is because of iatrogenic vaginal axis deviations which can shift intra-abdominal forces to different compartments of the vagina.
  ◦ Patient's own tissue is weak or absent.
    ▪ Augmenting of repair may create a "bridge" between patient's own tissue.
  ◦ Patient has specific dysfunction of connective tissue, nerve, or muscle.
  ◦ To avoid constriction of the vagina with plication.
    ▪ This is especially important high in vagina (i.e., proximal), since the sidewalls are further apart and plication of levators is likely to lead to narrowing and dyspareunia.
  ◦ To increase strength of repair as there continues to be strain on surgical site.
- Currently, many experts will augment their repairs for patients who have
  ◦ Recurrent POP (especially same-site recurrence)
  ◦ Patients whom they feel have higher risk of recurrence (based on risk factors) or who have had several recurrences
  ◦ Advanced POP (stage 3 or 4)
  ◦ Certain type of defects (e.g., central endopelvic tissue defect encountered during anterior prolapse evaluation)
- If using graft materials, try to use good technique by minimizing dissection, bleeding, contamination, and length of incision over graft (use straight incisions instead of U-shaped incisions).
- Additionally, use as little graft as possible to achieve repair without leaving the graft on tension.
- Normal wound healing consists of three stages:
  ◦ Hemostasis
  ◦ Inflammation
  ◦ Remodeling
    ▪ In migration of endothelial cells (capillaries → angiogenesis reduces infection as immune cells and antibiotics are able to reach implant)
    ▪ In migration of fibroblast cell (deposition of collagen and other proteins)
    ▪ Transitional connective tissue = granulation tissue (has lots of capillaries and collagen)

    ▪ With time, collagen reorganizes and capillary density decreases
    ▪ New tissue appears like surrounding tissue histologically
- Remodeling can occur with biological grafts.
- Remodeling does not occur with synthetic meshes, instead
  ◦ A capsule may form around mesh fibers.
  ◦ Mesh integration = tissue in-growth does occur within synthetic mesh (tissue in-growth ↑ remodeling).
  ◦ Much more data are needed on safety and efficacy of grafts used for POP.

BIOLOGICAL MATERIALS USED IN FPMRS

- Cadaveric fascia involves an extensive screening process prior to tissue harvest. A thorough sterilization process prior to use of fascia is described below.
  ◦ Advantages: (1) no harvesting necessary, (2) decreases morbidity, and (3) decreases operating time.
  ◦ Disadvantages: (1) expensive, (2) risk of infection, (3) low erosion risk, (4) autolysis (up to 20%, especially cadaveric fascia lata): tissue rejection and early failure risk, and (5) processing may weaken tissue.
  ◦ Solvent dehydrated: Hypertonic solutions to osmotically rupture cells and destroy bacteria and viruses. Hydrogen peroxide is then used to oxidatively destroy most proteins. Sodium hydroxide can be used to destroy viruses, eradicate DNA and RNA, and inactivate prions (if present).
  ◦ Freeze-drying changes tissue to acellular fibrous mesh and reduces the risk of viral infection.
  ◦ Cadaveric fascia may also be prepared by (1) using povidone-iodine solution followed by hypertonic saline, and finally ascorbic acid, (2) dissolving lipid layer walls using isopropyl alcohol, and (3) using gamma radiation to kill bacteria by disrupting the nucleic acid.
  ◦ Cadaveric fascia lata used today is either fresh-frozen, solvent dehydrated, or freeze-dried and irradiated as described earlier.
- Autologous
  ◦ Advantages: (1) low incidence of rejection, (2) no autolysis when compared with cadaveric fascia, (3) ability to harvest long strip of tissue, (4) has no risk of viral transmission, (5) very low risk of infection, and (6) very low risk of erosion.
  ◦ Disadvantages: (1) similar to cadaveric fascia, in that tissue width, length, and strength (50%) are lost over time. Tissue strength can be maintained by

harvesting wider samples, (2) harvesting of rectus fascia requires long abdominal incision with its associated morbidity (e.g., incisional hernia and infection) and recovery time, (3) patients with incontinence and POP may have inherent weakness in their tissue collagen, elastin, and so on. Obtaining autologous tissue to repair or augment innate weakness in tissue may not be effective, and (4) additional operative complexity for surgeon.
  ○ Rectus abdominis fascia for sling was first used by A.H. Aldridge in 1942.
  ○ Undergoes necrosis (2 weeks) → neovascularization (3-8 weeks) → fibroblast proliferation, collagen deposition, and remodeling (at 12 weeks).
  ○ Autologous rectus fascia and fascia lata are the most commonly used biological materials today.
• Both cadaveric and autologous fascia have been noted to have isolated, unexplained early sling failure (i.e., fragmentation, breakage, absorption, or softening of fascia so as to render recurrent early SUI).
• Sources of fascia
  ○ Rectus abdominis fascia
    ▪ May be autologous or cadaveric.
    ▪ Harvesting requires a large abdominal incision.
    ▪ Autologous rectus fascia has same strength as cadaveric fascia lata (solvent dehydrated) and dermal graft.
    ▪ Good tissue remodeling.
  ○ Fascia lata
    ▪ May also be autologous or cadaveric.
    ▪ Its use was proposed in order to eliminate problems of rectus fascia. Autologous fascia lata is thicker and stronger than autologous rectus fascia (therefore increased strength) and uses small incision to harvest.
    ▪ Disadvantage: Harvesting autologous tissue requires second operative site which (1) prolongs OR time, (2) is associated with its own pain, risk of infection, hematoma/seroma, and slightly longer hospital stay, and (3) surgeon may have less knowledge and comfort with thigh anatomy versus abdominal wall anatomy.
    ▪ Cadaveric fascia lata has disadvantages of antigenicity of the material, potential loss of tissue strength, and risk of transmission of viral infections (hepatitis B virus [HBV], HIV).
    ▪ Fascia lata samples obtained more laterally on the thigh are stronger than those more centrally located on the fascia lata of thigh.
• Vaginal wall patch
  ○ Advantages: (1) readily available and (2) no need for long incision or second operative incision.
  ○ Disadvantage: (1) weaker than fascia or synthetic material, (2) thin, (3) theoretically risk of

contamination from vaginal bacterial environment, and (4) stretchable and plastic nature of vaginal mucosa whose intended function is to accommodate childbirth rather than to serve as a support structure.
  ○ Tissue failures found to be more frequent because tissues have already weakened over time due to stress (e.g., childbirth) causing loss of collagen and elastin. This explains the low success rate of vaginal patch sling over time.
• Cadaveric dermal allograft (Hydrix HD [Caldera] and Repliform [Boston Scientific])
  ○ A prehydrated acellular dermal allograft.
  ○ Stringent screening and processing of donor dermis which meets requirements of Food and Drug Administration (FDA) and American Association of Tissue Banks (AATB).
  ○ Advantages: (1) strong, (2) soft, (3) pliable, and (4) random collagen fibril orientation resists suture pull-through.
  ○ Harvested skin must be free of abrasion, puncture wounds, and hair.
  ○ Most acellular dermal allografts are prepared using frozen skin retrieved from tissue banks: slow, initial freeze and thaw of dermis → epidermis and dermal cells are delaminated and removed so only collagen and elastin framework remains → bacterial destruction, viral and prion inactivation, and "decellularization" are accomplished using low and high pH treatments → a buffered solution is used to remove the residual chemical before preservation with lyophilization.
• Porcine
  ○ Dermis (DermMatrix [Carbon Medical Technologies] and InteXn [American Medical Systems])
    ▪ Acellular collagen matrix
    ▪ Advertised advantages: (1) strong, (2) flexible, (3) good tissue in-growth, (4) resist suture pull-through, (5) no erosion, and (6) no rejection
  ○ FortaFlex Technology (Organogenesis Inc.)
    ▪ Acellular collagen matrix
    ▪ Tissue → acid + base → rinse → cross-link technology → package → gamma radiation to sterilize
    ▪ Advertised advantages: (1) strength, (2) low suture pull-through, (3) good integration into host tissue and remodeling at 6 months, (4) no foreign body response elicited, and (5) no calcification of implant
  ○ Small intestine submucosa (porcine acellular collagen matrix)
    ▪ Remove mucosa and muscularis externa from intestinal wall of pigs → acellular extracellular matrix (ECM) (90% Type I collagen) remains → freeze-dry → ethylene chloride → sterilized → packaged

- Absorbable, soft, and pliable
- Used to augment and reinforce during POP surgery:
- Pelvicol (C.R. Bard)—porcine acellular collagen biomesh
  ○ Site-specific posterior repair with Pelvicol augmentation had high success rate at 6 months (94%)
  - PelviSoft (C.R. Bard)-porous Pelvicol which optimizes tissue in-growth and revascularization
  - Used as midurethral sling in SUI correction surgery
    - PelviLace (C.R. Bard)-Pelvicol transformed into sling tape
  - Long-term data are needed on safety and efficacy after POP surgery
    - Symphasis for POP and Strasis for SUI (Cook)-porcine acellular collagen biomesh
      ○ Data: biomesh implantation → time = 0–1 month: tissue in-growth (e.g., capillary, fibroblast, and inflammatory cells) → time = 3 months: differentiation between tissue and Symphasis is difficult (therefore, Symphasis in incorporated instead of being encapsulated) → time = 12 months: implant cannot be seen and inflammation is resolved.
      ○ Advertised advantages: (1) strong, (2) acellular, (3) nonimmunogenic, (4) non-cross-linked, and (5) inexpensive.
      ○ More data are needed on efficacy of Strasis after pubovaginal midurethral sling for treatment of SUI.
  - Allows good tissue in-growth before it is completely absorbed
  - May be weaker in tensile strength compared to fascia (more data are needed)
- Bovine pericardium acellular collagen matrix (Veritas [Synovis])
  ○ Cow heart pericardial tissue → screened → proprietary processing (decellularizes and cap free amine groups) → radiation sterilized → wet, ready-to-use, non-cross-linked acellular collagen.
  ○ Advantages: (1) not cadaveric, (2) advertised as "very" acellular (i.e., very little DNA) therefore minimal immune response by host, and (3) suture holds.
  ○ Disadvantages: assessment of strength and long-term data needed, potential for calcification (depending on use of glutaraldehyde to cross-link)
  ○ Advertised for use in SUI surgery and POP surgery.
  ○ Allows fibroblast proliferation and angiogenesis after implantation in rabbit. In a few months, it is histologically indistinguishable from host tissue (i.e., successful remodeling).
  ○ Veritas undergoes slow resorption by host's fibroblast enzymes as new tissue is being formed (tissue in-growth and remodeling).

○ 6-month study in 10 patients with POP grade III was successful (POP-Q score, no infection, breakdown, rejection, or nonhealing area). Long-term follow-up is needed to establish safety and efficacy.
○ Three compartments (anterior, posterior, and apical) prolapse repair by abdominal sacrocolpopexy using Veritas → follow-up data are needed on safety and efficacy.
- Relative tensile strength (autologous fascia lata is strongest → porcine small intestine is weakest)
  ○ Autologous fascia lata > autologous rectus fascia = cadaveric fascia lata (solvent dehydrated) = dermal allograft
  ○ > cadaveric fascia lata (freeze-dried)
  ○ > porcine small intestinal mucosa

SYNTHETIC MATERIALS USED IN FPRS

- Advantages: (1) readily available, (2) cheaper, (3) strong, (4) no risk of viral infection, and (5) decreases OR time because no harvesting needed and they are ready-to-use.
- Disadvantages: (1) foreign body inflammatory reaction potential, (2) higher risk of erosion (average of 5% for urethral and vaginal erosions with slings and meshes). Erosion rate comparison: polyester coated with collagen (ProteGen was recalled in 1999) 50% > GORE-TEX 20% > Mersilene 0.9%, (3) risk of fistula formation, and (4) industry push to use new products that have limited data on safety and efficacy.
- Synthetic mesh risk of erosion depends on several factors:
  ○ Infection
  ○ Foreign body inflammatory reaction
  ○ Healing environment (blood, nutrient, oxygen flow, and waste exchange)
  ○ Mesh characteristics (rigidity, pore size, inflammatory response created, monofilament vs. multifilament)
- Polypropylene and polyester mesh are the most commonly used synthetic materials today.
- Macroporosity is better because it increases the (1) ability to ward off infection and (2) has better tissue in-growth potential (pore size > 75 μm necessary for in-growth of capillaries, fibroblasts and their secreted collagen, polymorphonuclears [PMNs], and macrophages).
- Permanent meshes—very strong
  ○ GORE-TEX mesh (multifilament, expanded polytetrafluoroethylene; W.L. Gore & Associates, Inc.)
    - Used by general surgeons for abdominal hernia repairs.
    - Advantages: (1) soft, (2) comfortable, (3) retains suture, and (4) low immunogenicity.

- Disadvantage: (1) infectious risk, (2) erosion risk, and (3) multifilament mesh (regardless of pore size) may increase risk for infection as bacteria can enter between filaments but immune-fighting cell cannot.
- Surgeon can minimize infection risk by avoiding vaginal approach to POP.
- Large pore size = 800 μm.
- Increase risk of infection.
- Erosion has occurred.
- Minimal inflammatory reaction.
- Poorly incorporated or healed into human tissue.

○ Marlex (monofilament polypropylene) or ProLite (Atrium)
- Monofilament mesh has advantage of not having small spaces between fibers which may allow bacterial colonization.
- Stiffer than other meshes.
- Erosion has occurred.
- Produces intense inflammatory reaction.
- Adheres and forms scars onto tissue.
- Potential for fistula formation.
- Large pore size = 600 μm.

○ Prolene (monofilament polypropylene; Ethicon)
- Double-woven mesh similar to Marlex in material.
- Same as Ethicon Prolene suture material.
- Fiber diameters may vary by manufacturing company.
- Larger pore size (1008 × 1350 μm) therefore (1) lowest risk of infection (since immune cells can enter pores to fight bacteria), (2) theoretically better collagen deposition (since fibroblast can enter pores), tissue in-growth, and remodeling.
- Some polypropylene meshes may have even larger pore size (e.g., Uretex [C.R. Bard]: 1550 × 1250 μm).
- Polypropylene mesh is very resistant to infection.
- Soft and flexible.
- Prolene tape is used in most midurethral slings (e.g., tension-free vaginal tape [TVT] and transobturator tape [TOT]; see Table 14-1) → knitted mesh with uniform elasticity. Gynecare TVT has > 7 years of data on both efficacy and safety. Prolene tape material and barb-like edges → allow friction between tape and tissue (i.e., Velcro-like effect which makes suture anchoring unnecessary for these slings).
- Prolene mesh used for POP surgery.
  - Gynemesh PS (Ethicon): (1) thinner, softer, more flexible, and stronger than predecessor, Prolene mesh, (2) less suture pullout, (3) porous, (4) induces minimal tissue inflammation, (5) low infection rate, (6) repair of mostly stage III POP either vaginally or abdominally shows satisfactory outcome (≈70% have stage 0–1 at 1 year

follow-up in both groups; 100% have objective improvement in POP-Q at 1 year follow-up); (7) has been used for sacral colpopexy, (8) long-term data are still needed for safety and efficacy.
- Posterior intravaginal slingplasty (IVS Tunneler) (TYCO) for management of apical POP: transverse incision is made in vaginal apex → two stab incisions at level of anus on buttocks → curved needles passed from buttock, through ischiorectal fossa, perforating levator ani, and out just distal and inferior to ischial spine → then needle tip brought through vaginal apex → polypropylene mesh arms are connected to needle and needle is retracted as mesh is positioned → mesh is attached to vaginal apex to mimic level I support. In other words, two new synthetic meshes are placed which mimic the uterosacral ligaments.

○ Mersilene (multifilament PETP; Ethicon)
- Small fiber interstices (<10 μm) increase risk of infection (Why? Because bacteria able to enter but immune system cells [PMNs, WBCs, and macrophages] are too big to enter.)
- Tears at lower strength and has lower tensile strength than Prolene mesh.
- Easier suture pullout than Prolene mesh.

COMBINATION (SYNTHETIC + BIOLOGICAL) MATERIALS USED IN FPMRS

- Pelvitex (C.R. Bard)
  ○ Polypropylene mesh coated with hydrophilic porcine collagen.
  ○ Theoretically, the collagen coating allows the body to more readily accept the implant (good tissue in-growth) while maintaining the strength and durability of the synthetic mesh.
  ○ Used for tissue augmentation and reinforcement in POP surgery.
  ○ More studies are needed to establish safety and efficacy.
- Apogee (American Medical Systems)
  ○ Polypropylene mesh (IntePro) only or porcine dermis (InteXēn) only or a combination, "Apogee System," contained in one package to allow the surgeon to perform multiple repairs.
  ○ Designed to save preparation time in OR.
  ○ Used to correct symptomatic posterior vaginal prolapse: precut InteXēn is used to augment posterior wall repairs.
  ○ Used to correct symptomatic apical vaginal prolapse: polypropylene mesh arms are connected to

porcine graft material using provided clamp → transverse incision is made in vaginal apex → two stab incisions at level of anus on buttocks → curved needles passed from buttock, through ischiorectal fossa, perforating levator ani, and out just distal and inferior to ischial spine → then needle tip brought through vaginal apex → polypropylene mesh arms are connected to needle and needle is retracted as mesh is positioned → leaving biological graft to augment posterior repair; the graft is attached to synthetic arms which mimic level I support.

- ○ Theoretically, it may be used via vaginal, abdominal, or laparoscopic approach.
- ○ Controlled studies are needed to establish safety and efficacy.
- Perigee System (American Medical Systems)
  - ○ Polypropylene mesh (IntePro) or porcine dermis (InteXēn) or a combination, "Integraft," contained in one package.
  - ○ Designed to save preparation time in OR.
  - ○ Transobturator anterior vaginal prolapse repair: prepare porcine dermis graft or polypropylene mesh and polypropylene arms (×4) using provided clamp → mark incision sites (superior and inferior sites on medial obturator foramen) → anterior vaginal wall is incised in midline normal fashion and dissected laterally to inferior pubic ramus → ± reduction of cystocele by anterior repair in standard fashion → mark skin sites (two on each side) → curved needles are inserted for two superior sites (outside-in and needle exits lateral to urethra) → polypropylene arms with sheath are connected to needle and pulled out of skin as needle is rotated out → same steps are performed for the inferior arms except needle pointed at ischial spine but exits along arcus tendineus fascia pelvis (ATFP) → tension of arms is adjusted so that mesh or graft is in contact with endopelvic fascia without tension (this mimics level II support).
  - ○ Controlled studies are needed to establish safety and efficacy.
- Hybrid slings
  - ○ T-sling with Centrasorb: used in SUI surgery; consists of two polypropylene "arms" which hold onto tissue; the arms are connected to each other by monofilament, polydioxanone center. Designed to reduce erosion rate while maintaining efficacy.
  - ○ BioSorb: used in SUI surgery; encompasses a self-fixating polypropylene sling and suburethral biological graft of the surgeon's choice. Designed to reduce erosion rate while maintaining efficacy.
- Absorbable meshes
  - ○ Dexon (multifilament polyglycolic acid)
  - ○ Vicryl (multifilament polyglactin 910)

- ■ High success in laparoscopic posterior repair (80–90% success at 1 year)

BIBLIOGRAPHY

Alexander JW, Kaplan JZ, Altemeier WA. Role of suture material in the development of wound infection. *Ann Surg.* 1967;165:192–199.

Anderson JA. *Implantation Biology: The Host Response and Biomedical Devices.* Boca Raton, FL: CRC Press; 1994:113.

Badylak S, Kokini K, Tullius B, et al. Morphologic study of small intestinal submucosa as a body wall repair device. *J Surg Res.* 2002;103:190–202.

Balique JG, Alexandre JH, Arnaud JP, et al. Intraperitoneal treatment of incisional and umbilical hernias: intermediate results of a multicenter prospective clinical trial using an innovative composite mesh. *Hernia.* 2000;4(Suppl): 10–16.

Bidmead J, Cardozo L. Sling techniques in the treatment of genuine stress incontinence. *Br J Obstet Gynaecol.* 2000;107: 147–156.

Falconer C, Soderberg B, Blomgren B. Influence of different sling materials on connective tissue metabolism in stress urinary incontinent women. *Int Urogynecol J.* 2001;12(Suppl 2): s19–s23.

Fitzgerald MP, Molenhauser J, Brubaker L. Failure of allograft suburethral slings. *BJU Int.* 1999;84:785–788.

Game X, Mouzin M, Vaessen C, et al. Obturator infected hematoma and urethral erosion following transobturator tape implantation. *J Urol.* 2004;171:1629.

Handa V, Jensen JK, Germain MM, et al. Banked human fascia lata for the suburethral sling procedure: a preliminary report. *Obstet Gynecol.* 1996;88:1045–1049.

Hiles MC, Badylak SF, Lantz GC, et al. Mechanical properties of xenogeneic small-intestinal submucosa when used as an aortic graft in the dog. *J Biomed Mater Res.* 1995;29:883–893.

Hodde J. Naturally occurring scaffolds for soft tissue repair and regeneration. *Tissue Eng.* 2002;8:295–308.

Hodde J, Badylak SF, Brightman AO, et al. Glycosaminoglycan content of small intestinal submucosa: a bioscaffold for tissue replacement. *Tissue Eng.* 1996;2(3):209–217.

Iglesia CB, Fenner DE, Brubaker L. The use of mesh in gynecology surgery. *Int Urogynecol J.* 1997;8:785–788.

Jarvis GL, Fowlie A. Clinical and urodynamic assessment of the porcine dermis bladder sling for the treatment of genuine stress incontinence. *Obstet Gynecol.* 1985;92:1189–1191.

Law NW, Ellis H. A comparison of polypropylene mesh and expanded polytetrafluoroethylene patch for the repair of contaminated abdominal wall defects: an experimental study. *Surgery.* 1991;109:652–655.

Martin JN, Brewer DW, Rush LV, et al. Successful pregnancy outcome following mid-gestational uterine rupture and repair using GORE-TEX soft tissue patch. *Obstet Gynecol.* 1990;75:518–521.

Muir TW. Posterior wall prolapse: repair with graft augmentation. In: *The Ins and Outs of Pelvic Organ Prolapse Surgery.* Postgraduate Course. AUGS meeting; 2004.

Narducci PL, Narducci U. Anterior abdominal wall colpopexy using a polytetrafluoroethylene strip (GORE-TEX) for genital prolapse and preservation of vaginal function. *Ital J Gynecol Obstet.* 1988;1:97–101.

Nilsson CG, Kuuva N, Falconer M, et al. Long-term results of the tension-free vaginal tape (TVT) procedure for surgical treatment of female stress urinary incontinence. *Int Urogynecol J.* 2001;(Suppl 2):S5–S8.

Nilsson CG, Rezapour M, Flaconer C. 7 year follow-up of the tension-free vaginal tape (TVT) procedure for treatment of urinary incontinence. *Obstet Gynecol* 2004;104(6):1259–62.

Oelschlager BK, Barreca M, Chang L, et al. The use of small intestine submucosal graft in the repair of paraesophageal hernias: initial observations of a new technique. *Am J Surg.* 2003;186:4–8.

Olsson I, Kroon U. A three-year post operative evaluation of tension-free vaginal tape. *Gynecol Obstet Invest.* 1999;48(4):267–269.

Ostergard DR. Prolapse of the vaginal vault in the elderly; sacrospinous fixation with GORE-TEX. Presented at the 1991 Course on Stress Urinary Incontinence: Female Urinary Incontinence and Genital Prolapse Diagnosis and Therapy. Brescia, Italia.

Palma PCR, Dambros M, Ricetto CLZ, et al. Pubovaginal sling using the porcine small intestinal submucosa for stress urinary incontinence. *Int Braz J Urol.* 2001;27:483–488.

Snyder TE, Krantz KE. Abdominal-retroperitoneal sacral colpopexy for the correction of vaginal prolapse. *Obstet Gynecol.* 1991;77:944–949.

Stoll MR, Cook JL, Pope ER, et al. The use of porcine small intestinal submucosa as a biomaterial for perineal herniorrhaphy in the dog. *Vet Surg.* 2002;31:379–390.

Tunn R, Bettin ST, Fischer W. Tissue replacement by tension-free insertion of prolene tape (TVT technique according to Ulmsten) in urinary incontinence (UI): technical details, indications, specifications, results. *Scand J Urol Nephrol.* 1995;29:75–82.

Ulmsten U, Henriksson L, Johson P, et al. An ambulatory surgical procedure under local anesthesia for treatment of female urinary incontinence. *Int Urogynecol J.* 1996;7:81–86.

Ulmsten U, Johnson P, Rezapour M. A three-year follow-up of tension-free vaginal tape for surgical treatment of female stress urinary incontinence. *Br J Obstet Gynaecol.* 1999;106:345–350.

Weinberger MW, Osterdard DR. Long term follow-up of clinical and urodynamic evaluation of the polytetrafluoroethylene suburethral sling for the treatment of genuine stress incontinence. *Obstet Gynecol.* 1995;86:92–96.

Questions

1. The material (biological or synthetic) which is associated with the highest rate of autolysis is _____.
   (A) Mersilene
   (B) autologous rectus abdominis fascia
   (C) cadaveric fascia lata
   (D) vaginal wall patch
   (E) porcine small intestine submucosa

2. Commercially available product which has been used for vaginal repair of apical POP is _____.
   (A) Perigee (American Medical Systems)
   (B) IVS Tunneler (TYCO)
   (C) Pelvitex (C.R. Bard)
   (D) IntePro (American Medical Systems)
   (E) Symphasis (Cook)

3. A surgeon uses tissue from the thigh of a donor human body. The best term for this tissue graft is _____.
   (A) autologous
   (B) homologous
   (C) heterologous
   (D) xenograft

4. The most common reason to augment tissue during POP repair is _____.
   (A) weak native tissue
   (B) immunocompromise
   (C) central pubocervical fascial defect
   (D) poor wound healing
   (E) recurrent POP

Answers

1. *(C).* One of the disadvantages of cadaveric tissue is autolysis. This is especially pronounced (up to 20%) with cadaveric fascia lata. This may result from tissue rejection and leads to early failure of graft.

2. *(B).* The IVS Tunneler has been used for management of apical prolapses. It is purported to create a "neouterosacral ligament." The procedure is easy to perform and adds minimal amount of time to other POP repairs. Safety and efficacy remain to be seen as more data are necessary. Perigee System is for anterior POP repair. Pelvitex is polypropylene mesh coated with collagen. Theoretically, it can be used for any type of repair. IntePro is the polypropylene component of the Perigee and Apogee Systems. Symphasis is porcine small intestine submucosa graft. Theoretically, it may be used for any type of repair. More data are needed on all of the aforementioned products.

3. *(B).* The tissue described is a homologous allograft (i.e., graft using another human being's tissue, e.g., cadaveric dermis). Autologous graft uses one's own body tissues (e.g., autologous rectus fascia).

Heterologous graft uses animal tissue (e.g., porcine intestinal submucosa). Xenograft uses animal tissue. Allograft uses another human source.

4. *(E)*. Recurrent POP (especially same-site recurrence) and patients who have higher risk of recurrence (based on risk factors) are candidates for tissue augmentation. The type of material used to augment the repair (synthetic, biological, or autologous) is debatable.

51 ESSENTIAL INFORMATION ABOUT FEMALE PELVIC MEDICINE AND RECONSTRUCTIVE SURGERY AND APPLICATION TO OB/GYN SUBSPECIALTY FELLOWSHIPS IN THE UNITED STATES

Sam Siddighi

PAST, PRESENT, AND FUTURE OF FPMRS

It is paradoxic that it has taken so long for the field of gynecologic urology, which gave birth to the greater discipline of gynecology, to become a science in its own right.

PHILIP J DISAIA
(In: Ostergard's Urogynecology and Pelvic Floor Dysfunction, 2004)

UROGYNECOLOGY: TIME LINE OF MAJOR EVENTS

- *2000 B.C. Kahun papyrus*-is earliest description of disease of women including diseases of urinary bladder
- *1852 Marion Sims*—in 1835, he graduated med school; 1852 described successful *repair of vesicovaginal fistula* with silver wire suture; surgery accomplished by Sims position (knee-chest allows ballooning and opening of the vagina for better visualization of fistula), and Sims speculum (silver, duck's bill-shaped instrument which lifts the posterior vaginal wall toward ceiling while patient is in knee-chest position); 1855 founded small Women's Hospital in New York

City (where Waldorf Astoria Hotel currently stands). He is known as the "Father of Modern Gynecology" because of his lifelong teaching, handwork, and achievement, which established the connection between urology and gynecology

- *1905 William Hey* first to officially describe a female with suburethral diverticulum in the medical literature
- *1907 D. Von Giordano*—described the first sling operation using gracilis muscle flap
- *1909 George White*—first to describe a vaginal paravaginal repair in "cystocale, a radical cure by suturing lateral sides of vagina to white line of pelvic fuscia" in JAMA. Essentially, he described vaginal procedure for reattachment of the pubocervical septum to the ATFP.
- *1914 Wilhelm Latzko*—in 1863 graduated medical school in Vienna; 1908 extraperitoneal cesarean section; 1909 *pubiotomy* for management of dystocia; 1914 described *post hysterectomy vesicovaginal fistula* repair which in essence is a partial colpocleisis; became "extraordinary professor of obstetrics and gynecology" at University of Vienna
- *1918 Guy Hunner*—same time period and also at Johns Hopkins, described *Hunner's ulcer of the bladder* which is associated with *interstitial cystitis*
- *1919 Howard A. Kelly*—in 1882 graduated medical school; founded Kensington Hospital for Women in Philadelphia; believed that Obstetrics and Gynecology were too large to be combined into one field. Created the *first residency program in Gynecology* as innovation in surgery; professor of Gynecologic Surgery at Johns Hopkins, use of *air cystoscopy* (discovered by accident in 1893) in knee-chest position to visualize the bladder and ureteral orifices; *Kelly stitch (plication)* 1919 to fix damaged urethral sphincter; he also invented Kelly clamp and Kelly cushion. Considered by some as the founder of the specialty of Urology
- *1930* American Board of Obstetrics and Gynecology (ABOG) founded
- *1938 P. Johnson* described treatment of five patients with suburethral diverticula via complete excision of the diverticular sac
- *1942 AH Aldridge*—developed the rectus abdominis fascial suburethral sling, which after modifications, is the "traditional urethral sling" in use today
- *1948 Arnold Kegel*—the Kegel exercises-a professor of Ob/Gyn at USC/Los Angeles County Hospital; although he was not the first to describe pelvic and perineal muscle exercises, he was critical in standardizing and educating people about it
- *1948 K. M. Fugurnov*—described vaginal surgery for stress urinary incontinence (SUI), which is essentially the same as George White's paravaginal repair
- *1949 Victor F. Marshall, Andrew A. Marchetti, and Kermit E. Krantz* (MMK—urologist-gynecologist-gynecologist,

respectively)—shifted the focus of surgical approach for management of SUI from vaginal to abdominal. They performed the original retropubic urethropexy; theory of descent of urethra below pelvic diaphragm as cause of SUI. Retropubic urethropexies are still the gold standard for management of primary SUI

- *1956 Davis and Cian* introduced the positive-pressure urethrography for the diagnosis of suburethral diverticula
- *1959 Armand J. Pereyra*—First urethral needle suspension procedure which in essence is a vaginal retropubic urethropexy. It was used primarily when other vaginal surgeries were indicated. Thomas A. Stamey, Shlomo Raz, Dominic Muzsnai, and Rubin F. Gittes described modifications to the *Pereyra needle suspension procedure*
- *1960 A. Ingleman-Sundberg*—described partial denervation of the bladder at the hypogastric plexus through the vagina to treat refractory unstable bladder
- *1961 Goren Enhörning*—start of urodynamic studies
- *1961 John C. Burch*—described *Burch retropubic urethropexy* procedure, which attempted to eliminate problems of the MMK (procedure failures, osteitis pubis in 3%, predisposition to enterocele). However, Burch only eliminated osteitis pubis
- *1962 M. Tancer & R. Hyman*—described treatment of suburethral diverticulum by partial ablation in 11 patients
- *1965 Zoedler and Boeminghous* introduced *synthetic* pubovaginal sling for correction of SUI
- *1966 Jack Robertson*—modern cystoscope—used a modified culdoscope to perform cystoscopy to eliminate some of the problems encountered with the air cystoscopy (i.e., he used a better optical system, lens, eliminated need for knee-chest position, and made it an office procedure). The disadvantage of heat emission from light source still remained but this was resolved later with the invention of fiberoptics. J. Robertson is also known as the "Father of Urogynecology" as he was the first president of the Gynecologic Urology Society in 1979
- *1966 T. Jeffcoate and W. Francis*—bladder drills to manage urgency and urge incontinence
- *1968 Wayne Baden and Tom Walker* described the vaginal profile (now known as the Halfway or Baden-Walker), a classification system that grades pelvic organ prolapse
- *1969 Emil A. Tanagho*—performed key urodynamic study: showing midurethra as high-pressure zone (100 cm H_2O) in urethra and demonstrating that the pressure inside the urethra is derived mostly from the smooth muscle component, one-third from striated muscle component, and from the physical properties of urethral wall itself. Additionally, E. Tanagho modified the Burch by placing

sutures 1-2 cm away from urethra and avoiding dissection in the retropubic space to avoid trauma to the delicate urethra and its nerve, vessel, and musculature which could lead to sphincter incompetence (and thus, higher failure rate) after surgery

- *1970 H Spence and J Duckett*—described repair of a suburethral diverticula distal on the urethra by marsupialization
- Bob Shull-popularized the paravaginal defect repair and emphasized importance of obtaining good vault support (i.e., high onto the uterosacral ligaments) when doing any pelvic prolapse repair. He was also the president of the American Urogynecologic Society (AUGS) in 1996
- *1976* International Urogynecology Society was founded in Mexico
- *1976 Stuart L. Stanton*—Professor and program director of first certified fellowship (certified by the Royal College of Obstetricians and Gynaecologists) in Pelvic Reconstruction and Urogynecology at the University of London, St. George's Hospital
- *1978 Donald R. Ostergard* started the first fellowship in Urogynecology in the United States. Also published the first edition of his monumental textbook, *Urogynecology and Pelvic Floor Dysfunction*, in 1980. He was president of the Gynecologic Urology Society in 1984 (which later became known as AUGS)
- *1980 AUGS* held first meeting in New Orleans
- *1981 A. Cullen Richardson*—described treatment of SUI and cystocele in patients with paravaginal defect and SUI by attaching the pubocervical fascia to the arcus tendineus fascia pelvis (ATFP) or the *white line* as described earlier by George White
- *1984* Neuropathy theory of incontinence
- *1986 John OL DeLancey*—using histologic sections, described the paraurethral anatomy in detail in 1986. Then in 1989, went on to explain the anatomy and embryology of the lower urinary tract and also described the existence of the pubovesical ligament. In 1994, described the structural support of the urethra and how it relates to SUI (aka the hammock hypothesis). President of AUGS in 1995
- *1989 B. Shull and W. Baden*—published their experience with paravaginal defect repair for SUI and cystocele
- *1991 T. Vancaille and W. Schuessler*—first reported the laparoscopic retropubic urethropexy for the correction of SUI
- *1995 U. Ulmsten and P. Petros*—impairment of pubourethral ligaments at midurethra and the Integral Theory; first description of the minimally invasive, outpatient tension-free vaginal tape sling (TVT) which revolutionized the treatment of SUI
- *1996 Richard C. Bump*—headed a committee that described the pelvic organ prolapse quantification

(POP-Q) system to standardize the terminology of female pelvic organ prolapse and pelvic floor dysfunction to improve research and communication between physicians. This system was adopted by the International Continence Society (ICS), AUGS, and Society of Gynecologic Surgeons (SGS) the same year

BIBLIOGRAPHY

Aldridge AH. Transplantation of fascia for the relief of urinary incontinence. *Am J Obstet Gynecol.* 1942;44:398–411.

Burch JC. Urethrovaginal fixation to Cooper's ligament for the correction of stress incontinence, cystocele, rectocele, and prolapse. *Am J Obstet Gynecol.* 1961;82:281–190.

Enhorning G. Simultaneous recording of intravesical and intraurethral pressure. *Acta Chir Scand Suppl.* 1961;276:5–12.

Giordano D. Vintieme Congres Francais de Chirurgie; 1907:506.

Hunner GL. Elusive ulcer of the bladder. Further notes of a rare type of bladder ulcer, with a report of twenty-five cases. *Am J Obstet.* 1918;78:374–395.

Ingelman-Sundberg A. Vaginal partial resection of the inferior hypogastric plexus. In: Youssef AF, ed. *Gynecological Urology.* Springfield, IL: Charles C Thomas Publishing Co; 1960.

Jeffcoate TNA, Francsi WJA. Urgency incontinence in the female. *Am J Obstet Gynecol.* 1966;94:604–618.

Kelly HA. Medical gynecology. New York: Appleton; 1908.

Latzko W. Postoperative vesicovaginal fistulas: genesis and therapy. *Am J Surg.* 1942;58: 211–228.

Marshall VF, Marchetti AA, Krantz KE. The correction of stress incontinence by simple vesicourethral suspension. *Surg Gynecol Obstet.* 1949;88:509–518.

Pereyra AJ. Simplified surgical procedure for the correction of stress incontinence in women. *West J Surg.* 1959;67:223–226.

Richardson AC, Edmonds PB, Williams NL. Treatment of stress urinary incontinence due to paravaginal fascial defect. *Obstet Gynecol.* 1981;57:357–362.

Robertson JR. Office cystoscopy: substituting the culdoscope for the Kelly cystoscope. *Obstet Gynecol.* 1966;28:219–220.

Sims JM. On the treatment of vesico-vaginal. *Am J Med Sci.* 1852;23:59–82.

Speert H. *Obstetric and Gynecologic Milestones.* Pearl River, NY: Parthenon Publishing Group; 1996.

Spence HM, Duckett JW. Diverticulum of the female urethra: clinical aspects and presentation of a single operative technique for cure. *J Urol.* 1970;104:432–437.

Tanagho EA, Meyers FH, Smith DR. Urethral resistance: its components and implications. I. Smooth muscle component. II. Striated muscle opponent. *Invest Urol.* 1969;7:136–149.

Tanagho EA. Colpocystourethropexy: the way we do it. *J Urol.* 1976;116:751–753.

Tancer ML, Mooppan MM, Pierre-Louis C: Suburethral diverticulum treatment by partial ablation. *Obstet Gynecol.* 1983;62(4):511–513.

Ulmsten U, Petros P. Intravaginal slingplasty (IVS): an ambulatory surgical procedure for treatment of female urinary incontinence. *Scand J Urol Nephrol.* 1995;29:75.

SOCIETIES RELATED TO FPMRS

- Gynecologic Urology Society began in 1979 with Jack R. Robertson as its first president (hence, he is known as the "Father of Urogynecology"). Currently, the GUS is known as the AUGS (see below)
  - Jack R. Robertson 79–80, C. Paul Hodgkinson 80–81; Hugh M. Shingleton 81–82; W. Glenn Hurt 82–83; Douglas J. Marchant 83–84; Donald R. Ostergard 84–85; R. Peter Beck 85–86.
- *AUGS* began in 1986 with first president J. Andrew Fantl
  - J. Andrew Fantl 86–87; Richard O. Davis 87–88; Henry A. Thiede 88–89; Ernest I. Kohorn 89–90, David A. Richardson 90–91; J. Thomas Benson 91–92; Charles deProsse 92–93; John Higgins 93–94; Alfred Bent 94–95; John O. L. DeLancey 95–96; Bob Shull 96–97; Richard Bump 97–98; Mickey M. Karram 98–99; Nicolette Horbach 99–00, W. Conrad Sweeting 00–01; Peggy Norton 01–02; Linda Brubaker 02–03, Michael Aronson 03–04, Stephen Young 04–05.
- Vaginal Surgeons Society began in 1974 with Wayne F. Baden as its first president.
- *SGS* began in 1981 with Abe Mickal as its first president
- *ICS* originally known as the Continent Club and founded by Eric Glen in 1971. Peter Caldwell was the first president of the ICS, which held its first meeting in 1971. The goal of the ICS is to "study storage and voiding function of the lower urinary tract, its diagnosis, and the management of lower urinary tract dysfunction, and to encourage research into pathophysiology, diagnostic techniques and treatment."

TODAY AND TOMORROW

- Currently, the field of Obstetrics and Gynecology has four official, major subspecialty fellowships: Maternal Fetal Medicine (MFM), Gynecologic Oncology (GynOnc), Reproductive Endocrinology and Infertility (REI), and Female Pelvic Medicine and Reconstructive Surgery (FPMRS). Other fellowship opportunities also exist in family planning, breast, laparoscopy, and critical care. Three of the four major subspecialty fellowships are boarded by the ABOG. As of 2005, FPMRS is certified by ABOG and the American Board of Urology (ABU) and written/oral board examinations will follow soon. It is expected that in a few years, after an adequate number of accredited, 3-year fellowship programs are able to meet the requirements of the ABOG and ABU, there will be a written as well as an oral board examination in FPMRS. As of now, there are only 23 ABOG-approved, 3-year fellowship programs in FPMRS. There are also several noncertified, 3-year fellowship programs (few of which have been in existence before some of the certified fellowship programs). One 2-year fellowship and several 1-year programs also exist. Additionally, physicians with residency training in Urology can enter this field in an official manner, either by applying to the FPMRS fellowship programs (for a 2-year fellowship) or by applying to a separate 1–2-year fellowship in Female Urology.

- Discounting specialty "turf" politics, reasons why it has been difficult to attain an adequate number of ABOG certified programs are (1) Some 3-year programs in FPMRS have not applied for certification by the ABOG and ABU, (2) it can be difficult for certified programs to maintain their ABOG/ABU certification. For example, one of the well-respected 3-year fellowship programs in FPMRS, lost its certification due to the inability to recruit a second fellowship trained urogynecologist. The ABOG hopes "to create a cadre of academic teachers to educate young generalists and specialist in obstetrics and gynecology"(P. DiSaia). In the next few years this will become a reality as new programs emerge and meet the requirements of the board. The goal is to have at least one, well-trained urogynecologist in the department of Obstetrics and Gynecology and/or department of Urology of all tertiary-care centers across the country.

- In the past, "turf" battles have existed between urologists and gynecologists because of confusion over which specialty should manage certain conditions of the lower urinary and genital tracts. The "turf" politics are not unique to our two specialties (e.g., ENT vs. facial plastic surgery, OMFS vs. facial plastic surgery, general surgery and colorectal surgery, and so forth) The "turf" politics have resulted in fragmentation of our and other specialties. They have also made it difficult to develop a board examination for the subspecialty of FPMRS. It makes no sense to have such resistance since effective management of these patients requires a multidisciplinary approach. Consider the following facts:

1. Historically, the gynecology and urology were closely associated and one developed through the other (see time line above under Marion Sims and Howard Kelly)
2. "Embryologically, anatomically, and functionally, the lower urinary tract and genital tract are intimately associated" (W. Glenn Hurt. In:

Urogynecologic Surgery. 2nd ed. Lippincott William & Wilkins; 2000:6).

3. Neither gynecologists nor urologists are adequately trained in the field of FPMRS. To become a female urologist, graduating urology seniors must strengthen their knowledge of genital anatomy and receive training in pelvic prolapse surgery, and management of certain vulvar and vaginal conditions. Similarly, the graduating senior gynecologists must strengthen their knowledge of the management of urinary incontinence (also fecal incontinence), and receive additional training in the recognition, evaluation, and management of certain conditions of the bladder and ureter below the pelvic brim.

4. According to the statistics listed below, there is absolutely no need for turf battles since there is plenty of business for those interested in managing problems of the lower urinary tract and pelvic floor. However, there is a shortage of well-trained physicians to take care of the countless numbers of patients with these disorders.

- The good news is that this is beginning to change. There are 23 nationally accredited programs in FMPRS, which are certified by both the American College of Obstetrics and Gynecology and the ABU. Currently, the top centers in the country manage lower urinary tract and pelvic floor dysfunction via a multidisciplinary approach which involves FPMRS specialists, female urologists, colorectal surgeons, gastroenterologists, physical therapists, trained physicians assistants and nurse practioners, and others related to and/or trained in the specialty.

- Currently, there is a lot of interest in the field of FPMRS because of the rising demand. This interest will continue to flourish into the future. The "baby boomers" are aging. According to the National Center for Health Statistics and various other sources, the life expectancy for a woman was 79.8 years in 2001 and it is rising. Today 13% of people are over age 65 and that number will increase by 25% by the year 2030. Since women outlive men by ≈7 years, a larger percentage of the population will continue to be female by the year 2030. It is estimated that 7 million new surgeries and 2 million repeat surgeries for pelvic dysfunction will be needed annually by the year 2030. Fifty percent of women will have a bladder control problem during their lifetimes. One in every nine woman will undergo surgery for pelvic organ prolapse or incontinence by age 80. Even nulliparous college women who are not usually thought of as having pelvic dysfunction or incontinence experience these problems. Additionally, there is increased awareness among physicians of specialties other than obstetrics and gynecology about incontinence, pelvic organ prolapse, and pelvic dysfunction. Therefore more referrals are being made to gynecologists, female urologists, and urogynecologists. More women are also coming forth with their symptoms, perhaps, because of greater awareness, less shame, and physician screening.

- With the statistics being as such, there is no wonder why industry has such an interest in FPMRS. New pharmaceutical drugs, surgical instruments, anatomical models, incontinence products, tissue augmenting materials, pelvic floor dysfunction evaluation devices, and centers for behavioral and physical rehabilitation of the pelvis are emerging. The National Institutes of Health have noticed this need and have provided significant funding for research in this area. The Urinary Incontinence Network (UITN), which consists of investigators from nine centers and the Pelvic Floor Disorders Network (PFDN), which consists of investigators from seven centers across the United States is currently ongoing. The results of these trials will provide valuable information. In the near future, the field Obstetrics and Gynecology will require more practitioners who are well trained in FPMRS, and therefore job security and strong income potential for the fellowship trained urogynecologist.

APPLYING FOR FELLOWSHIP

- Applying for FPMRS fellowship can be a daunting task, but it is definitely "do-able." To increase your chances of being accepted, you must try to complete your application well before the deadline, which is usually before June 1 of the year prior to starting fellowship. Deadlines for Baylor and Brown may be earlier. Although most programs participate in the NRMP (National Intern and Residency Match Program), there is no centralized application system yet, so you have to complete every application separately. Acceptance to FPMRS fellowship is becoming very competitive for several reasons: (1) there is only one spot annually per program, (2) as of 2005, there are only a few programs (see list on next page) and many applicants (Tables 51-1 and 51-2) (3) only few programs are ABOG and ABU accredited and it is hoped that soon the specialty will become boarded as more programs meet accreditation requirements, (4) some programs do not participate in the match, (5) some programs have "internal" candidates, (6) some programs will interview gynecologists as well as urologists straight out of residency or after many years of practice in the community, and (7) subspecialties are becoming popular again. Nevertheless, do not be discouraged. If you start early and do your best, you have a shot at getting in. Do not make the mistake of putting all of your eggs in one basket. Make sure you apply to many programs if you want to increase your chances of getting accepted somewhere. Request an application well in advance of the deadline so you can have enough time to complete all of the applications, request letters of recommendation, and give yourself ample time to provide supporting documents. Applications deadlines are variable each year but are usually between June and mid-August of the year preceding start of fellowship. Brown may have an earlier deadline for application. Additionally, try going to the AUGS meeting 1 and/or 2 years prior to the time of your application so you can meet some of the key people in the field. FPMRS is a small community of physicians so this is truly possible.

- What kind of information is required in the application? Besides basic identifying information (name, address, telephone, e-mail, and so forth), you have to provide information about your undergraduate, medical education, and residency training. Dates and scores of examinations such as United States Medical Licensing Examination (USMLE) (or National Board of Medical Examiners [NBME]/National Board of Osteopathic Medical Examiners [NBOME]/Federation Licensing Exam [FLEX]/Medical Council of Canada Examination [LMCC]) and Council of Resident Education in Obstetrics and Gynecology (CREOG) are important. Non-U.S. citizens must provide proof of permanent immigrant status (e.g., green card) or an appropriate visa (e.g., J-1, F-1, H-1B) and examination scores such as Foreign Medical Graduate Examination in the Medical Sciences (FMGEMS) or any of the above. Additionally, you should include your state license number and Drug Enforcement Administration (DEA) number if you have them. If you have been denied a license, had a complaint filed against you to the board, or have had your license suspended or revoked you should include a letter explaining your situation. You should also include a letter of explanation if you have had gaps in your education or have been denied hospital privileges. Finally, if you have been fined, placed on probation, convicted, or imprisoned, you have a lot of explaining to do!

- You must also include a curriculum vitae and a personal statement. In your CV you may want to include any of the following: (1) a description of basic science and clinical research projects, (2) presentations at regional or national meetings, (3) peer-review publications, (4) books or manuscripts written (if any), (5) teaching experience, (6) community service, (7) awards, (8) languages spoken and fluency, (9) postgraduate medical education such as teaching appointments or practice experience, and (10) anything else that distinguishes

TABLE 51-1 2006 ABOG and ABU Accredited Fellowship Training Programs in FPMRS in the United States*

PROGRAM NAME	CONTACT INFORMATION	PROGRAM DIRECTOR	ASSISTANT INSTRUCTORS/DIRECTOR(S)	DURATION (YEARS)	SPOTS/YEAR	NRMP	COMMENTS/HIGHLIGHTS
Albert Einstein College of Medicine	Attn: Wilma Greston, Montefiore Medical Center, 3332 Rochambeau Ave., Bronx, NY 10467, Off: (718)-920-5233, mikhailgyn@aol.com	Magdy Mikhail	G. Lazarou, K. Powers, H. Rosa, M. Guess	3	1	Y	4 x B9-Gyn calls/mo, 3 weeks of vacation/yr, 4 full-time urogyn faculty, 3 clinical sites; strong office urogynecology experience; urology, colorectal surgery rotations, vascular surgery research facility available, 1st year basic science research (9 mo), minimally invasive experience avail., 3 months of elective time
Brown Medical School	The Center fo Women's Surgery, 695 Eddy Street, Providence, RI 02903, Off: (401) 453-7560 Ext. 107, dmyers@wihri.org	Deborah L. Myers	C. Rardin	3	$2/3^{\dagger}$	Y	1 weekend round/mo, no Ob call, 4 weeks vacation/yr, 2 week research "Boot Camp," start of fellowship, 1 day/wk of research x 3 years, minimally invasive surgery avail., 1 month urology and colorectal surgery rotation, teaching focus, D. Myers: trained by R. Scotti; designed clay pelvic model as teaching tool, trained L. Arya
Cleveland Clinic Foundation	9500 Euclid Ave., Desk a81, Cleveland, OH 44195, Off: (216) 445-6586, walterm@ccf.org	Mark D. Walters	M. Paraiso, M. Barber	3	$1^{\dagger}$	Y	No Ob call, $1/4$ B9-Gyn coverage, 3 weeks vacation/yr; strong research focus with 3-month research rotations/yr; one clinical site, organized lectures and journal club, cadaver lab avail; 1st year devoted to laparoscopy leading to degree in minimally invasive surgery in addition to FPMRS. June Alllyson Foundation Research Award x 2 years, Dr. M. Walters: well-known in FPMRS, authored numerous articles, Urogyn text book co-author with M Karram
Cooper Hospital/University Medical Center—Robert Wood Johnson Medical School	3 Cooper Plaza, Suite 221, Camden, NJ 08103, Off: (856) 342-2965, boardman-eileen@cooperhealth.edu	Kristine Whitmore	T. Grody, B. Vakili, J. Maccarone, A. Holzberg, R. Caraballo	3	1	Y	Few Ob calls per month in Camden, vacation xxx, surgical volume, 4 full-time urogyn faculty, surgical film production technology; opportunity to learn urologic surgical procedures (e.g., bladder augmentation, ureteral repair, and reimplantation), 2nd year research focus in 2 x 2 blocks, ongoing comparison studies funded by industry, colorectal and geriatrics rotations, K. Whitmore: internationally known urologist and expert in Interstitial Cystitis
Duke University Medical Center	Box 3192, Courier RM 239, Baker House, Durham, NC 27710, Off: (919) 684-4647, amund002@mc.duke.edu	Cindy Amundsen	A. Weidner, J. Wilkinson	3	1	Y	No ob call, B9-Gyn back-up call covering resident patients, 24/7 call for private attending patients; 2 months with G. Webster in first year (Female Urologist), optional MPH in second year; 2 month rotations in colorectal, urology, and neurology; some focus on research in 2nd and 3rd years, also 3rd year 1x/wk Gyn clinic at VA, 8 fellows graduated; C. Amundsen: Female Urology fellowship training, interested in Rx refractory urge incontinence (e.g., Botox, Interstim)

(Continued)

TABLE 51-1 2006 ABOG and ABU Accredited Fellowship Training Programs in FPMRS in the United States (Continued)

PROGRAM NAME	CONTACT INFORMATION	PROGRAM DIRECTOR	ASSISTANT INSTRUCTORS/ DIRECTOR(S)	DURATION (YEARS)	SPOTS/ YEAR	NRMP	COMMENTS/HIGHLIGHTS
Good Samaritan Hospital	Tristate Urogynecology, 375 Dixmyth Ave., Cincinnati, OH 45220-2489, Off: (513) 872-4171, mickey_karram @trihealth.com	Mickey Karram	S. Kleeman	3	1	Y	1 optional, paid Ob call per month, 4 weeks vacation/yr, 3 months research blocks in first 2 years, urology rotation 6 months first 2 years, 3rd year focus on electives, research, Colorectal Surgery; rotations avail, high volume of surgical cases; 12 fellows graduated since 93, da Vinci technology, research dept/ many ongoing projects, active cadaver lab, Karram: formally trained 2 years at UCLA-Harbor, Professor, authored major texts, >100 papers, many chapters, Editor in Chief Int J Urogyn, Teaches and hosts at annual Hawaii, Las Vega, and Philadelphia Female Urology and Urogynecology International Seminars Gynecology conferences
Indiana University	Methodist Hospital, 1633 N. Capitol Ave.,Suite 436, Indianapolis. IN 46202-1227, Off: (317) 962-8152, DougH22@aol.com	Douglass S. Hale	M. Mutone	3	1	Y	Ob call and vacation NA, strong laparoscopic experience, da Vinci utilized, innovative research projects, dedicated research assistance, Colorectal and Urology rotations; D Hale: fellowship at Indiana by Benson completed in '95; interest in evaluation and treatment of POP and Interstim
Loyola University Medical Center	2160 S. First Avenue, Maywood, IL 60153; Off: (708) 216-2170, lbruba1@lumc.edu	Linda Brubaker	M. FitzGerald, K. Kenton, J. Wheeler	3	1	Y	Call schedule NA, 3 weeks vacation/yr, 3 full-time urogyn faculty, surgical volume, diverse surgical experience, ample research opportunity, active in medical and surgical management of pelvic floor dysfunction, strong urology experience, colorectal surgery rotation, 1 of 7 sites for the PFDN; L. Brubaker: trained x2 yrs at Rush Presbyterian, St. Luke's Med Ctr, Professor, numerous papers, presentations, lectures about POP, incontinence, research methodology, co-author of texts Office Urogynecology, Operative Gynecology, Female Pelvic Floor: A multidisciplinary approach, on advisory committee for IC
Magee-Women's Hospital, University of Pittsburgh	300 Halket Street, Pittsburgh, PA 15213, Off: (412) 641-1441 or -1440, aweber@mail.magee.edu	Anne M. Weber	H. Zyczynski, P. Moalli, C. Ghetti	3	1	Y	No Ob call, daily urogyn call in monthly segments x 4 months/yr, 3 weeks vacation/yr, Master's of Science in Clinical Research integrated over 3 yrs and mandatory, several ongoing projects,1 of 9 sites of UITN; A. Weber: trained at Cleveland Clinic, coordinator of PFDN (1 of 7 sites), coauthor of Incontinence 2004 and Office Urogynecology

Institution	Address	Director	Faculty				Notes
Mayo Clinic Rochester	200 First Street, SW Rochester, MN 55905, Off: (507) 266-3262, fields.sherry@mayo.edu	John B. Gebhart	C. Klingele	3	1	Y	Gyn-Onc call 1-2/month, 3 weeks vacation/yr, Master' in Clinical Research recommended during yr. 1, many years of surgical tradition, "Mayo way", Plastic Surgery & ICU rotations required, ample and diverse surgical cases, Gebhart trained by T. Lee at Mayo
Mayo Clinic Scottsdale	13400 East Shea Blvd., Scottsdale, AZ 85259, Off: (480) 301-8090 or -6884	Javier F. Magrina	J. McGreena, J. Cornella, N. Itano, J. Heppell, Young-Saddock	3	1	Y	B9-gyn/Gyn-Onc call 1 out of 3–4 weeks, 3 weeks vacation per year, strong Gyn-onc management experience, large surgical volume, laparoscopic and robotic (da Vinci) surgery, years of surgical tradition—"Mayo way," Urodynamics performed by Urology, 4–6 weeks rotation with urology and colorectal in 3rd year, ≥2 research conferences funded during fellowship; P Magtibay: trained at Mayo-Scottsdale for fellowship, has additional 3 years of training in Gyn-Onc
National Capital Consortium, Washington, DC	6900 Georgia Ave., NW Washington, DC 20307-5001, Off: (202) 782-8433, john.fischer @na.amedd.army.mil	John R. Fischer	J. Buller, J. Clemons, other staff NA	3	1		30 days vacation per year, 5 urogynecologists on faculty, Rotations at Walter Reed and Washington Hospital Center, rotations in neurophsiology, Urology, Colorectal, and laparoscopic surgery, research opportunities avail.; J Fischer is a Lieutenant Colonel in United States Air Force, trained at Indiana University
New York University School of Medicine	550 First Ave., New York, NY 10016, Off: (212) 263-6362, robert.porges @med.nyu.edu	Robert F. Porges	C. Kwon, S. Smilen	3	1		4 Ob calls per month, xxx vacations/yr, diverse patient population, rotations at Risch, Bellvue, and St Peters in New Jersey, 3 full-time urogyn faculty members; R. Porges: ex-president of Vaginal Surgeons Society 1977–1978, co-author of text Pelvic Support Abnormalities, extensive experience in vaginal surgery
University of Alabama at Birmingham	618 20th St., South, NHB 219 Birminghum, AL 35233-7333 Off: (205)934-7874 Fax: (205)975-8893 evarner@uabmc.edu	R Eduard Varner		3	1	Y	not available because newly approved program
University of California Los Angeles	100 West Carson Street, Bld D-3, Box 489, Torrance, CA 90509-2910, Off: (310) 222-3592 or -3868, narenderbhatia @hotmail.com	Narender N. Bhatia	L. Betson	3	1	N	5 x ½ day calls (monetary compensation), 4 weeks vacation/yr; location of 1st formal urogynecology fellowship in the US with D Ostergard as director, flexible curriculum, N. Bhatia: well-respected in the field, authored numerous articles and chapters, trained by D. Ostergard, has trained numerous urogynecologists, current research interest in electrical nerve stimulation, emphasis on basic science research

(Continued)

TABLE 51-1 2006 ABOG and ABU Accredited Fellowship Training Programs in the United States *(Continued)*

PROGRAM NAME	CONTACT INFORMATION	PROGRAM DIRECTOR	ASSISTANT INSTRUCTORS/ DIRECTOR(S)	DURATION (YEARS)	SPOTS/ YEAR	NRMP	COMMENTS/HIGHLIGHTS
University of California San Diego	Women's Pelvic Medicine Center, 9350 Campus Point Drive, Suite 2A, La Jolla, CA 92037, Off: (858) 657-8435, aribant@ucsd.edu	Charles W. Nager	K. Luber, S. Menefee, M. Lukacz, M. Albo	3	1	Y	Q week Ob calls per month (≈1-2 nights/mo), vacation time NA, 4 full-time urogyn faculty, 1 of 9 sites of NIH Urinary Incontinence Treatment Network (UITN), CREST course (research training), >1 yr devoted to research, strong urology experience with Albo; C. Nager: trained under S Stanton for 1 year at St. George's Hospital in London, preceptorship under D Ostergard, authored many papers and chapters
University of Michigan Health System	1500 E. Medical Center Drive, Room L4100, Women's Hospital, Ann Arbor, MI 48109-0276, Off: (734) 764-8429	John O.L. DeLancey	D. Fenner, E. McGuire	3	1	Y	No Ob call, 2 weeks vacation per year, flexible curriculum, research emphasis and numerous anatomy research opportunities, 1 of 7 sites PFDN, collaboration with school of Biomechanical Engineering. Strong experience in urology with McGuire; J. DeLancey: Norman F. Miller Professor, world authority on clinical anatomy of female pelvis (anatomy, histology, MRI studies), interest in effects of aging and childbirth on pelvic floor anatomy
University of North Carolina at Chapel Hill	CB #7570, MacNider Bldg, Chapel Hill, NC 27599-7570, Off: (919) 966-4717, ecwells@med.unc.edu	Ellen Wells	A. Visco, A. Connolly, M. Jannelli	3	1	Y	B9-Gyn calls 3 (weeknights) + 1–2 (weekends) per month, 4 full-time urogyn faculty, research spread over 3 years but mainly during year 2, teaching focus, strong residency program, 1 of 7sites of NIH Pelvic Floor Disorders Network (PFDN), videourodynamics available, home of W Droegemueller, Wells has strong community-patient ties and teaching commitment
University of Pennsylvania School of Medicine	3400 Spruce Street, Philadelphia, PA 19143, Off: (215) 349-8401, larya @mail.obgyn.upenn.edu	Mark Morgan	Lily A. Arya, Najjia Mahmoud	3	1	Y	No Ob call. Home urogyn call 1/4 weekends, 4 weeks vacation/yr. 1 month rotation in Colorectal Surgery, 3 mo rotation in Urology. Basic science and Epidemiologic Research (funded) either in 2nd or 3rd year. Opportunity to earn a Master's Degree in Clinical Epidemiology is available. L. Arya was trained at Brown.
University of Southern California	Women's and Childrens, 1240 North Mission Road, Los Angeles, CA 90033, Off: (323) 226-3422 or -3419 or -3394	John J. Klutke	D. Duong	3	1	N	2 Ob calls/mo, 4 weeks vacation/yr, fellow has supervisory role in preop and postop care, 3rd year focus on research and electives, ongoing studies funded by industry, diverse cases, Klutke formally trained by C. Ballard, open to new techniques, interest in TVT vs. TOT

| University of Texas Southwestern Medical Center | 5323 Harry Hines Blvd. Dallas, TX 75235-9032, Off: (214) 648-7211, joseph.schaffer @utsouthwestern.edu | Joseph Schaffer | M. Nihira, M. Boreham, C. Wai, M. Corton, A. Word | 3 | 1 | Y | call schedule NA, 2 weekend rounds/ mo, 2 weeks vacation/yr, 4 full-time urogyn faculty, colorectal, urology rotation, 1 month elective, 1 month with B. Shull at Scott and White Hospital, 2nd year basic science research with A. Word, June Alllyson Foundation Research Award x 2 years, 1/9 site of Urinary Incontinence Treatment Network (UITN), Anatomy lab and Minimally invasive experience avail., Schaffer trained at Cleveland Clinic x 1 year fellowship |

ABBREVIATIONS: ABU = American Board of Urology
ABOG = American Board of Obstetrics and Gynecology
PFDN = Pelvic Floor Disorders Network
UITN = Urinary Incontinence Treatment Network
POP = Pelvic Organ Prolapse
IC = Interstitial Cystitis
NA = information not available
*Listed in alphabetical order.
†Brown has 1 opening every other year
‡Cleveland Clinic has 2 separate fellowship programs. Dr. Firouz Daneshgari is Director of a 2 yr fellowship for Urology-trained applicants at the Urological Institute
NOTE: Information contained in this table was compiled from several sources: (1) ABOG Web site, (2) AUGS Web site, (3) Multiple, lengthy interviews with faculty, fellows, residents, and/or staff by Sam Siddighi and/or each of the "collaborators" listed above this table, and (4) telephone and electronic mail questionnaires sent to various fellows, residents and/or staff. Great effort was made to be as accurate and unbiased as possible. Subjective terms were utilized minimally. The information contained in this table is meant to help the fellowship applicant and to serve as a comparison guide for the fellowship programs, directors, fellows, residents, and staff. The "Comments/Highlights" section contains more information for some fellowships vs. others because of the disparity of information provided by the fellowship representative(s). Extensive effort was made to be equally thorough and fair. Some programs did not provide much information.

TABLE 51-2   Nonaccredited Fellowships in Female Pelvic Medicine and Reconstructive Surgery in the United States

PROGRAM NAME	CONTACT INFORMATION	PROGRAM DIRECTOR	DURATION (YEARS)
Louisiana State University	Dept. Ob/Gyn, Section of FPMRS, 1542 Tulane Ave., New Orleans, LA 701112; Off: (504) 568-4866; Rchess@LSUHSC.edu	Ralph R. Chesson	3
Greater Baltimore Medical Center	6569 N. Charles Street, Suite 307, Baltimore, MD 21204; Off: (410) 828-3704	Alf Bent	3
Scott & White Hospital and Texas A&M USHSC COM	Dept. Ob/Gyn, Section of FPMRS, 2401 South 31st Street, Temple, TX 76508; Off: (254) 724-2677; bshull@mailbox.sw.org	Bob Shull	3
Evanston Hospital—Norwestern University	Evanston Continence Center, 1000 Central Street, Suite 730, Evanston, IL 60201; Off: (847) 570-2750	Peter K. Sand	3
Mount Auburn Hospital	Boston Urogynecology Associates, 300 Mount Auburn Street, Suite 302, Cambridge, MA 02138; Off: (617) 354-5452	Peter L. Rosenblatt	3
Oregon Health Sciences University	3181 W.W. Sam Jackson Parkway, Portland, Or 97201; Off: (503) 494-3107	S. Renee Edwards	3
Urogynecology Specialists of Kentuckiana @Norton Suburban Women's Pavillion	914 N. Dixie Ave., Suite 104, Elizabethtown, KY 42701; Off: (270) 763-1711; mheit@urogynspecialists.com	Michael Heit	3
Englewood Hospital and Medical Center/Mount Sinai School of Medicine/Winthrop Hospital	FPMRS, Ob/Gyn, North Annex 2nd Floor, Englewood, NJ 07631; Off: (201) 894-3515; Michael.Vardy@ehmc.com	Michael D. Vardy	3
University of Rochester	Dept Ob/Gyn, 601 Elmwood Avenue, Box 668, Rochester, NY 14642; Off: (585) 273-3313 or 3232	Gunhilde M. Buchsbaum	3
Atlantic Health System— Morristown Memorial Hospital	Division Urogynecology, Reconstructive Pelvic Surgery, 100 Madison Ave., Morristown, NJ 07962-1956; Off: (973) 971-7267; patrick.culligan@ahsys.org	Patrick Culligan	3
University of Louiville Health Science Center	Dept. Ob/Gyn, Urogyneoclogy Division, 315 E. Broadway, M-18, Louiville, KY 40202; Off: (505) 629-2184; sbtate01@louiville.edu	Susan Tate	3
University of California, Irvine - Medical Center	Center for Continence and Reconstructive Surgery, 101 The City Drive, Bldg 56, Orange, CA 92868; Off: (714) 456-8564; knoblett@uci.edu	Karen Noblett	3
Pelvic Health and Continence Center	7550 Fannin, Houston, TX 77054	Peter M. Lotze	3
Cleveland Clinic—Florida	Dept. Ob/Gyn, Section Urogynecology and Reconstructive Pelvic Surgery, 2950 Cleveland Clinic Blvd., Weston, FL 33331; Off: (888) 978-0004; davilag@ccf.org	Willy Davila	2–3
Johns Hopkins Medicine School	Dept. Ob/Gyn, 4940 Eastern Avenue, Baltimore, MD 21224-27805; Off: (410) 550-0335	Victoria Handa	NA
Boston Urogynecology/Mount Auburn Hospital	Dept. Ob/Gyn, Boston Urogyn, 725 Concord Ave., #3300, Cambridge, MA 02138; Off: (617) 354-5452; kafitzge@mah.harvard.edu	Kay Fitzgerald	NA
Institute for Females Hospital Pelvic Medicine/St. Lukes	2200 West Hamilton Street, Suikte 111, Allentown, PA 18104; Off: (610) 435-9575; milesmurphy@comcast.net	Miles Murphy	1–3
Women's Continence Center of Greater Rochester	500 Helendale Road, Suite 265, Rochester, NY 14609; Off: (585) 266-2360	Hilary Cholhan	NA
Emory University	69 Butler Street, Atlanta, GA 30303; Off: (404) 616-3366; radam@emory.edu	Rony Adam	NA
St. Lukes Hospital	701 Ostrum Street, Suite 102, Bethlehem, PA 18015; Off: (610) 954-4960	John W. Spurlock	NA
Women's Hospital Memorial Medical Center	701 E. 28th Street, Suite 212, Long Beach, CA 90806, Off: (562) 426-5630	Donald R. Ostergard	NA

NOTE: NA = not available.

you from other applicants (e.g., video production skills, medically related travel outside of the United States, other degrees, special talents, and so forth). What if you have done research but have not published a paper? A paper that has been published holds more weight than a research project completed. The following is the order of importance when it comes to completed research projects: paper published > in press > accepted > submitted > written > research done. The following is the order of importance of presentations: oral presentation > poster presentation. Regardless of the former, choosing an applicant is not a science.

- Spend some quality time on your personal statement because it is read carefully by most fellowships and may influence their decision to grant you an interview. You may want to answer the following questions in your personal statement. (1) Why do you want to go into the field of FPMRS? (2) What are your professional goals or where do you see yourself in your career in 5–10 years, and (3) What are your personal strengths and weaknesses.

- Three letters of recommendation are required (some places will require only two). One letter should be from the urogynecologist or gynecologist whom you have worked with extensively. One should be from the department chairman or residency program director. The last letter can be from an assistant/associate/tenured professor who knows you well. If you have been practicing in the community for many years, it may be difficult to get the above letters so you may get letters of reference from your colleagues or from someone with whom you have done research.

- Some programs (e.g., Mayo) will require additional documents such as official transcripts of all schools that you matriculated from undergraduate education onward, a dean's letter from your medical school, official score report from USMLE or NBME, and a copy of your medical school diploma (a valid Educational Commission for Foreign Medical Graduates [ECFMG] certificate will be required if you graduated from a medical school outside the United States or Canada). Some places will ask you for a recent passport type color photograph of your head and shoulders. Sending a photograph is always a good idea even if its not required because it can "humanize" your application and make them remember you better. Make sure you smile for the camera!

- Do not forget to send a stamped return postcard or to call the programs to make sure that they have received all of your application materials and that everything is in order. This is your responsibility, not theirs!

- A successful interview is critical to getting accepted to any fellowship in Obstetrics and Gynecology. If you have received an interview offer, there are some things about your application that are noteworthy. Remember your basic interviewing skills from medical school and residency interviews. If you are a bad interviewer, you may want to read a book or watch a video on interviewing before going to your interviews. Be well-groomed, communicate clearly, be energetic but cool. Do not be arrogant! The interviewers are probably more accomplished than you and they already know your accomplishments from your CV and application. Many times, they just want to see what kind of a person you are (your character, personality, how well you answer questions, how well you present yourself, and how well you fit in). They will ask you questions about things you have mentioned in your CV so know exactly what you have written. They may also try to put you in certain hypothetical situations to see how you react under pressure. Furthermore, they always will ask you if you have any questions. Do your homework and have some good questions prepared, even though many of these will get answered during the introduction or throughout the interview process.

- Who conducts these interviews? The fellowship program director, codirector(s), fellows, and other medical personnel who are involved in the fellowship (physicians assistants, nurse practitioners, researchers, other faculty member(s) all have some input about you. Typically, you will have five to seven, 15–30-minute interviews. The exceptions to this are Baylor and University of Southern California (USC) (three to four interviews per applicant) and University of Texas Southwestern (UTSW), which conducts ≈11 interviews per applicant. After your interview, the programs will meet and discuss all of the applicants. They will review your entire application once again, including notes made about you after the interview. They will rank you based on all of the above information. (Some programs may interview you at AUGS only or interview you at AUGS for a preliminary interview.)

MAKING YOUR RANK ORDER LIST

- If you are participating in the NRMP, you will have to make a rank order list. Making your list can be a frustrating endeavor because there are several excellent fellowships in existence. You will find yourself changing your list many times and even may make final adjustments just before the NRMP deadline. My two pieces of advice are these: (1) wait until you have finished all of your interviews to make your list, and (2) do some soul-searching to see what is really important to you. There is no magic formula. The program that is best for you may not be so good for someone else. Below is a list of some things (in alphabetical order) that applicants consider before making their rank list. None of these are of equal worth and for some people only one or two of these will be the most important factor(s) when making their final rank list.

CAREER GOALS:

Do you want to be an academician or a leader in the field of FPMRS? Do you want to be well trained and have a thriving private practice? Do you want to work for an Health Maintenance Organization (HMO)?

EDUCATION

Is this fellowship a place where you will get the best education either because of the people who are there, quality of teaching, the number of trained urogynecologists on staff, connections, or the work environment? Is it important to you that the person who is in charge of you is a full professor versus an assistant or associate professor?

FELLOWSHIP PERSONALITY

Do you see yourself getting along with the program director and others in the fellowship for the next 3 years? Do you have a connection with people in the fellowship when you were interviewing? How did you feel after your interview at this fellowship? Do you want to be at a regimented or structured program, in terms of schedule and expectations, or one that is more flexible?

FUTURE JOB OPPORTUNITY

Who are the graduates of this program and where are they now? Do the fellows have difficulty getting the job that they want? Does the program director help you establish yourself somewhere in the country?

GEOGRAPHY

Can you see yourself living in this city? Do you have family or personal obligations in a certain region that may influence your decision? Is it too expensive to live in this city? Can you save some money by living in this city for 3 years?

NAME

Is there someone in this fellowship that is world renowned, well published, and/or well respected in the field who will have positive influence on your career? Is this fellowship somewhere you have dreamed of going? Is there someone in this fellowship that you would love to learn from?

RESEARCH

Do you want to do basic science research or clinical research? How much time do you want to spend on research? What kinds of projects are interesting to you? Is there anyone in this fellowship that can help you publish papers?

TRAINING

Do you feel that you will be adequately trained in this field? Do you believe you will gain in your surgical skills in this fellowship? Do you believe that laparoscopic surgery is important in the future of Urogynecology? And if yes, does this fellowship provide opportunity to learn this skill?

WORK HOURS

How hard do you want to work during fellowship? Do you want to be at the country club, dog races, or somewhere in between? How is the call schedule? Do you want to do Obstetric call so you can collect cases for the boards or make some extra cash? Or do you want to have nothing to do with Obstetrics anymore? How much benign gynecology weeknight and weekend call do you have to take? Are you expected to be a research paper publishing machine? Do you have protected research time? Are you expected to function as a glorified resident? Are you only there to serve their needs?

UNTOUCHABLES

Do you have the opportunity to dissect cadavers and enter anatomy lab? Do you have the opportunity to work with industry if you so desire? Is the patient population such that you will see a variety of pathology in your 3 years? Does this fellowship offer an opportunity to learn advanced technologies? Does this fellowship offer an opportunity to rotate through urology, colorectal surgery, intensive care unit, plastic surgery, gynecologic oncology, or other specialty? What is the relationship of the urogynecology department with colorectal surgery and urology? Does this fellowship have elective rotation(s)? Outside rotations (e.g., another institution in the country or Africa to repair vesicovaginal fistulas)?

CONGRATULATIONS, YOU HAVE BEEN ACCEPTED

If you have been accepted then you may not be reading this, but if you are, here is a tip. Be positive. Help urogynecology fellowship graduates if you can. Good luck and see you at AUGS!

UROGYNECOLOGY AND FEMALE PELVIC RECONSTRUCTIVE SURGERY:
Just the Facts

BOARD EXAMINATION

QUESTIONS

1. Patient who is wearing a _____ pessary needs to be evaluated more often than usual.
   (A) Gehrung
   (B) donut
   (C) ring
   (D) Gelhorn
   (E) cube
2. The structure(s) which provide(s) the primary support to the female pelvis is/are _____.
   (A) white line
   (B) uterosacral ligaments
   (C) unfundibulopelvic ligaments
   (D) pubococcygeus muscle
   (E) pubic ramus

QUESTIONS 3 AND 4

A 54-year-old para 5 complains of low back pain and an unsightly bulge from the vagina for 1 year. She has a history of chronic constipation and has smoked 1 pack per week for the last 20 years. She had a splenectomy after a car accident 30 years ago and a supracervical hysterectomy 10 years ago for leiomyomas. Her vital signs are unremarkable. She is 5 ft 5 in. tall and weighs 225 lb. On observation, a mass protrudes from the vagina. The mass is 4 cm in width. The distance between the external urethral meatus and the posterior hymen is approximately 4.5 cm. The cervix appears to be 3.5 cm in length. Once the prolapse is reduced with the posterior blade of the speculum she is asked to Valsalva then cough (with a subjectively full bladder). Leakage occurs. The distance from the hymen to the top of the vagina is approximately 8 cm. A point, which is 3 cm inside, on the anterior vaginal wall and midline is marked with a pen. Now the patient is asked to strain, the marked point is now 3 cm outside the hymen and the anterior vaginal wall distal to this point is approximately 8 cm outside the hymen. The posterior vaginal wall is the mirror image of the anterior vaginal wall.

3. The patient was seen earlier in the week and on the chart you note that point Aa = 3.5 cm, based on your findings this value is _____.
   (A) incorrect → no decimal points are used in the pelvic organ prolapse quantification (POP)-Q system
   (B) incorrect → Aa = −3.0 cm
   (C) incorrect → Aa = +3.0 cm
   (D) incorrect → Aa = +8.0 cm
   (E) correct
4. Based on the above clinical scenario, which of the following is a true statement?
   (A) Her surgical history predisposes her to the prolapse described.
   (B) Bp = +4.5 cm.
   (C) The patient has *de novo* stress urinary incontinence (SUI).
   (D) The patient's body mass index (BMI) = 24.
   (E) The number "4" would not be found in any of the POP-Q slots.

QUESTIONS 5 AND 6

Choose the word above which best describes the sentence below. Each answer choice may be used once, more than once, or not at all.

(A) anterior
(B) posterior
(C) left lateral
(D) right lateral
(E) medial
(F) proximal
(G) distal
(H) oblique

5. The sacrospinous ligament suspension (SSLS) deviates the vaginal axis in a(an) _____ direction, thus predisposing the patient to prolapse of another compartment in the future.

6. The arcus tendineus fascia rectovaginalis (ATFRV) is situated in a(an) _____ direction relative to the arcus tendineus fascia pelvis (ATFP).

7. A 48-year-old para 2 who underwent an abdominal hysterectomy 2 months ago for a symptomatic fibroid uterus presents to your office with symptoms of persistent watery vaginal leakage for several weeks. Given your high index of suspicion you perform the tampon test, which is highly suggestive of a vesicovaginal fistula. During cystoscopy, the most likely location of the fistula is _____.
(A) dome of the bladder
(B) lateral bladder wall
(C) inferior to ureteral orifice
(D) superior to the interureteric ridge
(E) urethrovesical junction

8. A 48-year-old gravida 4, para 4 is seeing you at your office because she experiences loss of urine when she coughs, laughs, exercises, or gets up from a chair. This has been happening for the 2 years. She tells you that she is done with childbearing and is seeking surgical treatment. There is no POP noted on physical examination; however, the stress test is positive. She is in good health but has had some sort of continence surgery 8 years ago in Mexico. Urodynamic studies are consistent with SUI. You decide to perform the inside-out technique of the transobturator midurethral tension-free sling. The curved needle starts at the suburethral incision site, passes through the obturator foramen, then fascia lata, and eventually exits the skin. The most accurate anatomical relationship of the trocar before piercing the obturator foramen is described as _____.
(A) inferior to the perineal membrane
(B) inside the ischioanal fossa
(C) superior to the pubocervical fascia (PCF)
(D) inside the space of Retzius
(E) superior to the levator ani

9. The initial suture used to repair the vaginal part of the episiotomy repair should be placed above the vaginal apex to ensure _____.

(A) proper cosmetic result and approximation of tissue
(B) that retracted blood vessels are sutured
(C) a decreased risk of dyspareunia
(D) that the anal mucosa is avoided

10. A 41-year-old woman is undergoing a total abdominal hysterectomy and bilateral salpingoooophorectomy for endometriosis in supine position. While attempting to clamp the left uterine artery, the pedicle slips and hemorrhage ensues. A figure-of-8 suture is placed in the left parametrium and this is successful. However, the surgeon is concerned about injury to the left ureter. The next best step to diagnose ureteral injury is _____.
(A) intraoperative antegrade ureteral stenting
(B) dissection of the course of the ureter below pelvic brim
(C) intraoperative intravenous pyelogram (IVP)
(D) cystotomy with visualization of indigo carmine from ureteral orifices
(E) intraoperative cystoscopy with retrograde ureteral stenting

11. A 46-year-old gravida 4, para 4 has urodynamic SUI. While you discuss the risks of tension-free vaginal tape (TVT), you tell her that the most common perioperative complication is _____.
(A) injury to obturator neurovascular bundle
(B) injury to bowel
(C) injury to bladder
(D) long-term urinary retention
(E) inflammation of pubic symphysis

12. A 49-year-old woman presents to your office complaining of involuntary loss of urine with exertion. She says she wears a pad on a daily basis. She is healthy and has an unremarkable medical history. Her physical examination is remarkable for a small, nontender swelling in the distal, midline, anterior vaginal wall. Complex cystometry is consistent with urodynamic SUI. Cystoscopy shows a small diverticulum in the proximal urethra. Voiding cystourethrography is consistent with cystoscopic findings. The next best step in management of this patient is _____.
(A) positive-pressure urethrography (PPU)
(B) magnetic resonance imaging (MRI)
(C) marsupialization of diverticulum (Spence)
(D) diverticulectomy and TVT

13. The first test to distinguish between a vesicovaginal and ureterovaginal fistula is
(A) IVP
(B) retrograde filling of bladder with methylene blue
(C) computed tomography (CT)
(D) retrograde pyelogram
(E) plain x-ray

14. A 51-year-old female has just undergone complete evaluation for microscopic hematuria, which did not detect any abnormalities. She currently has no urinary symptoms. She is moderately obese, and has a history of hypertension controlled with lisinopril and metoprolol. She has worked in a meat-processing factory for the past 17 years, and has a 25 pack-year history of smoking. The next best step in management of this patient is _____.
    (A) observation
    (B) urine dipstick at annual physical examination
    (C) monitor blood pressure, and repeat urinalysis and cytology at 6 months
    (D) reevaluate if urinary symptoms develop
    (E) serum creatinine level and 24-h urine protein collection

15. A 34-year-old female presents with a variety of urinary symptoms that in some respects suggests a diagnosis of interstitial cystitis, but in other regards points to a diagnosis of urethral syndrome. Results of a urodynamic cystometric study further complicate the presentation with findings that are consistent with sensory-urgency-frequency syndrome. Despite numerous studies and tests, as well as a variety of different treatment modalities, the patient's symptoms have only slightly improved over the last several months. Assuming further diagnostic studies and treatment options exist, which of the following adjuvant therapies would be appropriate to recommend in the meantime?
    (A) vitamin B_6 supplements
    (B) herbal supplements
    (C) consultation with a mental health professional
    (D) light exercise
    (E) diet high in arylalkylamines

16. A 45-year-old gravida 2, para 2 is undergoing a vaginal hysterectomy for abnormal uterine bleeding unresponsive to conservative management. The surgery is begun and the posterior cul-de-sac is entered. While attempting to enter the anterior cul-de-sac, clear fluid emerges. The best way to rule out a bladder injury is by _____.
    (A) convert to laparotomy
    (B) administer intravenous indigo carmine and perform cystoscopy
    (C) perform an IVP
    (D) fill the bladder retrograde with dilute indigo carmine dye
    (E) dilate the presumed cystotomy site and identify Foley ball digitally

17. During a laparoscopic paravaginal repair for anterior vaginal wall prolapse, the surgeon notices the patient's right thigh moving as she attempts to dissect the tissue with her ultrasonic vibrating

device. The most likely nerve being stimulated is _____.
    (A) pudendal nerve
    (B) femoral nerve
    (C) genitofemoral nerve
    (D) obturator nerve
    (E) sciatic nerve

18. Which of the following patients might benefit from biofeedback therapy for their fecal incontinence?
    (A) A 42-year-old quadriplegic, who was injured 2 years ago in a motorcycle accident, is numb from the neck on down.
    (B) A 6-year-old boy whose parents are getting a divorce defecates in his pants when he hears them having a heated argument.
    (C) A 31-year-old, gravida 1, para 1 who over the last 6 weeks has developed fecal incontinence. She experienced a normal delivery of a 9 lb male infant. This has been very distressful to the woman.
    (D) A 73-year-old African-American woman, diagnosed with severe Alzheimer's disease, is incontinent of urine and stool.

19. A 45-year-old male was diagnosed with a suspected calcium stone measuring 1.3 cm on CT scan at the ureteropelvic junction. This is the patient's first incidence of urolithiasis and he has no other medical complications. There is no family history of stones. The patient's BMI is 23. Although in pain, he is stable. What is his best treatment plan?
    (A) observation
    (B) extracorporeal shock wave lithotripsy
    (C) ureteroscopic stone extraction
    (D) percutaneous nephrolithotomy
    (E) open stone surgery

20. A 24-year-old nulliparous female presents to your office with increased fullness in vaginal area. She is sexually active and uses oral contraceptives for birth control, but takes no other medications. She denies urinary or fecal incontinence, and does not complain of dyspareunia. On examination, you find a tall, lanky woman, with no abdominal tenderness, and a normal cardiac examination. Examination of the pelvis shows her cervix extending 0.5 cm beyond the hymenal plane, with no cervical motion tenderness and no vaginal discharge. Her past medical history is significant only for two prior episodes of nongonococcal pelvic inflammatory disease both treated with doxycycline. What other pathology should be investigated in this woman?
    (A) evaluation for possible Hashimoto's thyroiditis
    (B) evaluation for possible chronic pelvic inflammatory disease
    (C) evaluation for possible spina bifida occulta
    (D) evaluation for rheumatoid arthritis

21. A 35-year-old gravida 3, para 2 presents with a foul vaginal discharge 4 months after a vaginal delivery complicated by a third degree perineal laceration repaired at that time by her obstetrician. Vaginal examination and examination under anesthesia with a bivalve speculum shows a 2.0 cm rectovaginal fistula situated just above the external anal sphincter (EAS). Vaginal epithelium is pink and there are no signs of infection. The best surgical repair for this patient is _____.
    (A) transvaginal pursestring method
    (B) perineoproctotomy followed by a layered closure
    (C) conservative management (observation, a low-residue diet, and stool softeners)
    (D) rectovaginal fistula repair with a Martius bulbocavernosus muscle or labial fat pad
    (E) Latzko closure of rectovaginal fistula

22. You have evaluated a 70-year-old postmenopausal woman for POP. On examination, the patient is noted to have a stage 3 uterine prolapse based on the POP-Q system. On review of her medical history, she tells you that she suffered a myocardial infarction 1 month ago. The optimal timing of any elective surgical intervention for her POP (assuming cardiac clearance has been obtained) is _____.
    (A) there is no need to wait
    (B) 2–3 months
    (C) 4–6 months
    (D) 6–8 months
    (E) 12 months

23. A 58-year-old gravida 2, para 2 is seeing you in your clinic because she is concerned about the decreased frequency of sexual intercourse with her husband. She states that she has no problem becoming aroused during sexual relations and does not experience pain. She is satisfied when she has sex. She also states that her husband is not interested in having sex with her anymore. He is 60 years old, healthy, and on no medications. The patient's pelvic examination is unremarkable. The next best step in management of this patient based on the information given is _____.
    (A) paroxetine for patient
    (B) urology consult for husband
    (C) viagra for patient
    (D) couples therapy
    (E) androgen patch for patient

24. During an open abdominal sacral colpopexy, the anterior leaf of polypropylene mesh is left longer and under little tension in order to avoid _____.
    (A) overactive bladder
    (B) SUI
    (C) bowel herniation
    (D) mesh erosion
    (E) mesh avulsion

25. Of the following, _____ is the greatest risk factor for the development of a cystocele.
    (A) pelvis with narrow pubic arch
    (B) defect in fibrillin gene
    (C) Asian race
    (D) oral estrogen therapy
    (E) BMI of 28

26. When producing a urodynamics report, the bladder volume, patient position, and catheter size must be mentioned because these variables affect _____. (Choose the best answer.)
    (A) standardization efforts
    (B) patient comfort
    (C) cough leak point pressure (LPP) values
    (D) maximum urethral pressure values
    (E) functional urethral length values

27. A 54-year-old para 3 has classic symptoms of urge urinary incontinence, but complex cystometry in sitting position with coughing and Valsalva maneuvers has failed to demonstrate uninhibited detrusor contractions. The next best step would be _____.
    (A) ambulatory cystometry
    (B) video cystometry
    (C) reposition patient and place her hands in running water
    (D) perform heel bouncing then massage patient's back
    (E) repeat complex cystometry on another visit

28. The most potent alpha-adrenergic receptor blocker affecting urethral sphincter muscle is _____.
    (A) atenolol
    (B) tolterodine
    (C) naproxen
    (D) *Escherichia coli* endotoxin
    (E) phenylpropanolamine

29. Mountain dew, milk chocolate, certain puddings, and over-the-counter medications such as Excedrin all contain caffeine, which is known to cause detrusor overactivity. A true statement regarding caffeine is _____.
    (A) it is similar to furosemide in its mechanism of action
    (B) average caffeine consumption in the United States is 400 mg daily
    (C) patients with urge incontinence who reduced caffeine intake < 100 mg/day decreased their urgency by >60%
    (D) patients with high caffeine intake have a four-fold greater risk of detrusor overactivity than those consuming low amounts of caffeine
    (E) the average half-life of caffeine is 3 h

QUESTIONS 30–32

Match each of the descriptions below with the animal tissue that best describes it above. Each answer may be used once, more than once, or not at all.

- (A) cow
- (B) rabbit
- (C) human
- (D) cat
- (E) mouse
- (F) guinea pig
- (G) pig
- (H) horse
- (I) dog

30. The novel alpha-1-selective agent (ABT-866) is more specific for urethral sphincter muscle than phenylephrine (a nonselective alpha-1 antagonist). It may become a promising new drug for the treatment of SUI. ABT-866 was first tested in the _____ model.

31. Injectable agent which has been used for SUI (intrinsic sphincteric dysfunction [ISD]-type) is derived from _____(s).

32. Type of animal tissue commonly used in the United States when augmenting POP repairs.

33. After evaluation, a patient who has advanced POP (anterior compartment dominant) will undergo a pelvic reconstructive effort (by vaginal route) which includes all of the following: (a) total vaginal hysterectomy/bilateral salpingoooophorectomy, (b) midurethral sling (TVT), (c) vaginal vault suspension to high, ipsilateral uterosacral ligaments, (d) internal modified-McCall's culdoplasty, (e) anterior colporrhaphy, and (f) posterior colpoperineorrhaphy. The best order in which to perform this major surgery is _____.

- (A) a → b → c → d → e → f
- (B) a → c → d → e → b → f
- (C) a → d → c → e → b → f
- (D) e → a → d → c → b → f
- (E) a → c → d → e → f → b

34. An 80-year-old patient is seen in the emergency department because of colicky abdominal pain. She has history of hypertension and peripheral vascular disease. She had an abdominal hysterectomy 40 years ago and underwent an "injection in my urethra," for incontinence 10 months ago. After receiving the acute abdominal series of radiographs, a radiopaque area is noted in the pelvis. The urethral bulking agent used was most likely _____.

- (A) cross-linked bovine collagen
- (B) carbon-coated beads
- (C) ethylene vinyl alcohol_dimethyl sulfoxide
- (D) hyaluronic acid
- (E) chondrocytes

QUESTIONS 35–37

Match each of the statement(s) below with the percentage which most closely approximates it above. Each answer may be used once, more than once, or not at all.

- (A) 10%
- (B) 15%
- (C) 20%
- (D) 25%
- (E) 30%
- (F) 60%
- (G) 70%
- (H) 80%
- (I) 90%

35. At 1-year follow-up, rate of continence to solid stool after overlapping repair of the EAS in patients with intact pudendal innervation is _____.

36. The percentage of elite 20-year-old athletes who experience urinary incontinence while participating in their sport is approximately _____.

37. Of all the patients with mixed urinary incontinence undergoing a Burch urethropexy, _____ have improvement or resolution of their overactive bladder symptoms.

QUESTIONS 38–40

Match each of the statement(s) below with the word that best describes it above. Each answer may be used once, more than once, or not at all.

- (A) Urge
- (B) Stress (Hypermobile urethra-type)
- (C) Stress (ISD-type)
- (D) Overflow
- (E) Functional
- (F) Transient
- (G) Mixed
- (H) Bypass
- (I) Continuous

38. Involuntary loss of urine during intense sexual orgasm
39. Involuntary loss of urine as a result of spina bifida
40. Involuntary loss of urine as a result of fecal impaction

QUESTIONS 41–45

Match each of the statement(s) below with the word that best describes it above. If more than one answer seems reasonable, use the answer which is more specific. Each answer may be used once, more than once, or not at all.

(A) Squamous
(B) Transitional
(C) Columnar
(D) Cuboidal
(E) Neoplasia
(F) Metaplasia
(G) Pseudostratified
(H) Keratinizing
(I) Adenosis

41. Congenital proximal urethral diverticulum lined by unique epithelium
42. Bladder cancer resulting from long-term indwelling catheter
43. Urethral epithelium 5 mm proximal to meatus
44. Kidney (medulla) epithelium
45. Raised area within bladder with papillary texture

QUESTIONS 46–50

Match each of the word(s)/phrase(s) below with the derivative above. If more than one answer is correct, use the answer choice which is *later* in embryological development. Each answer may be used once, more than once, or not at all.

(A) Urogenital sinus
(B) Mullerian
(C) Mesonephric
(D) Gubernaculum
(E) Mesenchyme
(F) Cloaca
(G) Allantois
(H) Pectinate line
(I) Labioscrotal swellings
(J) Neural crest
(K) Endoderm
(L) Ectoderm

46. Superficial transverse perineal muscle
47. EAS
48. Early embryonic urine reservoir
49. Fimbria
50. Urethral diverticulum

ANSWERS AND EXPLANATIONS

1. *(E)*. The cube is usually the last option in pessaries. The six concave sides of the cube provide suction to the vaginal walls. This can lead to erosion within a few days. Therefore, the cube needs to be removed nightly.

2. *(D)*. The primary support of the pelvic organs comes from the pelvic floor muscles, mainly the levator ani. This muscle is made up of two components: pubococcygeus and iliococcygeus. Since only pubococcygeus is listed in the choices, D is correct. The "white line," or ATFP is important for level II support of the vagina. The uterosacral ligaments are important for level I support of the vagina. The infundibulapelvic ligaments (IP) ligaments do not provide much support to the uterus but are important because they contain vessels and nerves. The pubic rami, although a strong structure (bone) is not as important as the levator ani muscles for the support of the pelvic organs.

3. *(C)*, 4. *(E)*. Based on the clinical scenario, point Aa = +3 cm. Remember that points Aa and Ap are always between negative and positive 3 (thus eliminating choices D and E). Since her prolapse is outside the vagina, that eliminates choice B. A decimal point can be used in the POP-Q system as it is a quantification of POP. Based on the clinical scenario, the only measurement given as "4" is the width of the prolapse. The POP-Q does not take into account a diameter or width of a prolapse. Choice A is wrong because there are little data to prove or disprove that keeping a cervix (supracervical hysterectomy) is superior to removing it. If anything, the retention of a cervix and its urterosacral ligament may prevent future prolapse, but this is not proven. Point Bp is the mirror image of point Ba which as mentioned to be +8. Today, the patient has occult incontinence (aka potential or masked incontinence). This is not the same as "*de novo*." In the future, she is at risk for developing *de novo* SUI if she had her prolapse repaired without an anti-incontinence procedure. A patient who is 5 ft 5 in. has an ideal body weight of 125 lb. This patient is 100 lb above ideal weight and thus morbidly obese.

5. *(B)*, 6. *(H)*. SSLS deviates the vaginal posteriorly thus predisposing the vagina to anterior support defects in the future. On the other hand, the retropubic urethropexies deviate the vagina in an anterior direction thus predisposing to apical prolapse and enterocele formation in the future. The distal half of the rectovaginal fascia inserts onto a thickening of parietal fascia of the iliococcygeus called the ATFRV. This structure is actually connected to the ATFP, but is situated distal to the ATFP and goes in an inferior-oblique direction to attach to the perineal body.

7. *(D)*. Approximately 75% of vesicovaginal fistulas result from abdominal hysterectomies. Other etiologies include vaginal hysterectomy, urological procedures, radiation, foreign bodies, cancer, and obstetric trauma. Fistulous tracts can be small or several centimeters in diameter. Patients may present